Register Now for Online Access to Your Book!

SPRINGER PUBLISHING COMPANY

CONNECT™

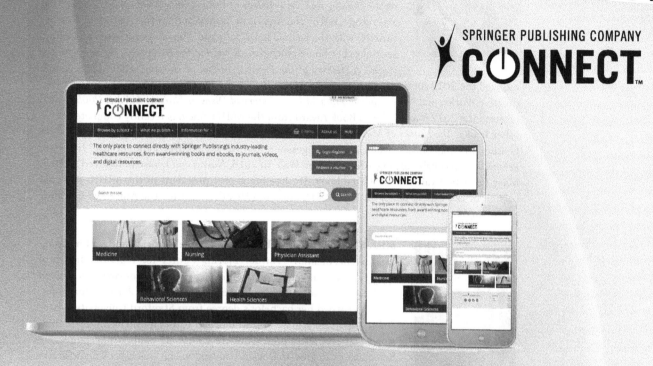

Your print purchase of *History of Professional Nursing in the United States, 1e,* **includes online access to the contents of your book**—increasing accessibility, portability, and searchability!

Access today at:
http://connect.springerpub.com/content/book/978-0-8261-3313-7
or scan the QR code at the right with your smartphone
and enter the access code below.

G5AY0PDC

Scan here for quick access.

If you are experiencing problems accessing the digital component of this product, please contact our customer service department at cs@springerpub.com

The online access with your print purchase is available at the publisher's discretion and may be removed at any time without notice.

Publisher's Note: New and used products purchased from third-party sellers are not guaranteed for quality, authenticity, or access to any included digital components.

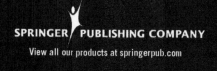

SPRINGER PUBLISHING COMPANY
View all our products at springerpub.com

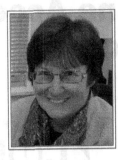

Arlene W. Keeling, PhD, RN, FAAN, is the Centennial Distinguished Professor of nursing at the University of Virginia School of Nursing, and associate director of the Eleanor Crowder Bjoring Center for Nursing Historical Inquiry. Formerly, she served as the director of the center. Dr. Keeling is the author of numerous articles on nursing history. She wrote *Nursing and the Privilege of Prescription, 1893–2000*, a book that was recognized by the American Association for the History of Nursing (AAHN) with the Lavinia L. Dock Award. She has coauthored and edited several other books, including *Rooted in the Mountains, Reaching to the World: A History of the Frontier School of Nursing, 1939–1989*, which received the 2012 *American Journal of Nursing's* Book of the Year Award for Public Interest and Creative Works, and *Nurses on the Front Line: A History of Disaster Nursing 1879 to 2005*, which received the 2012 Mary Roberts Book Award from the AAHN. She has recently completed three other books: *The Nurses of Mayo Clinic*; *Nursing Rural America: Perspectives From the Early 20th Century*, in collaboration with John Kirchgessner; and *Nurses and Disasters: A Global Historical Perspective*, in collaboration with Dr. Barbra Wall. In 2016, *Nurses and Disasters* received AAHN's Mary Roberts Award for an edited book. Dr. Keeling is past president of the AAHN, and past cochair of the expert panel on Nursing History and Health Policy for the American Academy of Nursing.

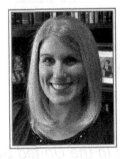

Michelle C. Hehman, PhD, RN, is a nurse historian and center associate for the Eleanor Crowder Bjoring Center for Nursing Historical Inquiry at the University of Virginia. Dr. Hehman's research has focused on the intersection of ethics and technology in early 20th-century nursing. She earned her bachelor's degree from Stanford University, where she was a 4-year scholarship athlete and team captain of the 2001 Division I National Champion Women's Volleyball team. While completing her master's degree at DePaul University, she was class valedictorian. Most recently she received her PhD from the University of Virginia. Her dissertation research received the Phyllis J. Verhonick Award from the University of Virginia School of Nursing, and the Theresa A. Christy Award from the American Association for the History of Nursing. She is also a member of Sigma Theta Tau International, the Honor Society of Phi Kappa Phi, and the Golden Key International Honor Society. Dr. Hehman has been working as a neonatal intensive care nurse for the past 10 years.

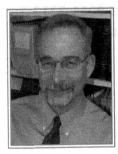

John C. Kirchgessner, PhD, RN, is a nurse historian whose research has focused on the nursing profession during the first half of the 20th century. His research explores the relationship between nurses and industry, specifically the work of nurses and the care they provided to West Virginia coal miners and their families. He has written and presented extensively on the West Virginia Miners Hospitals, the 1907 Monongah mine disaster, and public health in coal mining towns during the 1930s and 1940s. In addition, Dr. Kirchgessner has investigated how hospitals' nursing departments during the mid-20th century were often income generators for their perspective institutions and not the cost centers hospital administrators traditionally claimed. His research has been presented at international and national research meetings. He is an associate professor of nursing at St. John Fisher College Wegmans School of Nursing in Rochester, New York, and assistant director of the Eleanor Crowder Bjoring Center for Nursing Historical Inquiry at the University of Virginia. Dr. Kirchgessner coauthored *The Voice of Professional Nursing Education: A 40-Year History of the American Association of Colleges of Nursing*, has written book chapters, and has published in refereed journals. His most recent book, coauthored with Arlene Keeling, is *Nursing Rural America: Perspectives From the Early 20th Century*.

History of Professional Nursing in the United States

Toward a Culture of Health

Arlene W. Keeling, PhD, RN, FAAN

Michelle C. Hehman, PhD, RN

John C. Kirchgessner, PhD, RN

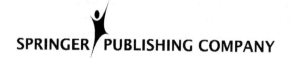

SPRINGER PUBLISHING COMPANY

Springer Publishing Company, LLC
11 West 42nd Street
New York, NY 10036
www.springerpub.com

Acquisitions Editor: Joseph Morita
Compositor: Westchester Publishing Services

ISBN: 978-0-8261-3312-0
ebook ISBN: 978-0-8261-3313-7
Image Bank ISBN: 978-0-8261-3096-9

An Image Bank is available from Springerpub.com/keeling

19 20 / 5 4 3 2

The author and the publisher of this Work have made every effort to use sources believed to be reliable to provide information that is accurate and compatible with the standards generally accepted at the time of publication. Because medical science is continually advancing, our knowledge base continues to expand. Therefore, as new information becomes available, changes in procedures become necessary. We recommend that the reader always consult current research and specific institutional policies before performing any clinical procedure. The author and publisher shall not be liable for any special, consequential, or exemplary damages resulting, in whole or in part, from the readers' use of, or reliance on, the information contained in this book. The publisher has no responsibility for the persistence or accuracy of URLs for external or third-party Internet websites referred to in this publication and does not guarantee that any content on such websites is, or will remain, accurate or appropriate.

Library of Congress Cataloging-in-Publication Data

Names: Keeling, Arlene Wynbeek, 1948– author. | Hehman, Michelle C., author. | Kirchgessner, John C., author.
Title: History of professional nursing in the United States : toward a culture of health / Arlene W. Keeling, Michelle C. Hehman, John C. Kirchgessner.
Description: New York, NY : Springer Publishing Company, LLC, [2017] | Includes bibliographical references and index.
Identifiers: LCCN 2017012991 (print) | LCCN 2017014412 (ebook) | ISBN 9780826133137 (ebook) | ISBN 9780826133120 (hard copy : alk. paper) | ISBN 9780826130969 (image bank)
Subjects: | MESH: History of Nursing | Nurse's Role—history | History, Modern 1601– | United States
Classification: LCC RT41 (ebook) | LCC RT41 (print) | NLM WY 11 AA1 | DDC 610.73—dc23
LC record available at https://lccn.loc.gov/2017012991

Contact us to receive discount rates on bulk purchases.
We can also customize our books to meet your needs.
For more information please contact: sales@springerpub.com

Printed in the United States of America by Bang Printing.

This book is dedicated to all nurses, for their contributions to the health of the people of the United States.

Contents

Foreword

As a historian and director of the Eleanor Crowder Bjoring Center for Nursing Historical Inquiry at the University of Virginia, I congratulate Arlene Keeling, Michelle Hehman, and John Kirchgessner for their publication, *History of Professional Nursing in the United States: Toward a Culture of Health.* The book chronicles the history of nursing from the earliest English settlements to the present. It provides a comprehensive look at nursing, not only from the leaders' views but also from the grassroots perspective of those lesser-known nurses who carried out the work of nursing in homes, hospitals, and public health arenas.

The authors demonstrate how U.S. nurses have worked throughout their history to restore patients to health, teach health promotion, and participate in disease-preventing activities. Recounting those experiences in the nurses' own words, the authors bring that history to life, capturing nurses' thoughts and feelings during times of war, epidemics, and disasters, as well as during their everyday work.

Today the nursing profession is focused on addressing the social determinants of health in order to be agents for change in health policy and practice. This book shows that, historically, nurses have tackled infant mortality, poor nutrition, poverty, and the physical environment, and the relationship of these factors to poor health. It highlights how race, ethnicity, social class, gender, and access to care had large effects on people's health. It also details how nurses' roles expanded, as knowledge in technology and science grew, along with the legal and ethical dilemmas nurses encountered.

The nursing profession is faced with similar pressing issues today, including access to health care, care of those with chronic and infectious diseases, childhood nutrition, and antibiotic-resistant drugs. In this book, the authors describe and analyze the roots of these issues in the history of nursing, demonstrating how the problems have evolved in different contexts and how nurses responded to those variations in different settings and time periods. It fills a gap in the secondary literature on the subject of the history of nursing that can be useful in these times of great social change. It is a "must read" for every nurse in the United States!

Barbra Mann Wall, PhD, RN, FAAN
Thomas A. Saunders III Professor of Nursing
Director, Eleanor C. Bjoring Center for Nursing Historical Inquiry
University of Virginia
Charlottesville, Virginia

Preface

Any work of this magnitude requires an explanation of its scope—to borrow from Florence Nightingale in her work *Notes on Nursing*,[1] "What it is and what it is not." In one book, it is impossible to cover every aspect of the nursing profession's history, every opportunity it had or challenge it faced over more than 400 years of our nation's history. However, in order to provide readers with an introduction to the complex and multifaceted history of the largest profession in the United States, we have accepted the challenge. In this book, we provide a general overview of how nursing got to where it is today. We hope the reading of this book inspires nursing students, scholars, and historians to further investigate for themselves the topics that spur their interest.

"WHAT IT IS"

This book is a history of nursing in the United States from 1607, when a small company of Englishmen landed on the shores of Virginia, to the present. It is intended as an introduction to nursing history for undergraduate and graduate nursing students and to others who might be interested in how the profession developed in the United States. Using a social historical framework, the book describes and analyzes the history of nursing from a multidimensional perspective, situating it within the social, political, and economic context of particular historical periods, and including a discussion on how race, class, and gender mattered.

Incorporating examples from various areas of the country, the narrative covers nursing in cities, small towns, and villages from urban areas of the northeast to Florida in the south and Alaskan outposts in the northwest. Nurses' involvement in wars takes the reader briefly to other continents, including Europe, Asia, and Africa.

The book uses examples of nursing education, nursing leadership, and changes in nursing practice throughout the narrative. Including other examples from public health, war zones, industry, missions, and hospital nursing, the book traces nurses' work in health promotion, disease prevention, and direct patient care over the past 400 years. To do so, we chose to highlight specific instances in which nurses worked to restore patients to health, taught health-promoting behaviors, or engaged in disease-preventing activities. In it we argue that nurses have long been involved in health restoration, health promotion, and disease prevention, both inside and outside the hospital setting. They have done so in rural, urban, and suburban settings, in war and in peace. We further argue that because of that long history and the holistic perspective on patient care that nurses have advocated, *nurses* are particularly well situated to take a leadership role in developing a culture of health in the 21st century.

The book captures individual nurses' experiences in their own words, gleaned from oral histories, diaries, letters, journal articles, and editorials. This feature, highlighting the personal experience in text boxes, is an attempt to engage the reader in the first-hand experience of a nurse in a specific setting, making history come alive. For example, one box captures a young mother's account of giving birth on the Overland Trail in the 1850s. Another uses Clara Noyes's own words to share her thoughts as she watched nurses set sail from New York Harbor in World War I. Because of their authenticity, it is important to note that the words used in the story boxes reflect the language of a specific person in the historical context in which he or she lived. Some words may not be considered appropriate in our multicultural society today. Nonetheless, these excerpts give voice to those who have long been silent in American history.

The authors recognize that much of the published nursing history to date has been told from the perspective of White, middle-class women. This book is an *attempt* to be more inclusive, recognizing the contributions of men and women of all races, including the work of African Americans, Native Americans, and Asian Americans. It also attempts to highlight nurses from all social classes—from African American slaves and granny midwives who were taught by their mothers and aunts, to upper-middle-class women who trained as professional nurses and provided leadership in nursing education or practice.

Woven throughout the history are examples of how race, class, and ethnicity influenced the context in which nurses worked. For example, private-duty nursing for elite White families on the Upper East Side of Manhattan differed from that of visiting nursing in immigrant neighborhoods on New York's Lower East Side. Nursing coal miners in West Virginia contrasted with the care of American Indians on the Cherokee and Navajo reservations or nursing the Inuit in Alaska.

The format of the chapters is consistent. Each chapter highlights select technologies, scientific achievements, ethical issues, and legal decisions that affected nursing during specific time periods. Each has "callouts"—short phrases that invite the reader to delve into the narrative. Each chapter concludes with questions for discussion that could be used in the traditional classroom or in an online class format.

"WHAT IT IS NOT"

The book is not a comprehensive history of health care through the ages. It simply cannot be. Although the book references nursing's historical roots in Europe, it is not a history of European nursing. It focuses on such leaders as Florence Nightingale, Theodore Fleidner, William Rathmore, and Ethel Fenwick only to note their influences on American nursing. In addition, the book does not cover the work of Catholic sisterhoods in Europe or the United Kingdom, except to recognize their origins and their immigration to America in the early 19th century.

Limited by the authors' expertise, page count, and time for its completion, the book does not detail the history of nursing in the New World prior to 1607. Lack of primary source material and the enormity of the time span precluded a discussion of Native American healers' work during the 17,000 years they inhabited North America before the English arrived.

The examples of selected technologies, medicines, legal decisions, and ethical issues that are included in each chapter are not meant to be all-inclusive. Incorporating every invention, newly discovered medicine, ethical dilemma, or legal precedent that affected the practice of nursing is beyond the scope of this book.

There are numerous other things the book is not. It is not a comprehensive history of nursing education or advanced practice. One narrative cannot adequately describe the entire history of diploma, associate degree, or collegiate education for nurses. Nor can it cover all the information on the stories of nurse-midwives, nurse practitioners, clinical nurse specialists, nurse anesthetists, public health nursing, nursing ethics, or nursing in war and disasters. Of particular note, the book is not a history of hospitals, medicine, technology, or pharmacy. Other books have been written on these topics. Instead, aspects of each of these subjects are included to situate nursing practice within the larger health care context. All that said, we hope that we have met the need for a book that introduces the reader to the world of nursing. Every nurse should know the historical roots of the profession, our cultural DNA.

NURSING IN THE COLONIAL ERA AND EARLY DAYS OF THE UNITED STATES, 1607–1840

Chapter 1 focuses on the home as the site of care. It begins with a discussion of health problems in Jamestown settlement and Plymouth Colony in the early 17th century. The chapter examines the roles family members and midwives played in the provision of nursing care in the early Colonial period, highlighting what little is known about nursing in the Revolutionary War and post–Revolutionary period. It goes on to describe the rise of almshouses, the founding of the Pennsylvania Hospital in 1751, and the establishment of a hospital in Williamsburg, Virginia, in 1783. Of necessity, because any history relies on primary sources, it highlights the words of male leaders and White women who kept diaries or wrote letters expressing their views.

The use of herbal medicines, teas, and home remedies is discussed throughout the chapter. The problems of obstetrics and infant welfare, infectious diseases and epidemics, and state-of-the-art medicine and science are also addressed. Highlights of a section on nursing care in the antebellum South include the role of the mistress of the plantation and the contributions of African American slaves. Medical boxes discuss variolation and the invention of the smallpox vaccine, and a technology box highlights the invention of the stethoscope.

THE ROOTS OF A PROFESSION, 1830–1865

Chapter 2 argues that nursing work changed from the commonly accepted notion that the family was the primary unit of care during illness to an organized system of "care by strangers" during the American Civil War, and that the medical and nursing situation in the military drew the nation's attention to the need for formalized nurse training. The chapter opens with a discussion on the flow of Nightingale's ideas from England to the United States in the mid-19th century. It goes on to describe nursing care on the Overland Trail during the great migration west, highlighting the work of wives and mothers using excerpts from women's diaries. In a transition segment, the chapter notes the reform of hospitals for the mentally ill in the mid-19th century, using St. Elizabeth's Hospital in Washington, DC, as an example.

The second half of the chapter discusses women's roles in both the North and the South during the American Civil War (1861–1865). It describes the work of Dorothea Dix, the Catholic Sisters of Charity and Mercy, and select middle-class women such as Mother Bickerdyke and Mary Livermore. This section also highlights the contributions of Black slaves, those of freed African Americans like Harriet Tubman and Sojourner Truth, and those of volunteer men like Walt Whitman. Referencing nurses in the Confederacy, the chapter focuses on the contributions of upper-class White women like Mary Chestnut, Phoebe Pember, and others who kept diaries.

The chapter follows the usual format for story boxes and other highlights. It uses direct quotes to document women's experiences with nursing care, weaving in some accounts of the use of herbs and teas to restore health. Medical/technology boxes include a brief description of horsehair sutures used in the Civil War and a list of drugs carried on wagon trains. A legal/ethics box explains Philippe Pinnel's moral therapy for the treatment of the mentally ill.

THE RISE OF A PROFESSION, "AN ART AND A SCIENCE," 1873–1901

Chapter 3 asserts that the creation of nurse training schools firmly established the notion that proper nursing required formal preparation and discipline. While nursing care continued to be viewed as women's work, the early nursing schools defied the conventional perception that sick nursing was tacit feminine knowledge and advocated for a trained nursing workforce. The chapter opens with a discussion of the need to establish formal nurse training schools in the United States in the late 19th century. It briefly examines changes in opportunities for women in the workplace and the difficulty of raising the social image of nursing at the time.

Most of the chapter focuses on founding the first three formal training schools in New York, Connecticut, and Massachusetts in 1873, followed by a description of the typical experience of pupil nurses at these and other early institutions. The origin and symbolism of nursing uniforms, caps, and pins are also examined and situated within the larger context of the image of nursing.

Specific to minorities in nursing, a discussion of early training schools for African American and male nursing students is also included. This section addresses some of the social and ideological factors driving the marginalization of these groups within the profession. For African American nurses, these included racial discrimination and segregation. For men, the cultural assumption that women were inherently better suited for the intimate work of nursing than men denied them access to the profession.

The chapter also discusses the rise of scientific medicine, using the origins of nurse anesthesia training at Saint Marys Hospital in Rochester, Minnesota, to illustrate the impact of science and technology on nursing practice. The chapter concludes by introducing the nursing education reform movement championed by Isabel Hampton, foreshadowing the establishment of nursing organizations and improvements in training-school curriculum. Medical/technology boxes highlight the invention of the thermometer, the discovery of chloroform, and Joseph Lister's theory of antisepsis.

VISITING NURSES IN CITIES, PARISHES, AND MISSIONS, 1886–1914

The central thesis of Chapter 4 is that nurses were aware of social factors influencing health, including poverty, inadequate housing, lack of job opportunities, and lack of education, and worked to address these. In relation to these issues, the chapter discusses the formation of the National Organization for Public Health Nursing, the Children's Bureau, and the Rural Nursing Service of the American Red Cross, emphasizing nurses' role in protecting the health of the public.

Chapter 4 opens with a discussion of nursing on Ellis Island and in cities of the northeast, demonstrating not only how nurses attempted to assimilate European immigrants into American culture, but also how nurses attempted to address the social factors influencing health. It includes the establishment of Visiting Nurse Associations, the founding of the Boston Floating Hospital, and the work of the Baltimore Lutheran Deaconesses.

Beginning in this chapter, the content of the medical/technology boxes becomes increasingly focused on scientific advances. Medical/technology boxes highlight the introduction of the autoclave in 1879, and infant formula testing in the late 19th century. The contents of the visiting nurse's bag, including medicines, are also highlighted. The 1906 Food and Drug Act is featured in a legal/ethics box.

PROFESSIONAL ORGANIZATIONS AND INTERNATIONAL CONNECTIONS, 1881–1920

Chapter 5 argues that the creation of national and international organizations advanced the professional status of nurses and that early nursing leaders recognized the power of an organized and united front. Through strategic planning, these organizations were able to enact meaningful change both within and outside of the sphere of professional nursing.

Opening with a discussion of the formation of the American Red Cross, this chapter focuses attention on the founding and development of the first nursing organizations. In addition to the American Red Cross (1881), the organizations discussed include the American Society of Superintendents of Training Schools in the United States and Canada (1893), the Nurses Associated Alumnae of the United States and Canada (1896), the International Council of Nurses (1899), and the National Association of Colored Graduate Nurses (1908). Each section describes the foundational purpose and goals of each society, and introduces early nursing leaders, including Clara Barton, Isabel Hampton, Lavinia Dock, Ethel Fenwick, Martha Franklin, and Adah Belle Samuels Thoms.

To illustrate the work of these organizations in action, the chapter takes the reader to Johnstown, Pennsylvania, in the aftermath of the 1889 flood, to the front lines of the international women's suffrage movement, and to southern states in the fight against racial discrimination in nursing state registries and licensure. Advancements in nursing education and research are also presented through the establishment of a graduate course in hospital economics at Columbia University Teachers College and the creation of the *American Journal of Nursing*. A medical/technology box highlights the progress made in communication technology through increased availability of the telegraph and telephone. An ethics box discusses the publication of *Nursing Ethics* in 1900, the first book on the subject.

ORGANIZATION AND INNOVATION IN THE EARLY 20TH CENTURY, 1898–1928

The central thesis of Chapter 6 is that at the turn of the 20th century, professional nurses had to distinguish themselves from untrained women who nursed. It opens with a quote from nurse leader Isabel Hampton Robb, calling attention to the need for the profession of nursing to organize after the Spanish–American War. It includes a description of nursing during that war, focusing on the care that Catholic Sisters and contract nurses provided for patients with typhoid and yellow fever, and noting in particular the part that African American fever nurses played. It follows with a discussion of the need for licensure and registration and goes on to describe the formation of the Army and Navy Nurse Corps.

The chapter also emphasizes the importance of innovation in nursing during the Progressive Era. It discusses the inception and establishment of school nursing in New York City, the rise of preventoria as an attempt to prevent tuberculosis in underprivileged children, and the inception and growth of industrial nursing, noting in particular nurses' work in mill and coal towns in the south.

Innovation in nurses' response to disasters is also discussed in Chapter 6. The nursing response to the 1900 hurricane in Galveston and the 1906 San Francisco earthquake are also addressed. The 1907 Monongah mining disaster in West Virginia is highlighted, particularly in relationship to the nurses' psychological support for rescuers and survivors.

New discoveries in medicine are emphasized in the relevant boxes. Medical and technology boxes in this chapter highlight the confirmation of the mosquito as the carrier of malaria, the discovery of the bacterium that causes tuberculosis, and the use of heliotherapy as treatment, the production of aspirin in 1900, and the discovery of insulin in the 1920s.

NURSES, SCIENCE, AND THE GROWTH OF HOSPITALS, 1910–1930

Chapter 7 argues that the transition toward hospitals as the preferred place for the treatment of illness profoundly affected the nursing profession. In particular, nursing's inability to claim authority over specific technical and practical aspects of hospital care would affect its professional status and economic prospects for years to come. The chapter examines numerous factors involved in the growth of hospitals during the early 20th century. Beginning with a discussion of the role of scientific discoveries and increased use of medical technologies, the chapter highlights the impact of the germ theory, antisepsis, and diagnostic tests on the practice of medicine.

Examination of the changes that occurred in nursing and medical education during this era includes a discussion of the 1911 Flexner report and the 1923 Goldmark report. The promotion of university-based medical and nursing education is also addressed, using Johns Hopkins University as the standard to which all schools aspired. Increased medical specialization is evaluated as a driving factor for hospital growth, particularly in surgery and obstetrics. Social and scientific forces behind the emergence of these specialties are individually explored, along with a discussion of their impact on nursing knowledge and practice.

Chapter 7 also explores the African American hospital movement, and the effects of racial discrimination and inequality on Black communities. An in-depth exploration of the unpublished 1925 Ethel Johns report, which examined the educational and professional conditions for African American nurses, provides a rich description of the cultural and institutional marginalization faced by these women in the early 20th century.

The chapter concludes with a discussion of the 1928 study *Nurses, Patients, and Pocketbooks*, on the grading of nurse training programs. This section explores how the growth of hospitals affected the nursing workforce from an economic perspective. The relationship between hospitals and nursing schools is also addressed, focusing on the inherent conflict of interest between patient needs, student needs, and hospital budgets.

Highlighted boxes are also included in Chapter 7. Medical/technology boxes highlight the adoption of the electrocardiogram into practice, increasing use of blood transfusions, and the introduction of the 1917 *Standard Curriculum for Schools of Nursing*. Ethics boxes discuss the publication of the American Nurses Association's 1926 Suggested Code of Ethics and the rise of eugenic philosophy in the Progressive Era. A legal box describes the Supreme Court's upholding of lawful forced sterilization in the *Buck v. Bell* decision.

NURSES IN THE NEWS: THE GREAT WAR AND PANDEMIC INFLUENZA, 1914–1919

The central thesis of Chapter 8 is that between the years 1914 and 1918 nurses fulfilled their patriotic and professional duties by volunteering during the Great War, both in Europe and within the United States. Rising to the challenges of the flu pandemic of 1918, they were instrumental in caring for the troops and the general public. The chapter describes U.S. nurses' participation in World War I beginning in 1917 with the American Red Cross call for volunteers. It includes a discussion of nursing on the home front with the challenges of pandemic influenza in the fall of 1918. Direct quotes from the war in France are excerpted from the letters of nurse Camilla Wills in Base Hospital No. 41.

The roles that nurse leaders Jane Delano and Clara Noyes played during the war are also discussed. Furthermore, the chapter includes a discussion of the formation of the Yale School of Nursing, the founding of the Vassar Training Camp, and the development of the Army School of Nursing in response to the nursing shortage during the war.

Highlighted boxes focus on discoveries during the war and the pandemic flu. Medical and technology highlights include the invention of Carrell-Dakin's solution for wound healing and Phieffer's discovery of a bacillus that he considered to be the cause of influenza. The invention and production of the Model-T Ford is highlighted, as nurses used the automobile to reach their flu patients during the epidemic.

NURSES, BABIES, AND PUBLIC HEALTH, 1920s

Chapter 9 asserts that in the 1920s, influenced by the opportunities provided by Sheppard–Towner funding, many nurses worked to promote the health of mothers and babies. The chapter opens with the National Organization of Public Health Nurses' 1920 endorsement of the Sheppard–Towner Bill, and goes on to examine the effects of that legislation on nurses' work in the areas of maternal and child care. Specific topics include the problem of high maternal and infant mortality, the origins of the Frontier Nursing Service in 1925, and the Frontier nurses' work in Appalachia.

The chapter draws attention to nurses' work with granny midwives in North Carolina, Mississippi, and Florida. Focusing briefly on the northwest, it includes a section on Red Cross nurse Stella Fuller's work in the remote territory of Alaska. The chapter also highlights nurses' work in the Indian Health Service in the 1920s, specifically using examples from their assignments on the Navajo reservation. In addition, it reports on Camilla Wills's experience in the Red Cross's Home Hygiene and Care of the Sick program in New Mexico.

Legal/ethics boxes highlight the Comstock Laws of the late 19th century, the Sheppard–Towner legislation of 1921, and the opening of Margaret Sanger's birth control clinic in Brooklyn in 1916. A medical/technology box highlights the widespread use of cod liver oil to promote health.

NURSING IN THE GREAT DEPRESSION, 1930–1940

Chapter 10 argues that nurses, some taking advantage of opportunities from federally funded initiatives, provided access to care for the poor in rural communities and in migrant camps. Teaching nutrition and well-baby care, dealing with epidemics, and promoting proper sanitation, nurses worked toward achieving a basic level of health despite difficult circumstances. In some instances, nurses collaborated with social workers and the Red Cross to respond to flood disasters; others worked beyond the boundaries of the traditional scope of nursing practice, assuming responsibilities for diagnosis, treatment, and referral—responsibilities usually reserved for physicians.

The chapter describes nursing during the Great Depression. It opens with a discussion of the crisis in unemployment of private-duty nurses and goes on to describe various new opportunities that presented to nurses in the 1930s. Among these were jobs in migrant camps, on passenger trains and airplanes, and in hospitals. In particular, the chapter focuses on opportunities for nurses provided by the federal government under the New Deal.

Chapter 10 also addresses developments in the field of anesthesia, national organization within the specialty, and legal challenges to nurse anesthesia practice. Medicine/technology boxes feature the discovery of Prontosil and the development of cyclopropane anesthesia, while a box on legal/ethical issues focuses the reader's attention on the passage of the 1935 Social Security Act.

NURSING IN WORLD WAR II: OVERSEAS AND AT HOME, 1940–1945

The central thesis of Chapter 11 is that World War II provided the nursing profession with opportunities and challenges both in the war zones and on the home front. Beginning with the Japanese attack on Pearl Harbor, the chapter discusses nursing in the war zones in Europe and the Pacific during World War II. Highlighting the work of nurses in specific evacuation hospitals, it provides data to support the argument that nurses were innovative and creative in the provision of care, and resilient in challenging situations. It then goes on to describe nursing on the American home front, providing evidence that nurses adapted to the demands of a wartime economy, accepting work in industrial plants, in mission clinics, and under federally funded initiatives like the Emergency Maternal and Infant Care program. The work of both Japanese American and Caucasian nurses in U.S. government-run internment camps is highlighted, as is the role that nurse anesthetists played in military and civilian hospitals.

Here again, boxes are used to enhance the narrative and highlight specific advances in science, law, and ethics. A medical/technology box features the production and use of penicillin during the war. An ethics box offers a brief discussion of nurse Eunice Rivers's participation in the Tuskegee experiment when penicillin was withheld from African Americans diagnosed with syphilis. The Emergency Maternity and Infant Care Program, established in 1943, and the Bolton Act of 1943, which formed the U.S. Cadet Nurse Corps, are highlighted in legal boxes.

MID-CENTURY TRANSITIONS AND SHORTAGES, 1945–1960

With a focus on hospital nursing, Chapter 12 argues that nurses adapted to the science of care and the increasing use of technology in hospitals while trying to pay attention to the needs of the patient. The chapter explores many of the changes in the profession, in hospitals, and in science that occurred immediately after World War II. It includes a discussion of the nursing shortage, the impact of Hill–Burton funding on the rise of the modern hospital, and the changes that ensued in how nursing care was given. In particular, the increasing use of hospitals for obstetrical deliveries during the baby boom and the inception of intensive care nursing during polio epidemics are discussed. A brief description of nursing care during the Korean War is provided. The chapter also covers many of the strategies used by hospitals to combat the continuing shortage of hospital nurses, discussing the rise of associate degree programs and the use of licensed practical nurses and auxiliary personnel. The concepts of progressive patient care and team nursing are also introduced.

Dramatic changes in medicine and science, as well as advances in the profession, are highlighted in boxes. Science and technology highlights include the discovery of the Salk vaccine for polio, advances in dialysis, antipsychotic medications, and the identification of the double-helix model of DNA. A legal box highlights the 1948 Brown report, which recommended a minimum college degree for professional nurses.

SPECIALIZATION, WAR, AND THE EXPANSION OF NURSING'S SCOPE OF PRACTICE, 1961–1980

Chapter 13 argues that during the 1960s the profession grappled with its identity, its scope of practice, and the control of nursing education. The chapter opens with a discussion of the rise of coronary care nursing and its impact on nurses' scope of practice. It follows with a brief discussion of military nurses' work in the Vietnam War, using excerpts from later interviews with the nurses to highlight aspects of their experiences.

Situating nursing in the political and social unrest of the 1960s, the chapter includes a section on Nancy Milio's work in Detroit, Michigan, and her establishment of a community-based "Mom and Tots' Clinic." The chapter also discusses the shortage of physicians in rural areas, the development of nurse practitioner programs, and the inception of the American Association of Colleges of Nursing.

Once again, boxes highlight major achievements in science and law that affected the nursing profession. Medical/technology boxes highlight the emergence of cardiopulmonary resuscitation and the invention of cardiac monitoring equipment. Legal boxes include the passage of the Nurse Training Act of 1964, the enactment of Medicare and Medicaid legislation in 1965, the authorization of prescriptive authority to nurse practitioners, and the 1973 Supreme Court decision in *Roe v. Wade*.

CARING IN CRISIS, 1980–2000

The main thesis of Chapter 14 is that between 1980 and 2000, the response of nurses to multiple crises would reinforce the profession's vital role in the delivery of health care services both inside and outside the hospital. The period began with the publication of the American Nurses Association's (ANA) *Nursing: A Social Policy Statement* in 1980, which defined nursing and outlined the reciprocal relationship between the profession and society.

The majority of Chapter 14 is dedicated to describing the response of nurses to a number of national and international health crises. Over the course of two decades, nurses worked through the HIV/AIDS emergency, a nationwide nursing shortage, challenges with access to care in rural areas, and the Persian Gulf War. The commitment and caring of nurses throughout each crisis would not only demonstrate the profession's dedication to individual patients, but also reveal the potential of nurses to promote health in an increasingly complex system of care.

The chapter concludes with an introduction to the *Healthy People* initiatives, a federal health promotion and disease prevention program that began in 1979 and continues today. Moving national health goals toward preventive strategies rather than reactionary medical intervention signified a changing approach to health and wellness, something nurses had been doing for decades. Unfortunately, it would not be until the planning for the *Healthy People 2030* initiatives that a nurse assumed a high-ranking leadership position on the advisory committee.

Medicine and technology boxes in this chapter highlight the discoveries of antiretroviral therapy, the implementation of universal precautions, the emergence of drug-resistant tuberculosis, the use of surfactant for premature infants, and the creation of the acute care nurse practitioner specialty, the National Institute for Nursing Research, and the Magnet® Hospital Recognition Program for Excellence in Nursing Services. Legal boxes describe the significance of the ANA Social Policy Statement and the enactment of the Health Insurance Portability and Accountability Act and the Institute of Medicine publication *To Err Is Human*, the latter highlighting the alarming incidence and impact of preventable medical errors.

TOWARD A CULTURE OF HEALTH: NURSING IN THE 21ST CENTURY

Chapter 15, which concludes the book, argues that nursing's ability to reclaim its focus on health promotion and caring will be critical to its ability to provide for a culture of health in the United States in the years to come. Nurses are uniquely positioned to do so because of their long history in this regard.

Beginning with the 2001 attack on New York's World Trade Center, this chapter discusses significant events that had an impact on nursing during the first 17 years of the new century. Because there is so much new information in the 21st century and nurses and nursing organizations are making advances on all fronts, the chapter focuses only on select events of a historic nature, including the September 11, 2001, attack on the World Trade Center; military nursing in the Iraq War; the problems of the nursing shortage and an aging population; nurses' roles in the response to Hurricane Katrina in 2005 and the influenza epidemic in 2009; and the Flint, Michigan, water crisis that began in 2014.

Consistent with the format of other chapters, boxes highlight advances in law as well as ethical issues for nursing. Legal boxes include a focus on the Millennium Development Goals set by the World Health Organization, the passage of the Nurse Reinvestment Act in 2002, and the enactment of the Affordable Care Act in 2010. An ethics box highlights the difficult choices that nurses faced under extreme conditions during Hurricane Katrina. The chapter ends with "Reflections on History," highlighting the words of historian Julie Fairman in 2016.

Thus, beginning with the early settlers in America and tracing the history of nursing through the centuries, this book highlights turning points in the professional journey and gives voice to those who have long been silent. We invite you to turn the page and begin that journey for yourself, identifying your professional roots and learning lessons from the past. **Also available online from Springer Publishing Company is an image bank of all photographs found in this book. Readers can access this at www.springerpub.com/keeling.**

Arlene W. Keeling
Michelle C. Hehman
John Kirchgessner

NOTE

1. Nightingale, F. (1859). *Notes on nursing: What it is and what it is not.* New York: J. B. Lippincott Company; 1859 reprint of copy from the Library of Congress, Washington, DC.

Acknowledgments

After years of teaching undergraduate and graduate courses on nursing history, we were intrigued with the possibility of creating a textbook on the history of the profession in the United States that would not only provide an overview of the major events and milestones, but also give some grassroots accounts of nurses' experiences in the field. We also wanted to situate nursing history within a larger social, political, and economic context of the history of the United States and include issues of race, class, and gender. In addition, we realized that the history of American nursing would need to include highlights of technology, science, medicine, ethics, and the law.

To write a history of nursing of this length and complexity required a team effort, and we need to thank all those who helped bring this project to fruition. First and foremost, we would like to thank the University of Virginia's dean, Dorrie Fontaine, for providing sabbatical time for Dr. Keeling to complete the work. We are especially grateful to Drs. Barbra Mann Wall and Barbara Brodie for their support and advice and to the Eleanor Crowder Bjoring Center for Nursing Historical Inquiry at the University of Virginia for its wealth of archival sources and administrative assistance. In particular, we would like to acknowledge the contributions of Linda Hanson, whose organizational skills and knowledge of the center's collections facilitated the work. She not only located photographs to illustrate the book, but also identified primary source documents to help us give voice to nurses who were diverse in culture, class, race, and ethnicity. Accolades must be given to Doris Rikkers for her ability to edit our work from proposal to completed manuscript. Her extensive knowledge of the production process and organizational skills kept us on track. We are also grateful for the vision and photography skills of Jennifer Elizabeth Byrne. She provided expertise with the selection of photographs and their enhancement. We would also like to thank Emma Duvernay for using her talent to provide us with ideas for a preliminary design and for her willingness to take a last-minute trip to Flint, Michigan, to document the water crisis there.

Special thanks go to the archivists across the United States who so generously gave their time, expertise, and patience to help document our research. Given the fact that this book is a compilation of years of research, we cannot acknowledge every archivist and his or her contributions. We would, however, like to recognize the assistance of Elisa Stroh at the Barbara Bates Center for the Study of the History of Nursing, the archivists at the Henry E. Huntington Library, the Bancroft Library at the University of California at Berkeley, the Stephen F. Austin archives at the University of Texas, the Pediatric History Center at the American Academy of Pediatrics, the West Virginia Archives, the University of Virginia Special Collections, the Sisters of the Holy Cross Archives and Records Department, the National Park Service Archives, and the Midwest Nursing

History Research Center. We are also indebted to archivists at the National Library of Medicine and the Library of Congress for putting many photographs and documents online.

In addition to using primary sources, we relied on published and unpublished histories of the profession. Therefore, we must acknowledge the contributions of our colleagues for the work they have done in the history of nursing and medicine. Their books and research articles informed our understanding of so many complicated issues related to nursing's history. Many are identified as sources for further reading. We would also like to recognize the University of Virginia School of Nursing graduate students for their papers, presentations, and doctoral dissertations. These not only provided us with source material for the book, but also gave us the impetus to compile their results into one source that could be shared widely. Their work is worthy of a read, providing unique, in-depth, and diverse perspectives on nursing's history. In this regard, we are particularly indebted to Beth Hundt for her work on St. Elizabeth's Hospital; Bridget Houlahan for her dissertation work on school nursing; Frank Hickey for his autobiographical history of Union Hospital on September 11, 2001; and Gwenyeth Milbrath for her papers and dissertation on the nurses of Pearl Harbor.

The perspective of those who were willing to read drafts of our material was particularly important to the development of the book, and special thanks go to the students of St. John Fisher College Wegmans School of Nursing. Undergraduate nursing students read Chapters 1 through 3 of the manuscript and provided constructive and very honest feedback. Our colleagues from the University of Pennsylvania Barbara Bates Center for the Study of the History of Nursing and their students also provided a critique of several early chapters. We thank them.

We are especially grateful to our families, friends, and colleagues for their support and patience. This project demanded a great deal of attention over many months. We would especially like to recognize Mike Hehman for his patience and support; Michael, Emma, and Matthew, who stood at the door of the study waiting for attention (and sometimes dinner!); and Pat and Vicky Chambers who provided unending babysitting hours for their grandchildren. We would also like to recognize Jenny and D'Arcy Byrne and their children, D'Arcy III, Gryphon, and L'Wren, who provided humor, love, concerts, and outings for relief from writing; Rich and Eric for their love and hospitality in Cape Cod; Preston White for his wonderful sense of humor and reminders that an "elephant can only be eaten in small bites"; Amy, Owen, and little Macsen for "Facetime" support; and David, Jen, Zadie, and Auden for providing brief weekend escapes to Chicago. Last but not least, we are indebted to Don for his loving support and willingness to keep the home fires burning in Rochester during our author meetings in Chicago and Charlottesville.

Finally, no project can be completed without funding, and for this we need to acknowledge previous funding from the National Institute of Nursing Research and the National Library of Medicine (G13), which provided resources to gather data on the history of nursing in coronary care units, the Frontier Nursing Service, and the Indian Health Service; numerous intramural grants from the University of Virginia School of Nursing Office of Nursing Research; and the Brunner Fellowship from the Barbara Bates Center for the Study of the History of Nursing at the University of Pennsylvania—all of which provided resources to research the 1918 influenza pandemic and nurses in migrant camps. More recently, funding from a "4VA" project, provided by the University of Virginia and James Madison University, allowed for the inclusion of Alaskan nursing and facilitated the completion of this book.

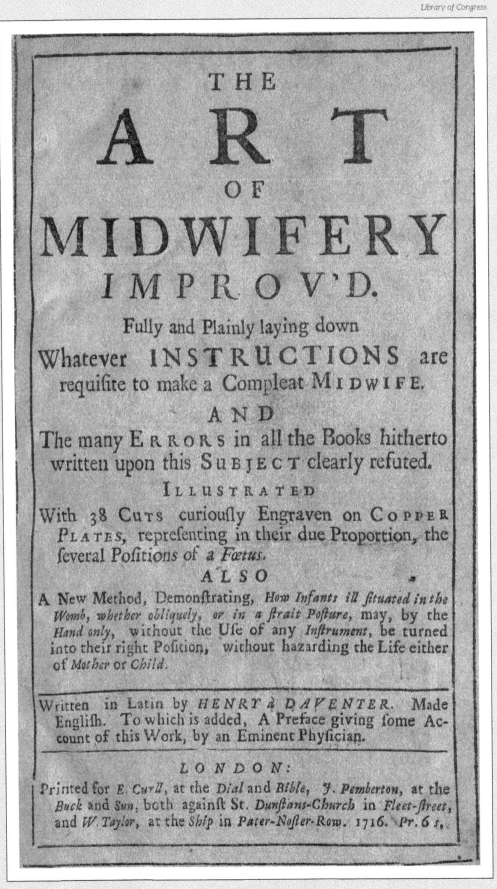

THE
ART
OF
MIDWIFERY
IMPROV'D.

Fully and Plainly laying down

Whatever INSTRUCTIONS are
requisite to make a Compleat MIDWIFE.

AND

The many ERRORS in all the Books hitherto
written upon this SUBJECT clearly refuted.

ILLUSTRATED

With 38 CUTS curiously Engraven on COPPER
PLATES, representing in their due Proportion, the
several Positions of a *Fœtus*.

ALSO

A New Method, Demonstrating, *How Infants ill situated in the
Womb, whether obliquely, or in a strait Posture*, may, by the
Hand only, without the Use of any *Instrument*, be turned
into their right Position, without hazarding the Life either
of *Mother* or *Child*.

Written in Latin by *HENRY à DAVENTER*. Made
English. To which is added, A Preface giving some Account of this Work, by an Eminent Physician.

LONDON:

Printed for *E. Curll*, at the *Dial* and *Bible*, *J. Pemberton*, at the
Buck and *Sun*, both against St. *Dunstans-Church* in *Fleet-street*,
and *W. Taylor*, at the *Ship* in *Pater-Noster-Row*. 1716. Pr. 6 s.

Cover of midwifery book.

CHAPTER 1

Nursing in the Colonial Era and Early Days of the United States

1607–1840

John C. Kirchgessner

"Our men were destroyed with cruel diseases as Swellings . . .
Burning Fevers . . . for the most part they died of mere famine.
There were never Englishmen left in a foreign Country in such
misery as we were in this new discovered Virginia."[1]

George Percy, 1625

In 1625, colonial leader George Percy wrote these remarks about the British colonists' experience during their first years in Virginia, a time in which they succumbed to illness and had no trained physicians or nurses to care for them. The newcomers might have turned for help to the Algonquian tribe living nearby, but instead, the colonists waged war with them. For thousands of years the Algonquians and other Native Americans had treated members of their own tribes when they, like the newcomers, experienced "cruel diseases." Basing their care on the restoration of "connectedness and wholeness," Native Americans treated their sick with natural remedies, rituals, and prayer. They used rest, good nutrition, and fluids to heal the body, and rituals and prayer to restore the spirit. The natives' care was "practical and sensible"; the English colonists who landed on the coast of Virginia in 1607 could have benefitted from their advice.[2]

Instead, the Englishmen invaded the Algonquian tribes' land, causing tension and hostilities between the settlers and the Native Americans, and leaving the colonists on their own to adjust to the wilderness and care for their sick. The colonists had few resources, and no physician, apothecary, or surgeon. Neither did they have any midwives, or even a woman who was not a midwife. The entire party was made up of men and boys employed by the London Company to establish English settlements in North America. Among them were two barber-surgeons whom the London Company *had* sent, assuming that a surgeon's skills would be necessary if the men suffered wounds and injuries during the Atlantic crossing or when they cut down trees to build a fort. The London sponsors, however, had not even considered disease as a serious possibility—most of the men in the company were young and healthy when they set sail from England.[3]

Based on previous experience with settlers on Roanoke Island in 1580 (in what would become known as the Lost Colony), the London Company had cautioned the colonists to avoid the lowlands of Virginia surrounding the Chesapeake Bay, warning them to avoid planting "in a low or moist place" because it would "prove unhealthful."[4] Ignoring the warning and establishing a fort in the marshy, mosquito-infested land on the banks of the James River, the colonists soon found the New World less than hospitable. Two thirds of the party died within the first year.

In 1608, a second supply fleet arrived in Virginia, bringing medical supplies, a physician, a surgeon, two apothecaries, and two women. Mistress Forrest, who came to join her husband, was accompanied by her personal maid young Anne Burras.[5] Together this small group of people with some knowledge of medical care would have to tend to the entire settlement.

More than a year passed before additional women arrived with the London Company's third supply fleet in August 1609. Soon more than 300 English colonists were living in Jamestown Settlement. These numbers placed an even greater burden on the food supply and other provisions. In fact, a lack of sufficient food became the limiting factor in the settlers' survival; severe malnutrition contributed to their susceptibility to disease. The settlers also began to experience illnesses resulting from drinking polluted and brackish tidal water. By September 1609, less than 2 years after their arrival, half of the original colonists were dead[6]; those who survived turned to each other for help.

Disaster struck in October when the Powhatans attacked James Fort, killing the settlement's livestock and any settlers who dared to venture outside the fortress. Those who were confined inside the fort faced rapidly dwindling supplies, unsanitary conditions, and the outbreak of disease. Winter brought further hardship. Known as the "starving time," only 60 settlers survived the winter of 1609 to 1610.[7] Desperate to survive, the remaining settlers ate what was available, consuming "everything from the horses brought by the Gates fleet to rats, snakes, mice, and roots dug from the forest."[8] Both men and women—whoever was left alive—cared for those who were weak and dying.

"The colonists were . . . so diseased . . . fainte, and desperate of recoverie."[9]

Sir Thomas Dale, 1611

By June 1610 another physician, Dr. Lawrence Bohune, arrived in Jamestown and found dwindling medical supplies and the settlers suffering from "fluxes and agues." With few resources, Bohune began to investigate "the medicinal properties of such plants as sassafras, rhubarb, and the gums of the local trees."[10] The daughter of the Powhatan chief, Matoaka (more widely known as Pocahontas), captured by the English settlers in 1609, no doubt provided help.[11]

Like the English colonists in Jamestown, the settlers who arrived on Cape Cod aboard the *Mayflower* in 1620 were on their own to care for others in their company when they became ill. In contrast to the Jamestown settlers, however, the pilgrims had in their company several leaders who had some training in aspects of medical care. They also had a few women in their ranks, some of whom may have had experience as midwives. Despite that medical expertise, more than half of the original company died during the winter of 1620 to 1621 after they had transferred from the Cape to the mainland. All were victims of an epidemic that swept the new colony of Plymouth, Massachusetts. The epidemic, likely the same disease (typhus, smallpox, or plague) that had destroyed many of the Native American tribes in the northeast a few years earlier, wreaked havoc among the settlers. One of their leaders, William Bradford, later recounted how care of the sick had been left to a handful of survivors, noting that "six or seven healthy persons" did all that was necessary.

From 1621 to 1630 additional ships arrived in New England; by 1630 the colony had grown to almost 300 people. All would be dependent on each other for survival. They would also need the help of Native American tribes long accustomed to the environment and its resources.

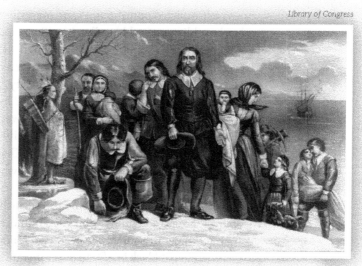

Pilgrims debark from the Mayflower in 1620 to settle colonial America at Plymouth, Massachusetts.

Other European nations had addressed the need for medical personnel for their newly established colonies even before the British arrived in America. In 1565, the Spanish government sent colonists to settle in an area that would become St. Augustine, Florida. Officials in the first wave of settlers included two surgeons and an apothecary. A century later, however, in 1697, the Spanish no longer supplied such personnel. According to one source, "small thatched hospitals were periodically erected, with convicts, soldiers or slaves being employed as nurses."[13] In contrast to the Spanish, the French colonies along the Gulf Coast fared much better; the Company of the Indies supplied them with medical personnel and assisted them in establishing hospitals.

> ### "A Rare Example" of Care
>
> *"There was but six or seven healthy persons, who . . . spared no pains, night or day . . . fetched them wood, made them fires . . . clothed them and unclothed them . . . in a word, did all the homely and necessary offices for them . . . a rare example and worthy to be remembered."[12]*
>
> William Bradford, 1621

CARE OF THE SICK AND INJURED IN THE EARLY 17TH CENTURY

Colonists arriving in the Americas brought with them techniques for caring for the sick and injured then in use in Western Europe. These, in turn, were influenced by ancient Greek beliefs as well as church doctrines. Epidemics, famine, and war were some of the factors that contributed to disease in the general population during this time and, more importantly, to the infant mortality rate during the 17th and 18th centuries.

European and Religious Influences

In the early colonial period care for the sick reflected the contemporary knowledge of health and disease and the methods of care customary in Western Europe. That knowledge, developed during the Renaissance, was in fact knowledge based on the rediscovery of the ancient beliefs of Galen, Hippocrates, and Aristotle. But how to care for the sick was also based on superstition. These beliefs (known as the Theory of the Four Humors) held that health was a balance of the four elements—fire, air, earth, and water—evidenced in the four cardinal fluids: yellow bile (fire), blood (air), black bile (earth), and phlegm (water).[14] Illness was viewed as an imbalance of any of the elements, or humors.

Beliefs about the causes of illness and the treatments varied. Because the Catholic and Protestant churches controlled medical training in Europe's universities, the cause of disease was often attributed to God's punishment for sin. In this case, prayer, fasting, and self-inflicted punishment were prescribed as cures. Some therapies included cupping, leeches, blisters, and bloodletting. These medical remedies often caused more harm to the patient, and sometimes resulted in death.

Some European religious orders nursed the sick. One of these religious orders was the Company of the Daughters of Charity of St. Vincent de Paul, Servants of the Sick Poor, which was founded in France in 1633 by Saints Vincent de Paul and Louise de Maril-lac. Unlike other religious women who were cloistered in convents and isolated from the outside world, the Daughters of Charity lived and worked among the poor. Later, in the early 19th century, the Daughters of Charity and other religious orders brought their nursing knowledge and skills to America where they established hospitals and provided urgently needed services.[15]

Sometimes, people blamed food rather than God for illness. According to one source: "Some food brought on good humors, and others, evil humors. For example, nasturtium, mustard, and garlic produced reddish bile; lentils, cabbage and the meat of old goats . . . begot black bile."[16] In other instances, people used food as a cure, making broths to counteract evil humors. For example, a common treatment for leprosy was a "broth made of the flesh of a black snake."[17]

Herbs were also considered as potential cures. Typical herbal remedies included cayenne, sarsaparilla, chamomile, and valerian root. In other instances, people used common household items like mustard, onions, honey, lemon, and porridge. They used mustard to make plasters or mix with bath water; onions to rub on the skin or hang in a sack around the patient's neck; honey and lemon to relieve sore throats; and "hot porridge" to treat cholera.[18]

Infant Mortality and Epidemics in Colonial America

From the earliest days of the colonization of America, children died in infancy at an alarming rate. The death of a baby in its first year of life is viewed as a reflection of the overall health and well-being of a nation, and in the 17th century infant mortality in the colonies has been estimated to be between 20% and 40%.[19] People living in isolated villages in rural New England fared somewhat better, with an average infant mortality rate of 15% or less. In contrast, infants living in cities or sea ports were at a much greater risk of dying in the first year of life.[20] Famines and war were contributing factors, as were maternal health, sanitation practices, and the availability of fresh water. There were, of course, yearly fluctuations in the infant mortality rate, with several contributing factors. Epidemics were commonplace and significantly affected the overall population's health and ultimately the infant mortality rate.

Epidemics were particularly threatening in America. Early English, French, and Spanish colonists suffered many of the same diseases they had experienced in their homelands; among these were respiratory and gastrointestinal infections, fevers, cancers, mumps, measles, diphtheria, scarlet fever, pertussis, dysentery, influenza, and small-pox.[21] Epidemics of any one of these diseases could be devastating to a community. A severe diphtheria epidemic swept through New England in 1735 and again in 1740, claiming more than 5,000 lives.[22] Each year during the summer months, infants and children were particularly at risk for a form of dysentery known as "bloody flux," "summer complaint," or "cholera infantum," usually caused by spoiled cow's milk.

While smaller, regional outbreaks of smallpox occurred every winter and spring in various locations throughout the colonies, epidemics of the disease involving large segments of the wider population struck approximately every 20 years.[23] In 1677, approximately one fifth of Boston's population died during a smallpox epidemic. By the late 18th century, as more colonists experimented with smallpox inoculations, epidemics became less common, but the disease was not completely eradicated.

Different regions within the new colonies faced a variety of additional diseases. In the marshlands of the south, colonists experienced yellow fever, malaria, and hookworm, while northerners had to deal with the ills associated with exposure to harsh, cold weather.[24] Cholera was endemic in cities and towns with poor sanitation and contaminated water supplies, regardless of the city's regional location. Later, the disease spread west with emigrants as they traveled on the Overland Trail.

CAREGIVER ROLES AND SETTINGS

Throughout the colonial period, care of the sick was delivered in the home. However, many citizens, particularly the poor and infirm, did not have family to care for them. Almshouses were established to house, feed, and care for the poor. Viewed as benevolent institutions, they were often crowded, filthy, and lacked adequate and nutritious food. Poor conditions and the inability to properly treat patients in almshouses would eventually lead to the establishment of the Pennsylvania Hospital and the Public Hospital for Persons of Insane and Disordered Minds in the mid-18th century.

Women as Caregivers

No matter the cause of disease, or the beliefs surrounding it, the majority of the care for the sick fell to women—wives and mothers or lay midwives who had been schooled in childbirth and herbal therapies by their mothers and grandmothers. As historians Barbara Ehrenreich and Deirdre English described, "The women were doctors without degrees . . . learning from each other, and passing on experience from neighbor to neighbor and mother to daughter."[25]

Colonial leader Cotton Mather (1663–1728), an influential Puritan clergyman and physician, praised the work of the women, noting how John Elliott's wife "obtained unto a considerable skill in physicks and chyryurgery [sic], which enabled her to dispense many safe, good, and useful medicines [to] some hundreds of sick and weak and maimed people."[26]

In the early years of the United States, midwives and laywomen continued to play an important role in healing the sick—a role that was passed down through the generations. Many of these women acted as pharmacists, offering their knowledge of the cultivation and medicinal use of herbal remedies. In pregnancy and childbirth, they acted as both abortionist and midwife, assisting women with family planning as well as delivering babies and offering postpartum care. As the "unlicensed doctors and anatomists of Western history," women healers performed a number of health services, "travelling from home to home and village to village."[27]

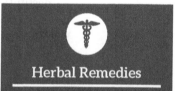

Herbal Remedies

"Many of the midwives' herbal remedies still have their place in modern pharmacology. They used ergot during and after labor . . . the drugs used today to stop post-partum hemorrhage. Midwives also used belladonna to inhibit uterine contractions when miscarriage threatened."[28]

Barbara Ehrenreich and Deirdre English, 2010

America's Almshouses

As Europeans settled in America and faced the problem of providing for the destitute, they adopted the methods that had been used to care for the poor and infirm in their homelands. Thus, they predominantly established almshouses for those without means or access to medical care at home.[29] Whether sponsored by churches, the government, or individual citizens, almshouses were social institutions and their mission was one of benevolence, particularly for the poor.[30]

Although they varied greatly in their size and conditions, almshouses were usually large facilities, often poorly managed, filthy, and unsafe. Food was inadequately prepared at best. In some cases, inmates were forced to "cook and forage" for their own food.[31] Living conditions were horrid. Residents lived in small crowded rooms; individuals often shared beds. In some instances, the dead were left for days before authorities removed them. The cramped, poorly constructed housing, lack of adequate and nutritious food, and poor sanitary conditions all contributed to the spread of disease within the institution. Other inmates or poorly paid former inmates provided what little nursing care was available.[32] Often these caregivers were slovenly, unkempt, and of poor character, and thus gave nursing a bad name. These institutions, which were designed to relieve the abysmal conditions in which the poor, infirmed, and destitute lived, ultimately served as a community's "catch-all."[33] In fact, admission to an almshouse served as a symbol of an individual's inadequacy to provide economically for himself or herself and his or her family, and inmates who once contributed to a community came to be viewed as the "undeserving poor."[34] By the mid-18th century, people in some towns and municipalities began to recognize the inadequacies of almshouses: They were incapable of providing safe and effective care for those who were acutely ill.

The Pennsylvania Hospital

In 1750, Philadelphia leaders were among the first to realize that the city's almshouses could not provide the care needed by those who were physically and mentally ill. Determined to address the issue, Benjamin Franklin and Dr. Thomas Bond appealed to the public and to government officials to establish a hospital. Using their political skills, Franklin and Bond convinced the citizens of Philadelphia and the Pennsylvania Assembly that such an institution was necessary. The men were successful; the Pennsylvania Hospital opened on February 10, 1752, with the initial intent to serve Philadelphians "who were destitute, ill, and worthy of society's compassion."[35] The new hospital was unique in that it was created to cure the sick. As Benjamin Franklin argued:

> Poor distempered persons, who languish long in pain and misery under various disorders of body and mind . . . cannot have the benefit of regular advice, attendance, lodging, diet and medicines . . . therefore often suffer for want thereof . . . which inconveniency might be happily removed by collecting the patients into one common Provincial Hospital, properly disposed and appointed, where they may be comfortably subsisted, and their health taken care of at a small charge, and . . . their disease may be cured and removed.[36]

Several important hospital policies differentiated the new hospital from Philadelphia's almshouses. Most importantly, only patients suffering from curable diseases would be admitted, while those with contagious diseases such as smallpox and yellow fever would be barred.[37] Second, those who were chronically ill were not admitted because they would take up beds needed for those who could be cured.[38] In addition, patients were held in the hospital no longer than was absolutely necessary; they were discharged as soon as they were considered cured. They were also discharged if they were "deemed incurable."[39]

"Susannah Brownholt was admitted 'with a Rottenness in the large Bone of the Leg.'"[40]

Pennsylvania Hospital Record, August 22, 1752

The Philadelphia Hospital's Board of Managers also made the decision to fund the voluntary hospital through the generosity of benefactors and through fees charged to patients who could pay. Originally, administrators envisioned the hospital to be an institution whose mission was to care for the indigent. Soon, however, those in charge realized that by admitting private patients when space was available, they could defray costs for those who were unable to pay.[41] In addition, the admission of middle- and upper-class citizens would help convince the public that it was acceptable to go to the hospital for a cure.[42]

In 1752, Pennsylvania Hospital had three "nurses." Elizabeth Gardiner served as a matron and another woman served as both a maid and nurse.[43] A male employee was also hired to care for the few mentally ill patients who were admitted to the hospital. For more than 100 years after its founding, untrained women and men provided the nursing care at the hospital. Often hospital trustees recruited former patients as nurses, most of whom were uneducated. As Francis Packard recalled, if patients "had shown some aptitude or desire to remain as attendants,"[44] they were offered positions in the ward. The hospital would not establish a training school for nurses until 1883.

Thus, the Pennsylvania Hospital evolved out of the societal need to provide care to the community's acutely ill citizens. At the same time, the hospital represented the beginning of a social movement that attempted to mold colonial society through charity. The hospital attempted to gain society's respect for the *worthy poor*—those citizens who had high moral values and a devout work ethic. Although Philadelphia established a unique way in which to care for

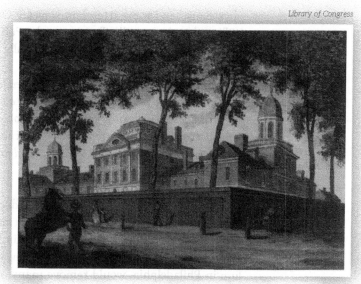

Starting from 1752, the Pennsylvania Hospital provided care to meet the medical needs of Philadelphia's poor.

its sick-poor, other cities and communities in the United States did not. For decades America's sick-poor had no choice but to seek care in almshouses.[45]

Williamsburg: The "Public Hospital for Persons of Insane and Disordered Minds"

In 1766, nearly a decade before the American Revolutionary War and 14 years after the establishment of the Pennsylvania Hospital, Virginia Governor Francis Fauquier spoke with the Williamsburg House of Burgesses about the need for a hospital in the city to house the colony's mentally ill. Describing them as "a poor unhappy . . . people" who were "deprived of their senses and wander about the countryside terrifying the rest of their fellow creatures," Governor Fauquier proposed the establishment of a public hospital in which the mentally ill could be cured.[48] Initially unconvinced, House delegates finally took notice after the governor confined some of Williamsburg's mentally ill citizens in the town's prison. On June 4, 1770, the delegates adopted an act to "Make provision for the Support and Maintenance of Ideots, Lunaticks, and other Persons of unsound Minds [sic]."[49]

Construction on the government-funded hospital began in 1771. It opened on October 12, 1773, with a staff of "a keeper, a matron for the female patients, two visiting

Dr. Benjamin Rush

Philadelphia physician Benjamin Rush, a 1768 graduate of the University of Edinburgh, was "perhaps the foremost American physician of the Colonial and early national era."[46] Influenced by the Age of Enlightenment, Rush subscribed to the idea that medicine should be based on empirical evidence rather than experience. He wrote extensively on cholera infantum (summer diarrhea), and diphtheria—both of which caused death in infants and children each year. Rush advocated the Theory of the Four Humors.[47]

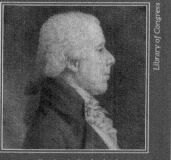

Benjamin Rush, the foremost American physician of Colonial America.

physicians," and some attendant slaves.[50] Originally intended to be a place to care for Williamsburg's mentally ill citizens, the Public Hospital was instead an institution that removed the severely and incurable mentally ill from society. In fact, it was set up as such:

> The building housed 24 cells, all designed for the security and isolation of their occupants. Each cell had a stout door with a barred window that looked on a dim central passage; a mattress, a chamber pot, and an iron ring in the wall to which the patient's wrist or leg fetters were attached. Neither harmless nor incurable people were admitted; the cells were reserved for dangerous individuals or patients who might be treated and discharged.[51]

Treatment during the first several decades of the Public Hospital's existence was focused on physical restraint, water treatments, bleeding, and blistering. It would not be until 1836, with the adoption of Phillip Pinel's "moral treatment," that the philosophy of care changed for the better. The new approach, already in use in the Friend's Asylum in Philadelphia, would remove many of the physical treatments and restraints in favor of providing a kinder environment, "firm but gentle encouragement" toward self-control, as well as "work therapy and leisure activity."[52]

NURSING IN THE REVOLUTIONARY WAR AND POST-REVOLUTIONARY PERIOD

The American Revolution called on individuals to care for the sick and injured, both in the field and at home. Most women remained at home and cared for their families and members of their local communities. Others followed the army, providing care near the battlefront. The nation's early leaders in the post–Revolutionary period believed the government had the responsibility to protect the public's health and general welfare.

Nursing and Medicine in the American Revolutionary War (1775–1783)

During the American Revolution, soldiers and laywomen (known as "camp followers") took care of the sick and injured in army camps. Both wives of army officers and "public-minded" women opened their homes to wounded soldiers and those undergoing smallpox inoculation. Without any formal training, the women fed the sick and injured, administered medications, washed clothes, and "attended to the hygiene" of those who were sick.[53]

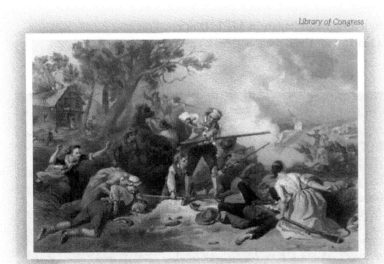

During the war, "public-minded" women with little nursing experience tended the sick and injured.

Throughout the winter months of the war, when the fighting and movement of troops was minimal, Martha Washington joined her husband in his winter encampment, often lodging in nearby farmhouses. Given the prevalence of smallpox among the troops, General George Washington insisted that his wife undergo inoculation for the virus before her first winter visit. He had seen enough of the ravages of the disease to take a chance on having her inoculated with a tiny amount of smallpox matter from an infected patient. Washington's fears were justified. As historian Jeanne Abrams has documented:

"Smallpox was one of the most feared diseases of the 18th century. In the spring of 1776, it wreaked havoc on the American army and killed more soldiers than combat."[54]

During those long winters of the war, Martha Washington comforted soldiers who were injured or sick.[56] Like most colonial women, she knew about the usefulness of rest, fluids, and herbal medicines to treat illness, and turned to "a variety of tonic cordials, rhubarb (a purging laxative), the opium-based laudanum, and the popular emetic, ipecac" when she deemed it necessary. She also used quinine bark and calomel, as well as her famous cure for pinworms: "whiskey, wormseed, rhubarb and garlic."[57] Mrs. Washington herself cared for her husband during his illnesses. In 1777, when the General contracted a sore throat that persisted for 10 days, Martha remained at his side treating his infected throat with "molasses and onions."[58]

Colonial Leaders and Health Beliefs

In the colonial period and early days of the United States, the nation's medical care was influenced by the beliefs of its founding fathers. Colonial leaders George Washington, John Adams, Thomas Jefferson, James Madison, and Benjamin Franklin were all followers of the Enlightenment. As such, they believed one key to the citizenry's happiness, contentment, and health was the government's promotion of the general welfare. Part of that responsibility was the protection of the public's health through preventive measures.[59] Among these were the endorsement of vaccination against smallpox, the recommendation that people exercise and have adequate nutrition, and the advice that certain foods were particularly beneficial to one's health.

The leaders were proponents of smallpox inoculation for all citizens, but in particular for their family members, employees, slaves, and the military troops. Each in his own way understood the importance of maintaining a healthy population in order for a plantation, city, colony, country, or army to be productive and to have continued success. Having seen the devastating effects of smallpox and its ability to spread through a community, General Washington understood the importance of smallpox inoculation—particularly for the health of the Continental Army but also for the health and productivity of the slaves on his plantation. Therefore, he insisted that both groups be inoculated.[60] Thomas Jefferson agreed, later advocating for smallpox inoculation for all Americans after hearing news of Edward Jenner's success with a cowpox vaccine in England.

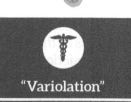

"Variolation"

For centuries, physicians in ancient cultures had experimented with live smallpox inoculation. The Chinese used powdered smallpox scabs inserted into the nostrils; the Turks scratched smallpox into tiny lesions on the skin. By the 1700s colonists in America adopted some of these informal and unscientific methods, performing "do-it-yourself" inoculations.[55]

The Discovery of Smallpox Vaccine (1788)

After observing that milkmaids were resistant to smallpox, in 1788 English physician Edward Jenner inoculated a healthy 8-year-old boy with matter from a cowpox lesion. After further experimentation, in 1798 Jenner published a small booklet on his successes, introducing the world to the preventive vaccination.[61]

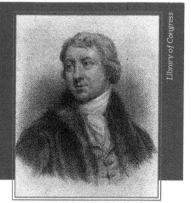

Edward Jenner, who introduced the world to the smallpox vaccination.

Both Thomas Jefferson and Dr. Benjamin Rush believed that citizens should do everything within their power to stay healthy. Both advocated rest, adequate nutrition, and exercise for the maintenance of health. They also recommended drinking hot chocolate as a health benefit. In 1785, Jefferson wrote about his belief, noting: "The superiority of chocolate both for health and nourishment will soon give it preference over tea and coffee."[63] Benjamin Rush concurred, prescribing a cup of weak chocolate with a biscuit as part of the diet for his patients being inoculated for smallpox.[64]

> "We should enable the great mass of the people to practice [smallpox vaccination] on their own families."[62]
>
> Thomas Jefferson, 1802

Martha Ballard, New England Midwife

While Martha Washington and other women followed the army during the war, providing care for soldiers, many colonial women stayed home, caring for their families and members of their local communities. Typical of these was Martha Ballard, a New England midwife who lived and worked in the small town of Hallowell on the Kennebec River in Maine. From January 1785 to December 1800 she documented her daily activities in a diary, writing about everything from "footing stockings . . . pickling meat, sorting cabbages" and spinning flax to assisting her neighbors in childbirth and illness. She also recorded the delivery of 814 infants.[65]

> "Called to Mrs. Shaw who has been ill some time. Put her safe to Bed with a daughter at 10 O'Clok this evening."[66]
>
> Martha Ballard, 1787

In August 1787 Martha Ballard delivered four infants in the small community. But she did more than "extract babies." In fact, Ballard functioned as "a nurse, physician, mortician, pharmacist and attentive wife."[67] During the late 18th century, physicians were scarce and those who were available usually practiced surgery.

Martha Ballard learned midwifery and nursing from her mother, her grandmother, and other women in the community by assisting them as they delivered babies and cared for the sick. That training was thorough. According to historian Laura Thatcher Ulrich, by 1785 Ballard "knew how to manufacture salves, syrups, pills, teas, and ointments, and how to prepare oil emulsions, how to poultice wounds, dress burns, and treat dysentery and sore throats," as well as treat a myriad of other conditions.[68]

Writing in her diary in August 1787, Ballard recounted the details of her daily activities, documenting her nursing and midwifery work:

> August 7: "Clear. I was Calld to Mrs. Howards this morning for to see her son. Find him very low. Went from Mrs. Howards to see Mrs. Williams. Find her very unwell . . . from thence to Joseph Fosters to see her sick Children. Find Saray and Daniel very ill. Came home went to the field and got some Cold water root. Then called to Mr. Kenydays to see Polly—very ill with the Canker. Gave her great Ease. Returned home after dark.

> August 16: "At Mr. Cowens. Put Mrs. Claton to bed with a son at 3pm. Came to Mr. Kenadays to see his wife who has a swelling under her arm. Polly is mending. . . . Called from there to Winthrop to Jeremy Richard's wife in Travil [labor]. Arrived about 9 O'Clok, Evin [sic] Birth Mrs. Claton's son"[69]

Sometimes Ballard stayed with families for a few days, providing direct care. At other times, pulled in several directions at once, she taught family members what to do for the patient, leaving "directions" for them before she left for another home or returned to her own family.

Diary Entry

August 23: "I set out to visit Joseph Forster's children. Met Eprhaim Cowen by Brook's Farm. Called me to see his Dafter [daughter] Polly and Nabby who are sick with the rash. Find them very ill. Gave directions."[70]

Martha Ballard, 1787

TRANSITIONS IN MEDICINE

Women who nursed have had to work within the context of the state of the art of medicine in any given era. Social and cultural boundaries directly influenced the care they provided to the sick and dying throughout the colonial and post–Revolutionary periods. However, these boundaries were often transcended, most notably on southern plantations. In the late 18th century, and for the first half of the 19th century, care was influenced by allopathy and homeopathy, two very different methodologies. It was these opposing philosophies that ultimately led to the reinvention of medical practice in the United States and the establishment of the American Medical Association.

The two types of physicians, allopaths ("regulars") and homeopaths, took different approaches to illness. "An Allopath would pour into those irritated, inflamed and bleeding bowels, cathartics, mercury, castor-oil, opium, astringents, such as sugar of lead, etc." And as they prided themselves on appreciable doses, the dose would consist of a considerable amount of the drug. A homoeopath, on the other hand, used remedies that acted more gently, "would remove the febrile irritation, control the spasms and severe distress, . . . gently, yet quickly and effectually."[71] In the 19th century some men began to question the regulars' practice. In fact, Thomas Jefferson, an advocate of using herbal medicines, advised aspiring medical students to "maintain a wise infidelity against the authority" of their allopathic instructors.[72]

Martha Washington at Mount Vernon

For years Martha Washington had followed the army during the Revolutionary War, serving as a nurse to her husband and the other men in the company. After the war, she returned to her role as mistress of Mount Vernon, a large plantation on the Potomac River across from Washington, DC. At Mount Vernon, Martha continued to nurse sick and injured family members, slaves, and any other individuals on the family's estate. As historian Jeanne Abrams notes, "Martha provided personalized medical care by 'watching' over her ill family members, sitting beside them, offering support and comfort, and administering food, drink, and medications."[73]

Martha Washington's lack of confidence in the contemporary medical treatments George Washington received during his final illness is one example of the public's growing doubt in the new scientific medical treatments espoused by physicians like Benjamin Rush. In December 1799, when more aggressive treatments were used to care for the president after he became acutely ill with a fever and sore throat, Mrs. Washington voiced concern when the president asked that one of the overseers at Mount Vernon bleed him. Nonetheless, working within the constraints of a hierarchical, male, and physician-dominated society, she agreed. That is not to say Martha did not attempt her own therapies. To relieve some of the discomfort in her husband's throat, Martha gave him syrup of molasses, butter, and vinegar.

Martha's concerns about the danger of harsh and invasive therapies

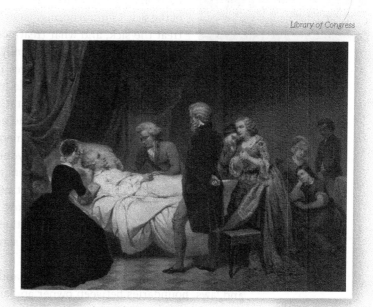

George Washington on his deathbed, 1799.

were valid. After his physician Dr. James Craik arrived, further bloodlettings occurred (a total of 32 oz. of blood was extracted from him in the fourth and final blood-letting). In addition, the president was given an emetic and an enema. Dr. Craik also "produced a blister on his throat in an attempt to balance the fluids in Washington's body . . . and ordered a potion of vinegar and sage tea prepared for gargling." In the end, neither the physicians' invasive treatments nor the home remedies given by his wife could save him. George Washington, the first president of the United States, died on December 14, 1799.[74]

Thompsonians and Botanicals

During the early 1800s, botanical therapies came to the forefront as a challenge to the more invasive practices of the regular physicians. The challenge was led by Samuel Thompson, a New Hampshire farmer, who had depended on a local woman "root healer" Mrs. Benton for care. Later, Thompson recounted how he had learned from the healer, writing: "When she used to go out and collect roots and herbs, she would take me with her." Those who adhered to Thompson's beliefs in botanical therapies soon became known as "Thompsonians."[75]

Exercise is "necessary for health, and health is the first of all objects."[78]

Thomas Jefferson, Letter to Martha, March 28, 1787

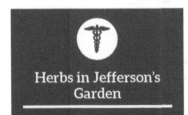

Herbs in Jefferson's Garden

Like many households in the early 1800s, Jefferson's garden included medicinal plants like marjoram (for cold symptoms), senna, rhubarb, and tansy (mild laxatives), and lavender, sage, mint, and thyme (for headaches, toothaches, and upset stomachs).

Thompson was not alone in his beliefs. Thomas Jefferson, author of the *Declaration of Independence*, second governor of Virginia, secretary of state under George Washington, and later the third president of the United States, supported the use of herbal medicines. He also supported the ingestion of wine and adherence to a regimen of daily exercise to promote health. Jefferson, who had a keen interest in medicine and knew more than most individuals about the topic, did not always agree with the use of harsh medical treatments like purges and bleeding used by the regular physicians. Instead, he relied on natural remedies, fluids, and rest—all with the goal of allowing nature to aid in recovery.[76] Jefferson did call on regular physicians and followed their advice when he felt it necessary. Usually this was in cases of "pleurisy, malaria and dysentery" among his family members or slaves.[77]

Cross-Cultural Exchanges in the Antebellum South

The institution of slavery, with its societal rules dictating how life was to be lived on both small farms and expansive plantations, also influenced the care of the sick. Cultural norms dictated who would request a physician, who would treat the sick, and what treatments would be used. It was a given that the planter and his immediate family, as well as White overseers, enjoyed all the freedoms of American citizenship. Slaves did not have citizenship status and were viewed as a commodity, an unchangeable fact until after the Civil War. Nonetheless, how slaves were treated varied from plantation to plantation; their care was dependent on several factors, most importantly the owners' and overseers' views toward their slaves. If owners viewed their slaves as mere property, they would often impose their European treatments for illness upon anyone who was ill, or tolerated the Blacks caring for themselves in their own way. If owners were more compassionate and caring, they viewed the slaves' health as their utmost responsibility and duty, acknowledging that effective treatment was important not only for the physical survival of the people, but also for the economic survival of their estate. In the latter case, owners often took into account the knowledge of the plantation slaves, even though it was illegal for Blacks to practice medicine.

While the institution of slavery demanded strict adherence to many customs, rules, and laws, boundaries between owner and slaves blurred when it came to maintaining the health of the plantation community. House slaves cared for their owner's family members, as well as their own. They participated actively in nursing care: doing the most menial tasks involved in caring for the sick, and also sharing recipes for cures. In turn, the mistresses of the plantation nursed the sick slaves.

The role that Southern women played in caring for their families' health was not greatly different from that of mothers and wives in New England and the Middle Atlantic states. The one distinct difference was the responsibility of the mistress of a large plantation. Her care extended beyond her immediate family members to everyone who lived on the estate, regardless of race and social status. The master of the plantation and the overseer may have been ultimately responsible for the well-being of their slaves, but the mistress usually attended to the sick slaves while the men were occupied elsewhere with plantation operations. As the daughter of one southern plantation owner remarked: "mother and grandmother were almost always talking over the wants of the Negroes . . . the principal objects of their lives seeming to be in providing [slaves with] these comforts."[79] In addition, it was not unusual for the mistress to protect the health of slave children as part of her routine domestic responsibilities. For example, a former slave from South Carolina, Emoline Glasgow, recalled that as a child her mistress gave her "mackaroot tea" as a worm remedy.[80]

Self-sufficiency on the plantation was critical for the well-being of everyone. Many plantations were miles away from the nearest physician, town, or city; reliance on those who were part of the "plantation family" was essential. Even if a doctor was in the vicinity, and the owner was willing to pay for professional care, the doctor sometimes was not available immediately, and hours or days could pass before the doctor's arrival. In the meantime, something had to be done to alleviate the pain and suffering of the slaves or family members. Someone White—the master, overseer, or mistress—had the responsibility to diagnose the problem and determine which drug was to be used, and at which dosage. Every household had a standard set of drugs available in their medicine chest, along with "accessories such as lancets, spatulas, scales, blister powders and paper for plasters, cupping instruments, mortars and syringes." Each household also had essential reference books, including "Simon's *Planter's Guide and Family Book of Medicine,* Ewell's *Medical Companion,* or South's *Household Surgery.*"[82] These provided help with the diagnosis, recommended treatments, and specific dosage of drugs.

Through trial and error the master and mistress learned what medicine and dosages worked best; if the combination was successful, it became the standard treatment for an illness until something better was found. Many recorded their findings and successful treatments in their personal journals or diaries. They also sought new options from newspapers, books, and almanacs.

The exchange of medical knowledge between slave owners and slaves was not uncommon.[84] Plantation mistresses relied on their past experiences and individual expertise in the use of herbs and other medicinal plants, the use of poultices and tonics, and the general principles used in home nursing care, but they also relied on the slaves' knowledge, sometimes discovering a better treatment than the one they had been using.

On larger plantations, hospitals of varying size and quality housed slaves who were severely sick, injured, or needed to be isolated from the general slave quarters. In these buildings the quality of care varied: Services were completely dependent upon the knowledge, skill, and experience of those in attendance. For the most part, other slaves and lay midwives cared for the sick. On smaller plantations, enslaved

> ### Treating Dysentery in a Slave Child
>
> *"I told [the slave child's] mother to give the tea made of the inner bark of Pine, Sweet Gum, and Dogwood."*[81]
>
> Mary Henderson, plantation mistress

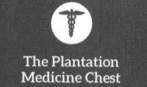

> ### The Plantation Medicine Chest
>
> "Plantation medicine chests were filled with ipecac from South America, jalap from Mexico, opium from the Far East, quinine from the Andes, and chamomile from Europe."[83] Other favorites were castor oil, calomel, laudanum, and camphor.

> *"Our Missus an' one of de slave' tend to the sick."*[85]
>
> A former slave from South Carolina

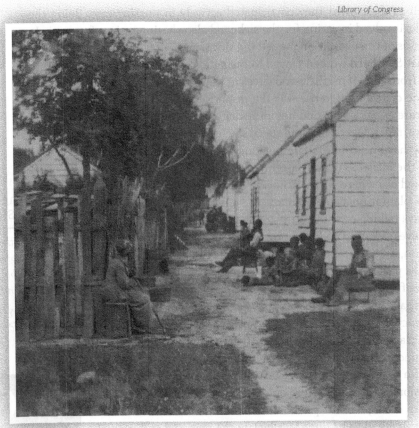

On smaller plantations, injured or sick slaves were cared for by their families in their slave cabins.

families cared for their own in their small cabins, some distance from the main house. For many slaves, prayer and song were as integral to healing as were herbal teas and poultices.

Black Slave Nurses and Midwives

On some southern plantations, one female slave was a gifted nurse and healer and thus became the primary attendant to all medical needs on the estate. Having secured the trust and respect of both Blacks and Whites, she used her knowledge of herbs and cures passed down through generations along with White remedies to restore health.

"Aunt Judy uster to tend us when we uns were sic' and anything Aunt Judy could'nt do 'hit won't wurth doin.'"[86]

"Uncle" Bacchus White, Former Slave, 1939

"Whenever any of de white folks 'roun' Hanover was goin' to have babies day always got word to Mr. Tinsely dat day want to hire me."[89]

Mildred Graves, Former Slave Midwife

A few Black slave nurses practiced their nursing skills beyond the boundaries of the plantation or household. Some town-dwelling slaves became well known for their care of others. One Black slave nurse, Jensey Snow, received high praise as well as her freedom because of her nursing skills. In 1825, Snow's owner, Benjamin Harrison, praised her for "several acts of extraordinary merit performed . . . during the last year, in nursing, & at the imminent risk of her own health & safety, exercising the most unexampled patience and attention in watching over the sick beds of several individuals of this town."[87] After obtaining her freedom, Jensey Snow continued to serve the public. She opened a hospital in Petersburg, Virginia— later known as "the Hospital of the well known nurse, Jinsey [sic] Snow."[88]

Black slaves worked as nurses alongside White women volunteers and doctors in the cities, especially when a yellow fever epidemic ravaged the community. During 1800 in Norfolk, Virginia, Blacks were forced to care for yellow fever victims. Sometimes their care was close to negligent, but at other times the Black nurses provided excellent treatment. During the 1855 yellow fever epidemic, 19 unnamed Black nurses traveled from their homes in Charleston, South Carolina, to Norfolk, Virginia, offering to provide care in the city hospital and in various homes, as it was widely recognized that they were somehow immune to the disease. Citizens who were nursed back to health responded to their care with appreciation.[90]

Black nurses were also appreciated for their midwifery skills, and it was common practice to use them for births on plantations as well as in the surrounding area. In fact, many slave owners allowed their slave midwives to provide services to both White and Black women outside the plantation. The fee the owner charged (and sometimes shared with the Black midwife) was more reasonable than the cost of a physician. As a result, a competent Black midwife was often in high demand.

Medical Care in the Wilderness

The care of the sick would soon extend beyond the boundaries of the 13 original states. In 1803, President Thomas Jefferson signed an agreement with France for the transfer of ownership to buy the territory that would become known as the Louisiana Purchase. Eager to find a river route to the Pacific Ocean, Jefferson appointed Meriwether Lewis and William Clark to explore and document the uncharted region. The expedition into unknown territory would be dangerous, and Jefferson, wanting to ensure the survival of the explorers, prepared them with medical knowledge.

Much like the pilgrims, Lewis and Clark would have to rely on their own knowledge and instincts to attend to their team's medical needs. Lewis had gained general knowledge of natural herbs and their uses from his mother, Lucy Lewis, a well-known herbal healer in Albemarle County, Virginia. She successfully nursed her family and members of the local community back to health with herbs, teas, and poultices. In addition, Lewis was schooled in basic medical practices from renowned physician, Benjamin Rush of Philadelphia. He was also given 11 rules by which to sustain his health, along with an extensive list of medical supplies to purchase before leaving the city.

Lewis and Clark set out in July 1803. Over the course of their journey, Lewis would serve as both the physician and the nurse on more than one occasion. Lewis's training would prove useful; he also sought help when he needed it. In early 1805 the wife of the team's interpreter, 16-year-old Sacagawea, went into labor. After a prolonged and intense labor, Lewis turned to Mr. Jusseaume, a fellow team member, for advice on how to hasten Sacagawea's delivery. Jusseaume suggested giving her a crushed portion of the rattle of a rattlesnake. As Lewis recalled:

> having the rattle of a snake by me I gave it to him and he administered two rings of it to the woman broken in small pieces with the fingers and added to a small quantity of water. Whether this medicine was truly the cause or not I shall not undertake to determine, but I was informed that she had not taken it more than ten minutes before she brought forth.[93]

Later that year Lewis would have to rely on his own medical knowledge to care for himself. In June Lewis was so sick with a high fever and violent intestinal pain that he could not eat. In his pain he considered what his mother, Lucy, would have done under

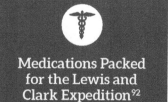

Medications Packed for the Lewis and Clark Expedition[92]

15 lbs. Best powder's bark
10 lbs. Epsom salts
4 oz. Calomel
12 oz. Opium
4 oz. Powder'd ipecacuana
8 oz. Powder jalap
8 oz. Powdered rhubarb
1 Flour of sulphur

these circumstances. Perusing his surroundings, Lewis saw an abundance of chokecherry, which gave him an idea. He requested that, "a parcel of the small twigs to be gathered stripped of their leaves, cut into pieces of about 2 inches in length and boiled in water until a strong black decoction of an astringent bitter taste was produced."[94] Drinking one pint of the concoction at sunset, followed by another dose an hour later, Lewis reported that he was "entirely relieved from pain" in just a few hours and was able to rest comfortably overnight.[95]

By September 1806 the expedition was over and deemed a success. Fortunately, no one had suffered from a broken bone or a wound that refused to heal. The company had, however, faced exhaustion, starvation, pain from venomous snakes, and infection from parasites, mosquitoes, and ticks. The men had also endured environmental hazards like flash floods, weather extremes, and the threat of death from accidents. In spite of this, Lewis's medical and nursing care had been enough to ensure the survival of the company.

The Ladies of the Benevolent Society—Charleston, South Carolina

As was evident in Lewis and Clark's exploration of the west in the early 19th century, place mattered in the care of the sick. Left alone to their own resources and skills as they crossed the wilderness, Lewis and Clark had to do what they could for their company. Meanwhile, citizens in cities and towns in the east had more resources available, including men with medical expertise, wealthy philanthropists, and benevolent organizations.

Class also mattered. The rich could afford to consult physicians and surgeons, while the poor often went without care or turned to each other for help. One notable exception was the care provided by the Ladies Benevolent Society in Charleston, South Carolina. The philanthropic society, organized in 1813 "by 125 women—the wives, sisters, and daughters of Charleston's wealthiest families," offered care to "anyone who did not fall within the purview of the almshouse, dispensary, or slave hospital and was unable to afford physician visits or hired nurses."[96] That care included the chronically ill.

Providing "an estimated 10 percent of the benevolent dollars spent in Charleston for the sick and needy," the ladies not only raised funds but also visited homes to distribute food and clothing. As historian Karen Buhler-Wilkerson documented: "The ladies visited every home that could be entered with propriety." They nursed the sick and provided them with "the simplest comforts: sugar, coffee, lamp oil, grits, wood, barley, soap and meat or chicken if ordered by the physician." Blankets were also provided. Medicines were obtained from the dispensary. The ladies also hired "nurses" to care for the sick. As one of the society's members wrote in her journal, "of what avail are medicines or proper nourishment, unless there be some kind hand to administer them in due season?"[97]

The Ladies Benevolent Society cared for all races, including Blacks, as long as they were freed. "Resorting to the great southern tradition of 'innocent because we did not ask,' the ladies concluded that they did not need to inquire how freedom was obtained. As long as the person was 'not held as a slave by any owner,' the ladies would visit them."[98]

By the mid-19th century, the Ladies Benevolent Society's work was winding down. Other groups, including the Sisters of Charity of Our Lady of Mercy, the Methodist Benevolent Society, the Howard Association, and the Young Men's Christian Association were also caring for the city's sick-poor.

Establishment of the American Medical Association

The early 19th century was a period of reinvention of medical practice and authority. Because very few formally educated European physicians had joined the settlers in America during the colonial era, medicine in America was not as advanced as it was in Western Europe, where educated European physicians had long established themselves as having the right to heal.[99] American physicians, however, quickly caught up with their European colleagues between 1780 and 1850. With their increasing reliance on new technologies and a scientific approach to medicine, as well as organizing local medical societies, the physicians began to establish themselves as legitimate healers.

In 1847, a group of elite physicians formed the American Medical Association, hoping to improve standards for medical education and practice. In addition, the American Medical Association explicitly stated that only physicians should have the authority to diagnose illness and prescribe for those who were sick.

Three factors that influenced the choice of who would be recognized as the healers in the United States were social class, race, and gender. This would ultimately lead to a medical profession composed for the most part of middle- and upper-class White males.[100] Until this time, both men and women had been considered legitimate healers. In fact, in many cases society preferred women healers, with their herbal remedies and gentle touch, to male physicians who bled and purged the sick.[101] However, as physicians began to assert themselves as the *true* healers (gradually accepting Black male physicians into their ranks) and as they associated modern medicine with modern scientific discoveries, women healers lost status and were viewed as practicing "people's medicine."[102] As physicians further established themselves as the healing profession, women healers—the people's healers—were forced to take on a different role within the American medical system. Rather than being associated with *curing*, as were male physicians, the nursing role was soon assigned the gendered notion of *caring*.[103]

Much would continue to change regarding the care of the sick in America, but the process would take time. During the years of the westward migration on the Overland Trail and during the American Civil War, direct nursing care of the sick remained in the hands of wives, mothers, sisters, aunts, and grandmothers. Physicians would administer invasive treatments, operate on the sick, amputate limbs, and prescribe medicines. Women would nurse their families and others back to health.

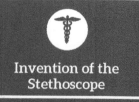

Invention of the Stethoscope

In 1819, French physician Rene Laennec developed the stethoscope, a hollow wooden monaural tube that transmitted sound from the patient's heart and lungs to the physician's ear. Initially invented to preserve propriety, the stethoscope allowed physicians to hear heart sounds without having to place their ears directly on a woman's chest. Stethoscopes would continue to be designed as a single earpiece until 1852.

For Discussion

1. Discuss the role of the midwife during the colonial period and early days of the United States.
2. How did the leaders of the new government affect change regarding principles of health?
3. Describe the care of the sick on plantations in the South.
4. Identify some treatments that were available for the sick in the colonial period. How were herbal remedies viewed?
5. Describe the Theory of the Four Humors.
6. What preparation did Meriwether Lewis have in the area of medicine and nursing care?

NOTES

1. George Percy, "The Experiences of a Virginia Colony," in *A Library of American Literature: From the Earliest Settlement to the Present Time, Vol. I*, eds. Edmund Clarence Stedman and Ellen Mackay Hutchinson (New York, NY: Charles L. Webster & Company, 1890): 35–36.

2. Volney Steele, *Bleed, Blister and Purge: A History of Medicine on the American Frontier* (Missoula, MT: Mountain Press Publishing, 2005): 22.

3. Sidney Negus, "Physicians at Early Jamestown," *The Virginia Journal of Science*, 8 (January 1957): 66.

4. Ibid.

5. "The Indispensable Role of Women at Jamestown," https://www.nps.gov/jame/learn/history culture/the-indispensible-role-of-women-at-jamestown.htm (accessed August 8, 2016).

6. "History," http://historicjamestowne.org/archaeology/jane/history (accessed July 25, 2016): para 2.

7. Ivor Noël Hume, "We Are Starved," http://www.history.org/Foundation/journal/Winter07/starving.cfm (accessed July 25, 2016): para 26.

8. Ibid.

9. Samuel Morison, *The Oxford History of the American People* (New York: Oxford University Press, 1965): 51.

10. Negus, "Physicians at Early Jamestown," 70.

11. Paula Gunn Allen, *Pocahontas: Medicine Woman, Entrepreneur, Diplomat* (San Francisco: Harper, 2004). Matoaka was more commonly known as Pocahontas.

12. William Bradford, "In These Hard and Difficult Beginnings," National Humanities Center Resource Toolbox, http://nationalhumanitiescenter.org (accessed October 2, 2016): para 1.

13. James H. Cassedy, *Medicine in America: A Short History* (Baltimore, MD: Johns Hopkins University Press, 1991): 7.

14. Susanne Malchau Dietz, *Women Religious and Nursing in the Renaissance: The Daughters of Charity and the Professionalization of Nursing* (Kolding, Denmark: University of Southern Denmark, 2011): 37.

15. Barbra Mann Wall, *Unlikely Entrepreneurs: Catholic Sisters and the Hospital Marketplace, 1865-1925* (Columbus: The Ohio State University Press, 2005): 18.

16. Barbara Ehrenreich and Deirdre English, *Witches, Midwives & Nurses: A History of Women Healers*, 2nd ed. (New York: The Feminist Press, City University of New York, 2010): 52.

17. Ibid.

18. Martha Libster, *Herbal Diplomats: The Contributions of Early American Nurses to Nineteenth Century Health Care Reform and the Botanical Medical Movement* (Naperville, IL: Golden Apple Publications, 2004): 174.

19. "Infant Mortality," http://www.encyclopedia.com/topic/Infant_mortality.aspx (accessed July 23, 2016): para. 3.

20. Ibid.

21. James H. Cassedy, *Medicine in America: A Short History* (Baltimore, MD: Johns Hopkins University Press, 1991): 4. Cassedy notes that measles, mumps, smallpox, and other infectious diseases that colonists brought with them from Europe were not known in the Americas and had devastating effects on the indigenous populations.

22. Stanford Shulman, "The History of Pediatric Infectious Diseases," *Pediatric Research* 5 (2004): 165.

23. Ibid.

24. Cassedy, *Medicine in America*, 4.

25. Ehrenreich and English, *Witches, Midwives & Nurses*, 48.

26. Cotton Mather, quoted in Libster, *Herbal Diplomats*, 94.

27. Ehrenreich and English, *Witches, Midwives & Nurses*, 25.

28. Ibid., 47–48.

29. Paul R. Huey, "The Almshouse in Dutch and English Colonial America and Its Precedent in the Old World: Historical and Archeological Evidence," *International Journal of Historical Archeology* 5, no. 2 (2001): 123.

30. John C. Kirchgessner, "A Reappraisal of Nursing Services and Shortages: A Case Study of the University of Virginia Hospital, 1945-1965" (dissertation, University of Virginia, 2006): 33.

31. Charles Rosenberg, *The Care of Strangers: The Rise of America's Hospital System* (New York: Basic Books, 1987): 22.

32. Kirchgessner, "A Reappraisal of Nursing Services and Shortages," 34.

33. Ibid., 33. Almshouses often housed the blind, crippled, alcoholics, mentally ill, and socially deviant, including criminals and prostitutes.

34. Dietz, *Women Religious*, 20.

35. Kirchgessner, "A Reappraisal of Nursing Services and Shortages," 30.

36. Benjamin Franklin, *Some Account of the Pennsylvania Hospital: From its First Rise, to the Beginning of the Fifth Month, Called May, 1754* (Philadelphia: B. Franklin and D. Hall, 1754): 5.

37. Ibid., 25. The regulation pertaining to the admission of infectious disease cases did state that this rule was in effect only until proper isolation facilities could be prepared.

38. Charles Rosenberg, *The Care of Strangers: The Rise of America's Hospital System* (New York: Basic Books, 1987): 22.

39. Cassedy, *Medicine in America*, 20.

40. Francis R. Packard, *The Pennsylvania Hospital of Philadelphia from 1751 to 1938* (Philadelphia: Pennsylvania Hospital, 1957): 54.

41. Kirchgessner, "A Reappraisal of Nursing Services and Shortages," 32.

42. William H. Williams, *America's First Hospital: The Pennsylvania Hospital, 1751-1841* (Wayne, PA: Haverford House Publishers, 1976): 15.

43. Susan Reverby, "A Caring Dilemma: Womanhood and Nursing in Historical Perspective," *Nursing Research* 36, no. 1 (January/February 1987): 5–11. In 18th century America, formal nursing education programs did not exist. Therefore, it was common for hospitals during this time to use domestic help, laundry help, and others as nurses when necessary.

44. Packard, *The Pennsylvania Hospital*, 114.

45. Kirchgessner, "Reappraisal of Nursing Services and Shortages," 32.

46. Jeanne Abrams, *Revolutionary Medicine: The Founding Fathers and Mothers in Sickness and in Health* (New York: New York University Press, 2013): 21.

47. Stanford T. Shulman, "The History of Pediatric Infectious Diseases," *Pediatric Research* 5 (2004): 163–176.

48. "Public Hospital," Colonial Williamsburg, http://www.history.org/almanack/places/hb/hbhos.cfm (accessed June 2, 2016): para 3.

49. Ibid., para 4.

50. Ibid., para 9.

51. Ibid., para 8.

52. Patricia D'Antonio, *Founding Friends: Families, Staff, and Patients at the Friends Asylum in Early Nineteenth-Century Philadelphia* (Bethlehem, PA: Lehigh University Press, 2006): 131.

53. Abrams, *Revolutionary Medicine*, 54.

54. Ibid., 55.

55. "History of Smallpox Vaccination," https://www.laff.org/smallpox (accessed October 6, 2016): para 1.

56. "Martha at the Front," *Mount Vernon,* http://www.mountvernon.org/george-washington/martha-washington/martha-at-the-front (accessed July 3, 2016): para 7.

57. Abrams, *Revolutionary Medicine,* 43–44.

58. Ibid., 53.

59. Ibid., 2.

60. Ibid.

61. Stephen Riedel, "Edward Jenner and the History of Smallpox and Vaccination," *Proceedings of Baylor University Medical Center,* 18, no. 1 (2005): 23.

62. Abrams, *Revolutionary Medicine,* 199.

63. Phillip Wilson and W. Jeffry Hurst, *Chocolate as Medicine: A Quest over the Centuries.* (Cambridge, UK: Royal Society of Chemistry, 2012): 79.

64. Ibid.

65. Laurel Thatcher Ulrich, *A Midwife's Tale: The Life of Martha Ballard, Based on Her Diary, 1785-1812* (New York: Vintage Books, Random House, 1990): 9–33 (quote 9).

66. Ibid., 39.

67. Ibid., 40.

68. Ibid., 11.

69. Ibid., 38.

70. Ibid., 39.

71. Abrams, *Revolutionary Medicine,* 44.

72. Libster, *Herbal Diplomats,* 4.

73. Abrams, *Revolutionary Medicine,* 44.

74. "Death Defied," *Mount Vernon,* http://www.mountvernon.org/george-washington/the-man-the-myth/death-defied-dr-thorntons-radical-idea-of-bringing-george-washington-back-to-life (accessed August 3, 2016): para 2. It appears by today's knowledge of viral and bacterial upper respiratory infections that Washington died from a particularly virulent case of epiglottitis, only 48 hours from the initial onset.

75. Libster, *Herbal Diplomats,* 43–44.

76. Abrams, *Revolutionary Medicine,* 174.

77. Ibid., 169.

78. Ibid.

79. As quoted in Todd L. Savitt, *Medicine and Slavery: The Diseases and Health Care of Blacks in Antebellum Virginia* (Chicago: The University of Illinois Press, 1978): 160.

80. Sharla Fett, *Working Cures: Healing, Health, and Power on Southern Slave Plantations.* (Chapel Hill: The University of North Carolina Press, 2002): 67.

81. Ibid.

82. Savitt, *Medicine and Slavery,* 155.

83. Fett, *Working Cures,* 67.

84. Ibid., 64.

85. Ibid., 67.

86. As quoted in Savitt, *Medicine and Slavery,* 180.

87. Ibid., 180.

88. Ibid., 181.

89. Ibid., 182–183.

90. Ibid., 243.

91. Ibid., 182–183.

92. "Lewis's Packing List," https://www.monticello.org/site/jefferson/lewiss-packing-list (accessed July 25, 2016): para 9.

93. As quoted in David J. Peck, *Or Perish in the Attempt: The Hardship and Medicine of the Lewis and Clark Expedition* (Lincoln: University of Nebraska Press, 2002): 134.

94. Ibid., 162–163.

95. Ibid.

96. Karen Buhler-Wilkerson, *No Place Like Home: A History of Nursing and Home Care in the United States* (Baltimore, MD: Johns Hopkins University Press, 2001): 5–6.

97. Ibid., 7.

98. Ibid., 11.

99. Ehrenreich and English, *Witches, Midwives & Nurses,* 64.

100. Ibid., 63.

101. Ibid., 64.

102. Ibid., 63.

103. Reverby, "A Caring Dilemma."

FURTHER READING

Abrams, Jeanne, *Revolutionary Medicine: The Founding Fathers and Mothers in Sickness and in Health* (New York: New York University Press, 2013).

Buhler-Wilkerson, Karen, *No Place Like Home: A History of Nursing and Home Care in the United States* (Baltimore, MD: Johns Hopkins University Press, 2001).

Clinton, Catherine, *The Plantation Mistress: Women's World in the Old South* (New York: Pantheon Books, 1984).

D'Antonio, Patricia, *Founding Friends: Families, Staff, and Patients at the Friends Asylum in Early Nineteenth-Century Philadelphia* (Bethlehem, PA: Lehigh University Press, 2006).

Ehrenreich, Barbara, and Deirdre English, *Witches, Midwives & Nurses: A History of Women Healers.* 2nd ed. (New York: The Feminist Press, City University of New York, 2010).

Fett, Sharla M., *Working Cures: Healing, Health, and Power on Southern Slave Plantations* (Chapel Hill: The University of North Carolina Press, 2002).

Libster, Martha, *Herbal Diplomats: The Contribution of Early American Nurses (1830-1860) to Nineteenth-Century Health Care Reform and the Botanical Medical Movement* (Naperville, IL: Golden Apple Publications, 2004).

Peck, David J., *Or Perish in the Attempt: The Hardship and Medicine of the Lewis and Clark Expedition* (Lincoln: University of Nebraska Press, 2002).

Rosenberg, Charles, *The Care of Strangers: The Rise of America's Hospital System* (New York: Basic Books, 1987).

Savitt, Todd, *Medicine and Slavery: The Diseases and Health Care of Blacks in Antebellum Virginia* (Chicago: University of Illinois Press, 1978).

Ulrich, Laurel Thatcher, *A Midwife's Tale: The Life of Martha Ballard, Based on Her Diary, 1785-1812* (New York: Alfred A. Knopf, 1990).

Wall, Barbra Mann, *Unlikely Entrepreneurs: Catholic Sisters and the Hospital Marketplace, 1865-1925* (Columbus: The Ohio State University Press, 2005).

Wilson, Phillip, and W. Jeffrey Hurst. *Chocolate as Medicine: A Quest over the Centuries* (Cambridge, UK: Royal Society of Chemistry, 2012).

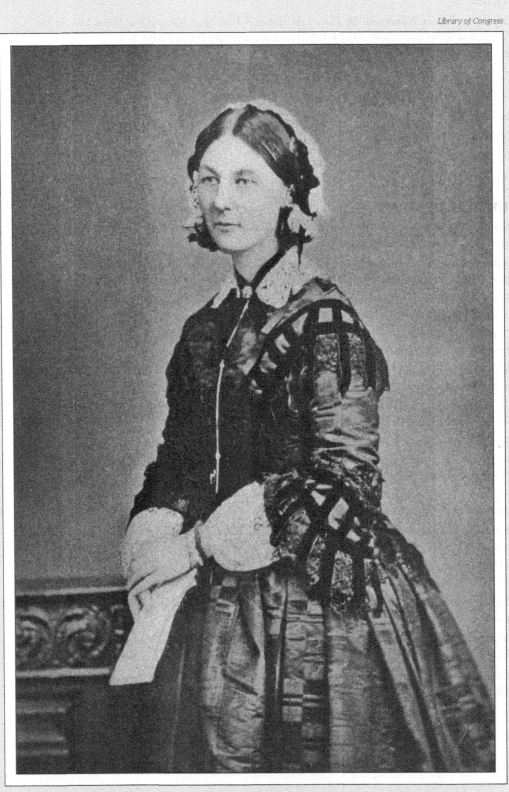

Florence Nightingale.

CHAPTER 2

The Roots of a Profession
1830–1865

Arlene W. Keeling

"Every woman, or at least almost every woman, in England, has, at one time or another of her life, charge of the personal health of somebody, whether child or invalid—in other words, every woman is a nurse."[1]

Writing these words in the introduction to her book *Notes on Nursing* in 1859, Florence Nightingale described the role of women in caring for the sick in the mid-19th century. Nightingale was writing about women in England, but the same could be said about the role that women in America played in the care of the sick during this time period.

WOMEN AS CAREGIVERS AND NURSES

Before 1873 when three training schools for nurses opened in the United States, women family members provided nursing care. As historian Patricia D'Antonio has argued: In an era when "women's domestic duties were tied tightly to notions about women's innate capabilities and their loving responsibilities . . . nursing was an almost unquestioned part of their lives."[2]

Women attended births, nursed the sick, and sat with the dying in the home. Whether in a small cottage in New England, a log cabin in the Midwest, a mansion on the Upper East Side of Manhattan, or a flat in the tenement district of a city like Boston, New York, or Chicago, nursing took place at home where most births, illness, and dying occurred.[3]

Sometimes, the location of caregiving extended beyond the physical walls of the women's primary residences. On Southern plantations, for example, women cared for the sick in slave quarters as well as in the "big house." During the great migration west in the mid-19th century, women provided care on the open plains, under trees along creek beds, or in covered wagons. During the American Civil War, religious Sisters and lay women volunteers not only took injured soldiers into their homes to care for them but also worked in tents and churches, in fields behind the lines of battle, on steamships, and in railroad cars. They also nursed the sick in makeshift city hospitals set up in factory warehouses and in hastily prepared "wayside hospitals" at railway intersections. Clearly, the place in which care was given began to change. Nonetheless, nursing was primarily *women's* work.

An exception to this status quo occurred during war, as it had in the Revolutionary War, when recuperating soldiers were expected to care for their injured comrades. During the American Civil War (1861–1865) convalescent Union and Confederate soldiers, both Black and White, served in this capacity. In the South, African American male slaves also provided care, not only to their masters, but also to entire hospitals filled with injured and sick soldiers. In other instances, freemen of color, trained as assistants to physicians in the North, worked as caregivers in Union hospitals.

For both females and males providing care, one thing was true. With the exception of the Catholic Sisters, the 100 or so female nurses who trained under the U.S. Sanitary Commission's nurse corps, and those slaves and freemen who had worked as assistants to surgeons prior to the war, *volunteers* gave most of the care. What was missing was skilled *professional* nursing.

Nursing on the Overland Trail

From the 1830s to 1867 when the transcontinental railroad was completed, between 350,000 and 500,000 North Americans migrated west, traveling the 2,000 miles by wagon train on overland routes across the American continent. Some sought adventure and free land; others crossed the country in search of California gold. Still others undertook the journey to improve the health of family members, particularly those with tuberculosis. During the cholera epidemic of the late 1840s many of the emigrants went west to escape the scourge in the east. Rather than escaping it, however, the emigrants carried the disease with them, leaving vibrio cholera in brackish streams and water holes along the way. Once in the water, cholera spread to the next group of travelers following them.[4]

For women, the great migration west challenged the prevailing societal norms that sharply distinguished between the spheres of men and women. In the mid-19th century it was commonly accepted that women's place was in the home, but on the Overland Trail women found themselves in a man's world—adapting to life in the open air and to chores they were not usually required to do.[5] Despite these realities, women attempted to maintain their separate sphere by adhering to the traditional female role. That role included such tasks as washing, mending, and cooking—even if it meant washing clothes in a creek, mending garments by candlelight, and cooking over fires of dried buffalo chips. It also included assisting other women in childbirth, supervising children, and caring for the sick. None of the chores that made up women's work were accomplished easily on the journey west, and all were made more difficult by pregnancy and the care of infants and small children. That burden was compounded when a child had an accident or became ill.

During sickness, the pioneer women did their best to restore the balance of the "humors" in the body. In the era before the germ theory, most people accepted the humoral theory of disease described centuries earlier by

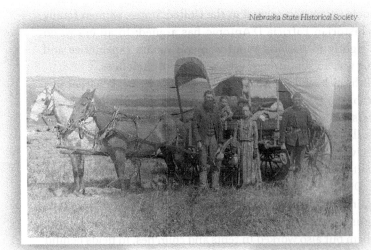

Nebraska State Historical Society

Pioneers on their way west.

Hippocrates, and later espoused by English physician Thomas Sydenham and 18th-century American physician Benjamin Rush. Diseases were thought to have their origins in an imbalance of one of the cardinal humors: blood, phlegm, black or yellow bile. As a result, treatments often included bleeding and the use of emetics and cathartics. While bloodletting and the use of harsh purgatives were left to physicians, the women used teas, roots, and other herbal medicines, all less invasive treatments.

Not every wagon train had a physician, and even when they did, most physicians had minimal training, usually in the practice of surgery. Given this reality, it is not surprising that the emigrant women cared for the sick themselves, relying on physicians to diagnose and prescribe for only the sickest individuals or for those who needed surgery or splinting of broken bones. Elizabeth Dixon Smith, a 38-year-old woman who traveled in 1847 with her husband and eight children, documented her preparations for the journey noting, in particular, the types of medicines a family might need:

> *June 3, 1847: Passed through St. Joseph on the bank of the Missouri. Laid in our flour, cheese and crackers and medicine, for no one should travel this road without medicine, for they are almost sure to have the summer complaint [dysentery, cholera, cholera infantum]. Each family should have a box of physicking pills, a quart of castor oil, a quart of the best rum and a large vial of peppermint essence.*[8]

In addition to caring for those who were ill, the women of the wagon trains treated routine discomforts that the westbound emigrants experienced as they crossed open prairies and then traveled along the Platte River and over the Rocky Mountains. Chief among the annoyances were blistering sunburns from long days on the prairie, hacking coughs from the endless dust, chills from the frigid nights, and itching and fevers that resulted from hundreds of mosquito bites.

On the Overland Trail, providing comfort through the alleviation of symptoms was the goal of treatment. The women dispensed gargles of sage tea, borax, and alum to treat sore throats; used syrup to relieve coughs; and coated mosquito bites with tallow. For cases of dysentery, they often used boiled rice and apples. In some instances, when the travelers drank bad water or ate spoiled food, the women turned to more radical therapies, considering that a purge was the only logical treatment. Amelia Knight recorded an incident in 1853 in which bad water caused them to be ill and purging was the "cure."

> *Friday, June 3: Came 21 miles today and have camped about opposite Scott's Bluffs. Water very bad—have had to use out of the Platte most of the time. It is very high and muddy.*
>
> *Monday, June 6: Still in camp, husband and myself being sick (caused by drinking the river water as it looks more like dirty suds than anything else), we concluded to stay in camp and each take a vomit, which we did and are much better.*[10]

Sometimes, a simple purge was not the answer. When the emigrants contracted cholera from contaminated water, purges served to further dehydrate them. In contrast, opium relieved pain and served to slow

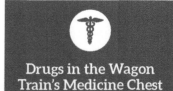

Drugs in the Wagon Train's Medicine Chest

Ipecac—to induce vomiting
Laudanum—a tincture of opium, morphine, and codeine
Lobelia—an herb with effects similar to nicotine
Calomel—a potent laxative
Jalap—a laxative
Castor oil—a laxative
Peppermint—for digestion
Pokeroot—for swollen glands and mastitis
Quinine—for fevers
Hartshorn—for snakebites
Citric acid—for scurvy[7]

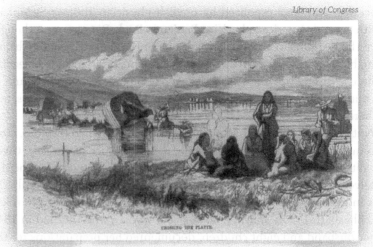

Pioneers crossing the Platte River risked cholera, losing supplies downriver, and ingesting water contaminated by the dead and other pollutants.

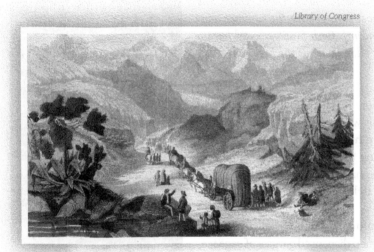

Pioneers in mountainous regions were susceptible to upturning their wagons resulting in numerous injuries.

down intestinal activity.[11] Neither treatment was curative and the outcome was often death. In that case, the most that caregivers could do was to wrap the body of fellow travelers to prepare them for burial.

For those who survived the trek across the plains, more hardships followed. As the pioneers neared the Rocky Mountains, the roads became increasingly treacherous. Steep descents down precipitous mountain slopes could cause pandemonium. Injuries were common as wagons tipped over or rolled out of control. Children fell out and were run over. Feet and hands got caught between the doubletree and the wagon box. Injuries ranged from cuts and bruises to sprained and broken limbs, and once again the women of the wagon train responded, bandaging and splinting as best they could or assisting the wagon train's physician to do so.

Mothers also had to care for sick children. Writing in 1848, Keturah Belknap described one instance:

> *My little boy [age 3] is very sick with Mountain Fever and tomorrow we will have to make a long, dry drive. . . . Must fill everything with water. We are on the brink of the Snake River, but it is such a rocky canyon we could not get to it if one' life depended on it. It's morning. I have been awake all night watching with the little boy. He seems a little better; has dropped off to sleep. . . . The sun is just rising . . . I have held the little boy on my lap on a pillow and tended him the best I could."*[13]

On the Overland Trail, the survival of the community was paramount. To get to California, Oregon, or Washington, the emigrants had to cross the western mountain ranges before the first snowfall. They could not afford to delay the journey for illness, births, or deaths. As a result, the goal of those who cared for the sick or for new mothers and their infants was to promote the functional status of the patients so that the journey could resume.

Working within their traditional role, women accepted the responsibilities of caregiving and maintaining the health of their families and fellow travelers. When they succumbed to illness themselves, or went into labor when other women were unavailable to help, men assumed the caregiving role.[14] One woman described her experience of giving birth prematurely, writing:

> *The ascent of the Sierras began now in earnest. The road was very rough, in many places covered with round boulders that made it almost impassable. I was obliged to lie down most of the day. . . . It was dusk when . . . the order was given to unyoke . . . Carl (the cook) brought me supper but I could not eat and spent the time in tears . . . I lighted my lamp and sat down to sew. I had been quietly at work making a small wardrobe out of some of the clothes . . . for I realized that I might need it before we arrived in California . . . There was only one more garment to finish . . . I sewed till about 10:00 . . . I woke my husband and told him the situation. . . . At three o'clock there came to us a dear little daughter, with no one near to help, comfort or relieve. After doing what he could for me, my husband wrapped the little one in a blanket and laid her in my arm. It had turned very cold and a dreadful chill came on. My husband put warm covers over me and tried to warm me by holding me in his arms. . . . My husband inquired of the first train that came past for some elderly woman to come in and see me, and the somewhat unexpected guest.[15]*

Women traveling west with the great Mormon migration beginning in 1846 had the support of "brothers and sisters" of the Mormon Church. This social network proved invaluable for pregnant women on the trail, as others in the group sometimes pushed her in a handcart if she was too weak to walk. At the forefront of Mormon doctrine was the importance of family, and motherhood was valued as a high and noble calling. Thus, other members of the community supported a woman in childbirth as best they could. According to one young girl, "I remember my mother going over with food and clothing to a lady who had given birth to a little baby in that cold and barren mountain retreat, far removed from every comfort."[16]

> *"These delicate emissions . . . caused a stoppage of six wagons for a few hours to prevent damage occurring to the mothers."[17]*
>
> Mormon Woman, 1850

Religious Groups, Charity, and Nursing in the Cities

While thousands of Americans were traveling to the West Coast of the United States on the Oregon, California, and Sante Fe Trails, the combination of an influx of immigrants from Eastern Europe and the rise of factories in the mid-19th century was changing the face of cities in the east. A host of social and environmental problems followed, most from overcrowding in tenement slums, a lack of indoor plumbing, and inadequate sewage and garbage disposal.[18] Epidemics of illness frequently erupted, and with no organized government infrastructure to address the social problems that were developing and the needs of a growing working class, members of churches and synagogues, as well as other newly formed volunteer organizations, responded to fill the gap.[19]

Catholic Sisterhoods were involved early in the mission for health. In 1832, the Catholic Sisters of Charity of Nazareth cared for the sick in Louisville, Kentucky, during the cholera epidemic that was sweeping the country. During the same outbreak the

Oblate Sisters cared for more than 200 patients in the Baltimore almshouse. A few years later, in 1843, the Irish Sisters of Mercy arrived in the United States and established a hospital in Pittsburg. Within a decade they left western Pennsylvania and set out to the west by stagecoach. After settling in Chicago, they established Mercy Hospital in 1852. Active in pioneer work in the Trans-Mississippi West, the Sisters of Mercy also opened institutions in Iowa and Nebraska. Another group of Irish Sisters of Mercy worked in San Francisco, setting up St. Mary's Hospital in 1854 after a cholera epidemic ravaged that city.[20]

About the same time, members of the Lutheran church were also working in Pittsburg. There, Lutheran clergyman William Passavant was determined to address the health and social needs of a growing labor force. Numerous Scottish and German immigrants were seeking work in the city's iron and glass factories. Through family and church connections in Germany, Passavant became aware of the work that Lutheran deaconesses were doing in Kaiserswerth. In that small town on the Rhine River, German clergyman Theodore Fliedner had established a penitentiary, an "Infant School," a hospital, an orphanage, and a seminary in the 1830s. Under Fliedner's supervision, the deaconesses played a major role in the town, providing care to orphans and the sick and teaching in the school. Using the deaconesses' work as a model, Passavant was determined to open a deaconess motherhouse and establish nursing services in the United States.

To begin his work, Passavant invited the Kaiserswerth deaconesses to establish a ministry in America. Responding to that invitation, four trained deaconess nurses, accompanied by Fliedner himself, arrived in Pittsburgh on July 14, 1849. Once there, the deaconesses took charge of the infirmary and in the first year provided care for more than 300 patients, some suffering from cholera, smallpox, and other infectious diseases.[22]

The groundwork was laid for the Lutheran deaconess movement to prosper in the United States. However, it would take several decades and financial support from wealthy benefactors before other visionary clergymen established Lutheran motherhouses in other U.S. cities.[23] The first American motherhouse was not organized until 1884 when the Lutheran Deaconess Motherhouse of Philadelphia opened, 35 years after the initial group of four Kaiserswerth deaconesses arrived in America.[24] The establishment of motherhouses in Milwaukee, Wisconsin, in 1893, and in Baltimore, Maryland, in 1894 soon followed. By 1900 seven Lutheran motherhouses had been established in locations where large numbers of German and Scandinavian Lutheran immigrants had settled.[25] Lutheran deaconess nurses ran all of them.

Dorothea Dix and the Asylum Movement

In the mid-19th century, other social reformers were turning their attention to the care of prisoners and the mentally ill. One of the most famous was Dorothea Dix, a native New Englander and teacher, who, having returned to Boston in 1841 after years away, volunteered to teach Sunday school to the female inmates in the East Cambridge jail. There she witnessed firsthand the inhumane conditions in which the insane were kept.[26] She was determined to help them, first by making public the reality of their life.[27] Dix spent months documenting the conditions in which the patients were kept. Afterward, she shared stories of the mentally ill housed "in cages, cellars, stalls, pens; chained, naked, beaten with rods, and lashed into obedience."[28] Her legislative successes led to the renovation of existing asylums in

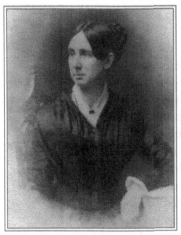

Library of Congress

Dorothea Dix, who publicized and revolutionized care of the mentally ill in New England.

Massachusetts and Rhode Island and the creation of a new and independent state-run psychiatric hospital in New Jersey.[29]

Dix adopted the principles of moral therapy, a philosophy that had its roots in the work of Philippe Pinel, a French physician and scientist. As historian Patricia D'Antonio described it: "The moral treatment of the insane was built on the assumption that those suffering from mental illness could find their way to recovery and an eventual cure if treated kindly and in ways that appealed to the parts of their minds that remained rational. It repudiated the use of harsh restraints and long periods of isolation that had been used [up to this time]. . . . It depended instead on specially constructed hospitals that provided quiet, secluded, and peaceful country settings."[30]

Adhering to the new principles of moral therapy, Dix worked with a network of superintendents of asylums who held similar convictions about reforming the care of the insane. The group, including physician Benjamin Rush, and Quakers William Tuke and Thomas S. Kirkbride, met in October 1844 to form the Association of Medical Superintendents of American Institutions for the Insane.[32] At their fourth meeting in May 1849 the superintendents concluded: "it is a deliberate conviction of this Association that an abundance of pure air . . . is essential in the treatment of the sick, especially in hospitals, and whether for those afflicted with ordinary disease or for the insane."[33]

Dorothea Dix agreed. While never herself a member of the Association of Medical Superintendents of American Institutions for the Insane, Dix developed strong personal and professional relationships with several members of the organization. Her correspondence with them included discussions of moral treatments for the insane, activities of the association, and her own legislative efforts.

Dix's moral authority, powers of persuasion, notoriety, and legislative successes fostered the association's construction of an empire of American asylums. She sustained her relationships with the superintendents for the rest of her life. At her burial in 1887 Dr. Charles Nichols, superintendent of the Government Hospital for the Insane, eulogized Dix with the words: "Thus has died and laid to rest in the most quiet, unostentatious way the most useful and distinguished woman America has yet produced."[36] Nichols was, of course, referring to Dix's work in reforming the care of the mentally

Moral Therapy

In his studies of the insane, Philippe Pinel found that traditional treatments for mental illness, such as corporal punishment, restraint, and isolation were ineffective. His observations led to the development of psychologically based therapy that incorporated the use of nature in the treatment of the mentally ill.[31]

Thomas Kirkbride's Vision

"Every hospital for the insane should be in the country, not within less than two miles of a large town . . . should have [at least] fifty acres of land, dedicated to gardens and pleasure grounds for patients. At least one hundred acres should be possessed by every State hospital . . . for two hundred patients."[34]

Thomas Kirkbride, 1854

"Asylums should be 'in a healthful, pleasant and fertile district of the country . . . the surrounding scenery should be of a varied and attractive kind.'"[35]

Thomas Kirkbride, 1854

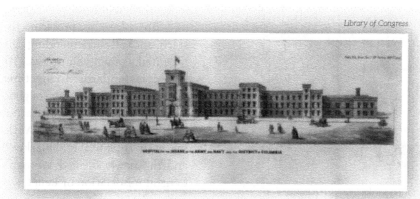

St. Elizabeth's Hospital, the first federally operated psychiatric hospital, opened in 1855.

ill. He was also referring to her leadership of the U.S. Sanitary Commission in the American Civil War.

NURSING IN THE AMERICAN CIVIL WAR, 1861 TO 1865

When the War Between the States broke out after the firing on Fort Sumter in April 1861, there were no trained *female* nurses to support the soldiers on either side. In fact, both the Union and the Confederacy were unprepared to treat the wounded and sick in the long and deadly conflict. Neither side expected that the war would last more than a few months, and neither had done much to prepare for hospitals, transportation of the wounded, or the recruitment of nurses and physicians. Despite this lack of preparation on the part of federal and state organizations, citizens in both the North and the South were well aware that care should be provided for soldiers at the front. By 1861 word had reached the United States of Nightingale's reformation of the British army's medical system in the Crimean War only a few years earlier. People on both sides had heard that there were new ideas about sanitation, nutrition, light, and air that should be used in the care of the sick. In 1859, the London Press had published Florence Nightingale's *Notes on Nursing*, a small book that outlined the basic tenets of nursing care. By 1861 Americans were reading it.

Union Nursing

Conditions in American military camps in 1861 were the opposite of what Nightingale advocated. As the soldiers mobilized and wrote letters home, their accounts of deplorable conditions, outbreaks of pneumonia and typhoid fever, and poor food in the overcrowded military camps soon reached their families. Determined to do something to help, a group of Northern women assembled in New York City and created the Women's Central Association for Relief. Afterward they sent representatives to Washington City to meet with U.S. President Abraham Lincoln and make their case for an organized system of care for the soldiers.

Responding to the representatives' pleas to organize the distribution of supplies being collected for the soldiers, Abraham Lincoln created the U.S. Sanitary Commission. He also directed Secretary of War Simon Cameron to commission Dorothea Dix as superintendent of women nurses of the army. She would manage all Union female nurses. Her first job was to find some. Unfortunately, Dix had no official corps of nurses from which to draw—in 1861 there were few trained nurses in the United States.

To solve this problem, the stern and often demanding Dix recruited women volunteers. Dix had high standards. To meet her criteria, women had to be of good health, of high moral character, and "plain" in appearance. Working with Dr. Elizabeth Blackwell and the newly formed Women's Central Association of Relief, Dix enlisted 100 women to train for a month under the direction of

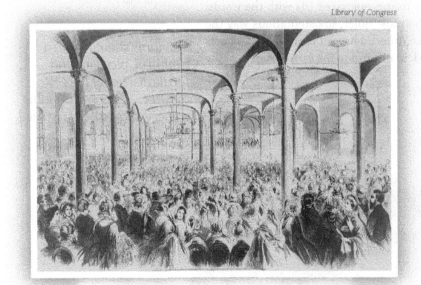

Library of Congress

The Women's Central Association for Relief representatives'
efforts led to the U.S. Sanitary Commission in 1861 to
improve health care for Union soldiers.

physicians at Bellevue and New York Hospitals. The nurses' role would be to supervise the care of sick and injured soldiers.

In addition to the lack of trained nurses, Dix had to contend with the fact that there were not enough military hospitals in place when the war started. In fact, all military hospitals were small post hospitals of about 40 beds each.[37] By June 1861 Dix had managed to set up a few makeshift hospitals in hotels and churches throughout Washington City and the surrounding area, including one at St. Elizabeth's, the hospital that had been established for the insane. Nevertheless, these were hardly enough to meet the needs of the 75,000 Union soldiers who had been mobilized.

Dix, however, was undeterred. According to her contemporary Mary Livermore, Dix's "whole soul was in her work. She rented two large houses, one as a depot for the sanitary supplies sent to her care," and another to shelter "nurses and convalescent soldiers." She hired two secretaries, purchased ambulances and "kept them busily employed," printed and distributed circulars, and "went hither and thither from one remote point to another in her visitations of hospitals."[38]

The inadequacies of the medical department's preparation became all too clear when thousands of wounded men poured into Washington after the Union defeat in the Battle of Bull Run (First Manassas) on July 21, 1861. Another plea for volunteers went out. A year later, even more nurses were needed as numerous battles took place during the spring and summer of 1862. Women from all classes and entirely different backgrounds responded; most had no formal training and had nursed only their family members. The result: Many of the volunteers were unprepared for the conditions and challenges they would face.

Mary Phinney, the upper-class widow of Baron von Olnhausen from Massachusetts, responded to the plea for nurses in August 1862.[40] After her arrival in Washington City, Phinney met with Dix, who assigned her to the Mansion House, a famous hotel the Union Army had appropriated for use

Bjoring Center for Nursing Historical Inquiry

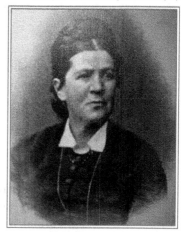

Mary Phinney, a volunteer nurse, who wrote home about patient conditions, hospital inadequacies, and her fellow medical care providers.

Library of Congress

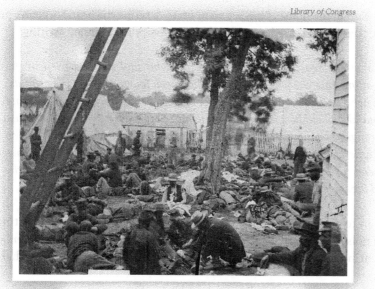

A Union field hospital was one of many understaffed and overfilled military care centers.

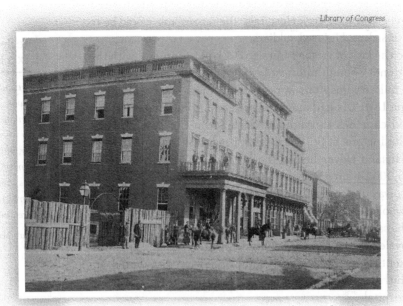

Mansion House Hospital, where Mary Phinney volunteered.

as a military hospital. Set in the outskirts of Washington in the Union-occupied town of Alexandria, the hospital attracted "political henchmen and their satellites, more eager for profit than for the binding up of wounds." The result was a corrupt hospital staff, inefficiencies, and disorganization. In addition, the medical staff of Mansion House hated female nurses—especially upper-class volunteers.[41]

"The operating room was literally a sea of blood."[44]

Mary Phinney

The day she arrived, Phinney had to "make her way through a double procession, one of seriously wounded men being taken in, the other of dead being carried out."[42] "With no . . . preparation," she was asked to assist that same night during surgeries "performed with little or no anesthetic, by surgeons who naturally brutal, had been made doubly so by the hurry of overwork and the magnitude of their seemingly endless task."[43]

Conditions in the ward were no better, as Phinney described in a letter to her family: "The ward was dirtier than you can know and had not one decent attendant," although it was the largest ward in the house. Phinney went on to describe the head surgeon's preference for a lower class "experienced nurse" and his contempt for Phinney, writing:

> About four weeks ago came a nurse (Mrs. R) who said she had been in the Crimea—at any rate she was English and had been fourteen years in hospitals. They gave her a back upstairs ward. She "of course" knows about bandaging and all that; but like all old hospital nurses is no nurse otherwise. . . . Last week just as I was congratulating myself how well all went and that the wards were so clean and orderly, up came Dr. S. and thundered out: "Madam, I intend to remove you. I intend Mrs. R to have this ward: this is the most important one in the house and I consider her the most splendid nurse in the country."[45]

Phinney went on to explain what happened next, writing: "Just as I was departing, we heard a fearful noise in the entry, and along was dragged my lady, by two officers, dead drunk and swearing like a trooper. So that's the way she took possession of her new ward!"[46]

Mary Phinney faced other challenges besides incompetent help, not the least of which was obtaining supplies. Phinney relied heavily on donations of blankets, knitted socks, bandages, and boxes of fruits and delicacies sent periodically to the front

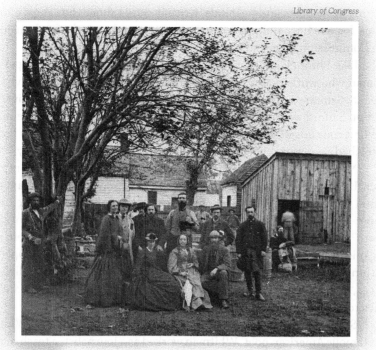

Volunteer nurses in 1862 attended to the innumerable
wounded soldiers after the Battle of Fredericksburg.

Observations of the Wounded

"Today has been such an awful day; bring in the wounded from Frederick [Fredericksburg]. The whole street was full of ambulances, and the sick lay outside on the sidewalks from nine in the morning until five in the evening. . . . The house was full . . . I have been so indignant all day—not a thing done for them. Not a wound dressed . . . they got dinner, but no supper."[48]

Mary Phinney,
December 15, 1862

by the soldiers' aid societies. As was true of military hospitals throughout the country, supplies and food for the patients in the Mansion House Hospital were hard to come by, especially in the case of fresh fruits and vegetables. Phinney acknowledged the importance of the "private" boxes from her hometown of Lexington, Massachusetts, writing: "It was such a delight to receive a box from Lexington, and the expectation of what had come was so great that I usually made a little feast for the men's tea . . . I never can enough thank that little band of good women who gave me the opportunity to do so much good. Their interest never flagged. Till the very end of the war every month brought comforts from them."[47]

After 6 months of determined caregiving Phinney had conquered the head surgeon's prejudice against women. In January 1863 she wrote:

> *You will be glad to know the change in Dr. S's treatment of me. I guess he finds it is creditable to him to have some ladies around. He is most polite when he meets me; and the night we were expecting the wounded he came to my door and asked me to go through my ward with him. It was nine o'clock but the rooms did look nice, the beds all so clean, and clothes for each man laid out, such bright fires and warm and cold water, sponges and everything else ready. He was so pleased and said he had found no other ward in such order.*[49]

Phinney's experiences in resisting physician prejudice, providing structure, organization, clean beds, and nutritious food for the wounded were not unique. Other women who volunteered also faced the surgeons' disdain and also managed to gain their respect.

After reporting to Dorothea Dix, Mary Ashton Livermore, another White, married "woman of genteel respectability," was assigned to the northwestern branch of the U.S. Sanitary Commission.[50] Organizing aid societies,

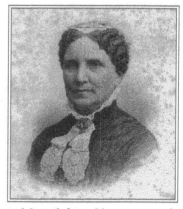

Mary Ashton Livermore made her name working for the U.S. Sanitary Commission.

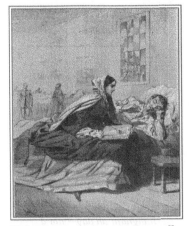

Volunteer nurses came from all backgrounds, but most had no formal training.

"Bearing the bandages, water and sponge, Straight and swift to my wounded I go."[53]

Walt Whitman

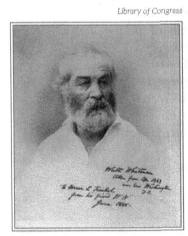

Walt Whitman, seminal American poet, volunteered as a nurse and visited more than 80,000 wounded and sick.

visiting army posts and hospitals, writing essays about the camps and hospitals for her husband's Chicago newspaper, and actively fund-raising for the Commission, Livermore gained a national reputation.

Like Phinney and Livermore, Mary Jane Safford was an upper-class woman who worked as a nurse, volunteering with the western division of the U.S. Sanitary Commission. After visiting her in Cairo, Illinois, Livermore praised Safford, writing that she "brought order out of chaos, systematized the first rude hospitals and with her own means, aided by a wealthy brother, furnished necessaries when they could be obtained in no other way."[51]

Not all upper-class women were inclined to help at the front, however. Unlike "mid-western women, free blacks, and Irish immigrants who found 'a ready path' into nursing work in the camps, most white, urban, upper- and middle-class women stayed away for fear of 'social contamination.'"[52] Remaining at home, these elite White women used their social organizations and church committees to serve the war effort. Operating within women's traditional sphere, they stitched garments, rolled bandages, made blankets, knitted socks, and prepared boxes of food and supplies to be sent to the front.

Some civilian men also volunteered. Among these was Walt Whitman, the famous American poet. Whitman worked as a journalist, a teacher, a government clerk, and a volunteer nurse during the war. As a hospital visitor, Whitman quickly found that he was of greatest service when he performed the smallest of tasks—writing letters for the soldiers, providing them with fruit and candy, or passing the time by playing games. Whitman's attention to the wounded was extraordinary. He estimated that over the course of the war, he had made "over 600 visits or tours, and visited over "80,000 wounded and sick."

Working on Their Own

Many women who volunteered to nurse could not meet Dix's criteria and worked outside of her jurisdiction. Among these were African American women—Sojourner Truth, Harriet Tubman, and Susie King Taylor. Defying the boundaries of time, place, gender, and race, these women not only cared for the soldiers, but also smuggled slaves to freedom using the complex Underground Railroad system, a network of safe houses and support operated by abolitionists.

Sojourner Truth, born a slave to Dutch-speaking parents, never learned to read or write English.[54] Nonetheless, she spent her life transporting family and friends from slavery to freedom in northern states and Canada, working through the Underground Railroad. During the Civil War, she worked for the Union as a nurse in Freedman's Hospital in the District of Columbia.

Harriet Tubman, born into slavery on the eastern shore of Maryland as Araminta Ross, worked most of her life helping slaves escape to the North. During the early days of the Civil War, Governor Andrew of Massachusetts, knowing "well the brave and sagacious character of Harriet," asked her to serve the Union as a spy, a scout, and if necessary, a nurse. For the remainder of the war, Tubman [her married name] worked with "untiring zeal for the welfare of the soldiers, both black and white." Gaining the confidence of the slaves by her cheery words and sacred hymns, Tubman obtained valuable information from them. She also nursed soldiers in Freedmen's Hospital, using roots and herbs to heal them when they were suffering malignant fever, smallpox, and other infectious diseases.[55]

Harriet Tubman in Her Own Words

"I'd go to de hospital . . . early eb'ry mornin'. I'd get a big chunk of ice . . . and put it in a basin, and fill it with water; den I'd take a sponge and begin. Fust . . . I'd thrash away de flies. . . . Den I'd begin to bathe der wounds, and by de time I'd bathed three or four, de fire and heat would have melted de ice . . . and it would be as red as . . . blood. Den I'd go an git more."[56]

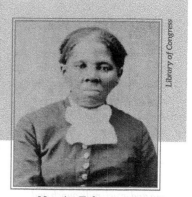

Harriet Tubman served as a spy and nurse during the Civil War.

Susie King Taylor was an escaped slave who served as laundress and nurse for the 33rd U.S. Colored [sic] Infantry on St. Simons Island, Georgia, in 1862.[57] Impressed by her ability to read, Union officers employed Taylor to teach English to young Black children and adults alike.

Besides the Black women, some White women also worked independent of the Sanitary Commission, outside of Dorothea Dix's jurisdiction. Among these was Mary Ann Bickerdyke, a New England widow known for her "skill as a nurse, the fertility of her resources, her burning patriotism, and her possession of . . . 'common sense.'"[58] Bickerdyke served under Union General Ulysses S. Grant on the western front, having been sent by her church to Cairo, Illinois, to investigate the medical situation in the military camps there.

In Cairo, Bickerdyke found appalling conditions. The city was filled with thousands of previously healthy young men, many now suffering from fevers, dying of measles and dysentery, and living in filth. Undaunted by her lack of military authority, and working against the strong objections of the surgeons in the camp, "Mother Bickerdyke" rallied the men, ordering them to chop kindling, build fires, and heat large kettles of water. In a whirlwind of activity, Bickerdyke arranged for clothes to be washed, soldiers to be bathed, bedding fumigated, and garbage removed. In fact, she made such an impact in so short a time that one surgeon complained that "a cyclone in calico" had struck the camp.[59]

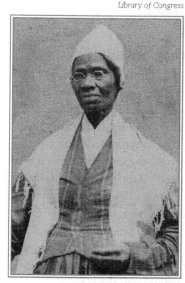

Sojourner Truth, notable abolitionist and women's rights activist, worked as a nurse in Freedman's Hospital.

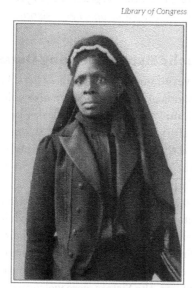

Susie King Taylor worked as a nurse for the 33rd U.S. colored infantry.

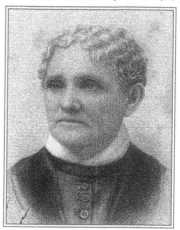

Mary Ann Bickerdyke's brief but significant time in Cairo, Illinois, revolutionized the medical conditions in military camps.

Library of Congress

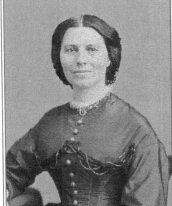

Clara Barton administered health care, sometimes in the middle of the battlefield while under fire.

"I thought that night if Heaven ever sent out an angel, she must be one."[63]

James Dunn on Clara Barton, 1862

Clara Barton

Soon after the Civil War broke out, Clara Barton, a Massachusetts woman who was working as a copyist in the U.S. Patent Office in Washington City, began an independent campaign to provide relief for the soldiers. She had refused to enlist in the military nurse corps headed by Dix, as she did not think herself "plain"—one of Dix's criteria for nurses. Instead, she served as a volunteer to Dix's nurses in a hospital ward set up on the top floor of the Patent Office. Later, working outside of the government's official nursing corps, Barton appealed to her New England friends and to local Washingtonians for contributions of woolen shirts, blankets, towels, lanterns, and camp kettles, as well as tobacco, whiskey, homemade jellies and other delicacies for the soldiers. Escorted by an older, married physician and friend, Barton visited military camps in Washington to deliver the items.[61]

On August 12, 1862, Barton received her first army pass authorizing her to take supplies to the battlegrounds of Virginia. Taking a leave of absence from her patent job, she made her way to Culpeper, Virginia, where she set up a makeshift field hospital and cared for the wounded and dying during the Battle of Cedar Mountain. It was at this time that Barton gained her famous title "Angel of the Battlefield," based on surgeon James L. Dunn's reflections:

I will tell you of one of these women, a Miss Barton . . . of Boston Massachusetts. I first met her at the battle of Cedar Mountain, where she appeared in front of the hospital at twelve o'clock at night, with a four mule team loaded with everything needed, and at a time when we were entirely out of dressings of every kind; she supplied us with everything; and while the shells were bursting in every direction, took her course to the hospital on our right; where she found everything wanting again. After doing everything she could on the field, she returned to Culpeper where she stayed dealing out shirts to the naked wounded, and preparing soup, and seeing it prepared, in all the hospitals. I thought that night if Heaven ever sent out an angel, she must be one, her assistance was so timely.[62]

Catholic Sisters: Working Outside the Convent

For every famous woman like Clara Barton who nursed in the Civil War, thousands of ordinary women also volunteered. According to historian Barbra Mann Wall, "among these lesser known women, the rank and file of nursing history," were the Sisters of St. Joseph and the Sisters of the Holy Cross. Their activities during the war "helped change the conventional view of nursing, the general public's image of the Sisters, and perhaps society's view of the Catholic Church."[64] Fourteen Sisters of the Philadelphia community of the Sisters of St. Joseph served in Union hospitals in Pennsylvania and on hospital ships in Virginia in 1862, while 10 others from the congregation in Wheeling, West Virginia, opened their own military hospital in 1864. Considering their nursing service as part of their religious duty, the nuns willingly endured hardships in order to care for the soldiers. Unlike laywomen volunteers, the Sisters were welcomed and trusted from the start.[65]

Sent by Father Sorm from Notre Dame to care for the sick and wounded soldiers of the Union Army on the western front, Mother Angela and the Sisters of the Holy Cross served in military camps in Illinois, Missouri, Kentucky, and Tennessee. At a time when most military surgeons opposed having women in their camps, referring to them as annoying and meddlesome, military officers welcomed the Sisters. Writing to the medical director in a Union camp in Louisville, Kentucky, General William Tecumseh Sherman praised Mother Angela's organizational skills. Mary Livermore also praised the Sisters' work, writing that Mound City Hospital, where the Sisters of the Holy Cross were employed as nurses, became "the best military hospital in the United States." As Livermore pointed out, the Sisters "by their skill, quietness, gentleness and tenderness, were invaluable in the sick wards."[66] As nurse historian Barbra Wall explained: The Sisters, empowered by their strong sense of mission, "moved beyond the boundaries of their convents and expanded their ministry to include the care of the sick."[67]

Union Nursing on Transport Ships

In addition to working in hospitals, Catholic Sisters nursed on steamboats commissioned by the Union Army to transport sick and wounded soldiers from battlefields in the South to hospitals in the North. By 1862 the Hospital Transport Service had seven ships working on the York and James River in Virginia, transporting casualties from battles of the Peninsula Campaign, the first large-scale Union offensive against the Confederate capital of Richmond. The Union also had other steamships on other rivers with several women assigned to each. The Sisters of St. Joseph nursed Union soldiers on the *Commodore* during their transport to Philadelphia, remained with them until they were settled in hospitals, and then returned to the ship.[68] Further inland, nurses worked on other hospital ships moving patients north to Ohio and Missouri. Four Sisters of the Holy Cross worked on the *Red Rover,* making frequent round-trip excursions on the Mississippi River from Cairo, Illinois, to Memphis, Tennessee, and New Orleans during 1863 and 1864. Ann Bradford Stokes, an escaped slave, assisted them.[69]

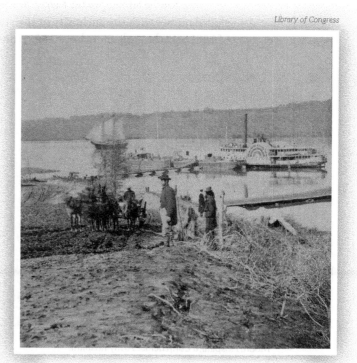

Steamboats served as mobile hospitals for the Union Army.

Nursing in the Confederacy

Like women of the North, thousands of Confederate women rallied to care for sick and wounded soldiers during the Civil War. Realizing that their survival depended on preserving a plantation economy and the production of cotton and tobacco, the women of the South immersed themselves in Confederate chauvinism when the war broke out in 1861. "Supporting the Cause" became their slogan. In a society in which separate spheres for men and women were the norm, women might not be allowed to fight the battle for secession themselves, but they could care for those who did. Soldier's Aid Societies soon sprang into existence throughout the Confederacy as the plantation mistresses and urban socialites converted their women's clubs and ladies aid societies to serve the war effort.

Unlike the women in the North, Southern women worked without the benefit of an official government organization, volunteering in makeshift hospitals in cities and towns across the Confederacy. After the battle of

"Every woman in the house is ready to rush into the Florence Nightingale business."[70]

Mary Boykin Chesnut, June 29, 1861

First Manassas, when the wounded Confederate soldiers deluged Richmond, Virginia, the need for organization and preparation became all too evident. Writing in August 1861, Mary Chesnut, an upper-class Southern woman who kept an extensive diary during the war, described the conditions at one of the city's warehouses that had been hastily converted to a hospital:

> But oh, such a day! Since I wrote this morning, have been with Mrs. Randolph to all the hospitals. I can never again shut out of view the sights I saw of human misery. I sit thinking, shut my eyes and see it all. . . . Gillands [sic] was the worst . . . long rows of ill men on cots. Ill of typhoid fever, of every human ailment—dinner tables, eating, drinking, wounds being dressed—horrors to be taken in at one glance. That long tobacco warehouse. . . . Then we went to St. Charles [General Hospital #8]. Horrors upon Horrors again—want of organization. Long rows of them dead, dying. . . . Awful smells, awful sights.[71]

It soon became apparent that the hospitals of the South needed the discipline of skilled nurses with the authority of the state behind them. Thus, during the last months of 1861 and the early months of 1862, the Confederate Government assumed the control and partial support of all the soldier's hospitals in the South. Despite this change, the women's relief societies were still entreated to supply food and clothing. As was true in the North, fresh fruits and vegetables were particularly needed. Mary Chesnut described one instance in which she simply did not have enough for all of the injured, writing: "Went to the hospital with a carriage load of peaches and grapes. When my supply gave out, those who had none looked so wistfully that I made a second raid on the market."[72]

With the advent of Confederate government control, however, other aspects of hospital organization changed drastically. Several women were made superintendents of hospitals. Among these was Sallie Thompkins, often called "Richmond's Florence Nightingale." When the government appropriated private hospitals, Sallie Thompkins (who had earlier established a hospital in Richmond) was allowed to maintain her hospital and was commissioned a "captain of cavalry, unassigned" by President Davis. Thus, Thompkins became the only woman in the Confederacy to hold military rank.[73] Other Southern women served as hospital matrons. On September 27, 1862, the Confederate Congress gave these positions official status, defining the functions of matrons, and assigning fixed salaries.

The matrons faced several major obstacles upon assuming their hospital responsibilities, however. One of the most significant obstacles was public prejudice against women serving in hospitals. Kate Cumming, an outstanding matron of the South who served with the Army of Tennessee, wrote: "There is scarcely a day passes, that I do not hear some derogatory remarks about the ladies who are in hospitals, until I think, if there is any credit due them at all, it is for the moral courage they have in braving public opinion."[74] That particular public opinion held that no self-respecting woman

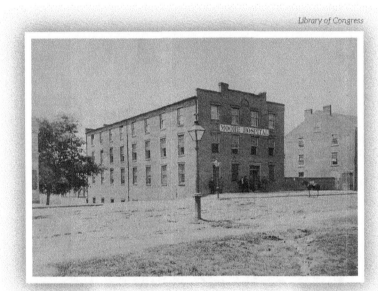

Moore Hospital, a Confederate Army hospital.

would be a nurse. As a result, lower class women were more likely to volunteer than were those in the upper classes. Phoebe Pember, chief matron of Chimborazo Hospital, a sprawling government-run institution outside Richmond, confirmed this fact, writing: "Very few ladies and a great many inefficient and uneducated women hardly above the laboring class" constituted the feminine portion of the hospital forces."[75]

Pember made other observations, writing in September 1862 that "sick or wounded men, convalescing and placed in that position, however ignorant they might be" were charged with caring for the sick.[76] Later, however, Chimborazo Hospital used hundreds of male slaves to work as nurses. They had been pressed into service for the Confederacy, with payment for their work going to their owners.[77]

At Chimborazo, Pember had to deal with red tape, the incompetence of key officials, internal strife, and shortages in supplies. Because of blockaded seaports, fuel, food, and medicines were unavailable. Soap and bandages were scarce. In some cases bandages were reused without being washed.[78] Pember remedied this situation as best she could, making do with what she had, imposing order and discipline.

Those hospitals in Richmond that could boast of excellent care for their patients were those in which the Sisters of Charity served. Doubtless the most skillful and devoted of the women who nursed in the Confederacy, the religious sisters constituted the only class of women in the South who possessed any formal training in nursing and hospital management.

Less efficient than the care provided by the Sisters was the care given by the Confederate women who boarded troop trains to help. Once on board, they bandaged and fed the soldiers. They also opened wayside homes to supply food and medicine to the thousands of wounded men left stranded by a railroad service devastated by the war. Mary Chesnut, who was in Columbia, South Carolina, in 1864, discussed her work there along with her reaction:

> Began my regular attendance in the Wayside Hospital. Today we gave wounded men (as they stopped for an hour at the station) their breakfast. Those who were able to come to the table do so. The badly wounded remain in the ward prepared for them, where their wounds are dressed by nurses and surgeons and we take bread and butter, beef, ham, hot coffee etc. to them there. . . . They were awfully smashed up—objects of misery, wounded, maimed, and diseased. I was really upset and came home ill. This kind of thing unnerves me quite."[81]

Overwhelmed with patients, Richmond hospitals transferred recovering soldiers to nearby cities. One of these was Charlottesville, home to the University of Virginia. There several hospitals were created in existing facilities. The largest was the Charlottesville General Hospital, a group of rented buildings scattered throughout the city. Pressed for space in these hospitals, the university was also used. Like other hospitals throughout the South, little preparation had been made for nursing care, and volunteer women filled in as best they could. Some, like the refined plantation mistress Ada Bacot, brought along her slave who took on the duties of changing straw in the bed sacks, cooking, and scouring floors, while Bacot attended to such tasks as writing letters for the soldiers.[83]

As the war progressed, it took its toll and those nursing the sick faced increasingly severe shortages of nearly everything. The Union troops destroyed railroads, burned barns and fields, and confiscated food, livestock, military, and surgical supplies. In addition, the Union blockaded seaports

"The rations became so small . . . every available article in our pantry was brought into requisition."[79]

Phoebe Pember

The Sisters of Charity

"At the almshouse, Dr. Gibson is in charge. . . . The Sisters of Charity are his nurses. That makes all the difference in the world!!. . . Everything was clean—and in perfect order."[80]

Mary B. Chesnut, 1861

Diary Entry

"Trains have been constantly [on the way to] Richmond Hospitals. Every lady, every child, every servant in the village has been engaged in . . . carrying food to the wounded as the cars stopped at the depot—coffee, tea, soups, milk and everything we could obtain."[82]

Judith McGuire, December 15, 1862

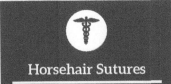
and declared medicines contraband of war. Food was particularly scarce. According to Phoebe Pember, "often there was not even enough dry corn-bread to satisfy the hunger of the patients," the only delicacies available were "dried apples for the convalescent and herbs and arrowroot for the desperately ill."[84]

The beginning of the collapse of the Confederacy occurred with General William T. Sherman's infamous "March to the Sea" after he burned Atlanta in 1864. Leaving the city in a broad expanse of fire, Sherman led his soldiers in two columns toward Savannah, Georgia, destroying everything in his path. On December 20, 1864, Sherman occupied Savannah, and a month later turned north to South Carolina. On February 17, Charleston was evacuated and Columbia went up in flames. By noon of April 2, 1865, Union troops captured Richmond, the capital of the Confederacy. Only 7 days later, on April 9, 1865, Confederate General Robert E. Lee surrendered to General Ulysses S. Grant at the McLean House in Appomattox, Virginia. After four long years of bloody conflict the Civil War had come to an end.

During the war more than 3,000 northerners had served as nurses; an estimated 1,000 Southern women had also done so. The women's success in organizing and restoring order in hospitals in both the North and the South would later be used as an argument for having trained nurses in cities and towns across the United States. Of equal importance, Clara Barton's work would lead to the organization of the American Red Cross.

For Discussion

1. Describe 19th-century women's role in caring for the sick.
2. What factors converged to change women's nursing role during the American Civil War?
3. How did race, class, and gender influence women's choices about work outside of the home in the 19th century?
4. Discuss differences between nursing in the Union and nursing in the Confederacy.
5. Discuss Dorothea Dix and Thomas Kirkbride's contributions to asylum reform in the mid-19th century.
6. What ethical issues surrounded the care of the mentally ill prior to the initiation of "moral therapy"?

NOTES

1. Florence Nightingale, *Notes on Nursing: What It Is and What It Is Not* (New York: J. B. Lippincott, 1859 reprint of copy from the Library of Congress, Washington, DC): preface p. i.

2. Patricia O. D'Antonio, "The Legacy of Domesticity: Nursing in Early Nineteenth-Century America," *Nursing History Review* 1 (1993): 229–246 (quote 229).

3. Ibid., 229.

4. Charles Rosenberg, *The Cholera Years: The US in 1832, 1849, and 1866* (Chicago, University of Chicago Press, 1962): 115.

5. Lillian Schlissel, "Women's Diaries on the Western Frontier," *American Studies* 18, no. 1 (Spring 1977): 87–100.

6. Martha Ann Morrison Minto, *Female Pioneering in Oregon: 1844*, Manuscript diary, Bancroft Library, University of California, Berkeley (Narrative recorded in 1878): 2–3.

7. Catherine Haun's diary in Lillian Schlissel, *Women's Diaries of the Westward Journey* (New York: Schocken Books, 1982): 168.

8. Kenneth Holmes, *Covered Wagon Women*, vol. 1, *Diaries and Letters from the Western Trails, 1840-1849* (Lincoln: University of Nebraska Press, 1983): 119. See also: John Unruh, *The Plains Across: The Overland Emigrants and the Trans-Mississippi West, 1840-1860* (Urbana: University of Illinois, 1979).

9. Helen Carpenter, as quoted in Holmes, *Covered Wagon Women*, 24–25.

10. Amelia S. Knight, Manuscript diary, the E. M. Huntington Library, California (1853): 43.

11. Volney Steele, *Bleed, Blister and Purge: A History of Medicine on the American Frontier* (Missoula, MT: Mountain Press, 2005): 80.

12. Jane Kellogg, "Memories," 1852, *Transactions of the Oregon Pioneer Association*, 1852, 59.

13. Keturah Belknap in Kenneth Holmes, *Covered Wagon Women*, 228–229. Mountain fever was probably Colorado tick fever.

14. Schlissel, "Women's Diaries," 87–100.

15. Virginia Ivins, *Pen Pictures of Early Western Days*, Manuscript, Graff Collection #2168, Newberry Library, Chicago (1905): 111–112.

16. Emily Evans, "In the Absence of Proper Medical and Surgical Skill: Childbirth and Nursing Care among the Mormon Pioneers, 1846-1866," *Windows in Time*, 18, no. 2 (October 2010): 6–9 (quote 7–8).

17. Ibid., 9.

18. Arlene Keeling, "Midway between the Pharmacist and the Physician: The Work of the Henry Street Settlement Visiting Nurses, 1893-1944," in *Nursing and the Privilege of Prescription, 1893-2000* (Columbus: The Ohio State University Press, 2007): ch. 1.

19. Washington Gladden, "The Church and the Kingdom," in *The Social Gospel in America 1870—1920*, ed. Robert T. Handy (New York: Oxford University Press, 1966): 102–118.

20. Barbra Mann Wall, *Unlikely Entrepreneurs: Catholic Sisters and the Hospital Marketplace, 1865-1925* (Columbia: The Ohio State University Press, 2005): 19.

21. Florence Nightingale, *The Institution of Kaiserswerth on the Rhine for the Practical Training of Deaconesses* (London: London Ragged Colonial Training School, 1851): 19–20.

22. Lisa Zerull, "Baltimore Lutheran Deaconess History" (PhD dissertation, University of Virginia, May 2010).

23. Ibid.

24. Herman Fritschel, *One Hundred Years of Deaconess Service 1849-1949* (Milwaukee, WI: Lutheran Deaconess Motherhouse, 1949): 113.

25. Zerull, *Baltimore Lutheran Deaconess History*, 129.

26. Alice Davis Wood, *Dorothea Dix and Dr. Francis T. Stribling: An Intense Friendship. Letters: 1849-1874* (Galileo Ghianniny Publishing, 2008).

27. Elizabeth Hundt, "St. Elizabeth's Hospital" (unpublished manuscript, University of Virginia, 2015).

28. Wood, *Dorothea Dix and Dr. Francis T. Stribling*, 20.

29. Ibid.

30. Patricia D'Antonio, *Founding Friends: Families, Staff and Patients at the Friends Asylum in Early Nineteenth Century Philadelphia* (Bethlehem, PA: Lehigh University Press, 2006).

31. Gerald Grob, *The Mad among Us: A History of the Care of America's Mentally Ill* (New York: Free Press, 1994): 27.

32. Gerald Grob, *Mental Institutions in America: Social Policy to 1875* (New York: Free Press, 1973).

33. Thomas Kirkbride, *On the Construction, Organization, and General Arrangements of Hospitals for the Insane* (Philadelphia, 1854).

34. John Curwen, "History of the Association of Medical Superintendents of American Institutes for the Insane" referenced in Elizabeth Hundt, "St Elizabeth's Hospital" (unpublished manuscript, University of Virginia, 2015).

35. Kirkbride, *On the Construction*, 7.

36. Francis Tiffany, *Life of Dorothea Lynde Dix* (Boston: Houghton Mifflin, 1891): 375.

37. Mary Livermore, *My Story of the War*, 1888 reprint (New York: Arno Press, 1972): 124, as quoted in Barbra Mann Wall, "Grace under Pressure," *Nursing History Review*, 77.

38. Ibid., 247.

39. Ibid.

40. James Phinney Munroe, *Adventures of an Army Nurse in Two Wars* (edited from the Diary and Correspondence of Mary Phinney) (Boston: Little, Brown, 1904).

41. Ibid., 36–37.

42. Ibid.

43. Ibid.

44. Ibid.

45. Munroe, *Adventures of an Army Nurse*, 44.

46. Ibid., 44–45.

47. Ibid., 49–50.

48. Ibid., 56.

49. Ibid., 61–62.

50. Jane Schultz, *Women at the Front: Hospital Workers in Civil War America* (Chapel Hill: University of North Carolina Press, 2004): 150.

51. Livermore, *My Story of the War*, 206.

52. Schultz, *Women at the Front*, 57.

53. Walt Whitman, "The Wound Dresser," https://www.poetryfoundation.org (accessed August 16, 2016): para 1.

54. Matthew Samra, "Shadow and Substance—The Two Narratives of Sojourner Truth," *Midwest Quarterly* 31, no. 2 (Winter 1997): 158–171.

55. Sarah H. Bradford, *Harriet Tubman: The Moses of Her People* (2012). Bedford MA: Applewood Books, reprint, 1961. First published in 1886. Auburn NY: W. J. Moses printer.

56. Ibid.

57. Schultz, *Women at the Front*.

58. Livermore, *My Story of the War*, 479.

59. Agatha Young, *The Women and the Crisis: Women of the North in the Civil War* (New York: McDowell and Oblensky, 1959): 92.

60. Livermore, *My Story of the War*, 483–484.

61. Stephen Oates, *A Woman of Valor: Clara Barton and the Civil War* (New York: Simon and Schuster, 1994).

62. James Dunn on Clara Barton, August 1862, https://www.nps.gov/anti/learn/historyculture/clarabarton.htm.

63. Ibid.

64. Barbra Mann Wall, "Grace under Pressure: The Nursing Sisters of the Holy Cross, 1861–1865," *Nursing History Review* 1 (1993): 71–87 (quote 71).

65. Barbra Mann Wall, "Called to a Mission of Charity: The Sisters of St. Joseph. *Nursing History Review* 6 (1998): 85–113 (quote 89).

66. Livermore, *My Story of the War*, 179.

67. Wall, "Called to a Mission," 102.

68. Ibid., 93.

69. Ibid.

70. C. Vann Woodward, *Mary Chesnut's Civil War* (New Haven: Yale University Press, 1981).

71. Ibid.

72. Ibid.

73. Sallie Thompkins, "Captain Sallie Thompkins Nurse and Officer," http://civilwarsaga.com, para 1.

74. "Kate Cumming: Journal of Hospital Life in the Confederate Army of Tennessee," *Daily Observations of the Civil War,* http://www.dotcw.com.

75. Phoebe Yates Pember, *A Southern Woman's Story: Life in Confederate Richmond* (Atlanta: Mockingbird Books, 1959).

76. Ibid., 18.

77. Barbara Maling, "Black Southern Nurse Care Providers in Virginia during the American Civil War" (dissertation, University of Virginia, 2009). See also: Grace L. Mullinax, "Chimborazo Hospital, October 1862–April 1865," *The Richmond Quarterly* 14, 1 (Fall 1991): 17–22.

78. Pember, *A Southern Woman's Story*, 83.

79. Ibid., 84.

80. Mary Chesnut, *A Diary from Dixie,* August 19, 1864, electronic ed. (New York: D. Appleton, 1905): 321.

81. Ibid.

82. Judith B. McGuire, *Diary of a Southern Refugee during the War by a Lady of Virginia,* 1862–1863, http://www.perseus.tufts.edu/hopper/text?doc=Perseus:text:2001.05.0028.

83. Barbara Maling, "Women Providing Nursing Care in Charlottesville during the American Civil War, 1861-1865," *Windows in Time: The Newsletter of the Eleanor C. Bjoring Center for Nursing Historical Inquiry* (University of Virginia) 15, no. 1 (2007): 6–10.

84. Pember, *A Southern Woman's Story.*

85. Casey Lawrence, "Sutures: The Historical Use of Horsehair during the Civil War," *Windows in Time: The Newsletter of the Eleanor C. Bjoring Center for Nursing Historical Inquiry* 24 (April 2016): 7.

FURTHER READING

Bostridge, Mark, *Florence Nightingale, The Making of an Icon* (New York: Penguin Books, 2008).

Clinton, Catherine, *The Plantation Mistress: Women's World in the Old South* (New York: Pantheon Books, 1984).

D'Antonio, Patricia O., "The Legacy of Domesticity: Nursing in Early Nineteenth-Century America," *Nursing History Review* 1 (1993): 229–246.

Evans, Emily, "In the Absence of Proper Medical and Surgical Skill: Childbirth and Nursing Care among the Mormon Pioneers, 1846-1866," *Windows in Time,* 18, no. 2 (October 2010): 6–11.

Maling, Barbara, "Women Providing Nursing Care in Charlottesville during the American Civil War, 1861-1865," *Windows in Time: The Newsletter of the Eleanor C. Bjoring Center for Nursing Historical Inquiry* (University of Virginia) 15, no. 1 (2007): 6–10.

Munroe, James Phinney, *Adventures of an Army Nurse in Two Wars* (edited from the Diary and Correspondence of Mary Phinney) (Boston: Little, Brown, 1904).

Oates, Stephen, *A Woman of Valor: Clara Barton and the Civil War* (New York: Simon and Schuster, 1994).

Pember, Phoebe Yates, *A Southern Woman's Story: Life in Confederate Richmond* (Atlanta: Mockingbird Books, 1959).

Schultz, Jane, *Women at the Front* (Chapel Hill: University of North Carolina Press, 2004).

Schlissel, Lillian, *Women's Diaries of the Westward Journey* (New York: Schocken Books, 1982).

Woodward, C. Vann, *Mary Chesnut's Civil War* (New Haven: Yale University Press, 1981).

Wall, Barbra Mann, "Grace under Pressure: The Nursing Sisters of the Holy Cross, 1861–1865," *Nursing History Review* 1 (1993): 71–87.

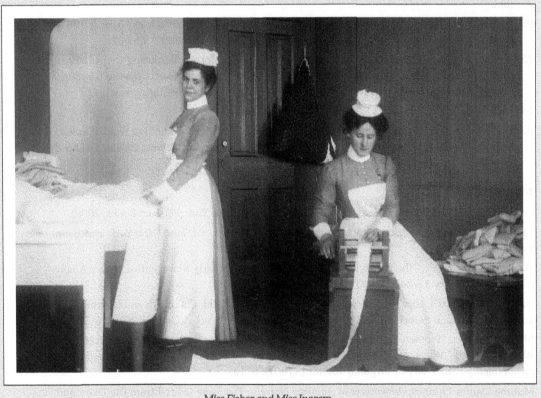

Miss Fisher and Miss Ingram.

CHAPTER 3

The Rise of a Profession: "An Art and a Science"

1873–1901

Michelle C. Hehman

"Nursing, in its more exalted sense, is as much of an art and a science
as medicine. . . . The organization of institutions for the training of
nurses [is] undoubtedly much needed, and they should be established
in every town and city in the United States. . . . We need good,
well-trained nurses by the thousands. Every community,
throughout the length and breadth of the land, should be
supplied with them, in order to do full justice to the subject."[1]

Speaking to his colleagues at the 1868 meeting of the American Medical Association, Dr. Samuel Gross campaigned for formal training for nurses, pointing out that no matter how educated or skilled the physician was, many patients would continue to perish unnecessarily unless "his efforts were properly seconded by efficient nursing."[2] With the exception of the instruction received by Lutheran deaconesses and Catholic Sisters, few training opportunities existed for American nurses in 1868. Some women, of course, had worked with the sick and injured in the American Civil War, but the majority of nursing was still performed by family members or inexperienced laborers. The dedicated work of Dorothea Dix's nurses and the efficient and organized care provided by Catholic Sisters in the Civil War challenged prevailing notions about women in nursing and advanced the idea that a good nurse was a properly trained nurse. After 1859, as word spread of Florence Nightingale's training school at St. Thomas Hospital in London, both physicians and the general public began to recognize the value of creating official nurse training programs in the United States.

While most sick nursing took place in the home, sociocultural changes occurring in the mid- to late 19th century also raised public demand for hospitals. The Industrial Revolution brought vast urbanization and immigration to major U.S. cities, and with it an ever-increasing number of poor citizens without the economic and family resources to weather unexpected hardship or illness. Hospitals developed in response to this growing need.

Classified as either public or voluntary institutions, the new hospitals sheltered the isolated and destitute members of the lower working class. Public hospitals evolved from the almshouses of the past, as supervisors needed a dedicated space to address the residents' medical issues. Traditionally regarded as dumping grounds for vagrants, prostitutes, and petty criminals, in addition to the disabled and chronically ill, almshouses sheltered those individuals whom society considered the "undeserving poor." In contrast, wealthy, upper-class philanthropists, looking to fulfill their responsibility for moral stewardship, established private hospitals for the "deserving and respectable poor." These barred certain individuals from receiving care, including those with venereal disease or consumptive illness.[3]

A national survey conducted by the American Medical Association in 1873 identified 120 hospitals, treating a combined total of more than 146,000 patients annually.[4] Not surprisingly, almost two thirds of the institutions were located in or near the nation's most populous cities, including New York City, Philadelphia, Brooklyn, Chicago, and Boston.

The quality of nursing care provided in hospitals varied widely, ranging from good in a few instances to downright dangerous in many others. Women employed as nurses in these institutions often came from the lower working class, either recruited through direct advertisement for cooks or laundresses or selected from former inmates and current patients who were able to care for others. Many nurses had little education, and their inability to read printed directions on medication bottles occasionally caused patient injury or even death.[5] Inadequate staffing and horrible working conditions discouraged many women from becoming, or even remaining, nurses. Stories of public drunkenness and sexual promiscuity further lowered the social image of nursing; thus, middle- and upper-class individuals considered the hospital to be no place for a respectable woman to visit, let alone work.

> "The condition of the patients and the beds was unspeakable. . . . Occasionally patients were found dead in the morning, who had been overlooked. Rats scampered over the floors at night."[6]
>
> Elizabeth Hobson, Visiting Committee for Bellevue Hospital, 1872

By 1872 a decline in the implicit value of nursing duties had already begun in the domestic sickroom, as social hierarchies and class distinctions dictated who performed the actual *work* of sick nursing in an increasingly commercialized economy. Upper- and middle-class women were expected to improve the lives of others in their primary roles as wife and mother, and became responsible for managing the home, developing manners and morality, and maintaining the health of their families. Seeking knowledge about the care of the sick, these ladies read a growing number of medical and nursing manuals, including Nightingale's *Notes on Nursing*, and attended lectures held by local physicians.[7] This information, however, was only intended to help them properly manage the working-class women, or professed nurses, whom they would hire to physically care for sick family members. As nurse historian Patricia D'Antonio described, "While a middle-class nursing mother had to know how to ventilate a room, how to prepare a nutritious diet, and how to keep her loved one comfortable in bed, the actual airing, cooking, turning, and bathing remained the purview of the hired help. Middle-class women would supervise such work; they would not *do* it."[8]

Power hierarchies and class divisions within the hospital closely mirrored those within the home, and individuals who worked for wages remained strictly within the servant realm. Nurses and hospital workers possessed as little authority as the patients, and these roles often overlapped as hospital matrons and superintendents frequently hired former patients as staff members.[9] In some instances, higher class women volunteered as nurses out of philanthropic duty, but nursing and other lower status jobs were only deemed acceptable when performed in a charitable capacity. A woman ceased to be a lady when she received money for those duties. Despite the gendered assumption that sick nursing was "women's work," choosing to become a hired nurse was simply not viewed as an appropriate career for a refined woman.

Supporters of formal nursing education knew that the image of nursing needed to change in order to attract educated women to the profession. The medical community as well as the general public had to endorse nursing as a respectable profession in order for them to financially support the schools and ensure their continued success by enrolling their daughters. Raising the social image of nursing to a level that mirrored those of other newly acceptable careers for young women became paramount. Literary works began to detail the stories of heroic nurses in times of war, beginning with Nightingale's iconic image as the "Lady with the Lamp" in the Crimea and continuing in works about volunteer nurses during the American Civil War.[11] Framing the need for educated nurses as a matter of great social importance, popular press articles also began to advocate for the establishment of nurse training programs. By the spring of 1871, the editor of the popular women's magazine, *Godey's Lady Book*, made the case for "lady nurses," writing: "Much has been lately said of the benefits that would follow if . . . the sick nurse were elevated to a profession which an educated lady might adopt without a sense of derogation. . . . Every medical college should have a course of study and training especially adapted for ladies who desire to qualify themselves for the profession of nurse."[12] Nurse training schools would only succeed in recruiting applicants with a higher social standing once the work of nursing became associated with respectable womanhood.

EARLY HOSPITAL-BASED TRAINING FOR NURSES

The first nurse training schools, based on Nightingale's model for St. Thomas Hospital in London, opened in the United States in 1873. Before that, however, a handful of physicians had attempted to improve the quality of care at their home institutions by introducing more formal practical instruction for nursing staff. As early as 1798, Dr. Valentine Seaman had organized a lecture series in connection with the Midwifery Department at the New York Hospital. Seaman instructed his nurse attendants on 24 subjects, including anatomy, physiology, and the care of children.[14] Unfortunately, the program was short lived, and instruction for nursing staff ended with Seaman's death in 1817.

In Philadelphia, Pennsylvania, in 1839, Dr. Joseph Warrington had founded the Nurse Society of Philadelphia in an attempt to improve obstetrical care offered to poor women. The society hoped to provide local mothers with "competent nurses" by "providing, sustaining, and causing to be instructed as far as possible, pious and prudent women for this purpose."[15] Warrington lectured nurses on sick room management and care of the postpartum mother and infant. After they had satisfactorily completed six supervised cases, Warrington awarded the nurses a signed certificate, making them eligible for private duty. By the time the Philadelphia Nurse Society Home and School opened in 1850, the society had employed nearly 50 nurses. It also extended nursing services to include some medical and surgical cases. Despite the society's growth, however, the demand for nurses in Philadelphia always exceeded supply, and in 1855 Warrington

A Negative Nursing Stereotype

In 1843 to 1844, novelist Charles Dickens published Martin Chuzzlewit and introduced the world to the character of Sarah Gamp, a private nurse. Dickens portrayed Gamp as a sloppy, drunken, incompetent, and immoral caregiver, and considered the character "a fair representation of the hired attendant on the poor in sickness."[10]

The Need for Educated Nurses

"There is a great want and demand for good trained nurses all over the world . . . this demand can only be supplied by training schools . . . any institution for nurses is only useful and desirable in proportion as it does properly train them."[13]

Fraser's Magazine, 1874

published a leaflet with Hannah Miller and Dr. Ann Preston, imploring more women to consider nursing.

Ann Preston and other female physicians became early advocates for the development of nurse training programs. After becoming the first female dean of a medical school when she founded the Female Medical College of Pennsylvania in 1850, Preston established the Woman's Hospital of Philadelphia in 1861. The hospital's purpose included caring for women and children, increasing access to clinical instruction for female medical students, and providing practical training for nurses.[16] Preston hoped to recruit "intelligent, benevolent and conscientious women" into nurse training.[17] Despite her attempts, the hospital rarely had enough pupil nurses to meet its needs. Little advancement was made prior to 1872, when a large endowment expanded the reach and capabilities of the program. That year, the Board of Lady Managers proudly claimed that graduates of the Woman's Hospital Training School had laid the foundation for the success of more prominent training schools, including New York's Training School for Nurses at Bellevue Hospital and the Connecticut Training School at New Haven Hospital.[18]

In 1862, another pioneering female physician, Dr. Marie Zakrzewska, was appointed chair of the New England Hospital for Women and Children in Boston, Massachusetts. The hospital, whose primary objective was "to provide for women medical aid by competent physicians of their own sex," also planned to offer practical training experiences for aspiring female physicians, as well as those interested in learning to nurse the sick.[19] In exchange for their service on the wards for at least 6 months, nurses at the hospital were provided with board and laundry services, a small wage, and practical instruction on the wards. Interest in the program remained low, however, with only 32 nurses receiving instruction under Zakrzewska in the first 10 years.

A new and larger hospital building opened in Boston on September 1, 1872, and the Board of Lady Managers reported a renewed focus on nurse training, admitting five "school nurses" to a year-long program of practical instruction.[20] Dr. Susan Dimock, the newly appointed head of the New England Hospital, had recently returned from 4 years of study in Germany, the last of which was spent at Kaiserswerth, where she was impressed by the system of nursing practiced by the deaconesses. Back in Boston, Dimock reorganized and took charge of the hospital's nurse training course, having pupils spend time rotating through each of the wards. Students spent 3 months apiece on the medical, surgical, and obstetric wards, 1 month on the pediatric ward, and 2 months on night duty. Physicians on staff gave lectures during the winter months, but no classwork or notes were required.[21] After satisfactory completion of the 12 months of practical training, the graduates received a certificate from the hospital. On September 1, 1873, the New England School awarded its first diploma to Linda Richards, who is considered the first trained nurse in the United States.

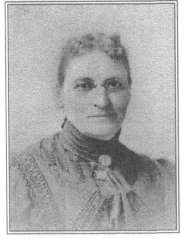

Linda Richards, who became the first trained nurse in the United States upon earning her diploma in 1873.

"Even though the course was far too short, and the advantages few, we five nurses of the first class were very happy, very united, and pretty well instructed."[22]

Linda Richards, 1907

THE FIRST NIGHTINGALE SCHOOLS

In 1873, three schools of nursing opened in New York, New York; New Haven, Connecticut; and Boston, Massachusetts. Despite the existence of previous nurse education programs, these schools are recognized as the first formal training schools in the United States because they were established using the Nightingale model at St. Thomas. Nightingale believed women were innately better suited to provide nursing care, and insisted that "the entire control of a nursing staff, as to discipline and teaching, must be taken out of the hands of men, and lodged in those of a woman, who must herself be a trained and competent nurse."[23] Schools that adhered to the Nightingale model would follow specific standards. A lady superintendent would lead each training school, and programs would be free of medical administration, directed instead by an independent women's nursing organization. The "Nightingale" schools also sought to recruit applicants who were well-educated, refined gentlewomen of excellent morals and chastity.[24] Faculty was to organize teaching around principles of proper sanitation, and emphasize technical skill and strict discipline for students. Preferably graduates would remain in the hospital setting, going forth to organize similar schools in other institutions and elevate nursing standards around the world. While few training schools adhered to every one of these standards, the Nightingale model served as an inspirational ideal to which formal training programs aspired.

> "We accept Ms. Nightingale's dictum as to what constitutes a training school."[25]
>
> Lavinia Dock, 1937

The Training School for Nurses at Bellevue Hospital

Attached to Bellevue Hospital, the Training School for Nurses opened in May 1873 and was soon identified as the "first" official nurse training program. The push to establish the school had begun a year earlier with the Visiting Committee for Bellevue Hospital, a group of women tasked by the State Charities Aid Association to report on the conditions of local hospital facilities and suggest methods of reform. After witnessing the deplorable surroundings and poor treatment hospital patients experienced in institutions throughout the city, the committee concluded that the creation of a training school for nurses would greatly improve the care provided at Bellevue and other New York hospitals. Bellevue house surgeon W. Gill Wylie traveled to Europe to examine nurse training schools in England, France, and Germany. He returned with a letter of support from Florence Nightingale, who wished the committee "God-speed with all [her] heart and soul in their task of reform."[26] Within 6 weeks of the publication of the visiting committee's final report, a sufficient initial endowment had been raised, and the Bellevue Training School officially began its work on May 24, 1873.

The first class at the Bellevue school contained a total of six probationary nurses, who were given charge of three units at the hospital.[28] They reported to Superintendent Sister Helen Bowden of the All Saints' Sisterhood, who previously was head of nursing at University College Hospital in London. Under Bowden's direction, the trainee nurses quickly demonstrated improved order, cleanliness, and overall patient care in the wards they administered. By the end of the first year, the "pupil" nurses were given privileges on two additional wards, and the number of applications from potential students surged. The school continued to grow in its second year as the new class had 29 probationers. In addition, the school provided service to three male surgical and three obstetric wards.[29]

> ### "Making a Good Nurse"
>
> "An American woman, with such an education and with her heart in the work, could be trained to become the best nurse in the world, for the race has quick wit, perception, and strong powers of observation. Let her, in addition to these qualities, acquire the habit of obedience, and you have all the elements for making a good nurse."[27]
>
> Elizabeth Hobson, Final Report from the Visiting Committee, 1872

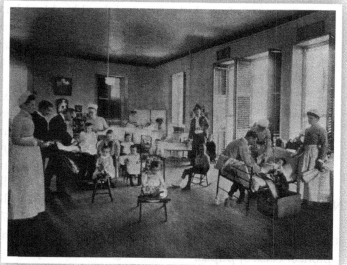

Students from the Training School for Nurses supervise patients on the pediatric ward of Bellevue Hospital.

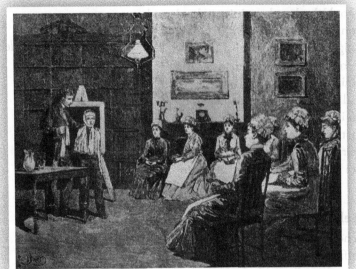

Students at the Bellevue Training School attended lectures on a broad range of subjects, including bandaging and wound care.

Pupil nurses graduated from the Bellevue school after 2 years of service at the hospital. After their first year, students became head nurses on the wards. They were also sent out to serve on private-duty cases. Initially, theoretical instruction at Bellevue was limited to teaching pupil nurses about basic cleanliness and attention to patient comfort, but quickly grew to include lectures from physicians and the assistant nursing superintendent. In 1876, students received "eight lectures upon circulation, respiration, digestion, diseases of women, and care of children; four lectures on obstetrics; ten on anatomy, physiology, and digestion; two on symptoms of disease and temperature; one on walking; one on hemorrhages; one on bedside manipulations."[30] By 1883, the total enrollment at Bellevue reached 64 students, and the training school directed nursing care in 14 wards at the hospital, each with 20 beds. In addition, students cared for a number of private-duty patients across the city.[31] The Bellevue school quickly established a reputation for training quality nurses. Indeed, the list of early graduates included Isabel Hampton Robb, Lavinia Dock, Edith Draper, Jane Delano, and Lucy Minnigerode; all of them became future leaders in the profession.

The Connecticut Training School for Nurses

Shortly after the Bellevue school began, New Haven Hospital in Connecticut also organized a training school for nurses, officially opening on October 6, 1873. Support for the establishment of a program had come earlier that year from both a hospital committee and a concerned citizen, Mr. Charles Thompson, whose "own family had suffered from the ignorance of the old fashioned nurse, and who was familiar with the European system of training schools."[32] A school charter was created on June 12, 1873, and the directors began the process of reviewing applications for admission. From the 21 women who applied, the Connecticut Training School accepted six students, the total number sanctioned by hospital trustees.

After illness detained two of the six applicants, the Connecticut Training School began its work with only four probationers and Superintendent Emily Bayard, an 1872 graduate of the Women's Hospital Training School in Philadelphia, Pennsylvania. The work proved challenging from the very first night, as one committee member recalled, "our four nurses and their superintendent found themselves at once plunged into hard work. The North ward was full of typhoid fever . . . and wards 1 and 2, East and West, were open and filled during the first week."[33] New Haven Hospital's total census at the time was 72 patients, but grew quickly to average more than 110 patients at any given time. The first class endured difficult working and living conditions, squeezing into small rooms on the top floor of an unfinished hospital expansion building and taking their "very poor" meals in the basement.[34] After word of their struggles traveled throughout the community, a number of applicants to the second class of trainee nurses withdrew their names from consideration.

"No class of nurses has ever had such demands made upon its endurance as this pioneer class of pupils."[35]

Mrs. Georgeanna Woolsey Bacon, Executive Committee Member for the Connecticut Training School, 1895

Unfortunately, getting approval to increase class size became difficult, despite the fact that hospital staff quickly praised the achievements made by the first students. Just 6 months after the school began, the Hospital Society reported, "In regard to the work undertaken by the school in the care of the sick and disabled, we find for it many general commendations. The physicians and surgeons report a decided improvement in the nursing, and speak strongly of the good already accomplished."[36] Despite having to care for every patient in the hospital as well as dozens of private-duty cases, two more years passed before the hospital board approved an increase in admissions to a total of nine student nurses, and another 7 years before yearly enrollment reached 12. An annual report from 1881 indicated the difficulty this placed on the training school and its students, stating, "The work was so hard many nurses broke down and were obliged to give up their profession . . . the school is thankful they are able to relieve suffering in the Hospital, but the school does not exist primarily for this purpose, but for the training of nurses for the public."[37]

Despite its challenges, the Connecticut Training School continued to flourish and establish itself as an early leader in nursing education. Within its first 4 years, graduates of the school were recruited to become superintendents of nursing at other hospitals, and second-year students began to nurse New Haven's poor citizens for free. Community confidence and appreciation for the nursing services of pupils and graduates continued to grow, and funding for a new dormitory was easily secured in 1881 in anticipation of larger class sizes. By 1895, the school had graduated a total of 285 trained nurses, and 31 hospitals around the country had recruited superintendents and assistants from among these alumnae. One early graduate, Ester Voorhees Hasson, would go on to become the first superintendent of the U.S. Navy Nurse Corps in 1908.

The Boston Training School for Nurses

On November 1, 1873, the Boston Training School for Nurses, the third Nightingale school to be established in the United States, began its work at Massachusetts General Hospital. Similar to the origins of the training school at Bellevue Hospital, the impetus behind the organization of the Boston school came from a concerned group of local philanthropists in the Woman's Educational Association. Unlike Bellevue, however, hospital trustees and house physicians considered the conditions at Massachusetts General Hospital to be of superior quality, and fought to keep the system unchanged. More than 11 meetings occurred over the summer of 1873 before hospital trustees and the training school committee approved the nurse training program on a probationary status.

Under this tentative agreement, four pupil nurses, two head nurses, and a superintendent assumed control over two wards inside "The Brick," as one building was referred to at the time. Often considered the "foul ward," hospital trustees chose The Brick because "it stands by itself, represents both medical and surgical departments, and offers the hard labor desirable for the training of nurses"[39] In exchange for hospital service of at least 2 years, students received room and board and a $10 monthly wage. Pupil nurses could not attend to patients "without previous training in moving and caring for persons in bed," and their training would involve "instructions in cooking and in the making of poultices and other appliances for the sick."[40] Highlighting the tensions between hospital staff and directors of the training school, as well as their deviation from the Nightingale model, the agreement also stipulated *shared control* over nursing students. Both the superintendent and hospital trustees maintained

Bjoring Center for Nursing Historical Inquiry

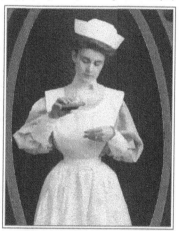

Nurse pouring medicine.

authority over student dismissal from the program, while physicians and surgeons held "exclusive medical jurisdiction" over instruction and activities of the pupils in the hospital.[41]

The Boston Training School experienced a challenging first year. Frequent leadership changes within the program stirred doubt about its effectiveness; the head nurses "were changed every day" and the school went through two superintendents in its first 13 months.[42] Students found classroom instruction lacking, as physicians at Massachusetts General refused to lecture to pupil nurses, leaving program directors asking staff from Boston City Hospital or other local doctors to come and teach instead. Finally, after convincing hospital trustees to allow the program to continue, the Boston Training School directors hired Linda Richards as superintendent.

On arrival, Richards found the routine and structure of ward work to be highly disorganized. She later described the illogical progression and rotation of students through their ward duties, saying:

> There was the strangest division of labor. For instance, a nurse would begin a day by washing poultice cloths and bandages, and it would often be two o'clock before her work was finished. She then went off duty for the afternoon. The second day the same nurse helped in the dining service and in washing dishes. After this was done, she was ready to do little incidental things as need arose. The third day she went into the wards, washed the patients' faces, made beds, swept floors, and did this, that, and the other duty until night. The fourth day she would act as head nurse. The fifth day she would begin as general utility nurse, but at nine go off duty to go to sleep, so as to be ready to go on duty that night. The sixth day she had to herself. Then the same rotation of service began again. . . . The doctors complained that nobody knew anything, and surely it was no wonder!"[43]

Superintendent Richards quickly rearranged practical instruction and increased the amount of direct training on the wards. Fully recognizing that the future of the Boston Training School rested upon her success, Richards remarked, "If I failed to prove that educated and trained nurses were superior to uneducated, untrained ones a death-blow would be given to the school in that hospital and serious injury would be sustained by the movement."[44] She requested new technologies for clinical use by her nurses: a watch to improve the accuracy of vital sign collection, and a thermometer, which had recently been redesigned to be more portable and less time-intensive. Richards also added a uniform requirement for cuffs and collars on all students to make them more easily identifiable in the hospital setting. Finally, she made affiliations with other organizations to allow pupils to rotate through the operating room, as well as the Eye and Ear Institute and the Boston Lying-In Hospital, thus providing the students with a richer clinical experience.[45]

Richards often took charge at night or supervised the most complicated patients to improve the nurses' training. Eventually she won over hospital trustees and staff physicians at Massachusetts General and the school was officially incorporated. In an 1876 Hospital Report, the trustees stated, "The incorporation of the nurses of the Training School into the service of the Hospital is a success. . . . Their employment is a mutual benefit to the School and to the Hospital, and with right notions of their duties, they will eventually prove a blessing to the sick of all classes in the community."[47] Linda Richards resigned from her position the following year, but by the end of her tenure, the training school had a total of 52 students providing

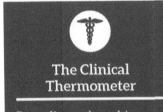

The Clinical Thermometer

Recording and graphing patient temperatures did not become routine medical procedure until the 1870s.[46] The practice had previously been impractical since the 1-foot-long mercury thermometer took 20 minutes to read a single temperature. This changed in 1866 when Thomas Albutt designed a more portable 6-inch thermometer that provided an accurate reading in just 5 minutes.

care for patients on all wards at Massachusetts General. The Boston Training School slowly achieved a reputation for excellence, and by 1895 had graduated 398 nurses, 58 of whom had been hired as superintendents or assistant superintendents at other hospitals around the country.[48]

LIFE AS A TRAINEE NURSE
Application and Acceptance

Looking to attract "women of a higher grade," the administrators stated the training school's admission requirements in a way that reflected the rigorous demands of student nursing, which tested a woman's strength of will as much as the strength of her body.[50] Candidates had to be young, healthy, and without any physical limitation. Most programs accepted applications from women between the ages of 25 and 35, although some extended the age limits to allow students from as young as 20 to a maximum age of 45 years. Training schools also automatically excluded all married women and those with living children, reasoning that a family would require an unacceptable level of commitment outside hospital life, and trainee nurses were expected to commit themselves fully to their hospital duties.[51] Two letters of reference were also required: one typically came from a physician confirming the applicant's good health and the other from a clergyman testifying to the candidate's moral character. Applications often included an overwhelming list of virtues expected from potential students, stating that nurses should be "honest, trustworthy, punctual, quiet, orderly, gentle but firm, cleanly and neat, patient, cheerful, and kindly."[52] Held to such high standards, only a small percentage of applicants were accepted for admission into the schools.

Upon acceptance, a probationer moved into the nurses' quarters in the hospital or the attached dormitories and surrendered herself to the hard work ahead during her 1-month trial with the school. Probationary students received room, board, and laundry services in exchange for their labor, but were not eligible for wages until they had survived the trial period and been promoted to junior nurse. Many left voluntarily; others were dismissed for some infraction of the rules. If the superintendent declared the student to be satisfactory at the end of the probationary period, she gave her a uniform dress, a plain white apron, and a muslin cap. The pupil-nurse subsequently signed a contract, promising to "faithfully obey" and be "subordinate to the authorities" in both the school and the hospital.[54]

Life as a trainee nurse in the late 19th century tested a young woman's physical, emotional, and intellectual limits. Standard schedules had students working 12 to 14 hours a day, 7 days a week, 50 weeks a year.[55] An hour each day and half the day on Sunday were allotted for study, rest, and recreation. Training schools were strict with this requirement, and as one student remembered, "It was as much of a misdemeanor for [a student] to be on duty when she should be off, as it was to fail to be on duty at the appointed time."[56] Some superintendents also expected their students to be present for daily prayer services, in either the morning or the evening, with mandatory church attendance on Sunday. Few opportunities existed for students to interact socially with one another outside of the hospital, although they were allowed to receive visitors or spend evenings with others until curfew, which was usually 10 o'clock.[57] Monthly wages varied across institutions, ranging from $2 to $14, and most schools had a tiered system whereby more senior students and head nurses received higher earnings.

"[Nurses] must see clearly, not to confound medicines; they must hear well, if a patient cannot speak above a whisper."[53]

Dr. William G. Thompson, 1883

Bjoring Center for Nursing Historical Inquiry

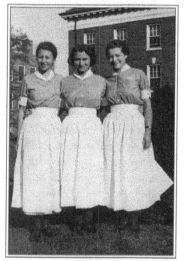

Probationary students had to be young, healthy, and of outstanding moral character.

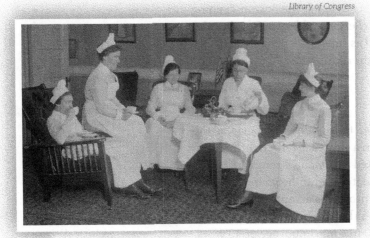

Typically, nursing students only had an hour every day and half of the day Sunday as leisure time.

"We were on the watch for stray bits of knowledge, and were quick to grasp any which came within our reach."[61]

Linda Richards, 1915

Diary Excerpt

"*August 5, 1888: A repetition of yesterday for medicines and temperatures- bathed fever cases with alcohol, also the backs of patients in bed. Dressed one with zinc ointment, made poultice for abscess. Washed patient with lotion for skin eruption.* *pm took four temps, gave milk to fever cases. Assisted with the evening medicines. . . . Every intervening moment during the day I was busy working and carbolizing various utensils in use in the ward.*"[63]

Mary N. Clymer, student nurse

In most training schools, class-room instruction in scientific theory was lacking. Instead, lectures and demonstrations were offered "from time to time," if at all.[58] On the rare occasion that lectures were given, students forfeited their daily hour of recreation time. As one early student recalled, "If the instruction given in the wards was meagre [sic] and would better be called experience, class-room instruction was likewise limited, there being but one class recitation and one lecture per week for each nurse. They were, however, always attended, no work nor ward emergency furnished adequate excuse for absence from class."[59] Pupil nurses often had difficulty staying awake during these presentations, which were usually held in the evening after students had spent a long day on the wards.[60] No standard course of study existed across the schools, and the topics covered were generally limited to the specialties of medical officers willing to offer didactic instruction to nursing students.

Likewise, head nurses, who were themselves only second-year students, provided meager supervision. Instruction occurred almost entirely through practical experience on the wards. Pupil nurses learned by example and repetition how to make and apply bandages, line splints, and cook and serve proper food for the sick. They also learned the best methods of controlling the environment of the sickroom, and became proficient in changing linens and administering sponge baths without disturbing patients in bed. Students were taught the proper manner for administering medications, including the procedure for the newly popularized hypodermic injection, but only learned the intended purpose of drugs after observing their effects on patients. Trainees also discovered the importance of keen observation, and were instructed to watch for changes in vital signs, sleep, appetite, or thirst and properly convey any disturbances to the head doctor. Students quickly understood their role was that of watchful handmaid for the physician in the care of the sick.[62] Opportunities to develop skills depended largely upon the types of hospital wards overseen by the training school, with the larger and specialty institutions offering valuable experience assisting with surgical operations, or with parturient women and their newborn children.

Regulations and Discipline

Success on the busy wards required swift, efficient work and strict adherence to a prescribed set of regulations. Designed not only to promote the specialized skills and moral character thought necessary for nurses, these rules also protected patients from inexperienced students whose responsibilities often exceeded their technical proficiency.[64] A rigid hierarchy determined individual duties and the level of accountability. The head nurse held full authority over every admitted patient on her ward, presiding over 20 to 30 cases at a time. One senior nurse and one junior nurse were assigned to each unit, along with a hospital orderly on the male wards to assist with heavy lifting and to maintain Victorian standards of propriety.

Physicians ultimately held the head nurse accountable for the diligent execution of all written orders, and the decision to delegate any and all required tasks rested upon her shoulders. More often than not, junior nurses were entrusted to bedside patient care, administering meals, changing beds, bathing patients, and applying dressings and poultices while senior nurses procured patient vital signs, gave prescribed medications, and documented information in the patient's record. The head nurse supervised all activities, ensured that tasks were performed to her standards, and corrected any perceived deficiencies.

Superintendents and head nurses in the early training schools took it upon themselves to mold students into an idealized version of the "proper" nurse, often through the use of militaristic discipline. Traits of self-sacrifice, dedication to duty, and complete obedience to superiors were stressed over individuality and independence, with overall behavior considered the measure of a student's moral character.[65] The overwhelming amount of work on the wards demanded stringent regulation, and many of the new students, who had come from middle- to upper-class families, had few disciplined work habits. To ensure that tasks were completed correctly and on time, head nurses and superintendents exacted complete and unyielding obedience from pupils under their supervision. As Florence Nightingale commented, "The whole organisation of discipline to which the nurses must be subjected is for the sole purpose of enabling the nurses to carry out, intelligently and faithfully, such orders and such duties as constitute the whole practice of nursing."[66]

The course of instruction in early American training schools encompassed a period of 1 to 2 years, with the majority eventually adopting the 2-year commitment. Hospital trustees soon realized that, in addition to a higher quality of patient care, association with a nurse training school provided a number of benefits, particularly by extending the length of the program. Head nurse positions were traditionally difficult to staff, but rather than rush first-year students into this challenging role, the addition of a second year ensured a consistent supply of experienced nurses throughout the hospital. Nursing students also proved to be cheap labor, often earning little to no income in

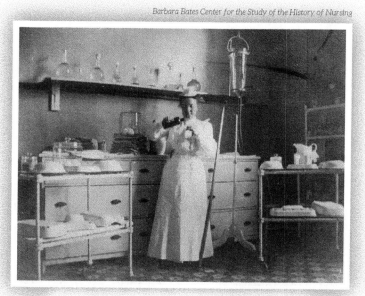

Head nurses taught primarily through example and were responsible for all of their students' activities.

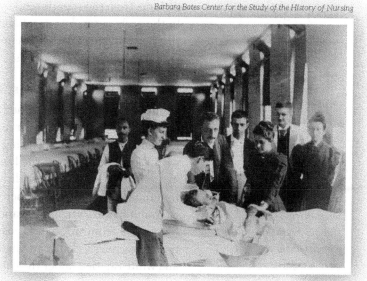

Primarily viewed as dutiful assistants to the physician, student nurses provided cheap labor for hospitals.

"It is not and cannot be democratic . . . to this end complete subordination of the individual to the work as a whole is as necessary for her as for the soldier."[67]

Lavinia Dock, 1893

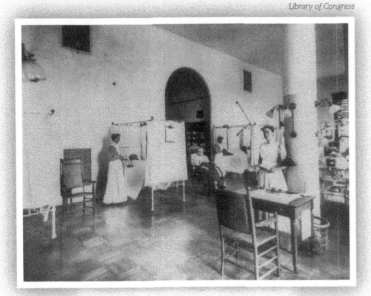

Nurses attend to patients on the women's ward.

exchange for lodging expenses and the education provided during the program. As program admissions increased, hospitals could replace their paid nursing positions with students, thereby decreasing costs while improving quality. Adopting a private-duty nursing requirement for students also generated income for the hospital board, as the facility demanded a percentage of wages earned by trainees in private homes.

Individual schools determined their own requirements for graduation, but many mandated that students perform recitations and examinations after the completion of their 2 years of service. Occasionally, a committee of the hospital medical staff presided over individual course examinations.[68] After successful completion of all requirements, graduate nurses received a diploma from the superintendent of the school, generally with little fanfare. In the early years, low enrollment numbers and rolling admissions meant that few students finished the program simultaneously, leaving no need for formal graduation ceremonies.

Nursing Uniforms, Caps, and Pins

Similar to the evolution of modern nursing practice, the development and endorsement of a uniform for nurses drew from both religious and military influences. The notion of using uniform dress as an identifier originated with Theodor Fliedner at the Kaiserswerth Deaconess Institute in Germany in the 1830s. Looking to establish deaconess nursing as a respectable vocation for unmarried women, Fliedner instituted a uniform policy that conformed to contemporary etiquette standards for female attire while distinguishing his nurses from untrained hospital workers. The image of the graduate nurse-deaconess, clad in an unadorned blue cotton dress, white collar, scarf, and white cap tied under the chin, became synonymous with caring, professional competence and an unquestionable moral character.[70] Identified by her uniform, a deaconess nurse could perform her duties in any setting without reproach, despite rigid social mores that discouraged most of the menial and intimate work of sick nursing.

Florence Nightingale, who studied at Kaiserswerth, also believed in the potential of uniform dress to help transform the image of nursing. During the Crimean War, Nightingale required her nurses to wear modest gray tweed dresses with long sleeves, full skirts, and a brown scarf embroidered with "Scutari Hospital." The plain uniform helped soldiers differentiate nurses from other women around the camps—including cooks, laundresses, and even prostitutes—and indicated the arrival of a competent caregiver.[71] At St. Thomas Hospital in London, student uniforms of plain wool and cotton reflected Nightingale's preference for simplicity and restraint. By avoiding the "fidget of silk and crinoline, [and] the rattling of stays and shoes" prevalent in contemporary women's fashion, nurses could maintain the quiet atmosphere necessary for healing and avoid any impediment to practical movement.[72] Since many middle-class Victorians also considered fashion an outward expression of individual moral values, with modest dress conveying order and self-sacrifice, the uniformed Nightingale nurse would represent respectability and quality of character.

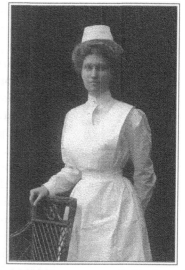

When the early American nurse training schools first started, no specific uniform requirement existed at any of the programs. Most suggested that students wear a simple calico or wool dress, usually crafted by a local dressmaker, along with removable aprons and cuffs that could be easily laundered. However, hospital trustees and superintendents quickly recognized the utility of standardized school uniforms: Student nurses would be easily distinguishable inside the hospital, and dress codes could become another means through which to control and discipline pupils. Indeed, an early report from the Bellevue Hospital Committee stated, "A uniform, however simple, is indispensable, and should be rigidly enforced. It is advantageous on the grounds of economy as well as neatness and its effect on a corps of nurses is the same as on a company of soldiers."[73] Unfortunately, many students, having come from higher class families, scoffed at the idea of standardized uniforms because they equated uniform dress with servitude.

Nurses were expected to dress demurely, often in long dresses with collars and cuffs, removable apron, and a white hat.

At the Bellevue Training School, student opposition to a uniform quickly faded when Euphemia Van Rensselaer, a member of the first class of trainees who hailed from a prominent family, appeared on the wards in a blue striped dress, white apron, and cap. As Lavinia Dock recounted the story, "So charming was she to behold, and so dowdy and insignificant did all the nondescript print dresses look beside her, that prejudice vanished and as rapidly as possible the uniform was adopted, and never again questioned."[74] Once the Bellevue school officially implemented its specific dress code, other programs quickly followed.

Despite differences in fabric color and details, student uniforms in the late 19th century shared a number of qualities and emphasized a similar silhouette. Dresses featured a high neckline, narrow waist, and full skirt that covered the ankles. Most of the dresses also had leg-of-mutton sleeves, full and loose at the upper arm and tapered at

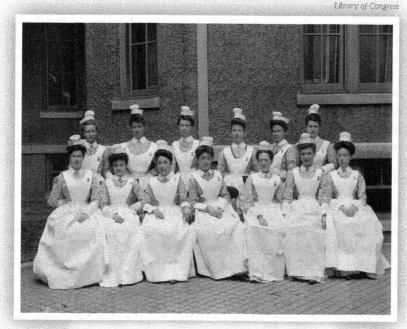

Providence Hospital nurses in their official uniforms, 1905.

The Importance of a Uniform in Nursing

"Nurses, of all others, should command respect and confidence, and they can only do this by appearing at all times modest and dignified. . . . The public overlooks in others what it condemns in a nurse, and for this reason the nurse must jealously guard her conduct, her dress, and her speech. The uniform of a nurse is an honorable distinction when worn with dignity."[75]

Clara Sanford Lockwood, 1901

the forearm and wrist. Completing the ensemble were a white apron, removable cuffs, and a white cap, with the uniformed nurse projecting an image of genteel femininity and respectability.

The practicality of the outfit, however, fell short in some ways: tight bodices and stiff collars impaired movement during physically demanding work, while long sleeves and elaborate cuffs could easily become contaminated. Despite scientific recognition of the relationship between bacteria and disease as early as the 1840s, it was not until the 20th century that the notion of the uniform as a barrier to contamination became widely popular. As historian Christina Bates described, "Personal hygiene was more of a moral than a medical imperative in bringing credibility and respectability to nursing. It was important for the nurse to look clean, but not necessarily to be clean."[76]

By the 1890s, student uniforms became a distinguishing characteristic for most nurse training schools, each identified by a particular color or fabric. The general public began to recognize school affiliation according to uniform dress, immediately attributing the prestige of the nurses' home institutions based on physical appearance alone. This presented some measure of external control over behavior, as student and graduate nurses alike endeavored to provide care worthy of their school's reputation.[77] Some programs also mandated different dress colors depending on the student's progression or status within the program, with probationers wearing light colors and more senior nurses wearing darker ones.[78]

In addition to a specific style and fabric for the dress, programs began to modify nursing caps to create their own distinctive style. Tracing their origins to the Catholic sisterhood and subsequently used to keep a nurse's hair clean and out of her face, caps became one of the few ways training schools could introduce a degree of fashion extravagance to the otherwise austere dress codes. Similar to the uniform dress, programs also began to use the cap as a way to signify rank or matriculation. Black bands were sometimes added to caps upon graduation, while other schools initiated capping ceremonies, whereby a probationer received her official school cap upon completion of her trial month in the program.

Nursing pins became a symbol of matriculation through a training school, awarded to graduates upon completion of program requirements. Precursors to nursing pins date back to the Crusades with the Knights Hospitalier, a religious order who cared for injured and suffering crusaders and identified themselves with a white Maltese cross worn over the heart.[79] Acceptance into the Knights Order was an honor, and the Maltese cross symbolized an individual's dedication to service. Nursing schools in England adopted the practice in the late 19th century, awarding gold and silver medals to outstanding nurses in each class, associating the award with excellence in nursing care. In the United States, training schools began awarding pins to all graduates, designing a unique symbol for their institution to distinguish its alumnae.

The Bellevue Training School Nursing Pin

Designed by Tiffany & Co. in 1880, the Bellevue Training School was the first to adopt an official pin. The design displays a crane in the center, representing vigilance, surrounded by a wreath of poppies, signifying the role of nurses to relieve pain and suffering. The outer unbroken circle of blue represents constancy, with the school's name "Bellevue" along the bottom.

AFRICAN AMERICAN HOSPITALS AND TRAINING SCHOOLS

As word spread of the success of these pioneer nursing programs, the number of formal training schools across the country grew exponentially. Records from the U.S. Census Bureau show a total of 15 nursing schools in the year 1880, growing to 35 schools by 1893, and ultimately reaching 432 training programs by the turn of the 20th century.[80] Nursing schools had increased professional opportunities available to young women in America, but only to those who reflected the social image of the ideal Nightingale nurse: middle-class women with a proper education, high moral character, and good health.

Unspoken in these standards was a strong racial bias, which severely restricted access to nurse training programs for women of color. Almost all schools refused to admit Black applicants, and the few programs that did often had strict quota systems that limited their acceptance.

After the Civil War, Black women across the United States fought against rampant racism and sexism, still finding themselves relegated to domestic work or other menial jobs with low wages, no status, and minimal respect. Even in Massachusetts, considered one of the more inclusive northern states with the most antidiscrimination laws, Black citizens continued to experience hostility, disenfranchisement, and discrimination by public and private institutions. The New England Hospital for Women and Children, however, demonstrated a commitment to inclusivity and equality almost from its inception. Early hospital reports proudly describe their racially and economically diverse patient population, celebrating equal access to treatment. The 1865 *Annual Report* remarked, "The hospital has represented striking contrasts the last month. In the lower ward, at either end of the little crib a tiny head protrudes. On closer view you find one of the little occupants is black, the other white. No antagonism is manifested except in position."[81] The hospital's approach to nursing also reflected this philosophy, considering the career "a high and noble work into which men or women fitted by nature and inclination may enter, without any loss of refinement or social position."[82] It is not surprising, therefore, that the hospital's nursing program graduated the first Black trained nurse in the United States, Mary Eliza Mahoney, in 1879.

Mahoney's graduation predates the existence of any school of nursing that exclusively trained Black women, a fact symbolic of the difficulty faced by African Americans and other minorities in their attempts to access nursing education programs.[83] Even at the New England Hospital for Women and Children, whose 1863 founding charter established a quota providing for the admission of one Black woman and one Jewish woman to each nursing class, no Black student had graduated prior to Mahoney in 1879.[84] Mahoney also had to work at the hospital to prove her character and work ethic before finally being admitted to the training school. The 16-month program was particularly challenging, as evidenced by the high level of attrition among Mahoney's own probationary class. Out of the 42 students considered during that year, only three other women graduated alongside Mary Mahoney on August 1, 1879.[85]

Mahoney's graduation paved the way for the admission of more Black nursing students, both at her home institution and at others in northern states. By 1899 Mahoney's program had trained and graduated five additional Black nurses.[87] Training schools at the New York Infirmary in New York City, Washington General Hospital in the District of Columbia, and the Women's Hospital of Philadelphia also graduated Black women from their programs. Martha Franklin, an early graduate of the school at the Women's Hospital of Philadelphia, would go on to found the National Association of Colored Graduate Nurses, the first nursing organization for Black women. Franklin, who completed the training program in 1897, became the second and final Black woman to graduate from the Women's Hospital; Anne Reeves had been the first, finishing the course of training in April 1888.[88] However, outside of these few instances, and particularly in southern states, Black women possessed very few opportunities to receive formal nurse training.

In the immediate post–Civil War era, African Americans experienced significant health disparities, suffering higher morbidity and mortality,

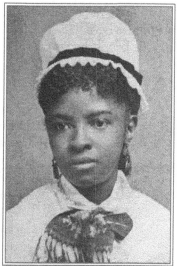

Mary Eliza Mahoney became the first trained Black nurse in the United States, graduating in 1879.

"Mary went to the hospital to work. She cooked, washed, and scrubbed and so got in. A woman doctor wanted her there, and that was the only influence she had."[86]

Miss Hawley, Friend of Mary Eliza Mahoney, 1954

increased rates of communicable diseases, and greater maternal and infant mortality. Poor overall health for Black Americans, combined with widespread segregation in many hospitals across the nation and restricted access to medical and nursing schools for students of color, provided the impetus behind the establishment of Black hospitals, medical colleges, and training schools. The first four Black nurse training programs began at Spelman Seminary in Atlanta, Georgia, in 1886; Dixie Hospital Training School in Hampton, Virginia, in 1891; Provident Hospital School of Nursing in Chicago, Illinois, in 1891; and Tuskegee Institute Nurse Training School in Tuskegee, Alabama, in 1892. Additionally, the first university-affiliated nurse training school began at Howard University in Washington, DC, in 1893. It should be noted that while the establishment of Black hospitals and schools increased access to care and opportunities for education, continued segregation and racial discrimination had profound consequences for all Black Americans. In particular, two Supreme Court decisions—*Plessy v. Ferguson* in 1896, which introduced the "separate but equal" doctrine, and *Cumming v. Richmond County Board of Education* in 1899, mandating segregation in schools—would provide legal precedent for sustained discrimination in education, housing, and health care for decades to come.

Spelman Seminary

"The colored people have long felt the need of a hospital where their sick can be properly cared for."[90]

Anna DeCosta Banks, 1899

Originally founded as the Atlanta Baptist Female Seminary, the college officially opened on April 11, 1881 as the first private school for Black women. The school was established through philanthropic support from John D. Rockefeller and his wife, Laura Spelman Rockefeller, and was later renamed Spelman Seminary in honor of Mrs. Rockefeller and her parents Harvey Buel and Lucy Henry Spelman, longtime activists in the antislavery movement.[91] Initially, the school focused its curriculum on training future teachers. School presidents held Spelman students to high standards of Victorian propriety, requiring freshly washed and ironed uniforms, with hats and gloves worn in public. In addition to theoretical instruction, students also learned domestic skills, such as sewing, cooking, and laundry. A nurse training program was added in 1886, and students carried out a 2-year course of study leading to a diploma upon completion.[92]

By 1901 the 31-bed MacVicar Hospital had become the school's infirmary and practice facility, and the nurse training program was extended to 4 years. Only the first year covered nursing theory, while the following three were spent on the wards at MacVicar Hospital or performing private-duty nursing around Atlanta. The small size of the hospital eventually presented a problem for administration, which decided to end the nursing program in 1927. As then president Florence M. Reed stated: "It had become apparent that first-class training could not be offered with the facilities provided by MacVicar Hospital. The hospital contained too small a number of beds; the variety of cases was too limited; and the equipment was insufficient for modern techniques."[93] During its existence, Spelman Seminary graduated 117 trained Black nurses.[94]

New York Public Library

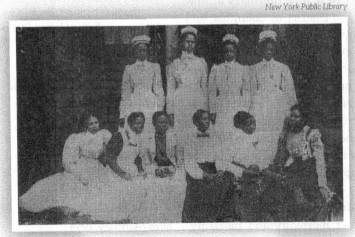

Trained nurses at Spelman Seminary, 1902.

Dixie Hospital and Hampton Training School for Nurses

At the Hampton Normal and Agricultural Institute, part of what would become Hampton University, teacher Alice M. Bacon opened the Hampton Training School for Nurses in 1891. Bacon, a White woman who had grown up in New Haven, Connecticut, and received a bachelor's degree from Harvard University, became dismayed when she heard that one of her Black students was denied entrance to a nurse training school because of her race. In response, Bacon raised enough funds to establish Dixie Hospital, a "little yellow-washed building" with 10 beds, and started a nurse training program for African American women on an "entirely experimental" basis.[95] With two students, a nursing superintendent and a resident physician, the Hampton Training School began its work in June 1891, caring for just one patient.

Describing the importance of the program, Bacon stated in 1892 that the first year had proven that "the colored woman, with a Hampton education behind her, can be trained into as good a nurse as any white woman."[97] The first class of students pushed through challenging conditions, having to live, sleep, and eat in whatever parts of the small hospital were not occupied by patients. Lectures, given by local physicians on a near weekly basis, were held either on the ward, in the kitchen, or outside the school depending on weather or convenience. Students and staff of Dixie Hospital cared for a total of 37 patients that year—20 men, 15 women, and two children—covering a variety of medical–surgical and maternity issues.[98] All patients were accepted, regardless of race, religion, or ability to pay, and students treated them either in the hospital or in their own homes based on available space or the communicability of the disease. In part, this was done because the hospital had no way to isolate infectious cases.

The hospital quickly gained a positive local reputation, caring for the community even in times of economic hardship. Clad in a gray uniform, white cap, and apron, the Dixie Hospital nurse gave compassionate and competent care for anyone in need of comfort, often receiving nothing but thanks, or perhaps the gift of food or a homemade quilt. During the first 10 years of its existence, nurses at the Dixie Hampton School cared for 1,087 patients, and 42 trained nurses graduated from the program. Class size had grown from two pupils to 20, with students ministering to 147 patients annually.[100] One of Hampton's first graduates was Anna DeCosta Banks, who would go on to help establish a nurse training school at Charleston Hospital in South Carolina where she served as a head nurse and superintendent. Later she would work as a visiting nurse for the Metropolitan Life Insurance Company.

> "There is need in the South for the trained colored nurse."[96]
>
> Alice M. Bacon, 1892

The First Hampton Training School Students

> "Our nurses have been kept busy, with plenty of work both inside and outside the hospital. . . . Sometimes two or three working together have fought day and night with death, when two or more of a family were down with typhoid fever, their interest never flagging, their courage and strength never failing, until all were tided over and brought safely back within the gates of life."[99]
>
> Alice M. Bacon, 1893

Barbara Bates Center for the Study of the History of Nursing

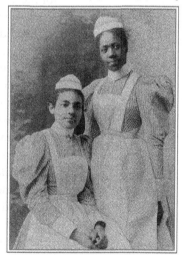

Graduates of Frederick Douglass Memorial Hospital School for Nurses, 1897.

MEN IN NURSING IN THE LATE 19TH CENTURY

By the time American physicians began to promote the idea of establishing nurse training schools, the number of men providing sick nursing care by choice rather than out of emergency or necessity had dramatically decreased across the world. A number of social changes have been attributed to the decline. The low social status of the hired sick nurse in secular hospitals translated into lower pay; traditionally, only working-class women accepted low-status and poor paying jobs, eventually increasing the gender disparity in nursing. Additionally, the Industrial Revolution increased the number and availability of factory appointments and jobs reclaiming natural resources, many of which required heavy physical labor and long hours away from home.[101]

Working-class men flocked to these positions on the promise of higher wages without the need for experience or education. Finally, variations in the number and makeup of religious orders that had begun in the Renaissance period, namely, a decline in monasteries and an increase in convents, meant that Catholic Sisters eventually replaced male clerics as caregivers in religious hospitals.[102]

As Florence Nightingale continually championed the superiority of *women* as nurses and caregivers, and the Nightingale model was implemented in nursing schools across the United States, the trained nursing workforce became increasingly made up of females. Unfortunately, Victorian gender norms and rules of propriety, which required that the intimate body work of sick nursing be provided only by members of the same sex, persisted well after the transition to modern nursing. A distinct quality gap emerged in the care being provided to male hospital patients, prompting requests for the establishment of nurse training programs for men. By the turn of the 20th century, a total of five nurse training schools for men had opened, located in or near some of the largest U.S. cities.

Bellevue Hospital established a training school for male nurses in 1888 in order to improve the care provided to its male patients. Named after D. O. Mills, a local dentist and philanthropist who donated the money to start the program, the first pupil nurses from the Mills Training School for Men cared for patients on a total of five wards throughout the male side of the hospital.[104] Initially one of the female head nurses directed the wards, but after the first Mills class matriculated, male graduates took over supervisory roles. Eventually Mills students and graduates staffed the entire male side of Bellevue Hospital. When the New York State Board of Examiners of Registered Nurses was first established in 1903, an early graduate of the Mills school, L. Bissel Sanford, was appointed to the board. Sanford is believed to be the first male registered nurse in the United States.[105]

THE RISE OF SCIENTIFIC MEDICINE

During the colonial period and the early 19th century, few legal or social obstacles existed for those desiring to practice medicine. Individuals with or without formal education or specialized training could present themselves as healers without consequence.[106] As late as the mid-19th century, medicine was viewed as an inferior career with limited prospects. Physicians had little political influence, only modest income, and limited social prestige, with some doctors lamenting their position in "the most despised of all the professions [to] which liberally educated men are expected to enter."[107]

The second half of the 19th century saw initial efforts toward standardization and refinement of the medical profession. The American Medical Association, created in 1848 to raise professional standards for doctors, made little progress in regulating and influencing medical practice across the country prior to the 20th century. Until the 1870s, wide variation in training standards for medical education persisted in the United States, and few states had licensing laws for physicians. Consequently, medical treatments did little to impact prevailing diseases, infant and child mortality rates remained high, and poor hospital conditions decreased physician popularity and usage among the general public.[108]

Discoveries, Bacteriology, and Technology

The development and application of the scientific method to medicine resulted in a number of medical discoveries in bacteriology, asepsis, immunology, anesthesia, and medical instruments during the last quarter of the 19th century. Germ theory and

Joseph Lister and Antisepsis

Joseph Lister, a British surgeon, revolutionized the prevention and treatment of wound infection. Lister soaked dressings in carbolic acid (phenol) before applying them to open wounds, and eliminated all instances of gangrene and sepsis following surgery or an open fracture over a 9-month period at the Glasgow Infirmary. The results were published in the medical journal *Lancet* in 1867, and physicians around the world gradually incorporated his antiseptic techniques.

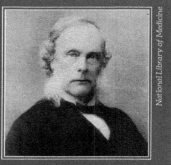

Joseph Lister, who made significant progress in antiseptic techniques.

antiseptic practices revolutionized medical understanding of disease and the application of advanced diagnostic instruments began to improve national health. Backed by scientific discovery and a monopoly over the use of new diagnostic technology, physicians began to enjoy a high level of social prestige that had previously eluded the profession. Medical leaders used their newfound social standing to further elevate their authority over health practice, bringing the ability to prescribe, diagnose, and treat under the exclusive control of the medical profession.[109] Moreover, the medical profession was able to "turn its authority not just into social privilege, but also economic power and political influence," eventually dictating the country's response to issues of public health, particularly child welfare and infant mortality.[110]

As physicians embraced new advances in science and technology, nursing became more challenging. When revolutionary scientific theories and diagnostic instruments found their way into the hospital, nurses needed to at least be familiar with the new knowledge and equipment to perform their duties effectively. However, physicians carefully controlled the transfer of technology between the medical and nursing fields, ensuring that doctors maintained authority. Even when nurses became the primary users of a new device, as in the case of the thermometer or urinary catheter, the technology never distinctively signified nursing because both doctors and nurses shared its use.[111] In many instances nurses did everything leading up to and preparing for the use of a technology, including a plan for postprocedural patient care, but the discrete act of using a specific device was reserved for the physician.

While physicians pushed the notion of modern nursing as just another tool in the arsenal of scientific medicine, nurses maintained a unique role in the provision of care. Nursing involved intimate bodily contact with patients as nurses attended to physical needs and comfort, provided treatment modalities and medications, and controlled the medical environment. As nurse historian Margarete Sandelowski has remarked, "While physicians were increasingly looking at their patients through microscopes and

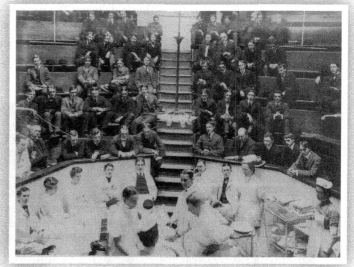

Barbara Bates Center for the Study of the History of Nursing

Medical students watch as Dr. Chalmers DaCosta performs surgery. Nurses stand waiting to hand over instruments, and observe the patient throughout the procedure.

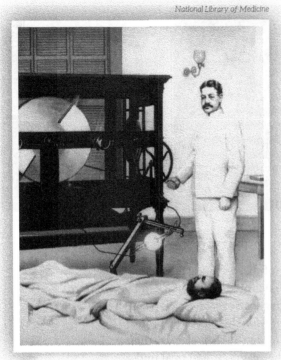

An illustration of a physician taking an x-ray.

X rays, listening to them through stethoscopes, and interpreting their conditions via laboratory assays and electrocardiograms, nurses continued to maintain more direct sensory and other physical contact with their patients."[112] Nurses used all of their senses in making clinical observations, needed strong and dexterous bodies and limbs to perform physically demanding work, and required effective critical thinking skills to interpret responses and anticipate changes. The work of nursing truly became both an art and a science, necessitating both physical skill and clinical knowledge to succeed.

Anesthesia at Mayo Clinic

For the administration of anesthesia, the characteristics celebrated in the model nurse, including a keen sense of observation, gentle hands, and a soothing voice, initially made nurses an ideal choice to control the procedure. In 1888, Dr. William Worrall Mayo hired Edith Graham, a graduate of Women's Hospital Training School in Chicago and the only professionally trained nurse in Rochester, to be his "anesthetist, office nurse, general bookkeeper and secretary."[113] A year later, after a tornado devastated Rochester, Minnesota, the Sisters of St. Joseph convinced him to open a hospital. Years later in 1915, it would become known as Mayo Clinic.

Shortly after Dr. Mayo hired Graham, he taught her how to administer anesthesia using the "open drop" method a German physician had taught him a few years earlier.[114] Like other surgeons, Dr. Mayo had noticed that too often patients died from chloroform poisoning because the medical student assigned to give anesthesia was so interested in observing the surgery itself that he would forget to observe the patient.[115] Mayo concluded that he would delegate the task of giving anesthesia to a specially trained nurse.[116]

Under Mayo's supervision, Graham quickly became adept at the open drop method of anesthesia delivery. The process was actually quite simple: A wire frame covered with gauze was placed over the patient's mouth and nose and the anesthetizer slowly placed drops of the anesthetic agent on the cloth until the patient lost consciousness. The key

Chloroform for Anesthesia

On November 8, 1847, Scottish obstetrician James Young Simpson discovered the anesthetic properties of inhaling chloroform vapors. Administration of chloroform for anesthesia required great skill, with a fine line between effective dosing and complete depression of the respiratory system. Early chloroform fatalities were widely publicized, but its successful use in 1853 by Queen Victoria while giving birth greatly increased the acceptance and popularity of the technique.

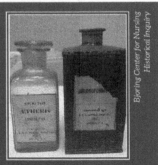

Starting in the mid-19th century, chloroform became popular as an anesthetic.

was in vigilant observation of the patient's response to ensure that the patient neither suffocated nor came out of the anesthetized state.[117]

Between 1889 and 1893, Dr. William and his brother Dr. Charles Mayo performed 655 surgical operations at St. Mary's Hospital. Of these, 98.3% were successful in that the patients left the hospital alive.[118] Edith Graham had given the anesthesia in every case.

As was custom during that time, Graham retired from nursing when she married Charles Mayo in 1893. That year, her friend and fellow nurse Alice Magaw assumed Graham's responsibilities, administering anesthesia using the German open-drop method.[119] Later, publishing a review of 14,000 cases in which she had assisted with anesthesia, Magaw was adamant that the open-drop method had demonstrated the best results:

> In my series of cases, the "open method" has been the method of choice. We have tried almost all methods advocated that seemed at all reasonable, such as nitrous oxide gas as a preliminary to ether (this method was used in 1,000 cases), a mixture of scopolamine and morphine as a preliminary to ether in 73 cases, also chloroform and ether, and have found them to be very unsatisfactory, if not harmful, and have returned to ether "drop method" each time, which method we have used for over ten years.[120]

The application method and skilled nursing care were essential to the patient's survival during surgery, and both depended on the nurse anesthetist's clinical judgment. For Magaw, whom Charles Mayo later called "the Mother of Nurse Anesthesia," putting patients to sleep was an art as well as a science. The nurse anesthetist had to monitor the patient's pupils, skin color, pulse, muscle tone, and facial expression, as well as the depth and effort of respirations, in order to judge the patient's response and adjust the dosage of the anesthetic agent accordingly.[121]

EDUCATIONAL REFORMS

By the turn of the 20th century, hospital boards had recognized the economic advantage of an association with a nursing school, as evidenced by the rapid increase in the total number of official training programs across the United States. Many of the newer training schools had been established at smaller hospitals or specialty institutions like tuberculosis sanatoria and insane asylums, which severely limited the range of practical experience available to students in the program. Nurse training programs exhibited a complete lack of standardization with regard to course length, lecture schedules, hospital ward rotations, private-duty experiences, and graduation requirements. All graduates could call themselves "trained" nurses, but no consensus standards regulated the meaning of the title.

Isabel Hampton, an 1883 graduate of the Training School for Nurses at Bellevue Hospital, believed strongly in improving and regulating educational standards for nursing students. Her vision of nursing as an honorable and respectable profession for women required a transformation of many of the currently accepted norms in the process and practice of nurse education. The reforms Hampton made while superintendent of two elite-nurse training programs demonstrated her ability to effectively lead change and inspire others toward her cause.

Despite a lack of administrative and leadership experience, Hampton was recommended for the position of superintendent at the Illinois Training School for Nurses, eventually assuming the role on July 4, 1886. Upon her arrival, Hampton found the

The Importance of Observation in Anesthesia

"The eyes give very early warning of danger. Some insist that the state of the pupils, the pulse, or change in respiration is sure indication of danger, but to rely upon any one of these signs would be folly; carefully watch all of these symptoms, not relying on any one of them."[122]

Alice Magaw, 1900

"The scope and breadth of experience in a large hospital, are what every nurse would choose if she could."[123]

Bertha Mayne, 1901

program already well established and yet in need of major reform. Improving the education of pupil nurses became her focus, and Hampton standardized the course schedule, began to use textbooks instead of lectures for elementary subjects, introduced a grading system, and extended the theoretical component of the program into both years when it had previously been restricted solely to the first year. She also divided students into junior and senior classes, and introduced a regular academic calendar, with a fixed schedule of classes, holidays, and a single graduation each year in June.[124] To broaden practical experience for trainee nurses, Hampton arranged affiliations with Presbyterian Hospital in addition to taking over more wards at Cook County Hospital. Finally, Hampton convinced the hospital board to terminate both the private-duty nursing requirement during the second year of the program and the monthly stipend provided to each student.[125]

Both of these changes were important to the future of nursing programs, proving that training schools were legitimate educational endeavors. Hampton seriously opposed private-duty requirements for students, believing they furthered their economic exploitation, interfered with academic studies, and endangered their health, as private patient assignments often required a nurse to be on duty for 24 hours straight, possibly many days in a row. She would later remark, "is it not poor economy and mistaken judgment . . . to sacrifice the health of one class of people [nurses] in trying to restore that of others [patients]?"[126] In discontinuing the provision of monthly stipends, the hospital board in Chicago showed that it had begun to view the school of nursing more as a legitimate educational institution than a vocational training program. As acting superintendent, Hampton found the change a welcome one, hoping to open the nursing profession to qualified women regardless of social class and economic means, attracting candidates for altruistic rather than monetary reasons.

Upon her appointment as superintendent of the newly established Johns Hopkins Training School for Nurses in 1889, Hampton immediately began improvements, much the same way she had instituted change in Chicago. She extended the program length from 1 to 2 years and standardized the theory portion of the curriculum through the introduction of examinations and grades. Significantly broadening the schedule of formal instruction, Hampton required students to hear a total of 66 lectures given by 13 physicians on a wide variety of topics during their first year alone.[128] Practical training in pediatrics, a rarity in American training schools, occurred through an affiliation Hampton arranged with the Thomas Wilson Sanitarium, a nearby vacation home for infants and children.

"It was a mistake to educate women for a profession, and at the same time pay the pupil a salary."[127]

Illinois Training School
Board Member, 1888

In 1893, Hampton published *Nursing: Its Principles and its Practice*, the first substantial work on trained nursing care. Hampton had hoped to fill the void of textbooks in the field of nursing, as Clara Weeks's *Textbook of Nursing for the Use of Training Schools, Families, and Private Students* (1885) had predominated in training schools, despite being intended for use by both nurses and the general public.[129] Hampton's text, written in the afternoons during her first years at Hopkins, detailed in its 480 pages all of the knowledge she believed a pupil nurse should learn over the course of her nursing education. In a review, a physician colleague remarked that the book should also be of use to doctors, as it specified "what a trained nurse of the present day may be expected to know and be able to do."[130] Hampton's text replaced the Weeks book and was widely used in schools for the next 20 years.

Isabel Hampton believed the educational needs of nursing students should always outweigh the economic needs of the hospitals they served, but recognized that individually, nurses held little power. Additionally, the strength and image of the profession relied on the quality of available nurse training; as graduate nurses made their way into the homes of the general public, their performance and abilities reflected upon nursing as a whole. Hampton's experiences as a superintendent would reinforce the need to standardize education throughout the training schools and prompt her to push for the establishment of national nursing organizations, a movement she spearheaded in 1893. The health of families and communities, however, could not wait on the establishment of these national societies. Local nurses with many different affiliations took it upon themselves to come together and minister to the needs of the sick through visiting nurse work.

For Discussion

1. What were some of the reasons behind the push to establish formal training programs for nurses?
2. Describe the social image of nursing in the early 19th century. How did this affect the quality of nursing care available at the time?
3. What were some of the standards required for training schools using the Nightingale model? Why was 1873 a watershed year for nursing education in the United States?
4. Describe the daily life of pupil nurses in the first nurse training schools. How and why did uniforms become an important symbol for improving the image of nursing?
5. How did the racial and social context of the time restrict access to nurse training programs for Black and male applicants in the late 1800s?
6. How did the scientific revolution affect the provision of medical and nursing care?

NOTES

1. "Report of the Committee on the Training of Nurses," *Transactions of the American Medical Association* 20 (1869): 162–163.

2. Ibid.

3. Susan Reverby, *Ordered to Care: The Dilemma of American Nursing, 1850-1945* (Cambridge: Cambridge University Press, 1987): 22.

4. J. M. Toner, "Statistics of Regular Medical Societies and Hospitals of the United States," *Transactions of the American Medical Association* 24 (1873): 314–333. The survey identified a total of 178 hospitals, but this number included 58 insane asylums, as discussed in Morris J. Vogel, *The Invention of the Modern Hospital: Boston, 1870-1930* (Chicago: University of Chicago Press, 1979): 137.

5. M. Adelaide Nutting and Lavinia L. Dock, *A History of Nursing: The Evolution of Nursing Systems From the Earliest Times to the Foundation of the First English and American Training Schools for Nurses*, vol. II (New York: G. P. Putnam's Sons, 1907): 380–381.

6. Elizabeth Hobson, *Recollections of a Happy Life* (New York: G. P. Putnam & Sons, 1916): 83–84.

7. Patricia D'Antonio, *American Nursing: A History of Knowledge, Authority, and the Meaning of Work* (Baltimore, MD: Johns Hopkins University Press, 2010): 13.

8. Patricia D'Antonio, "The Legacy of Domesticity: Nursing in Early Nineteenth Century America," in *Nurses' Work: Issues across Time and Place*, eds. Patricia D'Antonio, Ellen D. Baer, Sylvia D. Rinker, and Joan E. Lynaugh (New York: Springer Publishing, 2007): 43.

9. Reverby, *Ordered to Care*, 27.

10. Charles Dickens, *Martin Chuzzlewit* (London: J. M. Dent and Sons, 1907): xvi.

11. For a brief discussion of how popular literature about valiant war nurses helped change the social image of nursing, see Patricia O'Brien, "'All a Woman's Life Can Bring': The Domestic Roots of Nursing in Philadelphia, 1830-1885," *Nursing Research* 36 (1987): 12–17. See also:

Henry Wadsworth Longfellow, "Santa Filomena," in *Poems of Places: An Anthology in 31 Volumes,* ed. Henry Wadsworth Longfellow (Boston: James R. Osgood, 1876–1879); Louisa May Alcott, *Hospital Sketches* (Boston: J. Redpath, 1863); L. P. Brockett, *Woman's Work in the Civil War* (Philadelphia: Zieglar and McCurdy, 1867).

12. Sarah Hale, "Lady Nurses," *Godey's Lady's Book* 92 (March 1871): 188–189.

13. "Training-schools for Nurses," *Fraser's Magazine* 10 (December 1874): 706.

14. Nutting and Dock, *A History of Nursing,* 339.

15. As quoted in ibid., 341.

16. O'Brien, "All a Woman's Life Can Bring," 14.

17. Ibid.

18. D'Antonio, *American Nursing,* 2.

19. As quoted in Nutting and Dock, *A History of Nursing,* 348.

20. Ibid., 350.

21. Linda Richards, "At the New England Hospital," *American Journal of Nursing* 2 (1901): 88–89.

22. As quoted in Nutting and Dock, *A History of Nursing,* 351–352.

23. Ibid., 127.

24. Ethel Johns and Blanche Pfefferkorn, *The Johns Hopkins Hospital School of Nursing, 1889-1949* (Baltimore, MD: Johns Hopkins University Press, 1954): 13.

25. Nutting and Dock, *A History of Nursing,* 339.

26. Florence Nightingale, letter to W. Gill Wylie, as quoted in Nutting and Dock, *A History of Nursing,* 389.

27. As quoted in Lavinia L. Dock, "History of the Reform in Nursing at Bellevue Hospital," *American Journal of Nursing* 2 (1901): 95.

28. Elizabeth Hobson, *Recollections of a Happy Life* (New York: G.P. Putnam & Sons, 1916): 88.

29. W. G. Thompson, *Training-Schools for Nurses with Notes on Twenty-Two Schools* (New York: G. P. Putnam's Sons, 1883): 28–29.

30. Third Annual Report of the Managers of the Training School, 1876, as quoted in Dock, "History of the Reform in Nursing at Bellevue Hospital," 96.

31. Johns and Pfefferkorn, *The Johns Hopkins Hospital School of Nursing,* 41.

32. Margaret K. Stack, "Resume of the History of the Connecticut Training School for Nurses," *American Journal of Nursing* 23 (1923): 825.

33. Francis Bacon, "Founding of the Connecticut Training School for Nurses," *Trained Nurse* 15 (1895): 191.

34. Bacon, "Founding of the Connecticut Training School for Nurses," 192.

35. Ibid.

36. Ibid.

37. Stack, "Resume of the History of the Connecticut Training School for Nurses," 828.

38. Ibid.

39. Sara E. Parsons, *History of the Massachusetts General Hospital Training School for Nurses* (Boston: Whitcomb & Barrows, 1920): 21.

40. Mrs. Curtis and Miss Denny, "Early History of the Boston Training School," *American Journal of Nursing* 11 (1902): 333.

41. Parsons, *History of the Massachusetts General Hospital,* 22.

42. Ibid., 33.

43. Linda Richards, *Reminiscences of America's First Trained Nurse* (New York: M. Barrows, 1911): 27.

44. Nutting and Dock, *A History of Nursing,* 420.

45. Parsons, *History of the Massachusetts General Hospital,* 37.

46. Joel D. Howell, *Technology in the Hospital: Transforming Patient Care in the Early Twentieth Century* (Baltimore, MD: Johns Hopkins University Press, 1995): 52, 273.

47. As quoted in Parsons, *History of the Massachusetts General Hospital,* 41.

48. Curtis and Denny, "Early History of the Boston Training School," 335.

49. Parsons, *History of the Massachusetts General Hospital,* 39.

50. Elizabeth Hobson, Final Report Visiting Committee on Hospitals, as quoted in Nutting and Dock, *A History of Nursing,* 386.

51. "The 8th Annual Report of the Illinois Training School for Nurses, 1888-1889," 24, courtesy the Alan Mason Chesney Medical Archives of the Johns Hopkins Medical Institutions.

52. Thompson, *Training-Schools for Nurses,* 15.

53. Ibid.

54. "The 8th Annual Report, 1888-1889," 24.

55. Isabel Hampton, "Aims of the Johns Hopkins Training School for Nurses," *The Johns Hopkins Hospital Bulletin* 1 (1889): 6; Cynthia A. Connolly, "Hampton, Nutting, and Rival Gospels at The Johns Hopkins Hospital and Training School for Nurses, 1889-1906," *Image: Journal of Nursing Scholarship* 30 (1998): 24.

56. Mary M. Riddle, "Then and Now: A Contrast," *American Journal of Nursing* 28 (1922): 701.

57. Thompson, *Training-Schools for Nurses,* 20.

58. "The 8th Annual Report, 1888-1889," 25.

59. Riddle, "Then and Now," 702.

60. Janet Wilson James, "Isabel Hampton and the Professionalization of Nursing in the 1890s," in The Therapeutic Revolution: Essays in the Social History of American Medicine, eds. Morris J. Vogel and Charles E. Rosenberg (Philadelphia: University of Pennsylvania Press, 1979): 206.

61. Richards, *Reminiscences of America's First Trained Nurse,* 14.

62. Isabel Hampton, "Educational Standards for Nurses," in *Hospitals, Dispensaries, and Nursing,* ed. John S. Billings and Henry M. Hurd (New York: Garland Publishing, 1984): 31–33; Reverby, *Ordered to Care,*: 49–54; D'Antonio, *American Nursing,* ch. 2.

63. "Ward Notes, August 4, 1888 to November 19, 1888," Bates Center.

64. Reverby, *Ordered to Care,* 54.

65. Ibid., 50–51.

66. Florence Nightingale, letter to W. Gill Wylie, as quoted in Nutting and Dock, *A History of Nursing,* 389.

67. Lavinia Dock, "The Relation of Training Schools to Hospitals," in *Nursing of the Sick 1893* (New York: McGraw-Hill, 1949): 16.

68. Thompson, *Training-Schools for Nurses,* 16.

69. Riddle, "Then and Now," 703.

70. Irene Schuessler Poplin, "Nursing Uniforms: Romantic Idea, Functional Attire, or Instrument of Social Change?" *Nursing History Review* 2 (1994): 153–167.

71. Lynn Houweling, "Image, Function, and Style," *American Journal of Nursing* 104 (2004): 43.

72. Christina Bates, *A Cultural History of the Nurse's Uniform* (Gatineau: Canadian Museum of Civilization Cor., 2012): 22.

73. As quoted in Nutting and Dock, *A History of Nursing,* 400.

74. Nutting and Dock, *A History of Nursing,* 401.

75. Clara Sanford Lockwood, "Unprofessional Display of Uniform," *American Journal of Nursing* 2 (1901): 203.

76. Bates, *A Cultural History of the Nurse's Uniform,* 25.

77. Houweling, "Image, Function, and Style," 44.

78. Ibid., 45–46.

79. Mary W. Rode, "The Nursing Pin: Symbol of 1,000 Years of Service," *Nursing Forum* 24 (1989): 16.

80. U.S. Department of Commerce, *Historical Statistics of the United States: Colonial Times to 1970: Part 1* (Washington, DC: Government Printing Office, 1975): 76.

81. As quoted in Althea T. Davis, *Early Black American Leaders in Nursing: Architects for Integration and Equality* (Boston: Jones and Bartlett Publishers, 1999): 35.

82. *1874 Annual Report of the New England Hospital for Women and Children* (Boston: W. L. Deland Press, 1875).

83. Davis, *Early Black American Leaders in Nursing*, 33.

84. Mary Elizabeth Carnegie, *The Path We Tread: Blacks in Nursing, 1854-1984* (Philadelphia: J. B. Lippincott, 1986): 17.

85. Davis, *Early Black American Leaders in Nursing*, 41–42.

86. Mary Ella Chayer, "Mary Eliza Mahoney," *American Journal of Nursing* 54 (1954): 430.

87. Darlene Clark Hine, *Black Women in White: Racial Conflict and Cooperation in the Nursing Profession, 1890-1950* (Bloomington: Indiana University Press, 1989): 6.

88. Carnegie, *The Path We Tread*, 19.

89. Mary Elizabeth Pauline Lyons letter to Maritcha (May) Lyons, November 10, 1885, as quoted in Davis, *Early Black American Leaders in Nursing*, 192.

90. Anna DeCosta Banks, "Nurse Training in Charleston," *Southern Workman* 28 (1899): 224.

91. "History in Brief," *Spelman College*, http://www.spelman.edu/about-us/history-in-brief (accessed July 30, 2016).

92. Hine, *Black Women in White*, 9.

93. Florence Matilda Read, *The Story of Spelman College* (Princeton: Princeton University Press, 1961): 153, 214.

94. Carnegie, *The Path We Tread*, 21.

95. Alice M. Bacon, "The Dixie's Work-Is It Worth Continuing?" *Southern Workman* 23 (1893): 26.

96. Alice M. Bacon, "Report on Dixie Hospital and Training School for Nurses," *Southern Workman* 22 (1892): 108.

97. Ibid.

98. Harriet M. Lewis, "Medical Report of the Dixie Hospital," *Southern Workman* 22 (1892): 109.

99. Bacon, "The Dixie's Work-Is It Worth Continuing?," 27.

100. "The Dixie Hospital," *Southern Workman* 30 (1901): 524.

101. Chad E. O'Lynn, "History of Men in Nursing: A Review," in *Men in Nursing: History, Challenges, and Opportunities*, eds. Chad E. O'Lynn and Russell E. Tranbarger (New York: Springer Publishing, 2007): 24.

102. O'Lynn, "History of Men in Nursing," 23–24.

103. Russell E. Tranbarger, "American Schools of Nursing for Men," in *Men in Nursing: History, Challenges, and Opportunities*, eds. Chad E. O'Lynn and Russell E. Tranbarger (New York: Springer Publishing, 2007): 45.

104. *Bellevue: A Short History of Bellevue Hospital and of the Training Schools* (New York City: Alumni Association of Bellevue, 1915): 48.

105. Tranbarger, "American Schools of Nursing for Men," 45.

106. Lois N. Magner, *A History of Medicine* (New York: Informa Healthcare, 2007): 313.

107. "American versus European Medical Science," *Medical Record* 4 (1869): 133.

108. Philip A. Kalisch and Beatrice J. Kalisch, *American Nursing: A History* (Philadelphia: Lippincott Williams & Wilkins, 2004): 80–82.

109. Paul Starr, *The Social Transformation of American Medicine: The Rise of a Sovereign Profession and the Making of a Vast Industry* (New York: Basic Books, 1982): 123–130.

110. Ibid., 5.

111. Margarete Sandelowski, "Making the Best of Things: Technology in American Nursing, 1870-1940," *Nursing History Review* 9 (1997): 6.

112. Ibid., 15.

113. Jean Pougiales, "The First Anesthetizers at the Mayo Clinic," *Journal of the American Association of Nurse Anesthetists* 38, 3 (June 1970): 235–241 (quote 236).

114. Ibid., 236.

115. Judith Hartzell, *Mrs. Charlie, The Other Mayo: A Biography* (Gobles, MI: Arvi Books, 2000): 17.

116. Arlene Keeling, *The Nurses of Mayo Clinic: Caring Healers* (Rochester, NY: Walsworth Print Group, 2014): 18.

117. Arlene Keeling, "Prescribing Medicine without a License?": Nurse Anesthetists, 1900-1938," chap. 2 in *Nursing and the Privilege of Prescription* (Columbus: The Ohio State University Press, 2007).

118. Pougiales, "The First Anesthetizers," 236.

119. http://www.aana.com/resources2/archives-library/Pages/Alice-Magaw.aspx (accessed January 16, 2005): para 1. Magaw was so skilled in her technique that Charles Mayo would later name her "the mother of anesthesia" for her mastery of open-drop ether administration.

120. Alice Magaw, "A Review of over 14,000 Surgical Anesthesias," *Surgery, Gynecology, and Obstetrics* (December 1906): 795–799 (quote 795).

121. Arlene Keeling, *The Nurses of Mayo Clinic,* 19.

122. Alice Magaw, "Observations of 1092 Cases of Anesthesia from January 1, 1899–January 1, 1900," *St. Paul Medical Journal* 2 (May 1900): 306–311 (quote 307).

123. Bertha Mayne, "The Small Hospital and the Training-School," *American Journal of Nursing* 1 (1901): 260.

124. Isabel Hampton Robb, "My Association with the Illinois Training School," *Quarterly of the Illinois State Association of Graduate Nurses* (1908): 1–2; Grace Fay Schryver, *A History of the Illinois Training School for Nurses: 1880-1929* (Chicago: Board of Directors of the Illinois Training School for Nurses, 1930): 49.

125. Schryver, *A History of the Illinois Training School for Nurses,* 49.

126. Isabel A. Hampton, "Educational Standards for Nurses," in *Nursing of the Sick 1893* (New York: McGraw-Hill, 1949): 10.

127. Schryver, *A History of the Illinois Training School for Nurses,* 49.

128. Notebooks of Miss Emma O. Cleaver, Isabel Hampton Robb Archive, courtesy The Alan Mason Chesney Medical Archives of the Johns Hopkins Medical Institutions.

129. Clara S. Weeks-Shaw, *A Textbook of Nursing for the Use of Training Schools, Families, and Private Students* (New York: D. Appleton and Company, 1885).

130. "Notes on New Books," *Johns Hopkins Hospital Bulletin* 5 (April 1894): 55.

FURTHER READING

Carnegie, Mary Elizabeth, *The Path We Tread: Blacks in Nursing 1854-1984* (Philadelphia: J. B. Lippincott, 1986).

D'Antonio, Patricia, *American Nursing: A History of Knowledge, Authority, and the Meaning of Work* (Baltimore, MD: Johns Hopkins University Press, 2010).

Hine, Darlene Clark, *Black Women in White: Racial Conflict and Cooperation in the Nursing Profession, 1890-1950* (Indianapolis: Indiana University Press, 1989).

Nutting, M. Adelaide, and Lavinia L. Dock, *A History of Nursing: The Evolution of Nursing Systems From the Earliest Times to the Foundation of the First English and American Training Schools for Nurses,* vol. *II* (New York: G.P. Putnam & Sons, 1907).

Reverby, Susan M., *Ordered to Care: The Dilemma of American Nursing, 1850-1945* (Cambridge: Cambridge University Press, 1987).

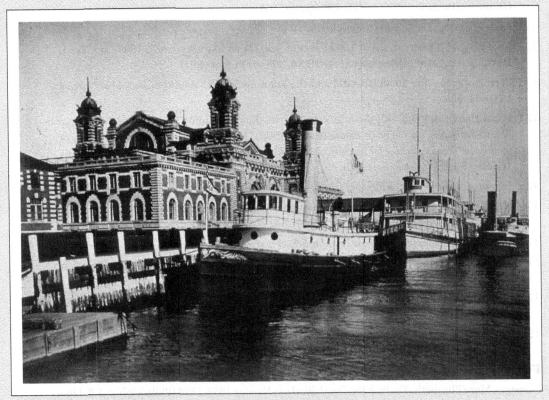

Ellis Island.

CHAPTER 4

Visiting Nurses in Cities, Parishes, and Missions
1886–1914

Arlene W. Keeling

"District or visiting nurse work covers that branch of nursing which cares for the sick poor in their own homes. . . . From the first years of its existence, when Fliedner at Kaiserswerth sent trained women into the homes of the poor, and William Rathbone saw the need of it in England, the character of this work has not changed; it still carries out the . . . principles of giving skilled nursing to the poor and the small wage earner . . . and teaching them to care for their own sick."[1]

Writing in the *American Journal of Nursing* in 1902, Harriet Fulmer, superintendent of the Visiting Nurse Association of Chicago, briefly described the history of visiting nurses in the United States. Fulmer not only recognized the German and English roots in the work of Theodor Fliedner and William Rathbone, but also described how American nurses made the idea their own as they set up district visiting nurse associations in cities and towns throughout the United States in the late 19th century. At that time, the nurses' work coincided with the work of elite and upper-middle-class women engaged in "municipal housekeeping"—the idea that women's influence could be extended from the home to the community. Those reform efforts, including an emphasis on sanitation, food safety, and the control of infectious disease, were designed to protect the health of the public. Woven throughout the reforms were the basic tenets of Progressivism.

Fulmer noted that in 1880 Albany was the first city to establish a visiting nurse association, followed in rapid succession by Boston and Philadelphia in 1886 and Chicago in 1889. She then explained that the visiting nurse services in the United States were originally formed to address the health care needs of the thousands of poor European immigrants who had settled in industrial cities of the northeast. These organizations, however, were not the only ones that responded to citizens' needs in the 19th century. Religious organizations, private insurance companies, ladies' aid societies, and other social clubs all took part in initiatives to treat those who were sick and teach preventive measures to ensure the health of the public.

NURSING THE IMMIGRANTS

Nurses had been providing care to immigrants from the time the newcomers first set foot on U.S. soil. Seeking religious freedom and economic opportunity, immigrants had been entering America for decades. Now, in the latter part of the 19th century, their numbers dramatically increased. Between 1880 and 1924, 25 million Europeans and a smaller percentage of Russians and Asians came to the United States. About half—particularly those holding second- and third-class tickets for the transatlantic crossing—entered the country through Ellis Island in New York Harbor, actually a series of small islands between New York and New Jersey. After being transferred by ferry from the Hudson River piers where their ships had docked, the immigrants arrived on Ellis Island. Having debarked the ferry, they crossed the docks and proceeded to the Great Hall, the central gathering place for immigrants approaching customs. At this location, the U.S. Marine Hospital physicians screened them for infectious diseases, mental illness, or disability. Health inspectors accepted those considered healthy enough to work, and detained or turned away those with serious defects or infection.[2]

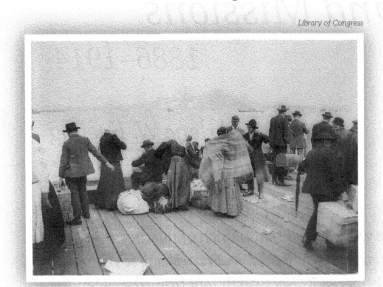

Library of Congress

Immigrants await transfer to Ellis Island for inspection after arriving in New York City.

Nurses, aides, and others worked with the health inspectors on Ellis Island, primarily after government hospitals opened on the islands. For the most part the nurses worked under the direction of the U.S. Public Health Service. Some nurses worked in Island No. 2's General Hospital, which opened in 1902 with 120 beds; they provided pediatric and maternity care, or circulated in the operating rooms, assisting with surgeries.

In 1911 a sprawling 18-ward, 450-bed contagious disease hospital opened on Island No. 3. Nurses also worked there, managing patients with measles, mumps, favus (a fungal disease of the scalp), tuberculosis, diphtheria, polio, trachoma, and other infectious diseases. By 1913 more than 25 nurses, both male and female, were employed in 22 buildings on the small islands.

Caring for newly arrived immigrants on Ellis Island was only the beginning of the public health work that nurses did on their behalf; visiting nurses also worked in urban tenement districts to help the newcomers with myriad health issues they faced. In the industrialized cities of the northeast, immigrants worked long hours in crowded factories with little lighting, clattering machines, and poor ventilation.

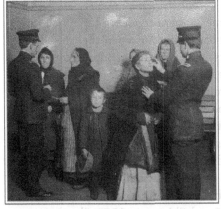

Library of Congress

Immigrant woman being checked for trachoma by a medical inspector.

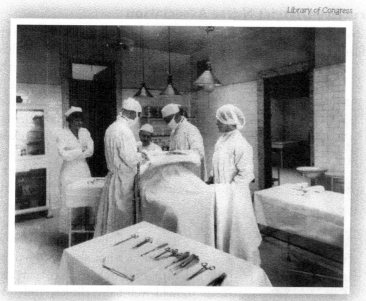

Ellis Island operating room.

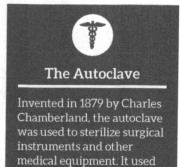

"Gleaming white iron beds lined the open wards; the mattresses sterilized by the newly invented autoclave."[3]

Lorie Conway, 2007

The Autoclave

Invented in 1879 by Charles Chamberland, the autoclave was used to sterilize surgical instruments and other medical equipment. It used high-pressure saturated steam to kill microorganisms.

As a result, many suffered from accidental injuries, hearing and eye problems, and lung conditions. High rents in the overcrowded cities forced multiple families to live together in tiny tenement flats, often without heating or plumbing, and with windows that opened to airshafts full of garbage. Refrigeration was scarce and milk often spoiled. Outside, the streets were unpaved and strewn with trash, animal waste, and rotten fruits and vegetables—the perfect breeding ground for infectious disease.

Each of the major U.S. cities had its immigrant districts with frequent epidemics of tuberculosis, measles, mumps, typhoid fever, whooping cough, cholera, and polio. Without an organized federal or state system of medical and nursing care, women's groups, churches, and other social organizations volunteered their help to improve health and sanitary conditions in order to prevent disease from "creeping uptown."[5]

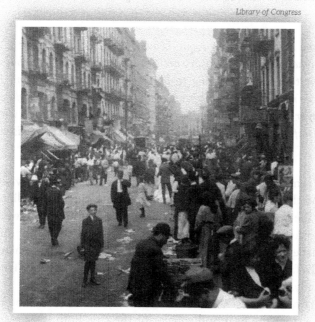

New York's Lower East Side, where immigrants lived in overcrowded tenements and worked long hours in poor conditions.

"The nurses, the ladies in white . . . were very nice. They talked to the children. They stroked their hair, and they touched their cheeks."[4]

Elizabeth Martin, Immigrant, 1920

Boston Instructive District Nurse Association

The Boston Instructive District Nurse Association originated in 1886 "to send out trained and skilled nurses" and to provide home nursing care to the city's sick poor.

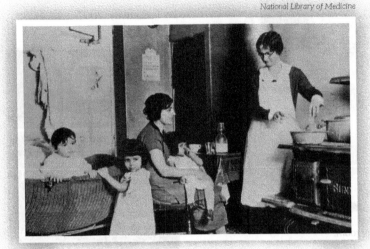

District nurse teaching mother about safe milk preparation.

Working from a small room in the Boston dispensary, nurses Calina Somerville and Elizabeth Rinker made more than 7,000 visits to 707 patients in the first year of the association's existence.[6] The next year, the association employed five nurses who were making more than 17,000 visits. By the end of 1889, the organization had six nurses on staff who made more than 26,000 visits a year.[7] The nurses not only cared for the sick but also provided mothers with prenatal and postpartum care, held well-baby clinics, and inspected children in nurseries and kindergartens. They also managed milk stations where they dispensed fresh milk and taught mothers who could not breastfeed how to wash baby bottles and prepare formula.

An important part of the nurses' work was the care of patients with infections and teaching the patient and family what to do when the nurse was not there. As the association's guidelines noted: "To one responsible member of the family, give thorough and careful instructions as to what shall be done between the visits of the nurses. These should include the following: Bath to reduce temperature . . . ventilation of room . . . nourishment given regularly . . . medicine exactly as ordered by doctor."[8] Before they could instruct others, however, the nurses had to follow strict rules themselves when they visited the home of a patient who had an infectious disease. The instructions for visiting a "contagious case" were particularly complicated and time consuming:

> *Remove hat and coat in an outer room. Leave bag with hat and coat . . . scrub hands. Thermometer and all necessary articles should be taken from bag at this time so as not to necessitate going to bag after entering sick room. Put on apron. . . . After necessary care has been given take off apron, fold right side in, roll in newspaper and leave in patient's room. Scrub hands thoroughly with soap and water. Disinfect thermometer. . . . Visit patient with infectious disease last in the day.*[9]

> *"The task of preventing an epidemic throughout the tenement or even the street is appalling."*[10]
>
> Boston District Nurse, Circa 1888

Promoting good nutrition was another aspect of the visiting nurses' role and the district nurses collaborated with the Boston diet kitchens to do so. The nurses were all too aware that for families who were very poor the choice was frequently "a question rather of food than of medicine." Any dispensary doctor could sign a "diet order" that a member of the invalid's family could have "filled free of cost," to ensure "fresh eggs and milk daily."[11] A third aspect of the nurses' role was to identify sick infants who needed pure milk and an escape from the heat and squalor of the city. Both were essential in the treatment of "summer complaint"—infantile diarrhea caused by contaminated milk.

In the late 19th century, before refrigeration and pasteurization of milk, an increase in the incidence of dehydration as a complication of summer diarrhea spiked infant mortality rates during the months of June, July, and August.[12] Caused by contaminated, sour milk to which milkmen added water and chalk, the illness was widespread. It was especially common among infants of poor women who were unable to breastfeed for a variety of reasons, including the need to work outside the home. The result—hundreds of children died.

In Boston in the 1890s, the nurse could refer mothers of infants with summer diarrhea to a physician who would give them a ticket to board the *Clifford*, a steamship that set sail daily

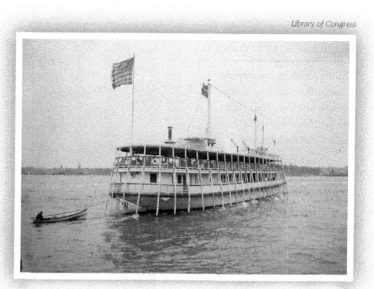

New York Floating Hospital in 1903, where inner-city children could access fresh air and a healthy meal.

from the docks on Boston Harbor. The ship would leave shore and anchor in the harbor for the day, returning in early evening. Its purpose was to provide sick infants with expert nursing and medical care in an open-air setting.

The Boston Floating Hospital, as the *Clifford* was soon named, had its origins on a particularly hot summer evening in 1893, when the Reverend Rufus Tobey noticed mothers "wearily carrying their infants back and forth across the South Boston Bridge, seeking relief from the heat of their downtown tenements." After talking with friends and philanthropic groups, Tobey decided to begin excursions on the harbor for indigent mothers and their sick infants.[13]

Tobey's plan was based on the successes of a floating hospital in New York City.[14] There the *Emma Abbot* sailed 3 days a week between July and September on the Hudson River, allowing inner city children and their mothers to "avail themselves of healthy sea breezes" and receive necessary medicines, fresh milk from clean bottles, and nutritious foods. Aboard ship children also received salt-water baths.[15]

Replicated in Boston in 1894, the excursions on the *Clifford* allowed mothers and their infants to escape the heat and disease of the tenement district, and benefit not only from the cool breezes of Boston Harbor but also from nutritious meals, health teaching, and skilled nursing and medical care on board the steamer.

On the Boston Floating Hospital, trained nurses worked with medical students from Harvard (and later from Tufts) to care for the infants, taking temperatures and bathing those with fevers, feeding them with donated breast milk or a variety of freshly prepared formulas, changing their diapers, and allowing them to spend time in the sunshine and fresh sea air on the open decks. Below deck, Dr. Alfred Bosworth of Tufts University led a group of physicians who experimented with "20 different kinds of food or combinations of food" to prepare infant formula, calibrating each formula to the needs of each infant.[17]

By 1900 nurses worked on the Boston Floating Hospital for a year at a time, receiving a certificate of completion from the medical staff for their

"By the end of the first season in 1894, eleven hundred children had been given the benefit of a day's medical treatment and outing on the waters of Boston Harbor."[16]

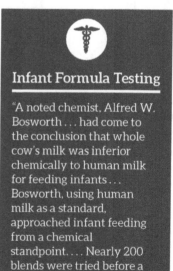

Infant Formula Testing

"A noted chemist, Alfred W. Bosworth . . . had come to the conclusion that whole cow's milk was inferior chemically to human milk for feeding infants . . . Bosworth, using human milk as a standard, approached infant feeding from a chemical standpoint. . . . Nearly 200 blends were tried before a final formula was considered successful."[18] (Later, this would be known as Similac.)

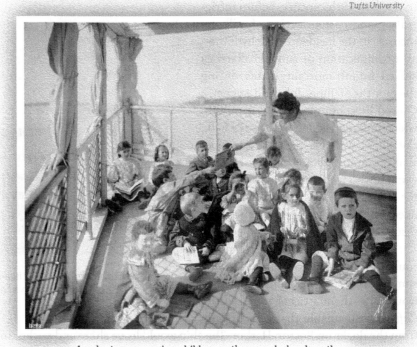

A volunteer supervises children on the open deck, where they receive sunshine and fresh air.

Formula Preparation

"Many formulas are prepared under the supervision of a graduate nurse. The infants are furnished with a different bottle at each feeding." [20]

Sarah Palmer, 1903

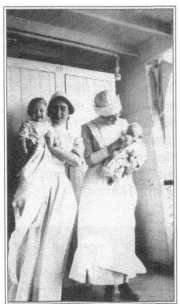

Nurses care for inner-city infants above deck.

Washing Baby Bottles

"To cleanse bottles: rinse in cold water, wash in hot soap suds, scald and then cool, fill with water into which you have put a pinch of soda." [22]

Nurse, Boston Floating Hospital

services. While on board, nurses taught the mothers principles of infant feeding, first and foremost advocating breastfeeding. If a mother could not nurse her infant herself, a nurse would provide her with bottles of donated breast milk, or bottles of formula to which breast milk, known for its antibacterial properties, had been added.[19]

In addition to providing the infants with feedings on the ship, the nurses taught mothers how to prepare formula, how to wash bottles, and how to store milk on ice between feedings when they were back in their own houses. The experiment worked: under expert medical and nursing care on a ship where there was fresh, cool air, babies began to thrive.[21]

Philadelphia Visiting Nurse Society

In 1886, the same year that the Boston Instructive District Nurse Association was founded, a group of women met to set up a similar organization in Philadelphia. Mrs. William Jenks led the women who named their association the "District Nursing Society"; a year later, however, they changed the name to "the Visiting Nurse Society of Philadelphia."

Working under a committee of elite "lady managers" and head nurse Miss Haydock, the Philadelphia District nurses made more than 380 visits during the first year. They assisted not only European immigrants, but also the many African Americans who had migrated to the city after the Civil War.[23] For the most part, the visiting nurses attended maternal and child cases. The nurses checked on expectant mothers, assisted physicians with home births, and followed mothers and babies in the first few weeks postpartum.[24]

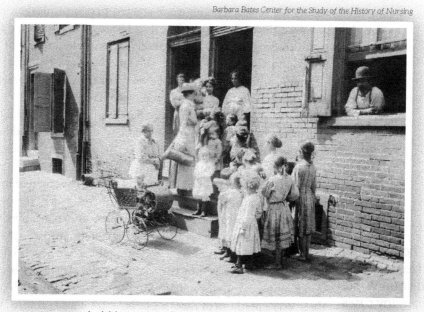

*A visiting nurse makes a home visit to a pregnant woman
and her children.*

Like their colleagues in Boston, the Philadelphia visiting nurses also made "sick" calls, caring for patients with illnesses like typhoid fever, diphtheria, and tuberculosis, all prevalent contagious diseases in the late 19th and early 20th centuries. Applying principles of contagion nursing, the nurses isolated these patients and taught patients and family members how to prevent the disease from spreading.

Health promotion and disease prevention soon became the focus of the visiting nurses' work. In 1903 the society cooperated with the city's Bureau of Public Charities to reduce the incidence of ringworm, pink eye, and nutritional disorders among school-children. From 1905 to 1908 the society stationed a nurse at the Starr Centre Association of Philadelphia, on the corner of 7th and Lombard, to help with maternity and childcare clinics, conduct vaccination drives, provide nutritionally sound "penny lunches," and distribute clean milk to Philadelphia's mothers.[25]

The nurses' work was important—particularly for the poor, and soon the visiting nurses referred infants for additional help, collaborating with physicians from the health department to do so. Identifying the problem was the first step and an investigation in Philadelphia showed the hospitals "to be sadly inadequate in their facilities for caring for the sick infants of the poor." As a result, the Department of Public Health and Charities of Philadelphia, under its director Dr. Joseph S. Neff, established "two refuges for babies on the recreation piers, situated on the riverfront." Visiting nurses and attending physicians sent sick infants to these "refuges" where "four trained nurses, two to each pier," would care for them around the clock. According to the final report, the "open air hospitals" proved to be "one of the most successful undertakings of the campaign."[26]

Chicago Visiting Nurse Association

Only 3 years after the visiting nurse groups in Boston and Philadelphia were started, the Chicago Visiting Nurse Association incorporated in 1889. It focused its attention on disease prevention and health promotion in the immigrant neighborhoods of the rapidly expanding Midwest city. The work started first on Chicago's north and south sides, then spread to the west and northwest, achieving the association's goal "to furnish visiting nurses to those unable to secure skilled attendants in time of illness, [and] to teach cleanliness and the proper care of the sick."[27] From the first, the association emphasized "the educational and preventive work" of the visiting nurses, particularly in cases of tuberculosis and among children and newborns.[28]

The Chicago Visiting Nurse Association had headquarters at Hull House where the nurses worked in concert with Progressive Era reformer Jane Addams, a founding member of the association and director of the settlement house. Located at 800 South Halsted in the middle of the immigrant slum districts, Hull House was established to ameliorate the effects of poverty in a city dealing with an overwhelming influx of European immigrants.[29] It was the perfect place for the nurses' work. The neighborhood surrounding Hull House was, according to Jane Addams, "inexpressibly dirty, the number of schools inadequate, sanitary legislation unenforced, the street lighting bad, the paving miserable, . . . and the stables foul beyond description." Hundreds of houses were not connected to the street sewer . . . many had no water supply except for a "faucet in the back yard." In such conditions, where there was a plethora of diseases to both treat and prevent, the nurses found an endless need for health education.[30]

Working from central headquarters, where they could receive telephone messages and applications for "relief and attendance on the sick," the Chicago visiting nurses started out "at 9 a.m. and at 1 p.m. each day," providing

> *"No food, no fuel, little bedding and less clothing seems to be their universal condition. . . . In many cases the sufferers might die for want of care were it not for these nurses."*[31]
>
> Woman's World, 1897

On District Nursing

"It is a hand to hand struggle against disease, poverty, and dirt, against the most pitiful ignorance and inherited prejudice. The nurse . . . goes from house to house, from one patient to another, mounting flight after flight of stairs, for it is curious but true fact that tenement house patients always live on the top floor of a very tall house."[33]

Miss Brent, paper read before the Congress of Charities, 1894.

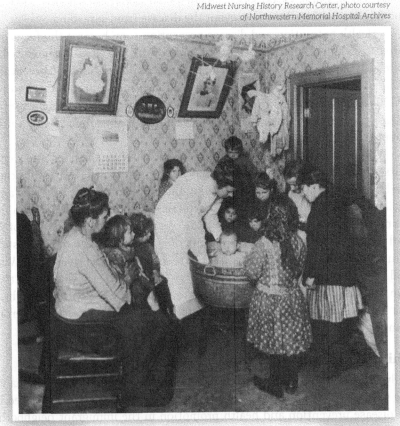

A visiting nurse demonstrates a baby bath in a home.

maternity and well-baby care, management of chronic illness, surgical dressing changes, and patient and family education. As was the case for other visiting nurses, much of the Chicago nurses' work involved mothers and babies. One newspaper article described the poverty and filth one nurse found when she arrived to care for a newborn: "Not a stitch of clothing was to be found on either mother or child, and the only bedding a mattress and an old quilt. The little one was rolled in a dirty rag, and, although only a few hours old, was already badly bitten by vermin."[32]

In the city of Chicago, visiting nurses worked hard to deliver quality care and communicate standards of preventive health and hygiene to immigrant families. Moving toward the American idea of health meant different things to different ethnic and economic groups, and the visiting nurses struggled to accommodate individual beliefs while introducing new concepts of wellness. The process was a constant negotiation, often hindered by language barriers, misconceptions, and economic constraints. Immigrant families living in the city came from all over the world, and nurses struggled to communicate. Nurses also struggled to help those with limited resources. As one nurse recalled, "Economy is one of the first lessons to be learned . . . the makeshifts a visiting nurse must use are sometimes laughable if not actually pitiful."[34] Infant beds, for example, were often too expensive to purchase but could be fashioned out of items like drawers or boxes found in the home.

Cultural beliefs about the nature of illness also proved challenging to the nurses' work, as many immigrants believed disease occurred through divine providence. Nurses worked to convince their patients that cleanliness and hygiene influenced the incidence and spread of disease. They also attempted, unsuccessfully at times, to promote ideas about quarantine when the patient had a communicable disease. The nurses' manual, instructing staff to value cultural differences when they could, was clear: "Respect racial and local traditions wherever you can. When these must be disregarded, let the family see that this is for the patient's welfare, not for their or your convenience."[36] In most case, both the nurse and the patient needed to compromise; it sometimes took months to develop a trusting relationship.

Baltimore Lutheran Deaconesses

In the latter part of the 19th century, nurses interested in caring for the community were not restricted to working with secular groups or in association with settlement houses. Working for religious organizations was another option. Catholic Sisters had long been involved in nursing activities. Since the beginning of parish nursing in 1849 by the Lutheran Deaconesses in Pittsburgh, nurses affiliated with the Protestant denominations also had opportunities. In 1884 a motherhouse for the Lutheran deaconesses was established in Philadelphia. Six additional Lutheran motherhouses soon followed in Brooklyn, New York (1885); Omaha, Nebraska (1887); Minneapolis, Minnesota (1889); Milwaukee, Wisconsin (1893); Baltimore, Maryland (1895); and Chicago, Illinois (1897). Each provided headquarters for different groups of Lutheran deaconess nurses.[39]

Working from the Baltimore motherhouse, six deaconesses provided nursing care to the citizens in that port city, a center for textile, iron, and steel manufacturing, and home to hundreds of newly arrived German immigrants.[40] As trained nurses, the Lutheran deaconesses offered a combination of physical and spiritual care. One of them was Jennie

"Prevention is the cheaper method of accomplishing our work. . . . It is false reasoning to send a nurse . . . to children who are ill from lack of clothing and nourishing food."[35]

Harriet Fulmer, 1909

"Let your visits be those of women to women; instead of reproving and fault finding, encourage, in Heaven's name, encourage."[37]

Edna L. Foley, 1926

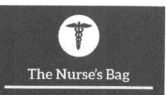

The Nurse's Bag

Visiting nurses carried leather bags full of supplies with them. . . . Larger than a traditional physician's bag, these heavy leather totes were . . . able to withstand the elements of a harsh Chicago winter. . . . Contents included soap, towels, scissors, forceps, antiseptic, gauze, cotton rubber sheets, wadding, Vaseline, thermometers, and patient records.[38]

Chicago Visiting Nurse, *Annual Report*, 1893

Christ, a young farm girl from Indiana who traveled to Kaiserswerth, Germany, to study parish nursing and then returned to the United States to work in Baltimore.

Writing in her journal on Wednesday, March 28, 1894, Jennie Christ described her feelings about her trans-Atlantic crossing—quite an experience for a Midwest farm girl:

I awoke early and . . . after a little primping and a goodbye to Mrs. Wenner, we left for the docks. I think there never was a girl on earth who had a homesick feeling more than I, as the S.S. blew that loud, long, hollow sort of a whistle, which only S.S. can, but I tried to be brave as possible. Many people stood on the pier. . . . What a flutter of white! And shouts of goodbye! It is impossible for me to describe the sensation I felt as we drifted from my native land. My duties may perhaps be difficult but I go with pleasure for I believe I ought to be thankful for this opportunity. We have had delightful sailing all day . . . I have felt no hint of seasickness yet, but I am a little fearful of it. I shall want to be on deck for the sight is so grand. One sees only wind, sky and waves so grand, majestic and beautiful. Our dinner at 6 o'clock was reasonably good. I sang and played a while and then retired.[41]

In Kaiserswerth for 1 year, Jennie Christ learned how to be a nurse. She also learned what it meant to be a deaconess, serving the patient in body, mind, and spirit.

"Little did I think that I would ever be sent out as a parish deaconess . . . God grant that some good may come out of the work which I have done here."[45]

Jennie Christ, York, Pennsylvania, 1897

Returning to the United States, Christ was first assigned to a German hospital in Philadelphia and later to the motherhouse in Baltimore where she worked for the next months. In Baltimore, requests for care were documented in the *Motherhouse Daily Record* and referred to as "home cases." These included patients with cancer, typhoid, crippling rheumatism, tuberculosis, and dysentery, among others. Like visiting nurses in other cities, in addition to caring for the sick and teaching about disease prevention, the deaconesses often addressed domestic issues and provided for the basic necessities of life.[42]

Besides working in Baltimore, the Lutheran deaconess nurses were sent out on assignment to Cumberland, Maryland; Richmond, Indiana; and places in New York and Pennsylvania. Altogether, over a 7-year period from 1897 to 1903, the Baltimore deaconesses served "more than 100 parishes."[44]

Henry Street Settlement Visiting Nurses

In 1895, the same year that the Lutheran deaconesses established their motherhouse in Baltimore, Lillian Wald and her colleague, Mary Brewster, founded Henry Street Settlement and Henry Street Visiting Nurse Services in New York City. Supported by philanthropists Jacob Schiff, Elizabeth Reed, and others, Wald opened the settlement house on the Lower East Side, in the heart of the immigrant tenement district. Decades later, in her 1922 radio speech, Wald spoke of its origins:

Library of Congress

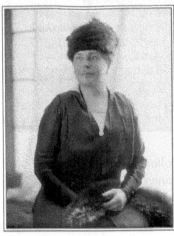

Lillian Wald in 1905, founder of the settlement on the Lower East Side, which provided immigrants with access to nursing care.

A sick woman in a squalid rear tenement, so wretched and so pitiful that, in all the years since, I have not seen anything more appalling, determined me within an hour to live on the East Side. . . . I induced my friend Mary Brewster to come with me, and we two together made up our minds not only that we would give our services as nurses but that we would live in the neighborhood in order to participate in its life and its problems.[46]

From its inception, Henry Street Settlement provided immigrants with connections to nursing care and social services.[47] Convinced that "the sickness they encountered in families was part of a larger set of social problems," the Henry Street nurses provided an impressive array of services, including safe places for children to play, ice, sterilized milk, medicine, meals, and "referrals for excursions to the countryside, or to one of the city's hospitals or dispensaries."[48]

"In one room I found a child with running ears which I syringed. . . . In another room, a child with summer complaint to whom I gave bismuth and tickets for a sea-side excursion."[49]

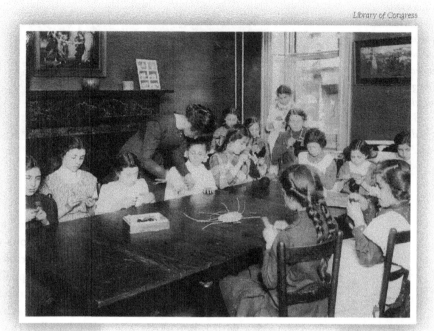

A volunteer teaches a knitting class at Henry Street Settlement to inner city children, 1904.

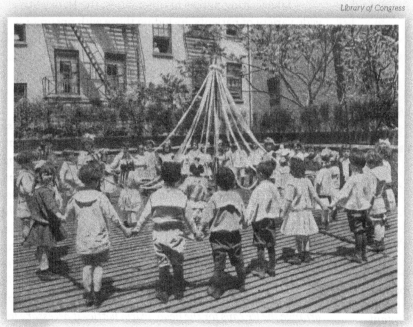

A group of children playing at a Henry Street Settlement playground.

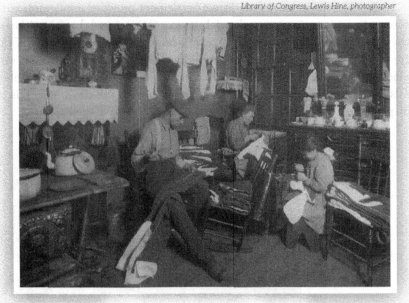

A child works in a Lower East Side tenement.

As was true in other industrialized cities, poverty, overcrowded and filthy living conditions, child labor, and tenement sweatshops created conditions that supported the spread of infection. The Henry Street Settlement nurses often served as case finders during epidemics, and what they found was appalling: Immigrant women who took home sewing work from the factories to supplement their incomes were themselves spreading disease.[50] Sometimes the women themselves were sick with tuberculosis when they handled the garments they were sewing; other times, infected children in the home contaminated the pieces.[51] Teaching the immigrants to isolate those who were ill became part of the nurses' job. Reporting child labor soon became another.

Like visiting nurses in other cities, the Henry Street nurses cared for a wide variety of patients, including those with pneumonia, typhoid fever, dysentery, thrush, colitis, scarlet fever, whooping cough, polio, influenza, diphtheria, measles, mumps, bronchitis, enteritis, tonsillitis, nephritis, burns, rheumatism, alcoholism, meningitis, tuberculosis, and cardiac problems. One nurse described her work during a home visit:

In amongst these pillows, covered by some and completely surrounded by others, is the patient, a child of two years. The temperature is 104.5 degrees, pulse 140, respirations 50. The fair curly hair is tangled and matted, the face and hands sticky with syrupy medicine, while the feet and legs are still soiled with the dirt of the street. . . . The nurse now begins her work. . . . First, the pillows and feather bed are removed; then the baby's over-abundant clothing is laid aside. . . . Next the cleansing soap and water bath is given, one of the cots in the front room put into correct position as to light and air . . . and the little one laid there clean and refreshed. . . . All this is preliminary to the more definite nursing work, which includes showing the mother how to give the alcohol sponge bath, swab the mouth, arrange the ice caps for the head, warm bottles if necessary for the feet, and give the medicines and nourishment. Simple bedside notes are left for the

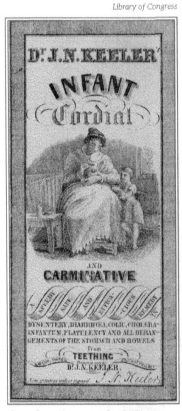

An advertisement for Infant Cordial, an over-the-counter remedy for multiple infant health problems.

doctor, showing the temperature, pulse and respiration, the general condition of the child, with a record of the work done by the nurse.[53]

The Henry Street nurses also visited pregnant women and followed both the mother and the baby after the delivery.[54] In short, visiting nurses were the "cornerstone of care for the sick poor at home," serving as "foot soldiers" in the modern campaign for public health.[55]

Much of the nurses' work centered on patient teaching, particularly about medicines, their dosage and administration, as well as which medicines to use and which to avoid. Before the Food and Drug Act of 1906, over-the-counter medications were not labeled for content of morphine, heroin, codeine, or opiates. Nor were these drugs restricted. In fact, mothers frequently used soothing cough syrups containing codeine for their sick infants. Some mothers gave their teething babies laudanum (containing opium) to calm them. Others gave it to their infants to keep them asleep while they worked. Overdoses were common.

By 1900 Henry Street Settlement employed 12 nurses "regularly engaged in systematic visiting nursing." That year the nurses made 26,600 calls.[57]

In a society regulated by Jim Crow Laws, even within the progressive environment of Henry Street Settlement, nurses adhered to the accepted practice of racial segregation. Working within these social boundaries, Lillian Wald invited Elizabeth Tyler to join her staff in 1906. Tyler had graduated from the Black Freedmen's Hospital in Washington, DC, and came to Henry Street on the recommendation of Jessie Sleet, a young Black nurse whom New York City officials had hired in 1901. Sleet had been working since then in "the Negro district" of Manhattan. Sleet, who had trained at the Providence Hospital in Chicago, had arrived in New York "filled with determination to work among the neglected ones of her own race." Within a few months, she had accomplished a great deal, fitting into the neighborhood, and gaining the community's trust. Writing in 1901, Sleet described her work:

> *I beg to render to you a report of the work done by me as district nurse among the colored [sic] people of New Yourk City during the months of October and November. I have endeavored to search out the families in which there was sickness and destitution. But I have never hesitated to visit anyone when I have felt that a word of advice or a friendly warning was all they needed. I have visited 41 sick families and made 156 calls in connection with these families, caring for 9 cases of consumption, 4 cases of peritonitis, 2 cases of heart disease, 2 cases of cancer, 1 case of diptheria, 2 cases of chicken pox, 2 cases of tumor, 1 case of gastric catarrh, 2 of pneumonia, 4 cases of rheumatism, and 2 cases of scalp-wound. I have given baths, applied poultices, dressed wounds, washed and dressed new born babies, cared for mothers.*"[58]

Sleet's experiment was a success and led to Wald's hiring of Tyler and another African American nurse, Edith Carter. In December 1906, the settlement added the "Stillman House Branch of the Henry Street Settlement for Colored People," to its service centers. Located in a small storefront in the San Juan Hill area, the Stillman House Branch nurses, Elizabeth Tyler and Edith Carter, served the needs of African Americans on Manhattan's west side.

The 1906 Food and Drug Act

The Food and Drug Act of 1906 required true statements on medication labels and the disclosure of "alcohol, opium, cocaine, morphine, chloroform, marijuana, acetanilide, chloral hydrate or eucaine" as contents. It did not, however, restrict pharmacists from dispensing these over-the-counter remedies, nor did it restrict the public from purchasing them and keeping them at home.[56]

"The work is fortunate indeed in the rare abilities of . . . Miss Tyler and Miss Carter. . . . They are both especially alert to . . . organized preventive work."[59]

"News," American Journal of Nursing, 1906

The Norfolk City Union of the King's Daughters

From its inception in the Northeast in the 1880s, the visiting nurse movement spread across the United States. In Virginia, Edith Nason, an "eminently qualified" graduate of St. Luke's Hospital in Chicago, accepted a position in January 1897 as a visiting nurse of the Norfolk City Union of the King's Daughters, a nondenominational women's organization in Norfolk, Virginia. Like other organizations, its purpose was to address the needs of poor Whites and Blacks in the burgeoning city. And, like other visiting nurses, the King's Daughters nurses provided direct care to the sick. Working from her room in the Young Women's Christian Association (YWCA), Nason began her service to the city's sick poor, seeing more than 1,700 patients her first year. Addressing social and economic needs of the poor in addition to providing nursing care, Nason and other King's Daughters nurses established a community supported milk and ice program, and began a seaside camp for children. To accomplish this they held fund-raising "tag" days in which donors to their cause would receive a tag to wear on their clothing signifying that they had given.[60]

In the opening decade of the 20th century the City Union of King's Daughters expanded its staff to include another graduate nurse and a student. By 1910 a Black nurse, Eva Davis, had joined the staff; another African American nurse soon followed. Both were needed—in the segregated city where African American infants died "at almost three times the rates of whites," the organization's nurses were needed to care for Black mothers and their babies. By 1913 the King's Daughters employed five White nurses and four Black nurses. That year the nurses made 8,423 visits to White patients and 7,851 visits to African Americans.[61]

Over the next decade, the organization continued to grow. By the mid-1920s the King's Daughters had a small complex of buildings from which to work, two Ford automobiles to transport the nurses on their home visits, and several health stations throughout the city.[62] The nurses were making a valuable contribution to the community's health.

Missionary Nurses in Alaska

While visiting nursing organizations were spreading throughout the lower 48 states, the situation was quite different in the newly acquired Territory of Alaska. This region in the late 19th century had no Lutheran motherhouses, no visiting nurse associations, and no public health nurses. Instead, the indigenous people sought care from local shamans, their own families, and community members, while White explorers and military men turned to the few military physicians in their isolated outposts. Roman Catholic and Protestant churches sent missionaries and educators to the isolated territory, but their goal was to educate and convert the indigenous people, not to provide for their health. Soon, however, both groups discovered that it was medical and nursing services that the Alaskan people needed most.

Churches of both denominations responded, sending missionary doctors and nurses. In 1885 three Catholic Sisters, all nurses, arrived in Juneau and set up a hospital. Three years later, the Presbyterian Mission at Sitka also built a hospital and employed a nurse and physician there. In 1897 Ann Dikey, an Episcopalian missionary, arrived to work in Skagway, "the gateway to the Yukon gold fields."[63]

Living and working in the isolated, remote, and often inaccessible areas of Alaska gave nurses an inordinate amount of professional autonomy. The scarcity of physicians was one factor, the climate and geography another. In spring and summer, water routes afforded access to care. In winter, when the rivers were frozen, dog sleds served as the only available transportation.[64]

With the discovery of gold in the new territory, prospectors flocked to Alaska shores. By the summer of 1900, more than 20,000 miners worked the Bering Sea Shores of Alaska's Seward Peninsula, further increasing the demand for medical services. In late June and early July 1900, a smallpox crisis in Nome brought the need for care to the forefront, and people turned to the Sisters of Providence for help. The Reverend Father Renee, the apostolic delegate to Alaska, wrote to them to persuade them to come.[65]

When it proved impossible for the Sisters to travel to Alaska, the reverend wrote again a year later, renewing his request for "two to three" Sisters. Recognizing that ice in the Bering Sea and the Alaskan Gulf would make any ocean voyage to Alaska impossible until spring, he wrote: "We shall expect them at the beginning of September. Otherwise it will be too late."[66]

"The population of Nome is unanimous in clamoring for a hospital and Sisters without delay."[67]

The Reverend Father Renee, 1901

A year later, after a 45-day trip from Montreal, Canada, to Alaska—a journey that involved the transcontinental railroad, a 9-day sea voyage, and a delay of 72 hours in quarantine for smallpox—Sisters Rodrique, Lambert, Napoleon, and Conrad arrived in Nome.[68] It was not the first time that Sister Conrad had been to the Northwest; at age 50 she was an experienced nurse who had set up other hospitals in Washington and Oregon. This was, however, the Sisters' first venture into the territory of Alaska, and finding no one to meet them, they made their way to the nearby church on their own, where the priests welcomed them. Determined to begin their work, within their first week the Sisters purchased a three-story building and began to set up Holy Cross Hospital, where they would live and work.

During their first year, the Sisters faced multiple challenges, not the least of which were the extreme temperatures, the dark days of winter, and a sense of isolation

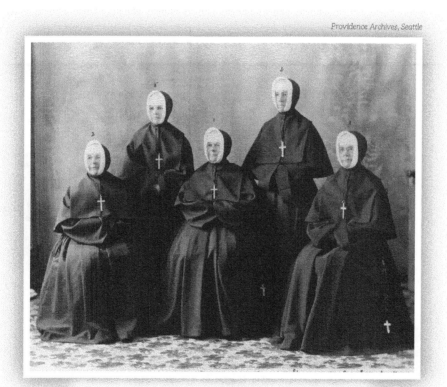

The five Sisters who settled in Nome, Alaska, in 1901 and cared for indigenous peoples and gold prospectors.

living at "the end of the world."[69] Within months, Sister Rodrique was forced to return to the states for health reasons, leaving them short one nurse.[70]

The remaining Sisters kept busy. Given the nutritional status, poverty, and living conditions of the indigenous people, contagious diseases ran rampant. Tuberculosis was endemic, epidemics of diphtheria, typhoid fever, and measles were all too commonplace. Accidents in homes, the gold mines, construction sites, and at sea were the facts of life. The Sisters cared for 190 patients during their first year.

In 1919 five new Sisters of Providence from the motherhouse in Montreal arrived in Nome, but were sent immediately to Fairbanks. There they assumed the administration of St. Joseph Hospital, replacing the Sisters of St. Benedict. Working under the leadership of Sister Superior Mondaldi, these Sisters of Providence served the people of the frontier-mining town of Fairbanks for more than 40 years.[72]

Missionaries of other religious denominations also made their way to the Alaskan territory. Among these were Archdeacon Stuck of Alaska and nurse Miss Woods. Both would be needed when a diphtheria epidemic swept through their mission station in 1907. Stuck wrote of his difficulties trying to manage alone before Woods arrived:

When I last wrote I had pitched my tent at the Chandalar Village, 65 miles north of Fort Yukon, and was ministering as best I could to the diphtheria patients while Mr. Knapp took the team and went back to get Miss Woods [RN]. . . . For the five days following I swabbed out throats two or three times a day, cooked beef tea and milk and rice, took temperatures, and did my best . . . I knew that five days was the least time in which Miss Woods could possibly

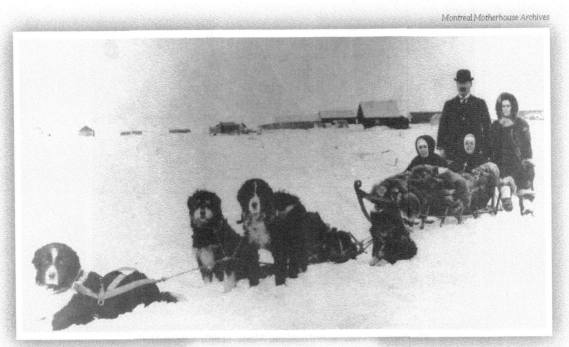

Montreal Motherhouse Archives

Sisters of Providence traveled by dogsled.

come. . . . When the five days were up, she came . . . I shall never forget how she 'bobbed up serenely' from that toboggan after her 35 miles' ride through the bitter cold, and took general charge in her placid, undemonstrative way.[73]

Anglican missionary nurses like Wood had to deal with more than the care of the sick. Faced with a lack of manpower, the missionaries often had to serve in multiple roles. Frigid weather and difficulties obtaining supplies only complicated the situation.

"Miss Woods is 'up to her eyes' at Fort Yukon all the time; school, mission, sick people, housekeeping; the two little scamps she has taken to look after . . . and now they talk of making her post-mistress."[74]

Archdeacon Stuck of Alaska, 1907

NEW ORGANIZATIONS

As the 20th century opened and more U.S. citizens migrated to Alaska, medical and nursing services increased. By 1918 when an influenza epidemic arrived in the territory, Alaska had a local chapter of the American Red Cross—one that had been initiated as part of the American Red Cross Rural Nursing Service. In fact, the 20th century would see a rise in several new organizations that would profoundly affect how nursing would be delivered in communities. In addition to the rural nursing service of the American Red Cross, these included the National Organization of Public Health Nurses and the Children's Bureau.

The Rural Nursing Service of the American Red Cross

Beginning in 1912, nurses could also work for the rural nursing service, part of the American Red Cross. The idea for a rural service originated with Lillian Wald. Based on her experience with Henry Street visiting nurses, as well as her knowledge of services in other countries, Wald "envisioned a well-organized structure within the American Red Cross" to provide nursing care to people in rural areas during times of war *and* times of peace. In a letter to her friend Jacob Schiff in 1910, Wald wrote: "It seems to me particularly appropriate for the Red Cross society to undertake . . . an extensive and systematically organized service of nursing for the scattered dwellers in rural regions, such as we now find well developed in Great Britain and in Canada. In the older countries, armies of trained nurses are sent into remote country regions to nurse, to educate, to bring scientific . . . sanitary messages to the public."[75]

That same year, Wald presented her suggestion at a meeting in New York City to promote camps for children with tuberculosis, part of a larger, international antituberculosis campaign initiated by the Red Cross. A few years later, long-time benefactor Jacob Schiff supported her plan at the annual Red Cross meeting. The plan called for the American Red Cross to organize a rural nursing service that would be "national in scope."[76] It included the establishment of a rural nursing service headquarters in Washington, DC, the utilization of trained nurses and traveling supervisors, and the development of local chapters led by community supervisors.[77]

With financial support from Schiff and others, in December 1911 the plan became a reality. The Red Cross appointed a committee on rural nursing. The committee brought together several notable Progressive Era leaders interested in nursing, Red Cross board members, philanthropists, public health service physicians, and nursing leaders Jane Delano (vice-chair), Lillian Wald, and Annie Goodrich. By February 1912 a subcommittee, including Jane Delano, Annie Goodrich, Lillian Wald, and Fannie Clement, had developed the standards for practice and education for rural nurses. Ten months later, on November 12, 1912, the American Red Cross Rural Nursing Service was established on a 1-year trial basis. Public health nurse Fannie Clement was named superintendent.[78]

During that first year, the committee developed a list of qualifications nurses would have to meet in order to work in the new service. The committee agreed that rural public health nurses needed additional education and experience beyond their training school education. To advertise the positions, the committee developed and distributed brochures outlining the criteria for becoming a rural nurse:

> An applicant must have had at least two years course of training in a general hospital . . . [plus] training or experience in visiting nursing or some other form of social service. . . . In states where registration is provided by law, an applicant must be registered . . . a knowledge of driving and riding horses, and more frequently the use of an automobile is necessary.[79]

Despite the advertising, the leaders found it difficult to find enough nurses to fill the rural positions. In 1913 Dr. Wickliffe Rose from the Rockefeller Foundation addressed the issue of recruitment, writing to Mabel Boardman at the American Red Cross:

> I would suggest that you may find it very difficult to induce young women who have become accustomed to city life to accept service for the rural districts. . . . You will find your best material in the country. In all our other work we find that people who have grown up in the country and who are now living in the country give us the best service.[80]

He was correct. Nurses who had grown up in rural areas were best suited for the job. The work required them to live and work within the community, travel some distance to see their patients, and do whatever needed to be done. Being comfortable in basic clothing and in the methods of rural transportation helped immensely.

The needs of each community directed the work of the rural nurse who needed to be skilled in all aspects of public health nursing. For example, in the lumber camps along New Hampshire's Pemigawsett River, one rural nurse found that she had to conduct classes in "Home Hygiene and Care of the Sick" for camp mothers. She also had to address specific problems, including unventilated housing, lack of immunizations among the laborers, and the high incidence of frostbite and communicable diseases. In South Carolina, another Red Cross nurse had "among various other duties," the job of inspecting "washerwomen," while three county nurses in Michigan were "devoted to school work, antituberculosis, and infant welfare nursing."[82]

Because of the varied responsibilities and the remoteness of the areas in which they worked, rural public health nurses required additional education. Topics such as communication, sociopolitical and economic factors, cultural understanding, and social awareness were particularly important. The minimum requirement was the completion of a 4-month course in public health nursing. Early on, the Committee on Red Cross Rural Nursing identified Teachers College at Columbia University in New York City as the exemplar for these new programs.

By 1913 the rural nursing service had demonstrated its success and changed its name to reflect an expansion of services to larger towns across the United States. It would now be known as the Town and Country

Rural Nursing in Maine

"My uniform consists of rubber boots, army breeches, short skirt, flannel shirt and sheepskin-lined coat. The mud is very deep, boats have a faculty of being wet inside as well as outside, and the highways and byways of Cranberry Isle are not yet paved or even very wide or well marked in any way . . . I am going to Islesford next week and then hope to have a horse for transportation."[81]

Christine Higgins, Rural Nursing Service, 1921

Nursing Service (1913–1918). In 1918 the Town and Country Nursing Service changed its name again, this time to the Bureau of Public Health Nursing. The name reflected a broader role and responsibility as these nurses supported additional populations scattered in towns, rural settings, and even large cities. This third title lasted until 1932, when it became known as the Public Health Nursing and Home Hygiene and Care of the Sick. It would keep that name until 1947 when the organization closed after years of losing funds, lack of qualified nursing staff, and increasing competition from various organizations.[83]

The National Organization of Public Health Nurses

In 1912 Lillian Wald and her colleagues Ella Crandall, Mary Beard, Edna Folley, and others established the National Organization for Public Health Nurses. Its major focus was to develop adequate numbers of public health nurses to meet the needs of the public and to link the emerging field of health nursing to larger public health efforts. Originally the organization included both nurses and lay people interested in public health, represented visiting and district nurses, and "2,500 poorly prepared and unsupervised colleagues in 900 agencies."[84] In fact, by 1910, more than 1,000 organizations across the United States were employing visiting nurses of some sort—including industries, social service agencies, and antituberculosis leagues.[85]

The organization's goal was to provide a central structure for the various groups interested in public health nursing and set standards for their work. As public health nursing leader Mary Gardner wrote: "For some years it has seemed to the nurses engaged in the different forms of visiting and public health nursing that a real danger exists in the phenomenally rapid growth of . . . this branch of nursing unless certain standards could be . . . established and maintained."[87] Elected as the organization's first president, Lillian Wald would lead the association in achieving this goal. Her first steps in that process were to establish standing orders for public health nurses and to communicate them through the *American Journal of Nursing* and the *Public Health Nurse Quarterly* (originally the *Visiting Nurse Quarterly*).[88]

The Children's Bureau

Concurrent with the development of the National Organization of Public Health Nurses in 1912 was the establishment of the Children's Bureau, a federal agency designed to address children's welfare throughout the United States. Once again Lillian Wald was involved with the process. In fact, Lillian Wald and social reformer Florence Kelley were the first to envision a federal agency whose sole focus would be the health and well-being of the nation's children. Years of activism and a strong lobby by Wald, Kelley, and other Progressive reformers would eventually push President William Howard Taft to sign legislation creating the U.S. Federal Children's Bureau.[90]

National Organization of Public Health Nurses

"The NOPHN is a general body, including in its membership all forms of public health nursing. It is concerned with developing standards of ethics and technique, maintaining a central bureau of information and issuing regular and occassional publications . . . [It] does not maintain nursing personnel as does the Red Cross."[86]

Library of Congress

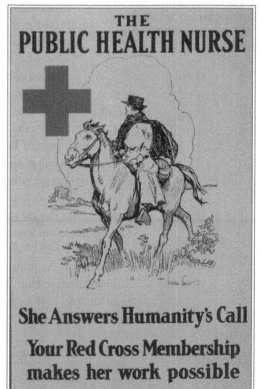

A poster for the National Organization of Public Health Nurses, which attempted to set nursing standards and organize public health nursing groups.

"We considered ourselves best described by the term 'public health nurses."[89]

Lillian Wald, 1941, National Organization of Public Health Nursing President

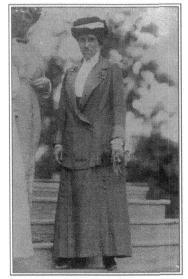

Julia Lathrop, the first chief of the U.S. Federal Children's Bureau, which, under her guidance, sought to reduce infant mortality.

The new legislation required the Children's Bureau to "investigate and report upon all matters pertaining to the welfare of children and child life among all classes of our people."[91] Julia Lathrop, the first chief of the U.S. Children's Bureau, searched for a manageable first project that would address a "pressing need" and establish "the scientific character of the bureau's work and its usefulness to the public."[92] After consulting with a number of influential reformers, including Lillian Wald, Jane Addams, and Edward Devine, Lathrop chose to focus the bureau's initial efforts on reducing infant mortality. A strong infant welfare campaign advocated for comprehensive birth registration, published baby-care pamphlets for parents, and conducted research on infant mortality. This first initiative provided the Children's Bureau with numerous opportunities for concrete action on behalf of children and the results were easily communicated to the public.[93] Infant mortality proved to be a much less controversial choice than child labor reform, despite the latter being the impetus behind the original establishment of the bureau.

In addition to being a primarily urban problem, the highest rates of infant mortality were largely ascribed to the immigrant poor. While the American Medical Association's 1857 report had acknowledged that high infant mortality affected city residents of all socioeconomic classes, it also proclaimed that, "among the suffering poor in our large cities, a fearful ratio of our infant mortality is found."[94] Initial research by the Children's Bureau on the social and environmental aspects of infant mortality reaffirmed the earlier conclusions on the relationships among race, class, and high rates of infant death.

Despite the admittedly "restricted and tentative character" of the initial survey, the results provided Lathrop with concrete evidence to support her requests for more funding to combat the "preventable waste" that was infant mortality.[95] As annual appropriations grew, so did bureau staffing, increasing from 15 to 76 people by 1915.[96] A larger budget and improved staff capacity enabled the bureau to broaden its focus to include other issues, including child labor, public education, special-needs children, and establishing child welfare standards.

Thus, by 1917 the nursing profession was well positioned to address the health of the nation, beginning with its youngest and most vulnerable citizens—infants and children. Before that, however, the profession had to address its own needs for organization and look beyond its national borders to collaborate with nurses around the world.

For Discussion

1. What was the influence of social class on the care of infants and children in the late 19th century? What ethical issues arise in this situation?
2. How did religious groups, visiting nurses, and other social organizations work to address the needs of immigrants in cities of the Northeast during the height of industrialization?
3. How did geography and the needs of the community influence rural nursing in the early 20th century?

(continued)

NOTES

1. Harriet Fulmer, "History of Visiting Nurse Work in America," *American Journal of Nursing* 2, no. 6 (March 1902): 411–425 (quote 411).

2. Alan M. Kraut, "Plagues and Prejudice: Nativism's Construction of Disease in 19th and 20th Century New York City," Part I in *Hives of Sickness: Public Health and Epidemics in New York City,* David Rossner, ed. (New Brunswick: Rutgers University Press, 1995): 68.

3. Lorie Conway, *Forgotten Ellis Island: The Extraordinary Story of America's Immigrant Hospital* (New York: HarperCollins Publishers, 2007).

4. Arlene Keeling, "Reflections on Immigration: The Nurses of Ellis Island," *Windows in Time: The Newsletter of the UVA Eleanor Crowder Bjoring Center for Nursing Historical Inquiry* 22, no. 2 (October 2014): 2.

5. Howard Markel, *Quarantine: East European Jewish Immigrants and the New York City Epidemics of 1892* (Baltimore, MD: Johns Hopkins University Press, 1997): 29.

6. Carrie Howse, " 'The Reflections of England's Light': The Instructive District Nursing Association of Boston, 1884–1914." *Nursing History Review,* 2009, 47–79 (quote 52).

7. Ibid., 52.

8. "Pneumonia," The Inventory of the Visiting Nurse Association of Boston Collection, Howard Gotlieb Archival Research Center at Boston University (hereafter HGARC-BU) Box 5, folder 1, 5.

9. "Technique for communicable diseases," Instructive District Nurse Association (hereafter IDNA) collection, HGARC-BU, Box 5, folder 1, 8.

10. IDNA collection, HGARC-BU, Box 5, folder 1.

11. IDNA collection, HGARC-BU, Box 5, folder 1: Mrs. W. T. Sedgwick, "Instructive District Nursing," reprinted from the *Forum* (Boston: Forum Publishing, November 1896): 297–307 (quote 303).

12. Stanford Shulman, "The History of Pediatric Infectious Disease," *Pediatric Research* 55 (2004): 163–176. For more on this topic see Rima Apple, " 'Advertised by Our Loving Friends': The Infant Formula Industry and the Creation of New Pharmaceutical Markets, 1870-1910," *Journal of the History of Medicine* 41, 1 (1986): 3–23.

13. Paul Beaven and James Baty, "A History of the Boston Floating Hospital," *Pediatrics* 19 (1957): 629–637.

14. For more on the floating hospitals in New York, see Cynthia A. Connolly, *Saving Sickly Children: The Tuberculosis Preventorium in American Life, 1909-1970* (New Brunswick, NJ: Rutgers University Press, 2008).

15. Sarah Palmer, "The Floating Hospital of St. John's Guild, New York City," *American Journal of Nursing* 4, no. 1 (October 1903): 4–8.

16 Beaven and Baty, "Boston Floating Hospital," 631.

17. Ibid., 629–638.

18. Ibid., 636.

19. Lucie Prinz and Jacoba Van Schaik, *The Boston Floating Hospital* (Boston: Tufts Medical Center, 2014).

20. Palmer, "The Floating Hospital," 4–8 (quote 7).

21. "The Mercy Ship," http://sites.tufts.edu/medicine/spring-2015/the-mercy-ship (accessed July 12, 2016): 1–4.

22. Prinz and Van Schaik, *The Boston Floating Hospital,* 26.

23. Karen Buhler-Wilkerson, *No Place Like Home: A History of Nursing and Home Care in the United States* (Baltimore, MD: Johns Hopkins University Press, 2001): 86.

24. Ibid., 30–33.

25. Archival Introduction to: "Visiting Nurse Society of Philadelphia Records, 1855-1987," MC-5, Barbara Bates Center for the Study of the History of Nursing.

26. S. W. Newmayer, "The Warfare against Infant Mortality," *Annals of the American Academy* (March 1911): 293–234.

27. "Notes on the History of the Visiting Nurse Association of Chicago," Chicago Historical Society, VNA collection, Box 1, folder 2, 1–4 (quote 1).

28. Ibid.

29. Jane Addams, *Twenty Years at Hull House* (New York: Macmillan, 1948). First edition: 1910.

30. Ibid., 48–49.

31. *Woman's World,* 1897.

32. Jane Addams, "Modern City," cited in *Twenty Years at Hull House.*

33. Harriet Fulmer, "History of Visiting Nurse Work in America," *American Journal of Nursing* 2, no. 6 (March 1902): 411–424 (quote 414).

34. Eliza Moore, "Visiting Nursing," *American Journal of Nursing* 1, no. 1 (October 1900): 17–21 (quote 18).

35. Visiting Nurse Association of Chicago, Superintendent's Report in the *Twentieth Annual Report* (Chicago, 1909): 40.

36. Edna L. Foley, *Visiting Nurse Manual* (Chicago: National Organization for Public Health Nursing, 1912): 23.

37. Edna Foley, "The Nurse's First Visit," *Public Health Nurse* 18 (1926): 530.

38. Visiting Nurse Association of Chicago, *Fourth Annual Report* (Chicago, 1893).

39. Lisa Zerull, *Nursing Out of the Parish: A History of the Baltimore Lutheran Deaconesses, 1893–1911* (dissertation, University of Virginia, May 2010).

40. Ibid., 77.

41. Jennie Christ Day Book, January 2, 1894–April 1, 1894. Cited in Zerull, *Nursing Out of the Parish,* 230.

42. Zerull, *Nursing Out of the Parish,* 223.

43. Ibid., 236.

44. Ibid., 239.

45. Ibid., 237.

46. Carole A. Estabrooks, "Lavinia Lloyd Dock: The Henry Street Years," *Nursing History Review* 3 (1995): 163.

47. Buhler-Wilkerson, *No Place Like Home,* 112.

48. Ibid., 105–107.

49. "Report of a Day in the Work of a Visiting Nurse, July 25, 1910," Lillian Wald Collection, Virginia Commonwealth University Thompkins McCaw Library for Health Science, Microfilm, reel 98, Box 85.

50. Marilyn S. Blackwell, "Keeping the 'Household Machine' Running: Attendant Nursing and Social Reform in the Progressive Era," *Bulletin of the History of Medicine* 74 (2000): 241–264; Karen Buhler-Wilkerson, "Bringing Care to the People: Lillian Wald's Legacy to Public Health Nursing," *American Journal of Public Health* 83 (1993): 1778–1786.

51. "The Treatment of Families in Which There is Sickness," Lillian Wald Collection, New York Public Library (hereafter NYPL), reel 29, 13.

52. R. L. Duffus, *Lillian Wald, Neighbor and Crusader* (New York: Macmillan, 1938): 43.

53. Buhler-Wilkerson, *No Place Like Home*, 170–71.

54. *Report of the Nurses' Work of the Settlement* (1905), LWC, Columbia University, Box 57, folder 1.3; Lillian Wald, "The Care of Sick Children in the Home," Paper presented to the Academy of Medicine, LWC, NYPL, May 10, 1917, 2.

55. Buhler-Wilkerson, *No Place Like Home*, 27.

56. Anne A. J. Andermanj, "Physicians, Fads and Pharmaceuticals: A History of Aspirin," *McGill Journal of Medicine* 2 (1996). http://www.v02n02/aspirin.html (accessed January 15, 2005): 1–9.

57. Lillian Wald, "The Nurses' Settlement," Official Reports of Societies, *American Journal of Nursing* 2 (1901–1902): 386–387.

58. Lucy Drown, "A Successful Experiment," *American Journal of Nursing* 1 (July 1901): 729–731 (quote 729).

59. "News," *American Journal of Nursing* 6, 12 (September 1906): 882.

60. Mary Gibson, "'The Prevention of Suffering Is as Much Her Work as Nursing': Origins of the City Union of the King's Daughters Health Work in Norfolk," *Windows in Time, Newsletter from the Eleanor Crowder Bjoring Center for Nursing Historical Inquiry* 16, 1 (February 2008): 7–10 (quote 7).

61. Ibid., 7–10.

62. Ibid.

63. Walter Hickel and Theodore Mala, *History of the Alaska Department of Health and Social Services* (Anchorage, AK: Frontier Printing, 1993): 2–29 (quote p. 8).

64. Lulu Welch, RN, quoted in Effie Graham, Jackie Pflaum, and Elfrida Nord, *With a Dauntless Spirit: Alaskan Nursing in Dog-Team Days* (Fairbanks: University of Alaska Press, 2003): 25.

65. John Shideler and Hal Rothman, "Pioneering Spirit—The Sisters of Providence in Alaska," (Anchorage, AK: Providence Archives, 1967): 13.

66. Reverend Father Renee, correspondence to the Reverend Mother General Mary Antoinette in Montreal, June 19, 1901. English translation of *Chronicles*, 1902–1908, Holy Cross Hospital. Providence Archives, Seattle, WA (hereafter PA-Seattle): 1.

67. Ibid.

68. Shideler and Rothman, "Pioneering Spirit," 22.

69. Ibid., 19–21.

70. *Chronicles* of Holy Cross Hospital, 38.

71. Ibid.

72. "History of Holy Cross Hospital," PA-Seattle 1.

73. "Nursing in Mission Stations," *American Journal of Nursing* 7, no. 9 (June 1907): 700–702: (quote 700).

74. Ibid., 701.

75. Lillian Wald to Jacob Schiff, 1910 correspondence, cited in Lavinia L. Dock, Sarah Elizabeth Pickett, Fannie F. Clement, Elizabeth G. Fox, and Anna R. Van Meter, *History of American Red Cross Nursing* (New York: Macmillan, 1922): 1213.

76. Ibid.

77. Sandra Lewenson, "Town and Country Nursing: Community Participation and Nurse Recruitment," in *Nursing Rural America*, eds. John Kirchgessner and Arlene Keeling (New York: Springer Publishing, 2015): 1–19.

78. Dock et al., *History of American Red Cross*, 1213–1215.

79. Ibid., 1236–1238.

80. Wickliff Rose, Letter to Miss Mabel Boardman, May 30, 1913, Rockefeller Sanitary Commission Microfilm, reel 1, folder 8 (American Red Cross Town & Country Nursing Service 1912–1914) cited in Lewenson, "Town and Country Nursing."

81. Elizabeth Fox, "Red Cross Public Health Nursing, Out to Sea," *Public Health Nurse* 13 (1921): 105–108 (quote 105).

82. Dock et al., *History of American Red Cross*, 1229–1231.

83. Lewenson, "Town and Country Nursing."

84. Philip A. Kalisch and Beatrice J. Kalisch. *American Nursing: a History* (4th edition) (Philadelphia: Lippincott-Williams and Wilkins, 2004): 176.

85. Introduction to the National Organization for Public Health Nursing (NOPHN) Records, 1913–53, MC83 Barbara Bates Center for the Study of the History of Nursing, University of Pennsylvania, 1.

86. Dock et al., *History of American Red Cross*, 1221.

87. Mary Gardner, "The National Organization for Public Health Nursing," *Visiting Nurse Quarterly*, 4 (July 1912): 13–18 (quote 14).

88. Edna Foley, "Standing Orders," *American Journal of Nursing* 13 (March 1913): 451.

89. Lillian Wald, "We Called Our Enterprise Public Health Nursing," foreword to *The Public Health Nurse in Action by Marguerite Wales* (New York: MacMillan, 1941): xi.

90. Kriste Lindenmeyer, *"A Right to Childhood": The U.S. Children's Bureau and Child Welfare, 1912–1946* (Urbana: University of Illinois Press, 1997): 9–18.

91. United States Department of Labor, *The Children's Bureau: Yesterday, Today, and Tomorrow* (Washington, DC: U.S. Government Printing Office, 1937): 1.

92. Helen Witmer, *A Research Program for the Children's Bureau* (Washington, DC: Children's Bureau, 1953): 8.

93. United States Department of Labor, *The Children's Bureau*, 30.

94. D. Meredith Reese, *Report on Infant Mortality in Large Cities* (Philadelphia, T.K. and P.G. Collins Printers, 1857): 14.

95. Ibid., 5.

96. United States Department of Labor, *The Children's Bureau*, 30.

FURTHER READING

Addams, Jane, *Twenty Years at Hull House* (New York: Macmillan, 1948). First edition: 1910.

Beaven, Paul, and James Baty, "A History of the Boston Floating Hospital," *Pediatrics* 19, no. 4 (1957): 629–638.

Buhler-Wilkerson, Karen, *No Place Like Home: A History of Nursing and Home Care in the United States* (Baltimore, MD: Johns Hopkins University Press, 2001).

Conway, Lorie, *Forgotten Ellis Island: The Extraordinary Story of America's Immigrant Hospital* (New York: HarperCollins Publishers, 2007).

Drown, Lucy, "A Successful Experiment," *American Journal of Nursing* 1 (July 1901): 729–731.

Gibson, Mary, "'The Prevention of Suffering Is as Much Her Work as Nursing': Origins of the City Union of the King's Daughters Health Work in Norfolk," *Windows in Time, Newsletter from the Eleanor Crowder Bjoring Center for Nursing Historical Inquiry* 16, no. 1 (February 2008): 7–10.

Hine, Darlene Clark, *Black Women in White: Racial Conflict and Cooperation in the Nursing Profession, 1890-1950* (Indianapolis: Indiana University Press, 1989).

Howse, Carrie, "'The Reflection of England's Light': The Instructive District Nursing Association of Boston, 1884–1914." *Nursing History Review*, 17 (2009): 47–79.

Keeling, Arlene, "Reflections on Immigration: The Nurses of Ellis Island," *Windows in Time: The Newsletter of the UVA Eleanor Crowder Bjoring Center for Nursing Historical Inquiry* 22, no. 2 (October 2014): 1–3.

Lewenson, Sandra, "Town and Country Nursing," *Nursing Rural America*, eds. John Kirchgessner and Arlene Keeling (New York: Springer Publishing, 2014): 1–20.

Markel, Howard, *Quarantine: East European Jewish Immigrants and the New York City Epidemics of 1892* (Baltimore, MD: Johns Hopkins University Press, 1997).

Palmer, Sarah, "The Floating Hospital of St. John's Guild, New York City," *American Journal of Nursing* 4, no. 1 (October 1903): 4–8.

Prinz, Lucie, and Jacoba Van Schaik, *The Boston Floating Hospital: How a Boston Harbor Barge Changed the Course of Pediatric Medicine* (Boston: Tufts Medical Center, 2014).

Rossner, David Rossner, ed. *Hives of Sickness: Public Health and Epidemics in New York City* (New Brunswick, NJ: Rutgers University Press, 1995).

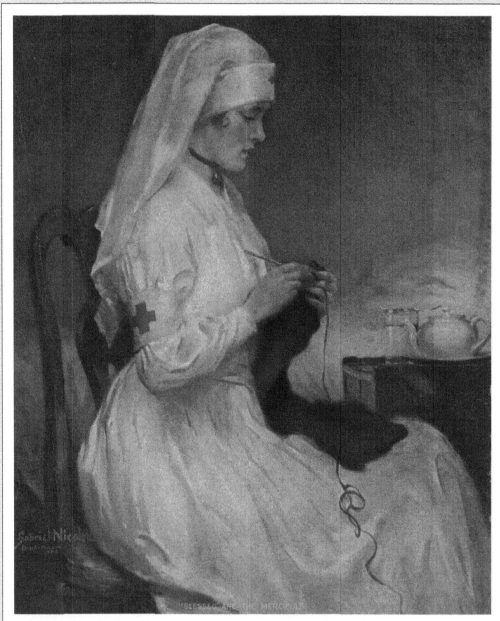

Painting of Red Cross nurse by Nikola.

CHAPTER 5

Professional Organizations and International Connections

1881–1920

Michelle C. Hehman

"Every civilized government is financially able to provide for its armies, but the great and seemingly insuperable difficulty is, to always have what is wanted at the place where it is most needed. . . . For these reasons the Treaty of Geneva and the National Committees of the Red Cross exist to-day. . . . It is only by favoring the organization of this Auxiliary Relief in times of peace . . . that a government may hope to avoid much of the needless suffering, sickness, and death in war."[1]

Reflecting on her purpose for establishing the American Red Cross, Clara Barton directly addressed the public in the preface of her written history on the organization, stating that its mission was "to assist in the prevention and relief of suffering."[2] Personal experience had taught Barton that conflict and disaster were unfortunate but common human events. She firmly believed, however, that a well-prepared Red Cross society could not only render immediate aid in times of emergency, but also mitigate the long-term destructive effects of these incidents. The application of certain core principles—preparation, organization, and strategic planning—proved invaluable to the American Red Cross from its very inception, as it began responding to natural disasters just days after the first chapter was established in 1881. Its relief efforts after the Johnstown flood of

1889 would solidify the reputation of the American Red Cross as a leader in emergency management.

These same principles of the Red Cross also drove early nursing leaders as they sought to unify and promote a fledgling profession. Recognizing the power and potential of organizations to bring members together and more readily enact change, a small cadre of elite nurses from around the world began to create societies to tackle the unique problems related to nursing education, job opportunities, and social prestige. Like the Red Cross, the new nursing associations used organization and planning to meet the needs of those they served. In addition, the changing social, cultural, and political climate of the early 20th century would push these societies beyond the sphere of professional nursing to address both the rising women's movement and continued racial discrimination across the country.

THE AMERICAN RED CROSS
Origins

Clara Barton became one of the most famous women in the country following the widespread publicity of her courageous efforts as the "Angel of the Battlefield" during the American Civil War.[3] After the war she engaged in a lecture tour, speaking to audiences about her experiences with soldiers, often tailoring her talk to describe a battle relevant to the particular community of veterans she addressed. The exhaustive schedule, in which she gave more than 300 lectures, left Barton physically drained. In 1869, she traveled to Europe in search of rest and recuperation, finding herself in Switzerland shortly after the start of the Franco-Prussian war. While Barton was in Switzerland, a member of the International Red Cross Committee invited her to join a relief group headed to the combat zones, and she eventually agreed. Fashioning a cross out of a red ribbon she had been wearing, Barton ministered to soldiers from both the French and German forces, as well as civilians in the city of Strassburg immediately after their surrender. This experience, more than any other, convinced Barton that the United States needed a Red Cross organization. She was appalled to learn that her country had twice refused to sign the Geneva Convention, a treaty that established the sovereignty of the International Red Cross during times of war.

"If I live to return to my country I will try to make my people understand the Red Cross and that treaty."[4]

Clara Barton, 1870

Returning to the United States in 1873, Barton began earnest efforts toward the establishment of an American Red Cross society and the ratification of the Geneva Convention by the U.S. government. In an 1881 address to the president and Congress, Barton recalled her experience with the Red Cross in Europe, contrasting that with her regrets from the American Civil War. Highlighting her disbelief in the United States absence from the Geneva Convention, she stated:

> These men had treaty power to go directly on to any field, and work unmolested in full co-operation with the military and commanders-in-chief; their supplies held sacred and their efforts recognized and seconded in every direction by either belligerent army. Not a man could lie uncared for nor unfed. I thought of the Peninsula in McClellan's campaign . . . of its dead and starving wounded, frozen to the ground, and our commissions and their supplies in Washington, with no effective organization to go beyond; of the Petersburg mine, with its four thousand dead and wounded and no flag of truce, the wounded broiling in a July sun- died and rotting where they fell . . . I thought of the widows' weeds still fresh and dark through all the land, north and south, from the pine to the palm, the shadows on the hearths and hearts over all my country. . . . Was this people to decline a humanity in war? Was this a country to reject a treaty for the help of wounded soldiers? . . . They needed only to know.[5]

Eventually receiving support from President James Garfield, Barton founded the "American Association of the Red Cross" on May 21, 1881, and was elected its first president. As outlined in the adopted constitution, the aim of the American Red Cross society was to "[o]rganize a system of national relief and apply the same in mitigating the sufferings caused by war, pestilence, famine, and other calamities."[7] In this way, Barton expanded the American Red Cross's purpose beyond that of its sister European Red Cross societies, enabling peacetime relief efforts in the event of natural disaster. This provision would come to be known as the "American Amendment" when the United States eventually ratified the Geneva Convention in 1882. As Barton argued, "seldom a year passes that the nation from sea to sea is not by the shock of some sudden, unforeseen disaster, brought to utter consternation . . . powerless, horrified, and despairing."[8]

Disaster relief would become one of the most important functions of the organization, which coordinated its first campaign in response to a devastating forest fire in Michigan in September 1881. The greatest early test of the American Red Cross's ability and effectiveness would come in 1889 after a devastating flood wave destroyed the community of Johnstown, Pennsylvania.

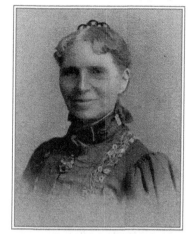

Clara Barton, who founded the Red Cross in the United States in 1881.

The Johnstown Flood

On May 31, 1889, the small industrial community of Johnstown, Pennsylvania, suffered one of the worst natural disasters the United States had ever seen. Situated on the Appalachian Plateau in a river valley junction, the thriving coal and steel town was prone to bouts of flooding. When snow melted too quickly in the mountains above or in times of heavy rain, Johnstown's approximately 30,000 residents prepared their homes to wait out the inevitable overflow of water into the streets. After multiple days of rain in late May, the river banks had crested and the lowest parts of the city already contained standing water. Townspeople began their typical precautionary measures; families brought their belongings to higher floors and readied themselves for the usual small flood.

Just 14 miles outside the city, however, members of an exclusive hunting and fishing club were also hard at work, frantically attempting to reinforce and relieve pressure on the questionably maintained South Fork Dam, the only barrier surrounding 20 million tons of water in Lake Conemaugh. When the dam finally gave way in the afternoon of May 31, the deluge of water steamrolled toward Johnstown, dragging any houses, barns, livestock, and people in its path. With "a sound as of an approaching railroad train," the massive flood wave crashed through the heart of the town, swallowing homes and businesses.[9] The wreckage bottlenecked at the Pennsylvania Railroad Company's Stone Bridge, creating a 40-foot-high, 30-acre-wide mountain of destruction that promptly caught fire. Water and any remaining debris barreled down the Conemaugh River to downstream communities. More than 2,000 people lost their lives in the flood wave. Survivors were trapped wherever they had ended up, waiting through a night of "indescribable horror" for the sun to rise and flood waters to retreat.[10]

Alarming newspaper headlines reported on a seemingly improbable level of destruction, noting that Johnstown had been "completely swept away" and that "thousands of lives are lost."[12] Even Clara Barton needed 24 hours and numerous reports to be convinced the event was not a hoax, after which she immediately began preparations for a Red Cross presence in Johnstown. Barton's Red Cross had already gained experience responding to disasters across the country, coming to the aid of communities during

"Its Basis Was Neutrality"

Speaking to a women's philanthropic society, Clara Barton articulated the importance of the Red Cross, saying, "Its basis was neutrality. . . . A Greek red cross on a field of white should tell any soldier of any country within the treaty that the wearer was his friend . . . The Red Cross means not national aid for the needs of the people, but the people's aid for the needs of the nation."[6]

May 31, 1889: A Night of "Indescribable Horror"

"The suppressed moans of the bruised, the agony . . . of separated friends and relatives; the cries of little children for food and water, which could not be supplied . . . the darkness and confusion . . . the sickening and stifling odors; the dying scenes on the wreckage about us, and in the conflagration at the railroad bridge . . . combined to make that night one of indescribable horror."[11]

Reverend David J. Beale, 1890

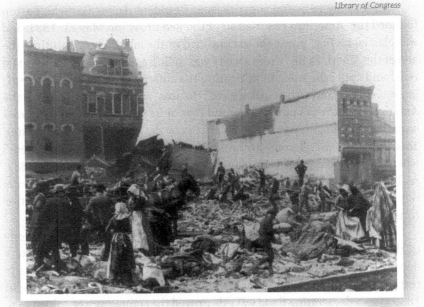

The aftermath of the Johnstown Flood in 1889, the biggest challenge Clara Barton's fledgling Red Cross had ever seen.

the Mississippi and Ohio River floods in 1882 and 1884, the Texas famine in 1887, and the yellow fever epidemic in Jacksonville, Florida, in 1888. Stepping off the train in Johnstown, however, Barton realized this would be the greatest challenge the organization had seen to date. Dr. Benjamin Lee, member of the Pennsylvania State Board of Health, described the aftermath of the flood wave:

> *Johnstown proper was partly a lake, partly several small streams, partly a vast sandy plain, and partly clusters of more or less ruined houses. Around, among, between, inside and on top of those houses, wherever the rushing torrent had been checked, were piled masses of wreckage; trunks of mighty trees, household furniture, houses whole and in fragments, bridges, locomotives and railroad cars, hundreds of tons of mud and gravel. . . . Not only was the work immense, but the difficulties in the way of its accomplishment were such as can scarcely be comprehended by those who did not see them.[13]*

Arriving on June 5 with a starting crew of 15 physicians and four trained nurses, Barton and the Red Cross began their work, speaking first with Johnstown residents to assess the immediate needs of the community.

The most basic human needs—those of food, clothing, and shelter—were the first priority. Volunteers erected living quarters and a kitchen department "from one mammoth tent," where anyone could come and receive assistance.[14] With dry goods boxes functioning as desks, Barton coordinated service to thousands over the course of her stay in Johnstown. Donated supplies quickly began pouring in from around the country. Out of a large pine warehouse built in the center of town, Barton took charge of organizing and distributing everything from hot meals and blankets, to cooking utensils, furniture, and lumber to Johnstown residents. Most families had lost everything, all local businesses had been destroyed, and state-collected relief funds would not be available for months. This left Barton and the Red Cross to fulfill urgent survival needs while cleanup efforts continued and before rebuilding could begin.

Learning from earlier disaster experiences, Barton aimed not only to provide immediate aid, but to assist townspeople to the point that they could be self-sufficient.

Focusing their efforts on long-term housing, multiple Red Cross "hotels" were established around the city, where Johnstown residents could stay rent free with "the only cost to the tenant being for fire, lights, and living."[15] The buildings resembled large apartments, and an appointed landlady operated the establishment like a bed and breakfast, offering meals for less than 25 cents. Knowing that the rebuilding process would take months, and possibly years, creating access to sufficient housing for the harsh Pennsylvania winter was an innovative health promotion measure. In addition to protecting residents from the elements, the hotels decreased the likelihood of families returning to unsanitary conditions in flood-ravaged buildings, and limited the potential spread of communicable diseases due to overcrowding.

"It occurred to us that the most important thing to do, next to feeding the hungry, was to provide proper shelter for these men and their families."[16]

Clara Barton, 1898

Many survivors also required medical attention. The only hospital in Johnstown, privately run for the Cambria Iron Company, was soon filled to overflowing. Volunteers established a large field hospital tent that could serve up to 40 people, in addition to four smaller tents for up to 10 patients each. The Philadelphia branch of the Red Cross, led by Dr. Robert Wharton and a hand-selected team of nurses, took charge of the medical work for injured survivors. Most of their patients had suffered broken bones, lacerations, bruising, and the effects of prolonged exposure depending on the time of their rescue.[17]

Personal accounts describe the immense emotional anguish felt by Johnstown residents who had lost so many family members, friends, and neighbors. Of the 2,209 people who had died in the initial flood wave, nearly 400 of them were children, and almost 100 complete families perished together.[18] Clara Barton saw individuals "stunned by the realization of all the woe that had been visited upon them," while another survivor discussed finding residents paralyzed in "nervous prostration."[19] Medical care addressed more than just physical ailments; as one journalist praised, "the [Red Cross] ministered to mind as well as body."[20]

Perhaps the biggest public health threat in Johnstown was that of water contamination. Lavinia Dock, who had recently returned home to Pennsylvania from nursing victims of the Jacksonville yellow fever epidemic, arrived and immediately began working with the Red Cross to implement sanitary controls.[21] Recovery of the dead would take months, and proper care, handling, and disinfecting of bodies were needed to ensure the safety of the surrounding water supply. It was not that easy, however. By the end of July, more than 200 cases of typhoid fever were reported in the flood zone. Responding quickly, medical workers contained the outbreak and only 40 fatalities occurred by the end of the summer.[22]

On October 24, 1889, nearly 5 months after their arrival, the Red Cross ended their efforts in Johnstown. More than 50 men and women had rendered aid and supplies, valued at more than $200,000, to upward of 25,000 residents.[23] The local *Tribune* published an editorial praising the work of Clara Barton, saying:

> *We cannot thank Miss Barton in words. . . . Picture the sunlight or the starlight, and then try to say good-bye to Miss Barton. . . . There is really no parting. She is with us, she will be with us always- the spirit of her work even after she has passed away. But we can say God bless you, and we do say it, Miss Barton, from the bottom of our hearts, one and all.*[24]

Growth and Change

The American Red Cross's first wartime relief campaign occurred during the Spanish–American War. A number of challenges during the conflict highlighted the need for an organized and dedicated group of trained nurses to care for soldiers during armed conflict. A government-led reorganization of the Red Cross in 1905 would provide ideal circumstances for the development of such a corps of nurses.

That year, Clara Barton transitioned out of the Red Cross presidency after 23 years of service, and Congress placed the organization under government supervision. State chapters could no longer function independent of the parent national organization, and would form through invitation only. The special purposes of the organization were updated and became: "To furnish volunteer aid in the sick and wounded of armies in time of war, in accordance with the spirit and conditions of the Geneva Convention. To continue and carry on a system of national and international relief in time of peace, and apply the same in mitigating the sufferings caused by pestilence, famine, fire, floods and other great national calamities."[25] Congress also formally protected the use of the Red Cross "brassard," and wearing the emblem was legally "reserved to the national societies and their workers on the battlefield."[26]

> "The necessity of being prepared for emergencies has been too often demonstrated to require argument."[27]
>
> American Red Cross Circular, 1905

A national committee was formed to help develop the Red Cross Nursing Service. Under the reorganization, nurses could join the Red Cross either through membership in a state society or through enrollment in the nursing corps. The committee's new priority was to increase enrollment of available nurses, so they enlisted the help of Isabel Hampton Robb (she married Dr. Hunter Robb in 1894) and the Federation of Nurses—a joint society composed of the Nurses Associated Alumnae of the United States and Canada and the American Society of Superintendents of Training Schools. Despite thorough research and the development of sound proposals by Robb and the federation, concrete action took many years. In 1909, the Committee on Nursing Service was officially founded in Washington, DC, with Jane Delano selected as the first chairman. Delano's concurrent appointment as superintendent of the U.S. Army Nurse Corps and national president of the American Nurses Association (ANA) afforded a crucial link between numerous nursing organizations at the time.

The outbreak of World War I prompted exponential growth in the American Red Cross. In 1914, total membership neared 17,000 among 107 local chapters across the country; by 1918 the Red Cross boasted 20 million adults and 11 million junior members among nearly 4,000 local chapters.[28] During the war, American citizens raised more than $400,000 in funds and material to support international Red Cross efforts that ministered to American and Allied forces, as well as civilian refugees.

The Red Cross Nursing Service also grew in size and status throughout the conflict. Tasked with supplying trained nurses to the U.S. Army and Navy Nurse Corps, the Red Cross enrolled 23,822 nurses during the war, of which nearly 20,000 were assigned to active duty overseas.[29] Red Cross nurses also played a key role on the home front, providing vital care during the worldwide influenza pandemic of 1918.

THE PROFESSION ORGANIZES ITSELF

As the United States transitioned from an agrarian economy to an industrial base in the late 19th century, advances in transportation and technology, access to education, and mass production of goods and services demonstrated America's emerging status as a leader in culture, industry, and scientific innovation.[30] The World's Columbian Exposition of 1893 in Chicago, named to celebrate the 400th anniversary of the arrival of Columbus in the New World, would serve to showcase the nation's new image as a global leader. International world's fairs and expositions, which had begun in London in 1851, had quickly become venues where technological advances and cultural standards could be presented to the masses. Displays of technology and industrial innovation from around the world dominated most of these shows, and inventors took advantage of a growing consumer and leisure culture to showcase and sell their products. Both medical and nursing leaders also used the atmosphere of the exhibitions to advance individual and professional ambitions. In particular, they viewed exhibitions as an attractive and convenient setting in which to organize large meetings and discuss pressing issues. The 1893 World's Columbian Exposition was no exception. It introduced the public to novelties like the Pledge of Allegiance, the Ferris Wheel, hamburgers, and Pabst Blue Ribbon Beer. It also resulted in a transformation of American nursing.

A series of congresses were held, aimed at opening and improving educational dialogue regarding the most pressing social concerns. The Congress on Hospitals, Dispensaries, and Nursing, a section of the International Congress of Charities, Correction, and Philanthropy, convened from June 12 to 17, 1893. Physicians from the Johns Hopkins Hospital dominated the special section on hospitals, and Isabel Hampton, superintendent of the Johns Hopkins Training School, was appointed chairperson of the meetings held on nursing. During the nursing sections, leaders from America and Western Europe presented papers, including Isabel Hampton, Lavinia Dock, and Isabel McIsaac. In addition, Hampton read a paper sent from Florence Nightingale to all attendees. Hampton had contacted Nightingale prior to the Congress, saying, "No such meeting of nurses would be complete without having an expression of your interest in us and your views."[31] Despite being unable to personally attend, Nightingale responded by sending both her paper and her "earnest hopes for the highest success" of the meeting.[32]

Hampton's paper, "Educational Standards for Nurses," denounced the lack of standards for training schools across the United States. Citing her success in reforming both the Illinois Training School and Johns Hopkins Training School, Hampton advocated for a 3-year course of study, standard entry and graduation dates, 8-hour workdays for students, and the end of private-duty requirements. Hampton criticized the economic exploitation of pupil nurses by hospitals, which typically utilized students for all their nursing needs and demanded of them 10- to 12-hour workdays. National labor reform campaigns had begun in the 1890s and aimed to restrict workdays to 8 hours and reduce exploitation of women and children. Unfortunately, provisions within the suggested legislation often exempted students from these limits because they were not technically employees.[33] In gaining support for widespread adoption of her proposed educational changes, Hampton hoped to standardize the path to becoming a graduate nurse and ultimately elevate the social perception of nursing quality and training. Changes of that magnitude, however, would require unity and a shared vision for the future of modern nursing.

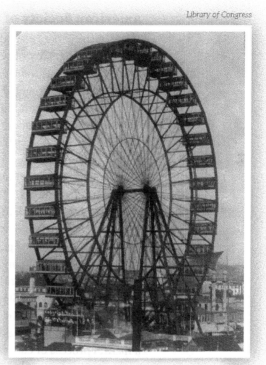

The world's first Ferris Wheel, at the 1893 World's Columbian Exposition.

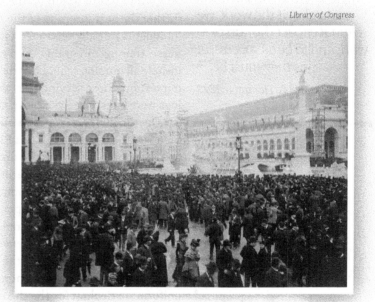

The crowds at the 1893 World's Columbian Exposition.

"A 'trained nurse' may mean then anything, everything, or next to nothing."[34]

Isabel A. Hampton, 1893

American Society of Superintendents

Many of the papers read at the 1893 Congress pushed toward an official professional status for nursing, part of which involved the development of national and international nursing organizations. A conflict arose over the subject. Nightingale and many religious orders of nurses struggled with the idea of a "professional" nurse, preferring to view nursing as more of a vocational calling or moral imperative. In contrast, many American and Canadian nursing leaders, including Hampton, understood the importance of pushing toward professionalization as a way to elevate nursing quality by regulating the use of the title "trained nurse." This would, in turn, improve the social standing of nursing and distinguish the work of nursing from that of medicine. As Edith Draper asserted during her paper presentation, "The needs for a national organization are becoming more and more strongly realized, until now our success for the future depends on our unity."[35]

During a discussion of the potential of nursing associations, Hampton outlined her own vision: creating an organization of superintendents, as well as establishing a national group for nursing alumni.[36] At the completion of the session, about 18 superintendents sat together and formed the American Society of Superintendents of Training Schools in the United States and Canada, later renamed the National League for Nursing Education (NLNE) in 1912. Impressed with Hampton's ability to facilitate her own goals at the Congress, Lavinia Dock later remarked, "Miss Hampton really went through a mental process of construction of the entire subsequent evolution of the nursing profession. She placed the papers so that certain ideas should be worked out, and waited almost breathlessly for the results."[37]

> "Until we can get superintendents united regarding the fundamental principles of the work, we cannot expect the nurses to work and to be as successful as they must be."[38]
>
> Isabel A. Hampton, 1893

The society's purpose was threefold: "To promote fellowship of members; To establish and maintain a universal standard of training; [and] To further the best interests of the nursing profession."[39] The Society of Superintendents initially restricted membership to superintendents of approved nurse training programs, but would eventually expand qualifications to include all nursing school instructors, public health nurses teaching student nurses, and those serving on state boards of nurse examiners. Society meetings were held once every year, the first scheduled for January 10, 1894, in New York City. Dues included a one-time initiation fee of $5, followed by an annual $1 membership fee.[40] Members elected Linda Richards, current superintendent at the New England Hospital Training School, as the first president.

In its early years, the Society of Superintendents focused on improving educational standards across all nurse training programs, and empowering superintendents in their ability to shape curriculum. Members supported the proposal to extend nurse training programs to 3 years, in conjunction with reducing student work hours to a maximum of 8 hours each day. The practicality of implementing these changes, however, remained in question for many years.[41] Additionally, the notion of a standard curriculum throughout nurse training schools dominated annual discussions. As early as 1895, members proposed a uniform curriculum for the theoretical component of nursing education, as well as standardized examinations for graduation. As nurse historian Sandra Lewenson comments, the standard curriculum would "uphold a professional nursing standard and prevent the unqualified from calling themselves nurses. Not unlike the other professional groups of medicine and law, uniformity of professional accreditation for nursing was desirable and obtainable."[42]

The society established a curriculum committee early on and tasked it with the responsibility of determining the contents of a basic nurse training program. The careful selection of theory and practical courses, overall program length, and the best methods for educating students all underscored the belief that elevating standards would lead to more knowledgeable and better prepared graduates, and eventually improve the quality of care delivered to patients across the country. After years of research and deliberation, the NLNE eventually produced the *Standard Curriculum for Schools of Nursing* guidelines in 1917.

Hospital Economics Graduate Course

The 1917 *Standard Curriculum* guidelines afforded superintendents a great deal of authority to improve their own programs, by either adding more instructors, increasing the overall theoretical component, or reducing clinical requirements for students on the wards. Superintendent duties were already multifaceted, however, and these changes only added to their complexity. As the persons in charge of both the instruction of student nurses and the provision of nursing care throughout their associated hospitals, superintendents frequently had to balance the educational needs of the students with the practical and economic constraints of patient care on the busy wards. Few nursing schools enjoyed absolute independence from regulation by hospital trustees and medical officers, rendering superintendents unable to unilaterally alter program structure or curricula, particularly if the changes proved costly or inconvenient for the hospital.

Presumably from their own experiences, members of the Society of Superintendents recognized that adequate preparation for the role of superintendent could not be found in basic nursing education. In addition to the qualities traditionally found in exceptional nurses—discipline, keen perception, tact, thorough understanding of nursing practice, and superior skill—nursing superintendents also needed to possess strong *teaching* abilities in order to be successful.[43] To increase the academic effectiveness and improve the administrative knowledge of nursing superintendents, Isabel Hampton Robb (now married to Dr. Robb) suggested the development of a postgraduate program at an institution directed at training teachers, such as the one at Teachers College, Columbia University, in New York City. Robb hoped that standardizing educational requirements for becoming a superintendent would generate a trickle-down effect, thereby creating more uniformity and standardization in the teaching methods and program outlines for training schools, which were primarily developed by superintendents. She even suggested that matriculation through such a course should become a new membership requirement in the Society of Superintendents.[44]

In 1899, a graduate course in Hospital Economics in the Department of Domestic Science at Teachers College opened to two graduate nursing students. The 1-year program featured courses in biology, psychology, education, hospital economics, domestic sciences, and social science. As Robb described the contents of the program, "Some of these courses are intended especially to lay the foundation for a scientific theory of education; others are directed towards the practical work of teaching, and yet others seek to give the intending teacher a better knowledge of the subjects to be taught."[46] Leading public health nurses Lavinia Dock and Lillian Wald volunteered as faculty, and Mary Adelaide Nutting became the first professor of nursing when she took over as head of the Department of Household Administration at Teachers College in 1907.[47]

> "It is one thing to graduate as a trained nurse, but quite another thing to enter upon the duties and responsibilities of a training school."[45]
>
> Isabel Hampton Robb, 1898

The Nurses Associated Alumnae

The formation of the Nurses Associated Alumnae of the United States and Canada occurred as the result of the coordinated efforts of a steering committee from the Society of Superintendents. Discussion on the importance of a national organization for all graduate nurses had begun at the 1893 World's Columbian Exposition, with Edith Draper clarifying the goals of such a society. She said, "By a national association we mean a society with legal recognition, that every nurse who is a member of the same will be guaranteed for by the association and entitled to its benefits; and that we will be a recognized profession just as doctors are."[48] For 3 years, the Society of Superintendents advocated for the establishment of more alumnae associations, which would be the basis for the desired national association.

In September 1896, at the Manhattan Beach Hotel in Brooklyn, New York, 12 delegates from alumnae associations of various training schools met with 12 members of the Society of Superintendents to found the Nurses Associated Alumnae of the United States and Canada. Isabel Hampton Robb was elected the first president. The members drafted a constitution and bylaws, indicating the purpose of the new organization: to improve educational requirements for training programs; to foster collegiality among nurses; and to establish a code of ethics.[50] Membership eligibility rested on individual affiliation with an approved alumnae association. Only alumni associations from training programs that lasted at least 2 years and were connected to a hospital of at least 50 beds would be granted approval.[51] The latter requirement of affiliation with a larger hospital would inadvertently lead to discriminatory practices within the association, as most African American hospitals had fewer than 50 beds.

The Nurses Associated Alumnae experienced substantial growth over the next decade. At the first annual convention in 1898, organization members hailed from 23 different training school alumnae associations, but by 1912 that number had grown to 142 alumnae associations in 31 states.[53] By that time, members had changed the name to the ANA.

During the 1910s and 1920s, the ANA worked with individual state nurses' associations to legislate the registration of graduate nurses, while the curriculum committee concentrated on standardizing curricula in existing nurse training schools. The association's attempts to create a code of ethics proved to be more difficult, as they disagreed over content and wording.[54] The first "suggested" code of ethics would not be submitted for organizational approval until 1926, and an official code would not be adopted until 1950.

The American Journal of Nursing

Despite the struggle to establish a code of ethics, ANA leaders succeeded elsewhere. They were able to move nursing forward toward the status of a recognized profession with the creation of a nurse-controlled journal. The need for a written forum, in which nurses could freely share ideas and information across the profession, arose early within the organization. A Committee on Periodicals, which Robb had established in one of her first acts as president, reported, "No sooner had the Society of Superintendents been formed . . . than the need of a journal managed, edited, and owned by the women of the profession began to make itself felt."[56] Robb approached Lippincott Publishers to discuss costs in January 1900, and discovered the association needed to raise funds from a joint stock company before proceeding.[57] After generating enough capital from shareholders of the American Journal of Nursing Company, the first issue of the *American Journal of Nursing* was printed on October 1, 1900. Circulation for the initial publication totaled only 581, but would grow to more than 23,000 by 1928.[58]

Robb envisioned the Nurses Associated Alumnae someday owning and maintaining the journal. Ideally this would occur right after the association generated enough revenue to fund the transfer of the journal's ownership

Nursing Ethics

In 1900, Isabel Hampton Robb published *Nursing Ethics: For Hospital and Private Use*, the first formal text on the subject. The book detailed the expected behavior for the probationer, junior, senior, head, and graduate nurse. One chapter was dedicated to outlining the qualifications necessary for women entering nursing, stating that they must be, "fit and becoming . . . mentally, morally and physically well poised."[55] The book reaffirmed Victorian standards for ideal feminine behavior, with themes reflecting a blending of morality and etiquette.

from individual shareholders to the association as a whole. Some disagreement arose between Robb and editor Sophia Palmer, who felt the American Journal of Nursing Company should remain incorporated and turn a profit for the original shareholders. During the struggle, Robb lamented that they should "never make money out of a magazine for our [nursing's] own personal benefit."[60] After some political maneuvering on both sides, a Journal Purchase Fund was created in 1905 to expedite the process of transferring ownership back to the Nurses Associated Alumnae. By 1912 the fund had amassed enough money and bought all rights to the periodical.

Nursing and the Women's Suffrage Movement

The origins of the women's movement in the United States date back to July 1848, when a group of broad-minded ladies met in Seneca Falls, New York, to discuss the rights of American women. Drafting a "Declaration of Sentiment," Elizabeth Cady Stanton skillfully tied the burgeoning reform movement to the Declaration of Independence and argued that "all men and women are created equal . . . [but] the history of mankind is a history of repeated injuries and usurpations on the part of man toward woman, having in direct object the establishment of an absolute tyranny over her."[61] The Seneca Falls Convention highlighted a number of institutional and social barriers that restricted independence for women, including a lack of educational and economic opportunities, an inability to control their reproductive futures, and an absence of legal and legislative representation. In the wake of the Civil War, however, activists chose to focus solely on gaining the right to vote. Unfortunately, little momentum was gathered for the cause, even among women themselves. In 1902, Susan B. Anthony and Ida H. Harper lamented, "In the indifference, the inertia, the apathy of women, lies the greatest obstacle to their enfranchisement."[62]

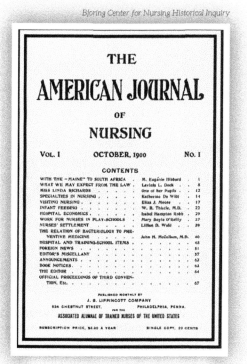

The first issue of the American Journal of Nursing, printed in 1900, which was created to share nursing ideas and information all across the profession.

"It will be the aim of the editors to present month by month the most useful facts, the most progressive thought, and the latest news that the profession has to offer."[59]

Sophia Palmer, 1900

The turning point came during the Progressive Era, as groups of educated middle-class citizens began reform campaigns aimed at improving a host of social problems. Inspired to political activism, "Progressives" sought to reform the nation at the local, state, and national levels by regaining control of their lives and their government. They believed that social problems such as racism, sexism, poverty, violence, and corporate greed could best be addressed by providing a good education, a clean living environment, and a safe workplace for all Americans. Viewing the government as a tool to be utilized for change, Progressives fought for housing and sanitation reform, federal inspection and regulation guidelines for consumer products, government oversight and intervention in big business, and an overhaul of labor practices. Labor reform drastically improved safety and decreased the exploitation of workers, particularly women and children. During this time, the campaign for women's suffrage finally gained the public support its early leaders had been seeking.

At the 1893 World's Columbian Exposition in Chicago, women found a welcome platform to highlight their current status in the United States. An entire Women's Building, designed by a female architect, sat prominently along the fairgrounds and showcased goods and services created by and for women. Bertha Palmer, president of the Board of Lady Managers for the World's Columbian Exposition, hoped to highlight the global

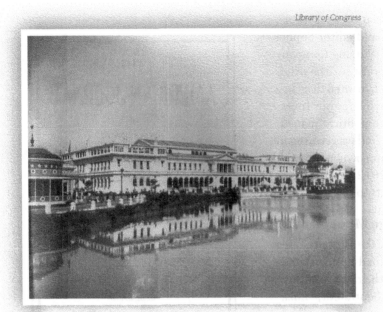

The Women's Building at the 1893 World's Columbian Exposition, which showcased the accomplishments and creations of women.

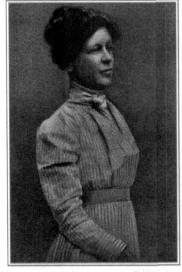

Lavinia Dock, an outspoken suffragist nurse.

"At the basis of all progress is the equality of citizens."[65]

Lavinia Dock, letter to
Isabel M. Stewart

struggles of women to achieve political, educational, legal, and economic equality. The ultimate goal was to provide an international forum for discussion of these issues. In her opening address, Palmer expressed her confidence that the fair would enable "the interchange of thought and sympathy among influential and leading women of all countries for the first time working together with a common purpose and an established means of communication."[63] Not surprisingly, the National Council of Women, a group concerned with the political and economic needs of women, used the World's Columbian Exposition as a meeting place to further the suffrage movement in the United States.

Initially, the major nursing organizations concerned themselves with issues specific to the profession. Early leaders focused on strengthening educational standards and uniting trained nurses across the country in an effort to elevate the overall status of nursing. As the issue of state registration moved to the forefront, however, nurses found themselves struggling to arouse interest from state legislators. Suddenly, the lack of voting rights for women had become a significant barrier to advancing the goals of nursing, or any other profession dominated by female workers. Lavinia Dock, the most outspoken of her colleagues on the issue of suffrage, gave her first of many opinions on the subject at the 1907 convention of the Nurses Associated Alumnae. She stated:

> [I] speak to you on a subject which is not strictly in the line of our profession but which presses itself upon me . . . I mean the subject of the political enfranchisement of women, which embraces the whole consideration of the many fields in which women are striving for a secure foothold, that they may live and express themselves and share those rights of life, liberty and the pursuit of happiness. . . . What I feel strongly is that our National Association might and should rise to a broader and more general consideration of large, general subjects than it has heretofore done.[64]

Not all nurses agreed with Dock nor supported the suffrage movement, and the issue came to a head at the 1908 annual convention of the Nurses Associated Alumnae in San Francisco. At the meeting, the president of the Women's Suffrage League requested that the association endorse "every well-directed movement which tends to emancipate the women of our land and give them their rightful place in government."[66] After only a brief discussion, the motion was dismissed by a large majority. Member reactions to the vote seemed mixed, although supporters of women's suffrage sent exceedingly critical letters to the editor of the *American Journal of Nursing*. Seeking to clarify the position of the journal, Sophia Palmer responded by stating:

The letters which are appearing in the Journal, and which come to the editors personally, on the suffrage question, are evidence of a misunderstanding of the Journal's position in this matter. This magazine is a professional journal, devoted to the interests of nursing. On every nursing subject it has a definite policy. On all other broad questions, its attitude is neutral.[67]

Palmer's reaction received as much criticism as the original vote. One nurse condemned, "As nurses, meeting all classes of people, we need all the *breadth* and *largeness* of vision we can get, and our Journal should be one of our chief sources for *getting*."[68]

Lavinia Dock expressed profound frustration with the whole situation, claiming she was disappointed for the first time with the Nurses Associated Alumnae since its founding. She outlined her beliefs on the women's suffrage movement by saying:

There are no reasons against political equality for women except selfish ones, and every good reason for it. . . . First, the patriotic reason: to deny the sacred duty of citizenship is to deny the foundation principle on which our democracy is built. As for the common sense reasons, they are on every hand. To help bring about more just and equal opportunities and equal pay for self-supporting women; to aid in the great child-saving crusade against the horrors of child labor; to carry good home-making and sanitary housekeeping into our city governments—why I could not count all the reasons![71]

Dock enthusiastically supported the campaign for equal voting rights, working to prepare for the 1913 New York City suffrage parade and joining the National Woman's Party. She led suffrage pickets from the National Woman's Party headquarters to the White House and was arrested on three separate occasions for participating in what were deemed "militant demonstrations."

"It is a significant fact that the same age that has produced the highly trained nurse has raised the cry of suffrage for women. The same evolutionary force that has moved womanhood to the intelligent combatting of disease and pain has impelled her also to study the remedying of every sort of public ill."[69]

M. Elena Dame, 1909

"As business or professional women we need to recognize the debt we owe to the women who have done things before us."[70]

Ada M. Stafford, 1908

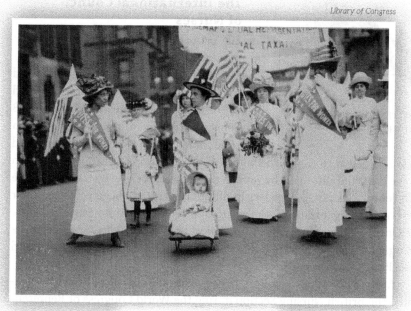

Library of Congress

New York Suffrage Parade of 1913.

Lavinia Dock Gets Arrested

Lavinia Dock was arrested multiple times, the most notable being after a months-long picketing campaign in front of the White House as one of the "Silent Sentinels." In August 1917 Dock and five other women were sentenced to a 30-day incarceration at Occuquan Workhouse in Virginia. The experience gave Dock an insider's perspective on the horrors of prison confinement, and she used her position and knowledge of public health to speak out against the unsanitary conditions affecting all inmates.

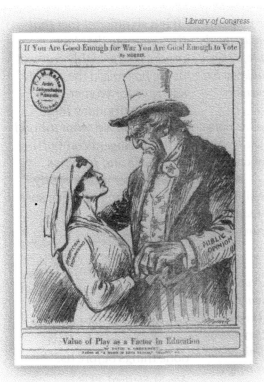

Finally, in 1915 the ANA officially endorsed the women's suffrage movement, passing the following resolution during its 18th annual convention:

WHEREAS, the enfranchisement of women—the recognition of the political rights of one-half the people of the United States to have a voice in the decision of questions of vital interest to them, such as peace and war, child labor, marriage and divorce, community property, etc.—is the foremost issue of the day; Therefore, be it resolved, that the American Nurses Association in convention assembled in San Francisco, June 25, 1915 endorse the Susan B. Anthony Amendment . . . and urge its passage by the 64th Congress.[72]

Five more years passed before women across the entire country legally possessed the right to vote. World War I had a profound impact on the suffrage movement, as women played a major role on the home front throughout the conflict. The heroic actions of nurses on the battlefield also were frequently cited as evidence in favor of granting voting rights to women. A drawing in the *Brooklyn Magazine* proclaimed, "If you are good enough for war you are good enough to vote."[73] The struggle to ratify the Nineteenth Amendment, which guaranteed U.S. citizens the right to vote regardless of their sex, lasted for years in both the U.S. Congress and state legislatures. Finally, on August 26, 1920, the amendment officially became part of the U.S. Constitution.

The International Council of Nurses

The primary sentiments of the women's movement—equal rights and representation for all citizens—spread far beyond the borders of the United States. Inspired by the message first presented at the 1848 Seneca Falls Convention and the strength to be gained through unity, women around

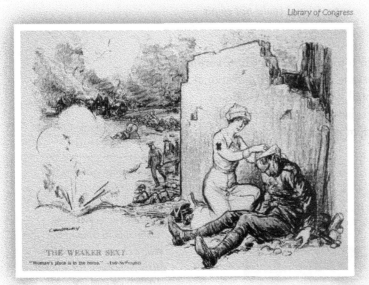

Drawings showing the positive effect of battlefront nurses' bravery helped further the cause of the suffrage movement.

"What could be more natural than that the women of all nations whose earthly work has to do with healing should aspire to forge a link?"[74]

Ethel Gordon Fenwick, 1901

the world began to establish their own organizations, seeking recognition for the contributions made by women throughout society. By the turn of the 20th century, as nursing leaders in different countries began creating their own national organizations, the vision of professional unity expanded globally. Once again amid the backdrop of world's fairs, the idea for a new nursing organization materialized, this time in the heart of British suffragist and nurse Ethel Gordon Fenwick.

At the 1893 World's Columbian Exposition in Chicago, Fenwick represented the British Nursing Section during the World Congress of Representative Women held by the National Council of Women. A year earlier, Fenwick had traveled to the United States to plan for the convention, where she met with Isabel Hampton and Lavinia Dock at the Johns Hopkins Training School for Nurses. Discussing the challenges facing nurses in their respective countries, Fenwick, Hampton, and Dock found common ground regarding the low social status of nursing, the lack of educational standards, and the exploitation of student labor by hospitals.[75] Fenwick would later recall that "the seed of the International Nursing movement, now so full of vitality, was then sown."[76]

Returning to the United Kingdom, Fenwick began writing about the ways she believed American nursing was superior, pushing her agenda for collaboration among nations as a way to strengthen the profession throughout the world. As nurse historians Nancy J. Tomes and Geertje Boschma explain:

> Fenwick saw the virtues of international combination largely in terms of strengthening the reformers' positions within their respective nations. By sharing ideas and strategies, they might better craft their national crusades to uplift nursing. If one country achieved a superior educational standard or legal protection for nurses, all the rest might cite it in their own battles, appealing to the spirit of national rivalry. In this fashion, international communication and cooperation would advance the whole of the nursing profession.[78]

After the meeting of the International Council of Women in London in 1899, Fenwick's goal was finally realized. Appointed to lead the council's professional section, Fenwick gathered leaders from various female professions to examine the contributions of women in the labor force. During a daylong session specifically on nursing, delegates from around the world discussed the overall status of the profession and supported "the greater strength which comes from union."[79] Once the meeting had adjourned, foreign nursing leaders were then invited to attend the second annual conference of the Matrons' Council of Great Britain and Ireland. Building on the momentum from the council's nursing section, Fenwick officially proposed the creation of an International Council of Nurses. She stated:

> I venture to contend that the work of nursing is one of humanity all the world over. . . . The work in which nurses are engaged in other countries is precisely the same as that in our own. The principles of organization would be the same in every country, the need for nursing progress is the same for every people, and my suggestion briefly is, therefore, that we should here and to-day inaugurate an International Council of Nurses, composed of representatives of the nursing councils of every country.[80]

A provisional committee was established and tasked with creating a constitution and bylaws, which were reviewed and ratified the following year. The purpose of the International Council of Nurses was twofold: to facilitate communication between nurses of all nations and to provide opportunities for these nurses to meet and discuss issues "relating to the welfare of their patients and their profession."[81] Members elected Fenwick as the council's first president, with Lavinia Dock appointed secretary and Canadian nurse Mary Agnes Snively treasurer. National nursing associations could join the council pending approval of the executive board, and the initial dues were 1 pound per year for each of the four delegates

---

"The future lies entirely in our hands. There may be associations of women for many causes, but none who may draw closer to the world's needs than that of the Trained Nurses' Association."[77]

Isabel Hampton Robb, 1899

"The nursing profession, above all things at present, requires organization; nurses, above all other things, at present require to be united."[83]

Ethel Gordon Fenwick, 1901

Preamble to the International Council's Constitution

"We, nurses of all nations, sincerely believe that the best good of our profession will be advanced by greater unity of thought and sympathy of purpose, do hereby band ourselves in a confederation of workers to further the efficient care of the sick, and to secure the honor and the interests of the nursing profession."[84]

chosen to represent their country on the International Council of Nurses' Grand Council.[82]

From the very beginning, Fenwick's aim was to see the International Council of Nurses organizing and uniting nurses from all over the world. Since only six countries were the first representative members—Great Britain, the United States, Canada, Australia, New Zealand, and Holland—extending the reach of the organization to "all over the world" would prove to be a lofty goal. Addressing this "ambitious scheme," in which Fenwick hoped to one day see "delegates of national councils from every civilized country on the face of the earth," she simply replied, "I like big things." Fenwick continued, "It is easy to predict that great importance will be attached to decisions arrived at by a body of nurses so representative of all shades of nursing opinion as those delegated to act on the International Council. It should ultimately become the deliberative assembly and supreme court of appeal to the nursing world."[85]

The delegates to the initial council were not only few in number, they also lacked diversity and shared a decidedly Anglo-American vision and mission. While nurses from Germany and Denmark also actively participated, the early essence of the International Council of Nurses mostly reflected the beliefs and values of nurses from England and its colonies.[86] The organization always aimed to elevate the status of professional nursing throughout the world, but "progress" was often measured through the lens of the mostly White Western women in leadership roles. Thus, their solutions to problems frequently reflected contemporary notions of colonialism, social elitism and class stereotypes, and racial and religious segregation. The International Council of Nurses was not unique in these circumstances, as the same could be said of many national and international organizations of the time. But as nurse historians Joan Lynaugh and Barbara Brush noted: "Nursing, so intimate in its work, faithfully mirrors both the unattractive and the uplifting aspects of the human experience."[87]

This is not to say that the International Council of Nurses failed to produce meaningful change in its first few decades. In fact, the organization made great progress in encouraging the exchange of ideas among nurses of different nations despite the inherent travel and communication challenges facing its members. The council had no base of operations, and delegates were individually responsible for expenses incurred traveling to and from international meetings. Official conferences were held only every 5 years, with one interim meeting usually held between the quinquennial gatherings. All communication between members and elected officials occurred via letter, and could be hampered by language barriers. Prior to the interim meeting in Paris of 1907, Lavinia Dock encouraged delegates to "put [their] pennies by and rub up on [their] French."[88]

The first few International Council of Nurses congresses were committed to developing nursing journals, improving educational standards, and encouraging states to regulate the title of professional nurse. At the 1907 Conference in Paris, France, Fenwick hosted an international press dinner, in which she invited the editors of major nursing publications to gather and discuss how best to promote the science and image of nursing. The editors represented prominent journals from a number of different countries, including the *British Journal of Nursing*, the *American Journal of Nursing*, *Unterm Lazaruskreuz*, and *La Garde-Malade Hôspitaliére*.[90] At the suggestion of Isabel Hampton Robb, an International Standing Committee on Education was formed at the interim

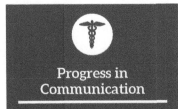

Progress in Communication

Well into the 19th century, the exchange of personal communication continued to be slow, taking days, weeks, or even months to reach far-off locations. The invention and mass availability of the telegraph and telephone in the late 19th and early 20th centuries dramatically improved individual messaging. Telegraph usage, which peaked at the turn of the 20th century, faded with the advent of the telephone, which enabled instantaneous communication. Telephones became more widely available after World War I with the development of a government-sponsored national telephone network and the completion of a transcontinental telephone line.

"We hope to unite ourselves in professional bonds with those of our own guild in other countries and become identified with women's work at large all over the world."[89]

Isabel Hampton Robb, 1900

congress in 1909. Delegates tasked this group with gathering information on the standard preparation of new graduate nurses in each of the affiliated countries. The eventual goal would be to develop a suggested standard curriculum and provide a unified definition of the training deemed necessary for successful nursing care. By the 1912 congress in Cologne, Germany, members moved their focus toward state registration and the fight for women's suffrage.

The outbreak of World War I halted progress at the International Council of Nurses. At the poorly attended 1915 interim Congress meeting in San Francisco, acting president Annie Goodrich lamented the "terrible tragedy" that had "cast such a shadow over everything."[92] During and immediately after the war, many of the international delegates were thrust into the conflict or were forced to deal with the resultant devastation in their home countries. As a result, the collegiality between members of the International Council of Nurses was severely interrupted, and a congress was not held for 10 years. By 1922, however, the organization had seen immense growth from its original founding group, with affiliated councils present in Belgium, Switzerland, India, Italy, Japan, South Africa, and China. All were dedicated to promoting health for citizens throughout the world.

The National Association of Colored Graduate Nurses

As professional nursing organizations gained social and political influence across the world, Black nurses struggled to find representation within and among these groups. All nurses in the United States faced similar problems, including widespread exploitation of students by hospital trustees, heterogeneous standards for nursing education, and overall low wages for graduates. But continued racial discrimination made these difficulties even more pronounced for Black nurses, who also faced restricted access to nursing education programs and job opportunities, received lower pay than White nurses, and saw alarming health disparities within their own communities.

Lack of representation for Black nurses in national organizations became yet another example of their marginalized status within the profession. Although the original membership requirements for the Society of Superintendents and the Nurses Associated Alumnae did not specifically preclude individual participation based on race, they did create barriers that disproportionately affected Black nurses. Initially, eligibility rested on membership in a recognized alumni association, which existed at very few exclusively Black training schools. Later, organizations limited acceptance to nurses belonging to state associations, which eliminated African American nurses from 16 southern states and the District of Columbia, as segregation laws in these areas prohibited them from taking registration examinations.[94] Since the majority of Black professional nurses lived and worked in southern states, they were effectively excluded from the more prominent nursing organizations, and left without a national platform to address their unique challenges. Even the Red Cross Nursing Service uniformly rejected the applications of African American nurses wishing to volunteer. Without the necessary Red Cross referral, Black nurses were then barred entry into the U.S. Army Nurse Corps.[95]

Concerned about the status of Black graduate nurses, Martha Minerva Franklin initiated an independent general study on the subject. In the fall of 1906, Franklin sent out 500 letters to graduate nurses, school superintendents, and nursing organizations, hoping to gather factual information to support the need for improvements in nursing

The 1912 Suffrage Resolution

"In the belief that the highest purposes of civilization and the truest blessings to the race can only be attained by the equal and united labours of men and women possessing equal and unabridged political powers, we declare our adherence to the principle of Woman Suffrage, and regard the Suffrage Movement as a great moral movement making for the conquest of misery, preventable illness and vice and as strengthening a feeling of human brotherhood."[91]

"It is not sufficient that the nurse should be the instrument for the relief of suffering; she must also be the harbinger of its prevention."[93]

Ethel Gordon Fenwick, 1909

education and employment opportunities for Black women.[96] Unfortunately, responses came slowly and were few in number, but Franklin was undeterred. No stranger to hard work and perseverance—she had been the only Black graduate in her class at the Women's Hospital Training School for Nurses in Philadelphia in 1897—Franklin remained committed to the cause. By 1907 she had collected enough feedback and determined the need for collective action. Franklin sent out another 1,500 letters, asking nurses to consider a national meeting to discuss the creation of an organization for Black nurses. Adah Belle Samuels Thoms, president of the Lincoln Hospital School of Nursing Alumnae Association, responded by sponsoring the meeting and inviting Franklin and all interested nurses to New York City. On August 25, 1908, 52 nurses met and formed the National Association of Colored Graduate Nurses (NACGN), the first association focused solely on the distinctive challenges facing African American nurses.[97]

"In man's struggle for liberty and truth, which are the outgrowth of social conditions, the burden is always borne by the few."[98]

Adah Belle Samuels Thoms, 1929

This first 3-day convention laid the foundation for the organization. After an opening address from Thoms, Franklin presented a paper outlining her study results. She discussed the merits of establishing a permanent national society to bring African American nurses together to promote higher educational standards and secure more professional, cooperative interaction with leaders of other nursing organizations. Attendees responded enthusiastically, and officially inaugurated the NACGN. Members established a constitution that outlined the group's purpose, bylaws, and code of ethics, then elected organizational leaders. Franklin was selected as the first president by acclamation. As outlined in its constitution, the objective of the association was, "To advance the standing and best interests of trained nurses, and to place the profession of nursing on the highest plane attainable."[99] The sole membership prerequisite was graduation from a recognized nurse training program, opening the group to all professional nurses regardless of race, class, or gender. After much deliberation, members agreed that the most pressing goals of the association were threefold: "To advance the standard and best interests of trained

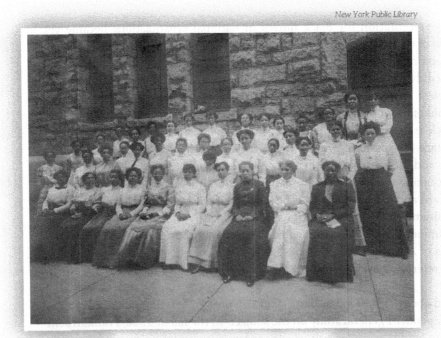

New York Public Library

The first meeting of the National Association of
Colored Graduate Nurses in 1908.

nurses; To break down discrimination in the nursing profession; and to develop leadership within the ranks of Negro [sic] nurses."[100]

In addition to the formation of the NACGN, the first meeting also included multiple sessions intended to promote education, research, and shared professional experiences. The papers presented covered a wide range of topics, and included "Community Nursing on St. Helena Island," "Obstetrical Nursing," "Professional Etiquette," "Settlement Work in New York City," "Massage," and "Training Schools for Nursing."[101] Much of the discussion centered on public health issues disproportionately affecting the African American population, namely, tuberculosis and high infant mortality. Most members understood and had themselves witnessed the effects of discriminatory practices in both northern and southern cities. Continued racial bias limited access to adequate housing and health care facilities for Black citizens, restricted job opportunities, and decreased available resources, which in turn aggravated many health problems in Black communities. Improving the overall health of African Americans became paramount to the organization. As the association's executive secretary Mabel K. Staupers remarked, "The members realized that if the health of [all] Americans were to be improved, every segment of the population must be given equal opportunity to receive adequate healthcare."[102]

Almost from the start, national and international nursing leaders recognized the important perspective and contributions of the NACGN and its members, with Lillian Wald and Lavinia Dock leading the way. On the last day of their 1908 meeting in New York, Wald hosted a luncheon at the Henry Street Settlement for association members, and continued providing support and mentorship over the years.[103] Dock took a vocal stance on race relations within the Nurses Associated Alumnae at its 13th convention in 1910, saying:

> I hope this association of nurses will never get to the point where it draws the color line against our sister Negro [sic] nurses, who are our sisters of the human race and are our coworkers in our profession . . . I do hope that in this one human problem, in dealing with the question of the negro race in America, that there, especially, we nurses will exercise and simply practice that one simple rule, to treat them as we would like to be treated ourselves.[104]

As secretary of the International Council of Nurses, Dock also invited the NACGN to select a delegate to represent the organization at the 1912 International Congress in Cologne, Germany, that year, facilitating contact with international nursing leaders for the first time. A collaborative relationship with the International Council of Nurses would continue for years, offering NACGN delegates a wider platform to discuss concerns specific to Black graduate nurses and encouraging cooperation among the various organizations.

Beginning in 1909, the association held annual conventions every August, the first in Boston, Massachusetts. Awareness of the organization began to spread to even the most rural regions, and by 1910, the conference boasted attendance from nurses in every section of the country.[105] Unfortunately, little constructive work occurred in the early years. Total membership remained low, and without a national headquarters, the significant distances between association members meant that most executive board meetings occurred via letter, thus limiting their ability to enact significant change. Things began to turn around after World War I, and by 1920 membership had grown to a total of 500 members. Most importantly, progress had been made in the fight toward equal opportunities for Black graduate nurses. Thanks to the relentless efforts of then

"Not for Ourselves, but for Humanity."[106]

NACGN Motto, 1916

president Adah B. Thoms, the NACGN established a national registry for Black graduate nurses.

State Registration for African American Nurses

Private-duty registries gained traction across the United States at the turn of the 20th century, with the intention of connecting graduate nurses with the patients and physicians in need of their services. As hospitals moved away from hiring individual nurses in favor of using students from their affiliated nursing school, graduate nurses found themselves relying on word of mouth and reputation alone as a way of securing private-duty employment, which often proved difficult. Particularly in large cities, centralized registries gained popularity since they assumed basic credentialing responsibility and afforded more steady employment for their affiliated nurses.[107] Alumni associations, commercial employment agencies, medical societies, and libraries all began to establish centralized registries, offering their services to graduate nurses for a fee. The situation was fraught with the potential for exploitation, and a number of nursing leaders cautioned against registries that were not organized and controlled by nurses themselves. State legislation seemed an obvious next step as a means of protecting the public as well as local nurses.

State nurses' societies, begun in 1901, established guidelines for nursing education, registration, and practice. Official legislation began in 1903, first passed in North Carolina and quickly spread across the county, with 40 states approving registration laws by 1914.[108] Each state set its own standards for registration and licensure, but most required that a nurse graduate from an approved training program and then pass an evaluation given by the state board of nurse examiners. Early licensing exams often contained both a written and a practical component, and the board of examiners usually included a combination of nurses and physicians. Because states determined their own qualifications and regulations, Black nurses frequently suffered legal racial discrimination. Some states outright refused to allow African Americans to sit for nurse registry examinations, while others administered a different test and awarded Black nurses a separate "Negro" license. Both scenarios drastically restricted employment opportunities and promoted unequal pay for African American nurses.

As early as 1909, the NACGN recognized that having states register nurses was a pressing issue for the nursing community, thus they actively fought for standard examination requirements across the country. Standards would succeed not only in eliminating the double standard for African American graduate nurses, but also in promoting the elevation of educational guidelines at traditionally Black nursing programs to conform to state licensure eligibility requirements.[109] One charter member of the association, Ludie Andrews, famously fought for equal registration opportunities for Black nurses in her home state of Georgia, where she was denied a license based on her race. In 1909, Andrews took legal action against the Georgia State Board of Nurse Examiners for their policy of administering separate examinations and certificates to African American nurses. According to nurse historian Darlene Clark Hine, Andrews believed that "the board's policy of issuing certificates to Black nurses based upon different standards and procedures from those applied to white examinees diminished their chances for employment by in effect branding them as inferior members of the profession . . . [and] that the special Negro certification granted to the state's Black nurses made it difficult for them to secure postgraduate education and employment in other states."[110] Andrews battled for racial equality for more than 10 years, even refusing the state's offer of an individual license. Finally, in 1920 she won the right for all nurses in Georgia to take the same licensing examination.

Despite this victory, many African American graduate nurses continued to face economic and professional uncertainty because of discriminatory legislative policies in state registration. In 1917, the NACGN began focusing its efforts toward a national registry for Black nurses. Addressing the National Medical Association, an organization specifically for Black physicians, in August of that year, association president Adah Thoms stated:

> The National Association of Colored Graduate Nurses proposes to establish a national registry which will be open to graduate, registered nurses only. This registry will be the means of aiding doctors and the public in securing the best nurses with the least exertion, and will likewise be a means of helping the nurses to secure desirable positions. Our object in establishing this registry is to raise the standard of nursing, for if doctors will employ only the best nurses, then only those who are determined to be the very best will enter the profession.[111]

At the association's 10th annual meeting in 1917, members elected a committee to form such a registry. By the next year Thoms reported that 12 nurses had received work as a direct result of the project.[112]

"We Are Moving Steadily Forward"

"As we look back over the years and see the progress that has been made by our race in the medical and nursing professions we are filled with pride to know that, despite the handicaps that beset us on every side, we are moving steadily forward . . . there is no power outside of ourselves that can keep us from sharing with the rest of mankind the liberty and freedom for which democracy stands."[113]

Adah Belle Samuels Thoms, 1917

Physician Response to Nursing Professionalization

The creation of national and international nursing organizations was not universally well-received, particularly by physicians. Both nursing leaders and prominent doctors of the time endorsed the notion of the ideal nurse as loyal and faithfully obedient to physicians. Consistent with the belief that nurses were skilled assistants, the physician was "primarily and ultimately responsible for the life and health of the patient" while the nurse's sole duty was "to obey orders, and so long as she does this, she is not to be held responsible for untoward results."[114] Medical leaders continually reinforced this tradition through endless papers and lectures. Even nursing school graduation speeches outlined the role of the nurse in relation to her superiors. Dr. Henry M. Hurd became a willing speaker at a number of graduation ceremonies, depicting nurses as "a physician's hands lengthened out to minister to the sick."[115] A clear hierarchy had been established in the delivery of care, and doctors refused to relinquish any of the social, legal, and professional authority they had fought so hard to acquire.

A number of physician leaders vigorously discredited early attempts by nursing organizations to gain professional independence and distinction at the turn of the 20th century. An article in the *New York Medical Journal* in April 1906 outlined the medical response to the notion of nursing as a true profession:

> A fundamental error obtains in attempting to designate the occupation of a nurse as a profession. It is a profession in no proper sense of the word, which "implies professed attainments in special knowledge, as distinguished from mere skill" (Century Dictionary). The work of a nurse is an honorable calling or vocation, and nothing further. It implies the exercise of acquired proficiency in certain more or less mechanical duties and is not primarily designed to contribute to the sum of human knowledge or the advancement of science.[116]

The author of the article, Dr. W. Gilman Thompson, had written an extensive history of the first American nurse training schools 20 years earlier, and still believed that the programs had produced immeasurable benefits to patients and hospitals. However, as nursing leaders began to advocate for state registry and a standardized curriculum, which included theoretical instruction in many of the courses taken by medical students, physicians criticized the need for either. Calling state registration "a folly with such a simple matter as nursing," Thompson stressed the danger of "a little knowledge" leading to "the overtrained nurse usurping much of the work which ought to be done by the house staff [medical residents]."[117] He urged his colleagues to demand physician involvement and oversight in the system of nurse training. Most importantly, Thompson believed that medicine needed to limit the scope of nurse study and practice. In fact, the debate on whether nursing fit the distinction of a true "profession" would endure for decades, and attempts by the medical profession to constrain nursing scope of practice continue even today.

However, contemporary realities in the early 20th-century United States demanded a well-trained and cohesive nursing profession to respond to the health needs of a nation undergoing dramatic transformations. Rapidly shifting social, political, and economic forces throughout the Progressive Era created a host of new challenges that directly affected the health of American citizens, both as individuals and as a whole. More than ever, organization and preparation would be needed for nurses to continue to advance health in the face of changing national demographics, revolutionary scientific discoveries and technological innovation, and new professional opportunities in a growing industrial economy.

For Discussion

1. How did Clara Barton become involved in the International Red Cross movement? What was the American Amendment and how did this affect the scope of American Red Cross relief efforts?
2. What were some of the key public health measures taken by the Red Cross during its response to the Johnstown Flood in 1889?
3. In what ways did the first nursing organizations hope to advance the profession of nursing? Describe specific improvements made by the NLNE, ANA, and NACGN.
4. Describe the impact of nurse participation in the women's suffrage movement. Do you think national nursing organizations have a responsibility to engage in political and social reform movements?
5. What were some of the reasons behind the formation of the NACGN? How did the issue of state registration negatively affect Black graduate nurses, and what was the response from the NACGN?
6. Why were some physicians opposed to the creation of nursing organizations?

NOTES

1. Clara Barton, *The Red Cross: A History of This Remarkable International Movement in the Interest of Humanity* (Albany, NY: James B. Lyon, Printer and Binder, 1898): 13–14.

2. Ibid., 14.

3. Clyde E. Buckingham, *Clara Barton: A Broad Humanity* (Alexandria, VA: Mount Vernon Publishing, 1977): 103.

4. Barton, *The Red Cross*, 62.

5. Ibid., 61–62.

6. Ibid., 96–97.

7. Buckingham, *Clara Barton*, 128.

8. Buckingham, *Clara Barton*, 136.

9. David J. Beale, *Through the Johnstown Flood* (Philadelphia: Hubbard Brothers, 1890): 29.

10. Ibid.

11. Ibid.

12. "Horrors of Horrors," *The Pittsburg Dispatch* (June 1, 1889): 1.

13. Beale, *Through the Johnstown Flood*, 182–183.

14. Barton, *The Red Cross*, 157.

15. Ibid., 162.

16. Ibid., 160.

17. Beale, *Through the Johnstown Flood*, 173–174.

18. Figures courtesy the Johnstown Area Heritage Association, http://www.jaha.org/Flood Museum/facts.html (accessed August 28, 2016).

19. Barton, *The Red Cross*, 136; Willis Fletcher Johnson, *History of the Johnstown Flood* (Philadelphia: Edgewood Publishing Co., 1889): 311.

20. Frank Connelly and George C. Jenks, *Official History of the Johnstown Flood* (Pittsburgh, PA: Journalist Publishing, 1889): 181.

21. Patricia D'Antonio and Jean C. Whelan, "Moments: When Time Stood Still," *American Journal of Nursing* 104 (2004): 68.

22. David McCullough, *The Johnstown Flood* (New York: Simon and Schuster, 1968): 233.

23. Barton, *The Red Cross*, 156.

24. As quoted in Barton, *The Red Cross*, 168.

25. "Editorial Comment," *American Journal of Nursing* 6 (1905): 280.

26. Ibid., 281.

27. "Editorial Comment: National Red Cross," *American Journal of Nursing* 5 (1905): 647.

28. Figures courtesy the American Red Cross, http://www.redcross.org/about-us/who-we-are/history (accessed August 28, 2016).

29. "World War I and the American Red Cross," http://www.redcross.org/about-us/history/red-cross-american-history/WWI (accessed August 28, 2016).

30. Louise C. Selanders and Patrick Crane, "Florence Nightingale in Absentia: Nursing and the 1893 Columbian Exposition," *Journal of Holistic Nursing* 28 (2010): 305.

31. Letter from Isabel Hampton to Florence Nightingale, January 31, 1893, Baltimore, Maryland. Photostat copy courtesy the Alan Mason Chesney Medical Archives of the Johns Hopkins Medical Institutions.

32. Letter from Florence Nightingale to Isabel Hampton, February 23, 1893, London, England. Photostat copy courtesy the Alan Mason Chesney Medical Archives of the Johns Hopkins Medical Institutions.

33. Cynthia A. Connolly, "Hampton, Nutting, and Rival Gospels at The Johns Hopkins Hospital and Training School for Nurses, 1889-1906," *Image: Journal of Nursing Scholarship* 30 (1990): 24.

34. Isabel A. Hampton, "Educational Standards for Nurses," in *Nursing of the Sick 1893: Papers and Discussions from the International Congress of Charities, Correction, and Philanthropy, Chicago, 1893* (New York: McGraw-Hill, 1949): 5.

35. Edith A. Draper, "Necessity of an American Nurses' Association," in *Nursing of the Sick 1893: Papers and Discussions from the International Congress of Charities, Correction, and Philanthropy, Chicago, 1893*, ed. Isabel A. Hampton (New York: McGraw-Hill, 1949): 149.

36. Janet Wilson James, "Isabel Hampton and the Professionalization of Nursing," in *Enduring Issues in American Nursing*, eds. Ellen D. Baer, Patricia D'Antonio, Sylvia Rinker, and Joan E. Lynaugh (New York: Springer Publishing, 2002): 71.

37. Lavinia Dock, "Recollections of Miss Hampton at the Johns Hopkins," *American Journal of Nursing* 11 (1910): 18.

38. Discussion on "The Benefits of Alumnae Associations," in *Nursing of the Sick 1893: Papers and Discussions from the International Congress of Charities, Correction, and Philanthropy, Chicago, 1893*, ed. Isabel A. Hampton (New York: McGraw-Hill, 1949): 157.

39. Isabel A. Hampton, "Introduction," in *First Words: Selected Addresses from the National League for Nursing 1894-1933*, eds. Nettie Birnbach and Sandra Lewenson (New York: National League for Nursing Press, 1991): xxvi.

40. Hampton, "Introduction," xxvii.

41. Sandra Lewenson, *Taking Charge: Nursing, Suffrage, and Feminism in America, 1873-1920* (New York: NLN Press, 1996): 61.

42. Ibid., 64.

43. Ibid., 66.

44. Isabel Hampton Robb, "Hospital Economics Course," in *Educational Standards for Nurses with Other Addresses on Nursing Subjects*, ed. Isabel Hampton Robb (Cleveland, OH: E.C. Koeckert, 1907): 127–134.

45. Ibid., 131.

46. Ibid., 130.

47. Lewenson, *Taking Charge*, 67.

48. Draper, "Necessity of an American Nurses' Association," 151.

49. Isabel McIsaac, "The Benefits of Alumnae Associations," in *Nursing of the Sick 1893: Papers and Discussions from the International Congress of Charities, Correction, and Philanthropy, Chicago, 1893*, ed. Isabel A. Hampton (New York: McGraw-Hill, 1949): 155.

50. Lorraine Freitas, "Historical Roots and Future Perspectives Related to Nursing Ethics," *Journal of Professional Nursing* 6 (1990): 197.

51. Lewenson, *Taking Charge*, 70.

52. Sophia Palmer, "Training School Alumnae Associations," *First and Second Annual Conventions of the American Society of Training Schools for Nurses* (Harrisburg, PA: Harrisburg Publishing, 1897): 56.

53. Lewenson, *Taking Charge*, 71.

54. Nancy Cadmus, "Ethics," *American Journal of Nursing* 16 (1916): 411–416.

55. Isabel Adams Hampton Robb, *Nursing Ethics: For Hospital and Private Use* (Cleveland, OH: E.C. Koeckert, 1900): 49.

56. As quoted in Blanche Pfefferkorn, "Improvement of the Nurse in Service: An Historical Review," *American Journal of Nursing* 28 (1928): 702.

57. Nancy Louise Noel, "Isabel Hampton Robb: Architect of American Nursing" (PhD dissertation, Teacher's College, Columbia University, 1978): 178.

58. Pfefferkorn, "Improvement of the Nurse in Service," 702.

59. "The Editor," *American Journal of Nursing*, 1 (1900): 64.

60. As quoted in Noel, "Isabel Hampton Robb," 180.

61. Seneca Falls Convention, "Declaration of Sentiments," in *The Concise History of Woman Suffrage*, eds. Mari Jo Buhle and Paul Buhle (Chicago: University of Illinois Press, 1978): 94.

62. Susan B. Anthony and Ida H. Harper, *The History of Woman Suffrage* (Indianapolis, IN: Hollenbeck Press, 1902): xxiv.

63. Bertha Palmer, "Address on the Occasion of the Opening of the Woman's Building, May 1, 1893," in *The Congress of Women*, ed. Mary Kavanaugh Oldham Eagle (Chicago: Monarch Book, 1894): 25.

64. Lavinia Dock, "Some Urgent Social Claims," *American Journal of Nursing* 7 (1907): 899–900.

65. Lavinia L. Dock, letter to Isabel M. Stewart, Feb. 2, 1951, as quoted in Teresa Christy, "Equal Rights for Women: Voices from the Past," *American Journal of Nursing* 71 (1971): 292.

66. "Proceedings of the Eleventh Annual Convention of the Nurses Associated Alumnae of the United States," *American Journal of Nursing* 8 (1908): 860.

67. "Editorial Comment," *American Journal of Nursing* 8 (1908): 956–957.

68. Ada M. Stafford, "The Suffrage," *American Journal of Nursing* 9 (1909): 359–360.

69. M. Elma Dame, "The Suffrage," *American Journal of Nursing* 9 (1909): 284.

70. Stafford, "The Suffrage," 360.

71. Lavinia L. Dock, "The Suffrage Question," *American Journal of Nursing* 8 (1908): 926.

72. "Proceedings of the Eighteenth Annual Convention of the American Nurses' Association," *American Journal of Nursing* 15 (1915); 1062.

73. "If You Are Good Enough for War You Are Good Enough to Vote," drawing by Morris, the *Brooklyn Magazine*, November 10, 1917. Image courtesy the Library of Congress.

74. Ethel Gordon Fenwick, "The International Council of Nurses: A Message from Its President," *American Journal of Nursing* 1 (2901): 786.

75. Nancy J. Tomes and Geertje Boschma, "Above all Other Things—Unity," in *Nurses of All Nations: A History of the International Council of Nurses, 1899-1999*, eds. Barbara L. Brush, Joan E. Lynaugh, Geertje Boschma, Anne Marie Rafferty, Meryn Stuart, and Nancy J. Tomes (Philadelphia: Lippincott Williams & Wilkins, 1999): 12–13.

76. As quoted in Tomes and Boschma, "Above all Other Things—Unity," 12.

77. Isabel Hampton Robb, "The Organisation of Trained Nurses' Alumnae Associations," in *Women in Professions: Being the Professional Section of the International Congress of Women, London, July 1899* (London: T. Fisher Unwin, 1900): 32.

78. Tomes and Boschma, "Above all Other Things—Unity," 14.

79. Mary Agnes Snively, "Discussion of Trained Nurses' Alumnae Associations," in *Women in Professions: Being the Professional Section of the International Congress of Women, London, July 1899* (London: T. Fisher Unwin, 1900): 33.

80. Fenwick, "The International Council of Nurses," 788.

81. Lavinia Dock, "The International Council of Nurses," *American Journal of Nursing*, 1 (1900): 115.

82. Ibid., 116.

83. Fenwick, "The International Council of Nurses," 787.

84. Ibid., 788.

85. Ibid., 789.

86. Tomes and Boschma, "Above all Other Things—Unity," 3.

87. Joan E. Lynaugh and Barbara L. Brush, "About This History," in *Nurses of All Nations: A History of the International Council of Nurses, 1899-1999*, eds. Barbara L. Brush, Joan E. Lynaugh, Geertje Boschma, Anne Marie Rafferty, Meryn Stuart, and Nancy J. Tomes (Philadelphia: Lippincott Williams & Wilkins, 1999): xiii.

88. As quoted in Daisy Caroline Bridges, *A History of the International Council of Nurses, 1899-1964: The First Sixty Five Years* (Philadelphia: J.B. Lippincott, 1967): 28.

89. Isabel Hampton Robb, "Address of the President," *American Journal of Nursing* 1 (1900): 103.

90. Bridges, *A History of the International Council of Nurses*, 29.

91. As quoted in Bridges, *A History of the International Council of Nurses*, 41.

92. As quoted in Bridges, *A History of the International Council of Nurses*, 50.

93. As quoted in Bridges, *A History of the International Council of Nurses*, 30.

94. Mabel K. Staupers, *No Time for Prejudice: A Story of the Integration of Negroes in Nursing in the United States* (New York: Macmillan, 1961): 17.

95. Lewenson, *Taking Charge*, 93.

96. Adah B. Thoms, *Pathfinders: A History of the Progress of Colored Graduate Nurses* (New York: Kay Printing House, 1929): 201.

97. Thoms, *Pathfinders*, 201.

98. Thoms, *Pathfinders*, 206.

99. Thoms, *Pathfinders*, 237.

100. Staupers, *No Time for Prejudice*, 17.

101. Althea Davis, *Early Black American Leaders in Nursing: Architects for Integration and Equality* (Boston: Jones & Bartlett, 1999): 79.

102. Staupers, *No Time for Prejudice*, 19.

103. Davis, *Early Black American Leaders in Nursing*, 90–91.

104. "Thirteenth Annual Convention of the Nurses Associated Alumnae of the United States: Minutes of the Proceedings," *American Journal of Nursing* 10 (1910): 902.

105. Thoms, *Pathfinders*, 207.

106. Thoms, *Pathfinders*, 226.

107. Jean C. Whelan, "'A Necessity in the Nursing World': The Chicago Nurses' Professional Registry 1913-1950," *Nursing History Review* 13 (2005): 49–75.

108. Darlene Clark Hine, *Black Women in White: Racial Conflict and Cooperation in the Nursing Profession, 1890-1950* (Indianapolis: Indiana University Press, 1989): 91.

109. Davis, *Early Black American Leaders in Nursing*, 87–88.

110. Hine, *Black Women in White*, 93.

111. Thoms, *Pathfinders*, 214.

112. Lewenson, *Taking Charge*, 92.

113. Thoms, *Pathfinders*, 215–216.

114. Isabel Adams Hampton Robb, *Nursing Ethics: For Hospital and Private Use* (Cleveland, OH: E.C. Koeckert, 1900): 250.

115. Henry M. Hurd, "Inauguration of the Johns Hopkins Training School for Nurses," *The Johns Hopkins Hospital Bulletin* 1 (December 1889): 7.

116. W. Gilman Thompson, "The Overtrained Nurse," *New York Medical Journal* 83 (1906): 845.

117. Thompson, "The Overtrained Nurse," 846.

FURTHER READING

Barton, Clara, *The Red Cross* (Albany, NY: James B. Lyon Printer and Binder, 1898).

Brush, Barbara L., Joan E. Lynaugh, Geertje Boschma, Anne Marie Rafferty, Meryn Stuart, and Nancy J. Tomes, *Nurses of All Nations: A History of the International Council of Nurses, 1899-1999* (Philadelphia: Lippincott Williams & Wilkins, 1999).

James, Janet Wilson, "Isabel Hampton and the Professionalization of Nursing," in *Enduring Issues in American Nursing*, eds. Ellen D. Baer, Patricia D'Antonio, Sylvia Rinker, and Joan E. Lynaugh (New York: Springer Publishing, 2002): 42–84.

Lewenson, Sandra, *Taking Charge: Nursing, Suffrage, and Feminism in America, 1873-1920* (New York: NLN Press, 1996).

McCullough, David, *The Johnstown Flood* (New York: Simon and Schuster, 1968).

Thoms, Adah B., *Pathfinders: A History of the Progress of Colored Graduate Nurses* (New York: Kay Printing House, 1929).

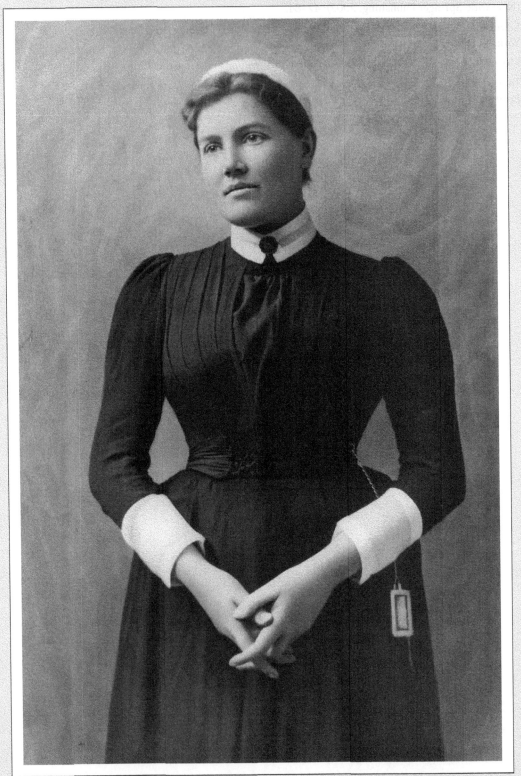

Isabel Hampton Robb.

CHAPTER 6

Organization and Innovation in the Early 20th Century

1898–1928

Arlene W. Keeling

"The past two years have shown the need for organization . . . for one can hardly doubt that the nursing of our soldiers during the Spanish–American war would naturally have fallen into our hands had our professional organization been completed earlier. . . . Today the need for a better organization of the nursing forces on a modern basis . . . is being as plainly demonstrated . . . as it was in the late Spanish American War."[1]

Speaking before an assembly of nurses at the Annual Convention of the Nurses Associated Alumnae on May 3, 1900, President Isabel Hampton Robb advised the audience to examine the state of nursing to better meet the needs of the profession and the public. It was the dawn of the 20th century and the fledgling nursing profession faced new challenges. In her speech, Robb called for the organization of military nursing, recalling the problem of finding nurses for service in the Spanish–American War just 2 years earlier. Next, Robb went on to justify both state registration and nursing licensure, describing how licensure could address the problem of distinguishing the "genuine trained nurse" from other "untrained nurses" who, as Robb put it, were "bringing private duty into bad odor."[2] Each of these issues was set in the context of changes at the turn of the 20th century, a period in which innovations in science, the rise of hospitals, discoveries of new drugs, natural and man-made disasters, racial discrimination, and the rapid industrialization of sections of the country presented both challenges and new opportunities to the profession.

ORGANIZATIONAL INITIATIVES AND REGISTRATION

One of the first challenges that the profession would face was that of supplying nurses for the war with Spain. That would be followed by the development of the Army and Navy Nurse Corps, an initiative identified as a solution to the problems of supplying nurses for future wars. Concurrent with these developments was the rising cry for the public registration of nurses—a proposal to protect the public from unlicensed and ill-prepared practitioners. Meanwhile, as the profession dealt with these issues, it also had to address the realities of private duty nursing and the need for specialized care for crippled and deformed children.

Nursing in the Spanish–American War

The Spanish–American War to which Robb referred had begun on April 25, 1898, and ended only a few months later on August 12, 1898. While 2,910 American military personnel died during the war, just 345 of those deaths occurred in combat. The remainder died of disease; more than 2,800 members of the regular army were devastated by diarrhea, dysentery, typhoid fever, yellow fever, and malaria. The military had been desperate for trained nurses to care for the soldiers,[3] as there were no *female* military nurses in the United States in 1898. In fact, the first uniformed trained nurses who served in the U.S. Navy during the Spanish–American war were *male* nurses who had graduated from New York City's Mills School for Men at Bellevue Hospital. The Mills school was one of the few general nursing programs in the country exclusively for men.[4] To make matters worse, no central organizing system within the military existed in 1898 to enlist nurses who did volunteer. In an effort to address this need, Isabel Robb, then president of the American Society of Superintendents of Training Schools, suggested "the Society offer itself to the government as the agent through which more and skilled nurses might be reliably secured."[5] Robb was too late in making the offer, however. By the time she visited Washington to discuss the matter, she discovered that U.S. Surgeon General George Sternberg had already placed physician Anita Newcomb McGee, vice president of the National Society of the Daughters of the American Revolution, in charge of selecting nurses for the army. McGee in turn had already established her own standards for the nurses' selection and suggested that the Daughters of the American Revolution act as an application review board. Thus, the Hospital Corps was founded, with McGee as its director.

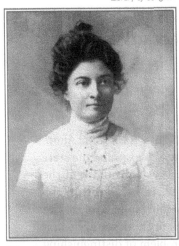

Physician Anita McGee, who set the standard for wartime nurses in the Spanish-American War and led the Hospital Corps.

Fortunately, McGee had set the standards high, insisting that any nurse who applied to serve in the war present a certificate of graduation from a training school for nurses. Nearly 5,000 women applied. Those who met the qualification of being a trained nurse between the ages of 30 and 50 years, and had submitted both a character reference and a certificate of good health, were put on a reserve list. They would be called when needed and hired under an army contract.[6]

The first "contract" nurses were appointed on May 10, 1898, and ordered to the General Hospital in Key West, Florida.[7] A month later, the United States entered the war in Cuba after U.S. Marines captured Guantánamo Bay and 17,000 troops landed at Daiquiri Siboney, the second largest city on the island.

Working outside military lines of authority, Red Cross director Clara Barton sailed from Florida to Cuba to help the citizens of Santiago. Barton's experience in the Civil War had given her "first-hand knowledge of the inefficiency of the governmental war machine" and she had no doubt that the supplies of firewood, flour, bandages, and clothes that she carried would be needed.[8] Her prediction was correct. On her arrival on July 1, Barton found scarce provisions and deplorable conditions for the care of the sick.

For the next 2 weeks, Clara Barton and the Red Cross nurses worked with the army staff to care for the sick and wounded in American and Cuban hospitals on the beaches of Daiquiri Siboney.[10] The Santiago troops were succumbing to yellow fever, a disease that caused the patient to exhibit "a high fever, often soaring to 104 degrees, flushed face, bloodshot eyes, and shaking chills" along with severe pain in the back and extremities.[11] The patient's recovery depended on "complete bed rest and stringent nursing care"—consisting of anything from the administration of mustard baths, laxatives, blistering, and cupping—to the "gentler approaches" of liquid nourishment, sponge baths, and waiting."[12] Nurses were urgently needed and Surgeon General Sternberg's mission was to find them.

Responding to the demand, Sternberg expanded his search for nurses to include African Americans, enlisting the help of five nurses from the Tuskegee Institute in Alabama. He also accepted the services of African American nurses from

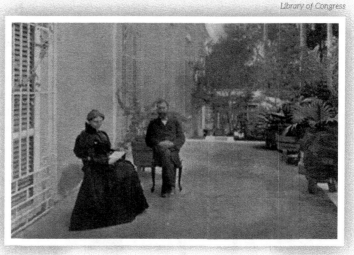

Clara Baron, director of the Red Cross, in Cuba.

"Men with fevers and flesh wounds were lying on coarse stubble grass in the tropical sun with no covering over them."[9]

Clara Barton, 1898

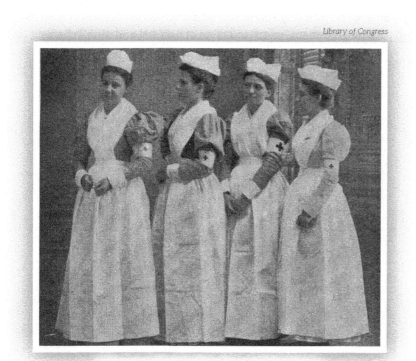

Nurses cared for the sick and wounded during the Spanish–American War.

"In view of the outbreak of yellow fever at Santiago . . . am now sending immune nurses, both male and female, for duty at the yellow fever hospitals."

George M. Sternberg, July 1898

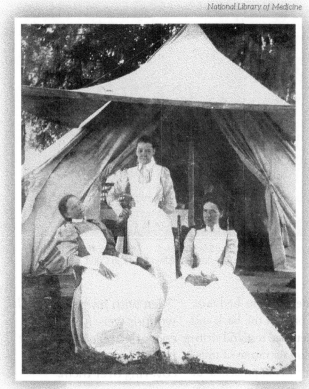

Nurses in front of a yellow fever hospital.

New Orleans—even those with no formal training. As survivors of the seasonal plagues of yellow fever that had long affected communities of the Deep South, Black nurses were considered to have special immunity to the disease, and thus were preferable to White nurses in the care of patients with yellow fever.[13] Thirty-two Black nurses volunteered.

To expand its ranks, the military also accepted nurses from Catholic Sisterhoods *despite* the fact that many were not graduates of nurse training schools. Of the 282 sisters who volunteered, including several from the Sisters of Mercy and the Sisters of the Holy Cross, 189 were from the Daughters of Charity.[14] With Providence Hospital in Washington, DC, as the nursing distribution center, the Daughters of Charity went to military hospitals throughout the United States. In most cases they were received with gratitude; their reputation for organization, order, and good work had preceded them.[15]

Twelve Sisters of the Holy Cross traveled from their motherhouse in Indiana to the Third Division Hospital at Camp Hamilton in Lexington, Kentucky. On arrival they found 600 men sick, one third of them with typhoid fever. The typhoid ward had minimal supplies, and the work was demanding. Battling typhoid fever required careful management of the ward environment, and the Sisters of the Holy Cross adapted two basic measures to stop the spread of the disease: "isolation and cleanliness."[17] Providing direct care was critical: The Sisters sponged feverish patients, fed them "restricted diets of beef tea and milk," changed linen,

"Well! At last I have gone to war, but this is not a war with Cuba but war with the typhoid cases!"[16]

Sister Valentina Reid, 1898

Experience in Coamo, Puerto Rico, 1898

"The nurses quartered in an old Spanish house . . . located in a banana grove. We drove to camp in mule ambulances. Put in long hours. . . . All water for any purpose hauled in barrels from a spring more than a mile away. Tents crowded—typhoid fever, dysentery and diarrhea— conditions bad: no ice, no diet kitchen."[19]

American Red Cross field nurse, 1898

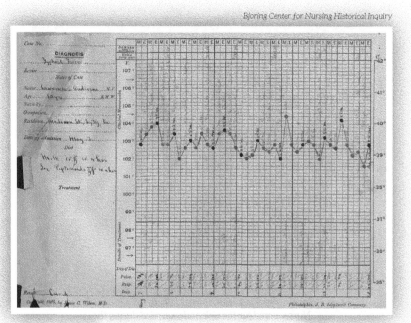

Fever chart for a patient with typhoid fever.

Clara Maass and the Mosquito Theory

Dr. Carlos Finlay's mosquito theory would be proven with the help of Clara Maass, a nurse from New Jersey who volunteered to be bitten by an infected mosquito while she collaborated with the international team in Cuba working to conquer yellow fever. Maass died in the experiment to prove the transmission theory. Her death confirmed that the mosquito was the vector of yellow fever.[22]

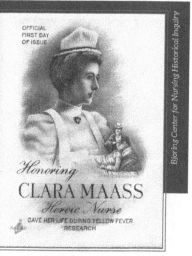

Clara Maass, who collaborated in the research on yellow fever.

and applied liniment to the patients' sore muscles to relieve the pain. Much of their time was spent taking temperatures and recording vital signs.[18]

Besides working in hospitals in the continental United States, the Sisters of the Holy Cross helped transport sick soldiers by ship from Puerto Rico back to the U.S. mainland. While in Puerto Rico, in addition to their work, the Sisters had to deal with both reptiles and insects, the worst of which were the mosquitoes. Sister Brendan recounted that experience, writing: "at night we were entertained by lizards, fleas, bedbugs and mosquitoes . . . fat enough to fry after feasting on us for two weeks!"[20] Unknown to the nurses and others at that time, mosquitoes were, in fact, the cause of the epidemic. Just 2 years later, U.S. Army physician Walter Reed proved that the mosquito was the carrier of yellow fever, accepting the theory originally proposed by Dr. Carlos Finlay in 1881.[21]

More than 1,700 female nurses served in general and field division hospitals during the 10-week-long Spanish–American War. Through their work they demonstrated the importance of trained nursing, organization, personal character, intelligent performance, and "executive ability, skill, and tact" to restoring soldiers to health.[23]

"Every medical officer with whom they [nurses] served has testified to their intelligence, and skill, their earnestness, devotion and self-sacrifice."[24]

Surgeon General
George M. Sternberg, 1899

The Army Nurse Corps

While most contract nurses had been subject to army control and regulations during the war with Spain, others had been paid by private sources and were under the control of private individuals and voluntary organizations, including the Daughters of the American Revolution and the American Red Cross. The arrangement, particularly the lack of a direct line of authority for the nurses, caused complicated administrative problems. As one contract nurse said of her stay in Tampa, Florida: "There seemed to be no organization. One never knew what would become of one next. All one's service seemed haphazard."[25] After the war, one thing was clear: The role of the army nurse had to be defined and regulated.

Determined to address this issue, Dr. Anita McGee, Isabel H. Robb, Anna Maxwell (chief nurse at the camp hospital of Chickamauga Park, Georgia), and Adelaide Nutting (nurse educator) used their influence to obtain federal legislation that would ensure a standing nursing service for the military. Congress passed the bill in 1901, establishing the Army Nurse Corps.[26] Appointed for 3-year periods, the nurses would serve under the Army Medical Department.

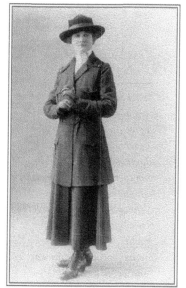

A member of the Army Nurse Corps, which was created in 1901.

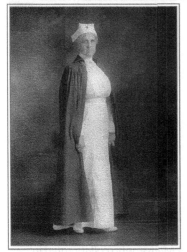

Jane Delano, superintendent of the Army Nurse Corps and later chairman of the National Committee on Red Cross Nursing Services.

Consistent leadership in the Army Nurse Corps was important and would change only once in the next decade. On March 15, 1901, Dita H. Kinney, a former contract nurse, was appointed the first superintendent of the Army Nurse Corps. Kinney served in that role until she resigned on July 31, 1909. The next month Jane A. Delano, an 1886 graduate of Bellevue Hospital School of Nursing, assumed the role of superintendent of the Corps, a position she would hold until 1912. Her term provided a significant link to the American Red Cross; in 1909, Delano had also accepted the position of chairman of the National Committee on Red Cross Nursing Services.[27]

The Navy Nurse Corps

In 1908, an act of Congress established the Navy Nurse Corps as part of the Bureau of Medicine and Surgery. Twenty female civilian nurses—some with experience in the Army Nurse Corps or as contract nurses in the Spanish–American War—made up the first cadre of navy nurses. They would work under the supervision of Esther Voorhees Hasson, formerly a member of the Army Nurse Corps.[28] Hasson had served during the Spanish–American War on the USS *Relief* and therefore had military experience both on land and sea.

Hasson's experience with other aspects of life in the military would serve her well. When she discovered that the government had made no provision for living quarters for the nurses, Hasson took it upon herself to solve the problem, leasing, furnishing, and financing a house for the nurses at 541 21st Street in northwest Washington, DC. Discovering that little had been done about uniforms, Hasson also designed the nurses' indoor uniform and the insignia for the Navy Nurse Corps. Moreover, Hasson established the requirements for nurses' eligibility for the Corps, ensuring that each nurse was "professionally, morally, mentally and physically fit" before she was accepted for duty.[29]

Both the Army and Navy Nurse Corps grew in size over the next decade. The increase in numbers of military nurses was timely, as nurses would be desperately needed when the United States entered the Great War in 1917. During those years of expansion, however, only a small percentage of the total number of American nurses served in the

Qualities of a Navy Nurse

"Above all [the Navy nurse] must possess in the highest degree the quiet dignity of bearing which alone can command respect from the apprentices or male nurses whom she must instruct. Although she possesses all else, and yet lacks this one quality, she had best seek another vocation at once as she would be absolutely useless for the work we wish her to do."[30]

Esther V. Hasson, 1909

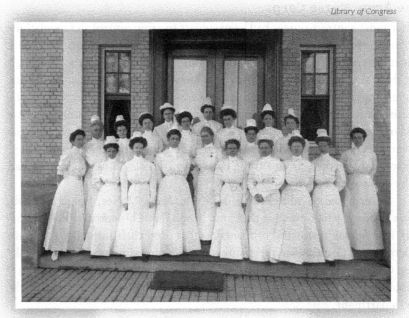

The original recruits of the Navy Nurse Corps.

U.S. military; the majority of training school graduates worked in "private duty" positions, giving care to individuals in their homes. A smaller number worked in hospitals, supervising student nurses on the wards and in the operating room. As they prepared graduates for private duty or hospital work, nurse leaders became concerned with the issues of mandatory licensure and state registration.

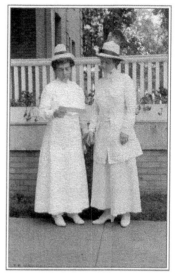

Navy nurses in 1909.

"Public Registration" for Nurses

Mrs. Bedford Fenwick, president of the International Congress of Nurses, was one of the first nurse leaders to address the issue of the legal regulation of the nursing profession with the goal of protecting the public. Speaking before an assembly of nurses in 1901, she called for state examinations and the "public registration" of nurses.

Responding to her recommendation, U.S. nurses turned their attention to making registration a reality. The first step in the process was to form state nurses' associations, and several states did so in 1901. North Carolina was the first state to pass a nurse registration act in 1903, followed by New Jersey, New York, and the Commonwealth of Virginia that same year. By 1912, 33 states had passed nurse practice acts, regulating the use of the title Registered Nurse, upgrading entrance requirements to schools of nursing, and increasing the length of programs of study.[32] Requirements varied by state, however, and no state *mandated* licensure. This problem persisted until the mid-20th century. In the meantime, graduates of nurse training schools who desired to work as private duty nurses simply placed their names on hospital directories, using the title of "graduate nurse."

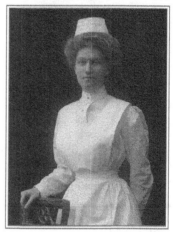

A private-duty nurse, who cared for her patients in their own homes.

Private Duty Nursing

In the late 19th and early 20th centuries, most nurses sought work on their own after graduation from training school. Although finding a position as a private duty nurse was challenging, they left the security of hospital work to student nurses and nursing supervisors. Enterprising nurses often announced

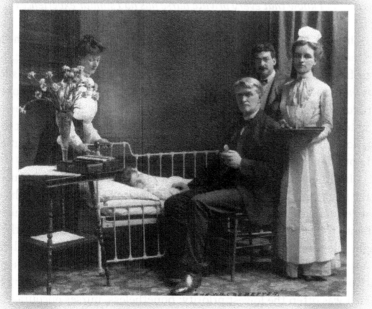

A private-duty nurse attends a patient with a physician.

The Need for Licensure

"It is the opinion of this International Congress of Nurses . . . that it is the duty of the nursing profession of every country to work for suitable legislative enactment regulating the education of nurses and protecting the interests of the public by securing state examinations and public registration."[31]

Mrs. Bedford Fenwick, 1901

Bjoring Center for Nursing Historical Inquiry

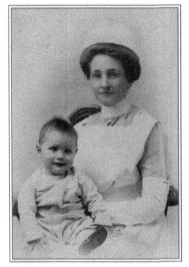

A private-duty nurse with a child.

Bjoring Center for Nursing Historical Inquiry

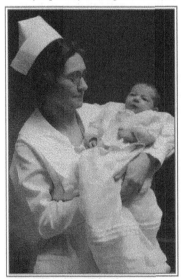

A private-duty nurse holding a baby.

their availability by notifying physicians, pharmacists, and patients that they were qualified and ready to care for patients.[33] This word-of-mouth method worked well in rural areas and small towns—but for the nurse living in a large city, advertising her availability for work was difficult. Early on, the profession recognized the value of a systematic method of hiring nurses through the use of hospital-based registries. These central directories, often administered by the alumnae association of the hospital nursing school, listed nurses who were seeking work. "Persons who wanted a nurse contacted the registry, which in turn sent out a suitable candidate." Given that the registry would only list nurses who met a certain school's standards, the system served as a "rudimentary credentialing process."[34]

Obtaining employment was only one aspect of the somewhat complicated reality of private duty nursing. While "private duty" provided the new graduates with a great deal of autonomy in their practice, the role also presented them with the challenge of fitting into a variety of households—from those of the very rich to those in the middle and lower classes. The nurse had to find her place in the household, establishing herself as a professional rather than a servant. Often this was not easy. As nurse educator Isabel Hampton Robb described the dilemma, the private duty nurse was "neither for the drawing room nor the kitchen."[35]

Mary Holleman described her experience in private duty, writing to the *American Journal of Nursing* in 1916:

> *Oh, the homes of the needy, where it is often almost impossible to procure necessary supplies and comforts for the patient especially when out in the country. Occasionally a nurse finds two, three or four sick people in such a home. In many instances we are obliged to resort to all kinds of improvising—our resourcefulness and originality being taxed to full capacity. . . . From personal experience I have in various instances found it necessary to scrub floors and furniture, . . . to wash the patient's bed clothes and towels or when there was practically no bed linen etc. to procure and use such suitable rags as I could find. Often I have found that unless I did the cooking there would be not food fit for any human being to eat . . . in one instance I actually milked the cow . . . I know that every private nurse has had similar experiences.*[37]

Indeed, private-duty nursing was difficult and exhausting—the length of time on any given case unpredictable, and the income sporadic. Nurses went from case to case, living in the homes of their patients for as long as they were needed. Sometimes the nurse remained with the patient for weeks, particularly if she was caring for a mother and her newborn.[38] Duties ranged from teaching the mother how to bathe, feed, and diaper the infant to cooking, doing laundry, and caring for other children in the family—duties that did not require the skills of a trained nurse.

In other cases, as in the care of a patient with terminal cancer, the nurse might be challenged to work to the limits of her training. She would change complicated dressings, feed and bathe the patient, try to relieve the patient's pain, and provide psychological support. As one case ended, the nurse might take a few days or weeks off, staying with family or friends, boarding in a rooming house, or living in a graduate nurses' club. Often the private duty nurse struggled financially, trying to make ends meet.[39] Taking care of herself was often the lowest priority; nonetheless, nurses encouraged their colleagues to do so.

By the mid-1920s, the setting for private duty nursing changed as more and more patients were admitted to hospitals when they were ill. In hospitals, most private duty nurses worked 12-hour shifts caring for their patients in private rooms.[41]

Fever Nursing

One of the most common jobs for the private duty nurse was "fever nursing." Since the colonial period, American mothers and midwives had taken turns caring for patients suffering from infectious diseases in which fever was the primary symptom. Before the advent of antibiotics and antipyretics like aspirin, those who nursed "fever patients" relied on herbal medicines, blankets, and sponging the patient with water or using mustard baths to break the fever. Writing on the topic "How to Bathe a Fever Patient" in the *American Journal of Nursing* in 1910, Minnie L. Crawford described the process, writing:

> *A warm mustard bath at 80, 100 or 105 degrees F. is well borne by nervous and peevish children, and is an excellent means of starting or favoring the elimination of toxic material. This bath is used mostly with children and is best prepared by placing an ounce of mustard in a muslin bag and throwing it into the bath. This bath will dilate the superficial capillaries, produce a sense of warmth, allay nervousness and insomnia, and also reduce the temperature.*[42]

Even 10 years after the Bayer Company began to produce aspirin in pill form, nurses relied on bathing patients to reduce fever. It was not until the mid-1910s that aspirin was marketed and used worldwide.

Nursing of "Crippled and Deformed Children"

Advances in the care of crippled children at the turn of the 20th century opened another new area of practice for nurses. Physicians and surgeons were beginning to use fresh air and heliotherapy as well as surgical procedures, braces, and splinting to address congenital orthopedic deformities in children. They also used these therapies for children who suffered the effects of tuberculosis (TB), polio, or malnutrition. Recognizing that children with deformities required care that included sun, fresh air, and proper nutrition along with the bracing of the joints for extended periods, Progressive Era reformers opened hospitals for the care of crippled children. In 1900, the New York State Hospital for Crippled and Deformed Children was established in Tarrytown on the banks of the Hudson River. Across the country in Seattle, the Children's Orthopedic Hospital opened in 1907 under the leadership of philanthropist Anna Clise.[44]

In these hospitals, nurses were responsible for the children's entire routine, including heliotherapy, medications, dressing changes, adjusting braces, feeding, and recreation. The nurses focused on providing the children with good nutrition, fresh air, and rest. Most important to the nurses, however, was providing the children with "daily attention and kind thoughtfulness."[45]

NURSING'S RESPONSE TO TRANSFORMATIVE EVENTS

At the turn of the 20th century, numerous other events would occur that demanded a response from individual nurses and the profession as a whole. Among these were the rise of school nursing, several significant natural disasters, the public's demand to care for premature infants, and novel

"A nurse should make an effort to fulfill her duty to herself by seeking to conserve her health, strength and energy."[40]

Nellie Miller, 1916

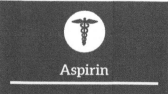

Aspirin

While salicylates had long been used to relieve inflammation, it was not until 1853 that French chemist Charles Gerhardt produced acetylsalicylic acid. In 1897, scientists at the German drug firm Bayer began to study acetylsalicylic acid as a less-irritating replacement for other salicylates. In 1899, the Bayer Company named the drug "aspirin," listed the product alongside their other drugs, and within 15 years, began selling it worldwide.[43]

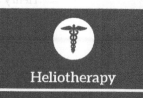

Heliotherapy

At the turn of the 20th century, physicians prescribed heliotherapy—exposure to sunlight—as treatment for scrofula (bone and skin) tuberculosis. Primarily used in sanatoria, the method called for keeping children on porches, gradually exposing them to sun and cool air. Once their acute symptoms had improved, the children moved outdoors for carefully timed sunbaths. In combination with a nutritious diet and fresh air, heliotherapy improved the symptoms of many children.[46]

programs to care for lower- and middle-class workers in industry. Working in the context of a society reeling from the widespread problems of TB and other infectious diseases, as well as the recurrent problem of juvenile diabetes, the profession would identify new and exciting solutions.

School Nursing

The beginning of school nursing in the United States in 1902 gave nurses a unique opportunity to expand their role beyond hospital work, private duty in the home, or district nursing. The role began in a demonstration project in New York City in an attempt to resolve the problem of children's absenteeism from school. The problem of absenteeism began in the late 1890s when health authorities began conducting medical inspections in the schools. Upon identifying conditions such as trachoma, pediculosis, impetigo, and ringworm in individual children, the health inspectors excluded the children from school. They would send a note along with the infected child to their parents, instructing them to have the child seen by a private physician. Many young immigrant parents often ignored the notes, either because they could not read English, did not understand the significance of the message, or had no money for a doctor. As a result, there was no assurance that a physician would actually treat the child or that the child would be isolated from others if the disease were contagious.[47] Meanwhile the child remained at home.

From her experience with visiting nursing in the immigrant neighborhoods of New York's Lower East Side, Lillian Wald understood the issues related to the lack of medical care for school children and the impact on the overall health of the community. At the same time, she also recognized the potential role nurses could play in promoting children's health. Using this knowledge, she proposed that nurses care for children with minor illness during the school day, and make home visits to those with serious disorders.[48]

In October 1902 Wald began a 1-month-long demonstration project, sending Henry Street nurse Lina Rogers into four neighborhood schools. The project was a success. By treating minor illness in the schools instead of sending the children home, Rogers substantially reduced absenteeism. City officials took note and within months a corps of 11 nurses, sponsored by the Board of Health and assisted by the Board of Education, began work in the New York City schools.[49] On average, each of the nurses visited four schools a day, treating children whom physicians had identified during their daily rounds.[50] Lavinia Dock of the Henry Street Settlement described the school nurse's role in 1902, writing:

> The school nurse should work with the physician, carrying out under his orders the treatment for simple cases, without excluding them from school, and following to their homes the more serious cases of eye, head, or skin trouble, seeing that they received medical attention, teaching the mother, when this should be necessary, and keeping a record of the time the child was absent, not allowing him to remain out of school longer than necessary.[51]

Only children "suffering from serious disorders too advanced to be cared for in the dressing-room were sent home."[52] Having treated the children at school, the nurse would make follow-up visits in their homes, speaking with mothers and "giving whatever advice was needed."[53] Within a year, the number of children excluded from New York City schools for health reasons decreased by 90%, causing some to remark that school nurses provided the "link needed to complete the chain of medical inspection."[54] By 1909, 141 nurses were working in the 458 schools of New York City, collaborating with the school principals and medical inspectors.[55]

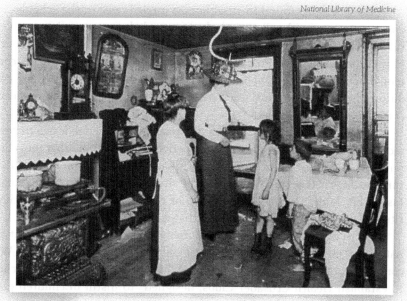

A school nurse on a follow-up visit to a student's home.

Within a few years, other state health authorities would implement school nursing in their city schools, often with the help of funding from the John D. Rockefeller Foundation. Rural schools would be their next target.

Many people held the conventional belief that rural children, with access to fresh air, clean water, and farm-fresh food, were healthier than urban children. In fact, the opposite was true.[57] At the turn of the 20th century, children living in remote rural areas of the country, where few families had sanitary privies or clean drinking water, "suffered greater morbidity and mortality than did children who lived in cities."[58] Nutritional deficits were commonplace as many impoverished children, subsisting on a diet of salt back and cornbread, had rickets and/or pellagra. Others had hookworm. Moreover, residents of isolated rural areas frequently lacked access to a physician or a nurse. As a result, children suffered from uncorrected skeletal deformities, dental caries, and vision defects.[59]

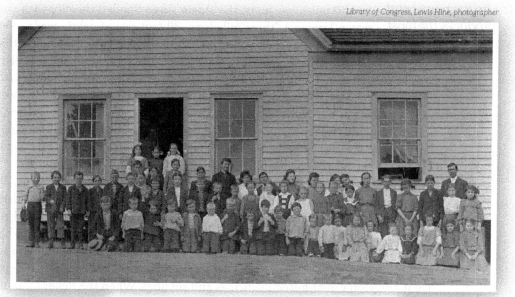

A one-room schoolhouse in High Shoals, North Carolina, in 1908.

"The school has been found . . . the best door of entry [to the home] and produces the most tangible results."[64]

Mary Gardner, Public Health Nurse, 1936

The problems found in rural homes carried over to the schools. The one-room country schoolhouses lacked proper lighting, screening, and ventilation; often the only source of heat was a wood stove and the only source of water a nearby well. Frequently children drank from a pail with a common dipper. Some schoolhouses even lacked an outhouse. Given these conditions, hookworm and malaria were endemic in rural areas; communicable diseases were also prevalent.[60]

Experts and nurses agreed that the role of the rural public health nurse required the best-educated and most experienced nurses, and that the school nurse was the most effective way to introduce principles of public health in rural settings.[62] One nurse explained the situation, noting: "In a great many cases, the children are the only means of reaching the homes, sometimes situated in such out of the way places that it is hard to find them."[63]

Word of the success of school nursing spread rapidly throughout the nation and public health nurses in other states soon adopted it. In rural Wisconsin, "county nurses" inspected school children and worked with teachers to establish Health Crusader Clubs, designed "to instill in children good health habits, such as brushing teeth, sleeping with the window open, and drinking three glasses of water a day."[65] In Hazard, Kentucky, a rapidly growing railroad town in Appalachia, the county nurse "examined all the school children."[66] In Michigan, the Kent County Board of Supervisors hired the first county school nurse in March 1915, and in North Carolina nurses "inspected 92,566 students and coordinated clinics for immunizations, tonsil and adenoid removal and dental treatments" during the years 1919 to 1921.[67] In some cases, school nurses provided the only source of health education and the only link between rural families and medical care.

Nurses and the Galveston Hurricane, 1900

Not all nursing opportunities presented in an organized fashion with demonstration projects as a way of introduction. Some new nursing roles, particularly in disaster relief, developed as a result of natural catastrophes. Such was the case on September 8, 1900, when a devastating hurricane struck Galveston, Texas, a wealthy port city located on a barrier island between Galveston Bay and the Gulf of Mexico. With 15-foot waves and winds close to 130 miles per hour, the storm surge flooded the city with chest-deep water, leaving a "three mile long, 30 foot pile of debris made of shattered houses, barns, shed and corpses." The city was in ruins; more than 3,600 homes, many owned by people in the lower classes, had been demolished. Between 6,000 and 12,000 people died.[68] When the storm hit Galveston's St. Mary's Infirmary, the Sisters of Charity of the Incarnate Word went about their usual work, but "when flying slates began crashing windows" they "took notice, moving patients away from windows" and later, when water poured in, moving them to higher floors.[69] By evening, the Sisters had taken in nearly 2,000 refugees. Most had been brought to the hospital by boats.[70]

Without a federal disaster plan and cut off from all communications, Galveston was initially alone in its relief efforts. The day after the hurricane, the city leaders formed a Central Relief Committee to begin the cleanup. With so many people dead and floodwaters inundating the city, burials were impossible—the bodies would have to be burned. Meanwhile, local physicians and nurses responded immediately, working in collaboration with the U.S. Army, the U.S. Marine Service, and the Galveston Health Department. Local drugstores distributed medicines and supplies. When the Relief Committee was finally able to send a message to the president and the people of the United States asking for help, volunteers came from all over the country. Six physicians and 20 nurses from Bellevue Hospital in New York were among those who volunteered, working wherever the Sick and Injured Committee assigned them.

The American Red Cross also responded. Arriving in Texas 9 days after the storm had hit, president of the American Red Cross Clara Barton and her assistant, Third Vice President Ellen Mussey, joined the relief efforts. First, because they could not get across to Galveston, they worked from tents and kitchens in Texas City, just across the bay. Accompanied by laymen rather than nurses, Barton and Mussey created an orphanage and worked with volunteers to distribute "food, clothing, and materials for shelter" to overwhelmed homeless citizens.[71]

Worn out from a lifetime of service, and easily fatigued at 78 years of age, Barton directed relief efforts from her hotel room after she and her team made their way to Galveston. On her recommendation, "committees were organized in every ward of the city and separate storerooms [were] established from which supplies could be distributed."[72] To ensure that African Americans were not overlooked in the socially segregated city, Barton created a separate Red Cross Auxiliary for Black people. Her intent was to make sure that they received their share of money and clothing, and "could determine for themselves the best way" to use the funds and donations. Unfortunately, the $397 collected for Blacks in Galveston paled in

Library of Congress

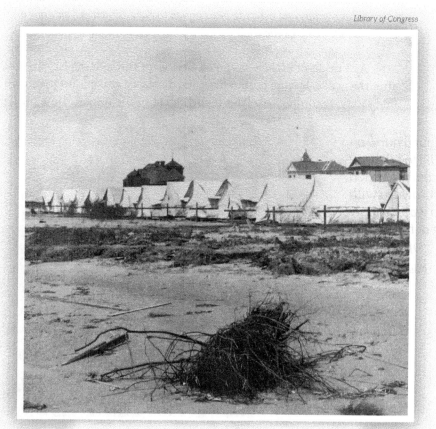

Aftermath of the Galveston hurricane of 1900, which destroyed thousands of homes and killed thousands of people.

comparison to the more than $1 million collected for White citizens.[73] It was a problem that would recur throughout the century: discrimination and unequal care for African Americans in the setting of natural and man-made disasters.

San Francisco Earthquake, 1906

Several years after the Galveston hurricane, another natural disaster, this time on the West Coast, also challenged nurses to respond. This time nurses were able to provide more care, as there were more survivors than after the hurricane. In 1906, an earthquake devastated San Francisco, a city of more than half a million people. The quake lasted almost 60 seconds and was felt up and down the West Coast. The death toll, from the quake itself and the fires that raged through downtown San Francisco afterward, destroyed 28,000 buildings, left half the city's population homeless, caused 225,000 injuries, and left more than 3,000 dead.[74] Nurse Lucy B. Fisher was among hundreds of nurses who responded. Later she related her experience:

> *The first vibration at 5:13 A.M. on the 18th day of April, [1906] awoke me . . . I stood gasping audibly . . . I felt that such a cataclysm meant nothing less than death. . . . I dressed quickly . . . and went in to the hall, where I met one of the nurses who belonged in the house. . . . It must have been half past six when we were walking down Polk Street, that our eyes were attracted by the sight of flames shooting high into the air from the heart of the business section of the city. It was a terrifying sight. We found on our approach to the Pavilion that its entrance was surrounded by a cordon, guarded by a force of policemen. . . . We said we were nurses . . . and were directed to the entrance. What a scene! The floor strewn with mattresses . . . nearly all occupied by patients. . . . My friend and I quickly took off our wraps and asked to be assigned to duty. "Pitch in," was our only order, and we followed it explicitly.*[75]

As a result of broken gas pipes, fire swept through the city for 3 days and 3 nights after the quake, leaving both nurses and displaced citizens on their own as they tried to find safety. According to a later report, most of the nurses "were on private duty at the

"We have put a nurse on Telegraph Hill to take care of the small unburnt portion which is overcrowded with people; no water supply except at the bottom of the hill."[80]

Miss Ashe, 1906

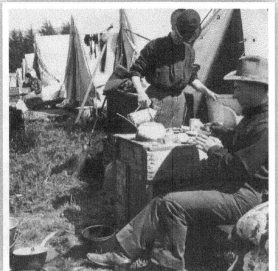

Library of Congress

The Presidio, a military base where more than 10,000 survivors of the 1906 San Francisco earthquake sought refuge and medical care.

time of the fire" and "rushed to the emergency hospitals."[76] At Golden Gate Park where thousands of citizens sought refuge, White Cross Society female nurses assisted the medical corpsmen at the temporary hospital.[77] The nurses, wearing long white smocks, "readied beds on mattresses on the ground, relieved pain with morphine injections, and gave strychnine hypodermically" for those in shock.[78] Other nurses worked at camps throughout the city, including the Presidio, a military base that included a 300-bed U.S. General Hospital and smaller post hospitals. There nurses worked 10- to 12-hour shifts 7 days a week to care for more than 10,000 survivors.[79]

In the days and weeks following the earthquake, hundreds of nurses joined the recovery efforts, working wherever they were needed. Some worked with a "hospital shore party" from the USS *Preble* at the Harbor Emergency Hospital, others at Children's Hospital or in rehabilitation camps outside the city. Still others set up headquarters to distribute donated funds to nurses who had lost everything and were themselves refugees.[82]

Nurses and the Monongah Mine Explosion

Twenty months after the San Francisco earthquake, nurses responded to yet another disaster, this time in Monongah, a small coal-mining town 6 miles from Fairmont, in West Virginia. While small in numbers of fatalities in comparison to the San Francisco earthquake, the Monongah mine explosion was the "deadliest mine disaster in American history," killing at least 361 miners and their sons.[84]

The explosion was thought to have been caused by the ignition of methane gas and coal dust after a faulty coupling pin broke and sent 14 coal cars plunging into Mine Six, ripping out rails and electrical wiring and allowing gas to circulate through the mines. Flames shot "more than sixty feet into the sky"; debris covered mine entrances, and cave-ins ensued. Inside, those who did not die immediately from trauma became victims of poisonous gas.[85]

Outside, doctors and nurses who had gathered at an emergency hospital in the local blacksmith shop stood by waiting for trauma victims, but none came. Only one of the men who had entered the mine that morning had survived. Instead, the medical teams cared for the exhausted volunteers. Some of the rescue workers battled fatigue from digging through the rubble; others suffered nausea and headaches from the after-damp in the unventilated mines. Sometimes the rescuers themselves had to be treated as they collapsed or lost consciousness.[86]

Nurses and physicians also cared for the 250 widows and 10,000 fatherless children in their grief. Many were in shock, and the nurses could only offer psychological support, blankets, hot coffee, and soup to those who had lost family members. Funerals were conducted continuously, the grief-stricken survivors standing over "the cold rows of open graves . . . in the snow-flecked West Virginia soil."[87]

The Monongah mine disaster brought a new reality to nurses who responded to emergencies: When there are no survivors, family members and rescue teams are the ones who need care. That realism would herald a new focus in disaster planning: In the future, medical and nursing personnel who specialized in the fields of psychiatry and psychology would be available at the scenes of disasters. Over the next 100 years, these specialists would be needed in numerous instances. One of the most memorable would be the attack on the World Trade Center in New York City on September 11, 2001.

Nursing Premature Infants

At the turn of the 20th century, the development of the incubator both improved the treatment of premature infants and provided a new opportunity for nurses to specialize

"The San Francisco nurses are working for little or nothing as the case may be, being thankful in many instances to secure shelter and food in return for their services."[83]

American Journal of Nursing, July 1906

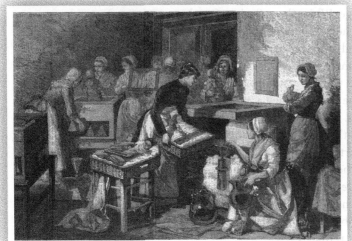

Paris Maternité Hopital, which used a basic incubator and
well-trained nurses to reduce infant mortality.

in the field of neonatology. For premature infants, whose deaths had historically been viewed as acceptable losses, the invention of the mechanical incubator signified a changing attitude toward treatment of these vulnerable newborns. By improving their chance at survival, incubator technology demonstrated that premature infants were worthy of medical and nursing intervention.[88]

First developed in France in 1880, the earliest incubators were little more than large wooden boxes that relied on hot water to warm the air inside. Caring for infants in these warming boxes was intensive and time consuming and the French relied on specially trained nurses to care for both the infant and the technology. In addition to their usual responsibilities of feeding, changing, and bathing the babies, the nurses had to change the water at least every 2 hours to maintain adequate temperatures. The French system worked by pairing the incubator with expert nursing care. Thus, premature infant mortality at the Paris Maternité Hospital decreased by almost half. Its success generated enthusiasm for the device throughout the world.[89]

Unfortunately, caring for premature infants was often prohibitively expensive for American hospitals and for individual families, particularly as incubator designs became more technologically advanced. Incubator-baby exhibits, in which visitors were charged a small admission fee to watch trained nurses care for live premature infants, emerged as a creative approach to offset the high cost of equipment and nursing care. The rise of mass culture entertainment in the early 20th century helped popularize the incubator sideshow phenomenon, and the exhibits quickly became a fixture along the midway section at World's Fairs and amusement parks like Coney Island. Exhibit buildings were designed to operate like small hospitals where premature infants received free care in exchange for being part of the display.[90]

Owners of the infant incubator sideshows employed one to two head nurses and up to 10 assistant nurses to work in three 8-hour shifts each day, depending on the size and capacity of the building.[91] For the duration of the show, nurses lived and worked at the fairgrounds, often for 3 to 6 months at a time. Each nurse claimed responsibility for no more than three babies while on duty, providing all care and feedings around the clock.[92]

Through a wall of glass windows, patrons watched as nurses changed, weighed, and bathed their charges. A

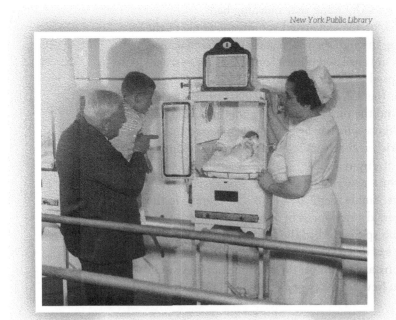

A nurse showing a patron the Infant Incubator
Exhibit in the early 20th century.

complete record of infant weight gain, as well as daily temperatures, feeding schedules, and infant growth was kept and placed atop individual incubators to display progress to visitors.[93] While the ethics of caring for newborns in fairground exhibits is questionable, their survival rates ranged from 82% to 90% at a time when infant mortality was at an all-time high.[94] Moreover, in addition to receiving excellent care, the infants on display drew attention to the social value of decreasing premature infant mortality.[95]

The better option for care of the premature infant was in hospital nurseries. The first long-term successful hospital unit for premature infants opened in Chicago, Illinois, in 1922. Under the direction of Dr. Julius Hess and head nurse Evelyn Lundeen, the Hortense Schoen Joseph Premature Infant Station at Sarah Morris Hospital for Children emerged as the preeminent center for the care of premature infants. In direct contrast to the carnival-like atmosphere surrounding the infant incubator sideshow exhibits, the "station" established premature care as a hospital-based specialty that placed trained and experienced nursing staff at the center of its treatment model. Focus shifted away from the technologic wonders of the mechanical incubator, and instead highlighted the necessity of employing skilled nurses to improve premature infant survival. Moreover, because of an annual endowment from a local philanthropic organization, nurses at the station were able to care for any baby, regardless of race, religion, financial status, or place of birth.[96]

All infant care activities, as well as the cleaning and maintenance of equipment and linens for the entire unit, fell to the nursing staff. Remaining vigilant at the infant's bedside, nurses monitored the babies for any change in color, appearance, or respiratory status. Feeding schedules for the infants, who were fed either every 3 or every 4 hours, governed most of the daily routine.[97] Using a variety of specialized techniques, including gavage, nasal spoon, and medicine dropper feedings, nurses provided sick and premature babies with the nutrition needed to ensure survival.

Nurses at the station accepted a great deal of responsibility for the infants' welfare, especially in the area of infection control. They were rewarded with the freedom to function fairly independently. Physicians and interns examined infants and wrote orders, but graduate nurses performed all treatments and were encouraged to report their own observations and clinical judgments. Indeed, the model of care promoted at the station involved a significant paradigm shift for the medical community at the time, one that placed complete control of the unit's daily activities directly in the hands of *graduate* nurses. The innovative approach proved successful, and by 1928 infant mortality rate at the station had dropped to 24%, while annual admission rates had increased from fewer than 20 infants in the station's first year to more than 100 infants in 1928.[99]

This innovative specialty role would lay the groundwork for other specialty roles in nursing, including in particular, those in the intensive care units that would be developed at mid-century.

Metropolitan Life Insurance Nurses

As preventive services in public health grew in city after city, so did the mix of government and voluntary initiatives. By the 1910s a wide variety of organizations employed visiting nurses. One of the most notable of these was Metropolitan Life Insurance Company. Lillian Wald first contracted with the company in 1909, offering to provide Henry Street nurses to its policyholders with the goal of keeping workers and their families healthy and reducing their mortality rate. Meeting this goal would also increase the company's profits.[101]

"The emergency treatments, the maintenance of a normal body temperature, the methods of feeding, and the close observance of clinical symptoms . . . are all responsibilities of the nurse."[98]

Evelyn Lundeen, Head Nurse, 1936

The Importance of the Nurse's Role

"Since it is our conviction that untiring, unremitting care has no substitute in the care of the premature infant, we have deemed it essential to give equal prominence to the role of the nurse."[100]

Evelyn Lundeen

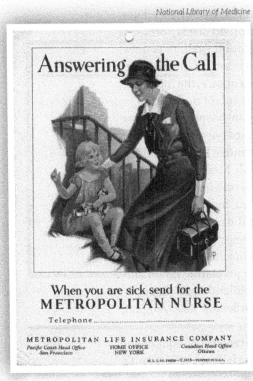

Answering the Call

When you are sick send for the
METROPOLITAN NURSE

Telephone...................................

METROPOLITAN LIFE INSURANCE COMPANY
Pacific Coast Head Office   HOME OFFICE   Canadian Head Office
San Francisco   NEW YORK   Ottawa

A poster for Metropolitan Life Insurance nurses, who cared for poor patients in tenement housing areas of cities.

"From the standpoint of prevention, [the nurses'] value consists in education, along sanitary and hygienic lines . . . [in] the homes that she visits."[106]

Lee Frankel, 1913

Met Life Insurance Nursing

"The company not only furnishes its policyholder with a visiting nurse, but it is also establishing a sanitarium for the treatment of tuberculosis patients and is distributing literature so that its policy holders may receive instruction in the care of the body and the preservation of health. It has instituted a concerted campaign to lower infant mortality."[107]

Nellie Linsay, 1911

Drawn to the work by the allure of "steady employment and relative professional autonomy," nurses "clamored to be accepted into the Metropolitan Visiting Nurse Service, promising to follow company rules."[102] Once employed, the nurses spent their days in the poor tenement districts of cities where their patients lived, walking through "muddy alleys, over rooftops, up flights of stairs or down into damp basements" to see their patients.[103] A typical day included eight visits, most of which were to patients with conditions like puerperal sepsis, respiratory illnesses, and communicable diseases.[104] Health teaching was a major part of their role. According to Lee Frankel, the president of the company, the Metropolitan Nursing Service was "a purposeful program which inspired the poor to learn self-help, thrift, and methods of self-protection against the ills of life."[105]

TB Nursing

For years, TB had been endemic in districts of large cities where poverty, inadequate sanitation, and overcrowding were the norm. For decades visiting nurses had been seeing TB patients in their homes, educating family members on their care and isolating patients as much as possible. Now, in the opening years of the 20th century, physicians were turning to Europe for new ideas on the treatment of TB. Having spent time in Europe visiting a sea–air hospital, John S. Ward, a board member of the New York Association for Improving the Condition of the Poor, returned with an idea to offer open-air treatment for children with bony TB or scrofula, "the swelling of the lymph nodes in the neck."[108] After he convinced the board of the idea, Ward opened Sea Breeze Hospital in June 1904 on Coney Island. At first the hospital consisted of open-air

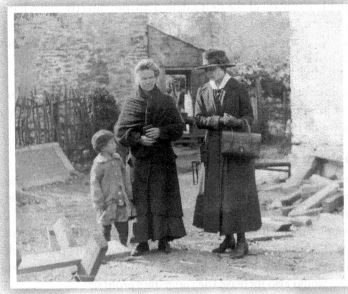

A visiting tuberculosis nurse walks with a patient.

tents facing the ocean. By November of that year, with cold weather setting in, the hospital built a permanent structure with windows and porches facing the ocean. In both structures, nurses were critical to the children's care.

By the turn of the 20th century, nurses' role in the care of the TB patient progressed from care and teaching in the patient's home to locating adult and pediatric TB patients and referring them to sanatoria. Edward Trudeau built the first TB cottages at Saranac Lake, New York, in 1906, making it possible to house patients who were severely ill with the disease. In these institutions, nurses treated patients by placing them for hours in the fresh air, and providing rest and nutritious foods. No antibiotic was yet available to cure them.

The Preventorium: Innovation in TB Prevention

In 1909, the idea was conceived that isolation would benefit children at high risk of contracting TB. The thinking was that isolation in a special "preventorium" would prevent the most vulnerable children from developing the disease. Nurses would provide the care and attention the children needed; thus another job opportunity presented itself for nurses.

With the 1908 discovery of tuberculin, a byproduct of the *tubercle bacilli* culture, doctors and nurses could use a simple test to identify children who had been exposed to TB but were not yet symptomatic. Referred to as "pretubercular," the children who had a positive test result could then be admitted to a preventorium, an institution in which they could be housed in better conditions, fed wholesome foods, and allowed to rest for long periods of time. During their entire stay in the preventorium, the children would be under the care of professional nurses. The whole program was based on the prevailing belief that "inadequate living environment, excessive crowding, overwork and insufficient nutrition clearly enhanced one's risk for developing tuberculosis." Removing the children from their situation was therefore a logical solution.[111]

The first preventorium opened in the Cleveland Cottage in Lakewood, New Jersey, in 1909. After considerable opposition from local citizens, however, it was moved a few miles away to a 170-acre farm in Farmingdale. In the new location, J. Palmer Quimby

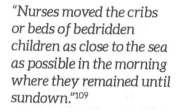

"Nurses moved the cribs or beds of bedridden children as close to the sea as possible in the morning where they remained until sundown."[109]

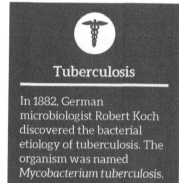

Tuberculosis

In 1882, German microbiologist Robert Koch discovered the bacterial etiology of tuberculosis. The organism was named *Mycobacterium tuberculosis*.

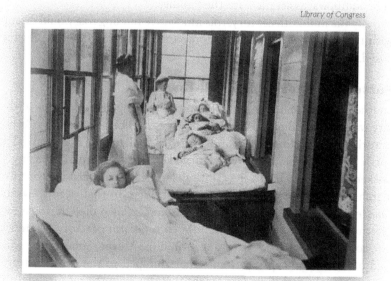

Library of Congress

Children rest at Lakewood Preventorium, which was created to ward off cases of tuberculosis in high-risk children through fresh air, nutritious meals, and nurse supervision.

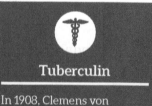

Tuberculin

In 1908, Clemens von Pirquet discovered that tuberculin, a by-product of the *tubercle bacilli* culture, could be used to identify individuals who were infected with TB before they developed actual symptoms. The discovery led to a new diagnostic category for TB: the "pretubercular."[110]

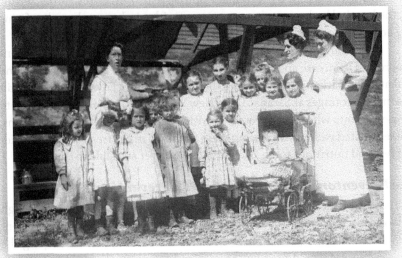

*Children being cared for at the preventorium at
Sea Breeze Hospital.*

The Tuberculosis Preventorium for Children, Farmingdale, New Jersey

"The institution was organized primarily for the care of poorly nourished, underfed children, exposed to tuberculosis infection in their homes . . . but who had no open disease. At this time no similar institution existed in this country. There was no place to send these children; in the summer some could be sheltered for a few weeks in fresh-air homes; in the winter a very few could be sent out of the city by unusual effort."[113]

J. Palmer Quimby

"The children are followed up by a special Department of Health nurse for years. . . . Our purpose is to permanently save every child that comes to us."[117]

Farmingdale Annual Report, 1912

The Industrial Nurse

"In fact, [the nurse's] main function should be to conserve the health and lives of the workers . . . her work should include . . . regular conference hours during the working day, regular inspection of sanitary conditions, special attention to diet, charge of the hospital, and regular group instruction in health and hygiene."[119]

Lillian Wald, 1917

served as superintendent of nurses, responsible for the nursing care of nearly 600 infants and children who were cared for each year at the institution.[112]

Soon after the establishment of the cottages in Farmingdale, at least 26 other preventoria opened throughout the United States and nurses were essential players in all of them. In the preventorium, nurses provided the pre-tubercular children with fresh air, rest, nutritious meals, and outdoor play. In fact, as historian Cynthia Connolly notes, the nurse had round-the-clock responsibility for the children's welfare, "from the day she fetched them from the railroad station until she returned them to their families two to three months later."[114] Nurses' responsibilities included "monitoring children's welfare, observing for illness, educating about hygiene, and supervising all aspects of life at the institution."[115] In addition the nurse served as the link between the children and their parents, communicating the child's progress, giving instruction in "cleanliness and hygiene and the proper disposal of sputum" and "obtaining aid or additional assistance" for the families.[116]

By the mid-20th century, this innovative nursing role would disappear. With the 1944 discovery of streptomycin as a cure for TB, the preventoria closed.

Nurses in Factories and Mill Towns

Another innovation in nurses' roles in the opening decades of the 20th century was that of industrial nursing. It was a role born of necessity. As manufacturing steadily increased and factories and textile mills spread from north to south, factory owners turned their attention to keeping their workers safe. New York's devastating Triangle Shirtwaist Factory fire on March 25, 1911, provided impetus for change. In that deadly sweatshop disaster, 123 poor immigrant shop girls and 23 men died during a rag bin fire that roared through an unventilated multistory factory where locked exit doors and a narrow fire escape prohibited escape. Some of the workers died of burns and asphyxiation. Others jumped to their deaths from the windows on the eighth floor, a height that not even the most modern 1911 fire-engine ladder could reach.[118]

In response to the disaster, Progressive Era reformers turned their attention to safety initiatives in factories in the large industrial cities of the northeast. Lillian Wald, director of Henry Street Settlement, was actively involved. She had witnessed firsthand the problems faced by poor immigrants working in factories and now advised nurses on their responsibilities to company employees. Her focus was to conserve their health and their lives.

Eventually nurses were employed in factories outside of large cities. By 1919 the U.S. Bureau of Labor began to establish sanitary and safety regulations for *all* U.S. industries, including factories and mills in smaller towns. The new regulations required that factory owners place guards over moving machinery parts, install proper lighting in workrooms and stairwells, and provide adequate fire escapes in all factories greater than three stories high. As labor regulations increased, some factory owners created welfare departments to provide workers and their families with child care centers, social work services, entertainment, and recreational activities. Some welfare departments began to hire professional nurses to address workers' medical needs, including "brown lung" (from cotton fibers in the unventilated factory rooms), hearing loss, fatigue, and nervousness, as well as TB, hookworm, and epidemics of infectious disease.[120]

Typical of the nurses' responsibilities was the task of staffing the first-aid room to care for employees injured or taken ill while on the job. The nurse also reported to the scene of every factory accident, and if no physician was available, they provided emergency treatment. In the cotton mills of the south, emergencies were commonplace and included crushed or amputated limbs, shock, eye injuries, burns, and fainting. In such emergencies, after determining the severity of the injuries the mill nurses decided on next steps; their actions were critical to the welfare of seriously injured workers.[121]

The industrial nurses' responsibilities were not limited to the factory. More often than not, the mill-town factory nurse provided care for the entire community. In that role, she taught hygiene and nutrition, counseled pregnant women and new mothers, and performed well-baby checkups. In addition, she dealt with epidemics of measles, scarlet fever, whooping cough, and other infectious diseases.[122]

Over the next 50 years, opportunities in industrial nursing would continue to grow as increasing demands for production created larger and larger industrial complexes. When women joined the ranks

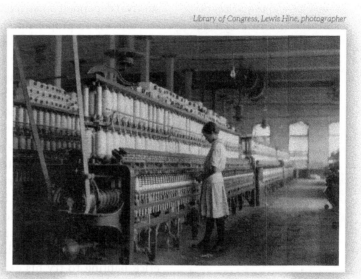

Library of Congress, Lewis Hine, photographer

A 14-year-old worker at Brazos Valley Cotton Mill in Texas in 1913.

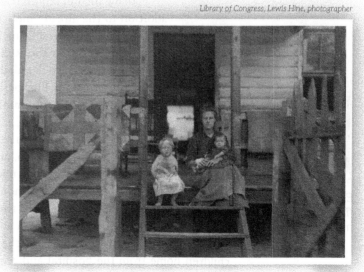

Library of Congress, Lewis Hine, photographer

Mill-town family on the porch in Matoaca, Virginia, in 1911.

of workers during World War II, the industrial nurses' role would expand once again to focus on the women's unique needs.

The Nurse and the Diabetic Child: Before and After Insulin

The discovery of insulin in the early 20th century initiated yet another innovative role for nurses. Before the use of injectable insulin, nursing a diabetic child was not only difficult and time consuming, but also futile: The juvenile diabetic often did not live for more than 2 years after diagnosis.[123] Management of the disease consisted of strict dietary control, restricting calories and carbohydrates (the Allen diet), and the close regulation of the patient's activity to match caloric intake.[124]

All in all, the nursing care of the diabetic had to be meticulous. In addition to managing diet and exercise, the nurse caring for a diabetic child in the preinsulin era had to test the urine for "diabetic acid with ferric chloride solution and recognize the odor of acetone" on the breath.[126] The patient's survival depended on strict control of blood glucose.

Access to proper nursing and medical care was critical. It was also a situation that was irrevocably linked to social class and privilege. If the patient and family had the means and the connections, they could obtain cutting-edge care. Such was the situation of Elizabeth Hughes, the young daughter of Charles Evans Hughes, one of the most famous politicians in the United States. Diagnosed with diabetes in 1919, 11-year-old Elizabeth required strict management of her diet and daily activities to keep her alive, so her parents hired a private-duty nurse, Blanche Burgess, to care for her. Having trained with the esteemed diabetologists Frederick Allen and Elliot Joslin, Burgess was an expert in the field of diabetes nursing. Once employed, she meticulously managed Elizabeth's daily food intake, monitored her for signs and symptoms of acidosis, and adjusted her daily activities to correlate with her energy level. In spite of this, Elizabeth's health declined. Determined to help her, Elizabeth's mother appealed to Canadian physician Frederick Banting to try his experimental drug insulin on her child. With his consent, she traveled with her daughter to Toronto for treatment, and in August 1922 Elizabeth became one of the first patients in the United States to receive an insulin injection.[127]

Using insulin required a new aspect to Burgess's care for Elizabeth. In addition to the already meticulous care she gave, Burgess now instructed Elizabeth to give herself insulin injections and to identify the signs and symptoms of insulin shock. Burgess also had to manage complications, as well as give Elizabeth detailed information on regulating her diet to match the insulin dose. In Elizabeth's case, since the pair traveled extensively, Burgess also had to communicate the child's progress to her parents and physician.

Not every family with a diabetic child could afford an experienced private duty nurse of its own, and as insulin became available to patients in middle and lower classes, a new role for nurses developed within the field of diabetes—that of the "Wandering Diabetes Nurse." This title was given to a nurse who worked outside the hospital, visiting patients in their homes as she was "free to wander in whatever direction diabetic patients might call her."[130] For the most part, the Wandering Diabetes Nurse followed diabetic children home from the hospital and remained with the family long enough to make sure the child's routine care was "sufficiently established." The nurse also made follow-up

Preinsulin
Management of
Diabetes

"The success of modern treatment of diabetes can be very largely measured by the strictness with which the diet and other regulations are carried out. . . . The nurse's notes will be of primary importance and these will include a record of the foods taken and actually consumed at the different meals . . . so that the physician can see the exact amounts of fat, carbohydrate and protein that have been consumed."[125]

Dietetics for Nurses, 1918

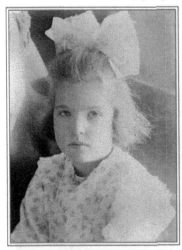

Elizabeth Hughes, one of the first patients to take insulin to treat her diabetes in 1922.

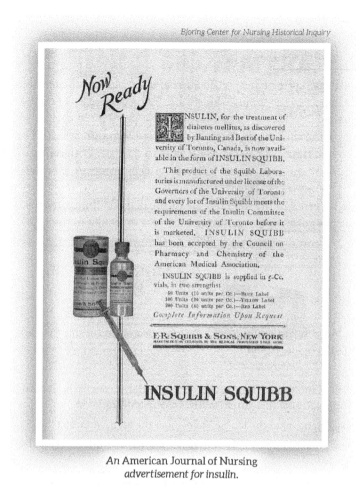

An American Journal of Nursing
advertisement for insulin.

The Discovery of Insulin

In Toronto, Canada, in 1921 Dr. Frederick Banting and his medical student assistant Charles Best experimented on dogs, testing Banting's theory about the function of the pancreas and the production of enzymes within it. They worked with support from John J. Macleod, a senior scientist. After positive results, in January 1922 the three went on to test the use of a substance called "insulin" on a 14-year-old boy with diabetes. The patient not only survived but also gained weight. The news of the successful treatment spread rapidly, and in 1923 Eli Lilly Drug Company prepared the first vials of insulin for medical use.[128]

visits and, in some instances, "made necessary contact with children's school teachers" to establish "a proper understanding of the restrictions surrounding a diabetic child." In summer, the Wandering Diabetes Nurses visited children in special diabetes camps set up for them.[131] Teaching the children how to manage the chronic illness was an essential component of her work.

Over the course of the century, subspecialty roles in nursing would continue to develop. The obesity epidemic, the graying of America, and the rising incidence of type 2 diabetes among U.S. citizens would all be contributing factors. Before that, however, other factors would create even more changes in the nursing profession. As the 20th century opened, the growth of hospitals, reforms in medical and nursing education, the rise of scientific medicine, and an increasing emphasis on medical and nursing specialization would revolutionize nurses' work.

"You will see a great change in Elizabeth. Her whole body is filling out and she is much stronger. Insulin is wonderful!"[129]

Blanche Burgess to
Mrs. Hughes, 1922

For Discussion

1. How did nursing in the Spanish–American War affect the development of the Army and Navy Nurse Corps?
2. Describe some of the factors that led to the inception of school nursing.

Teaching the Diabetic

"Even young children are taught to make the Benedict Test [a test for sugar in the urine] and to administer their own insulin, to weigh their food, to recognize unusual symptoms and to treat emergencies."[132]

Lovilla Winterbottom, 1931

(continued)

For Discussion (continued)

3. What were the nurses' primary responsibilities after the Monongah mine disaster?
4. What was the impact of the Triangle Shirtwaist Factory fire of 1911 on the rise of industrial nursing?
5. Describe some of the challenges of private duty nursing in the early 20th century.
6. What factors led to the rise of the preventorium in the early 20th century? What was nurses' role in the movement? Identify ethical issues in the preventoria movement.
7. What changes occurred in the nursing care of the diabetic child after the discovery of insulin? How did social class influence access to insulin in the 1920s?

NOTES

1. Isabel H. Robb, "Address of the President," *American Journal of Nursing* (hereafter *AJN*) 1, no. 2 (1900): 97–104 (quote 97–99).
2. Ibid., 102.
3. Barbra Mann Wall, "Courage to Care: The Sisters of the Holy Cross in the Spanish American War," *Nursing History Review* (hereafter *NHR*) 3 (1995): 55–77.
4. Richard Westphal, "Remember the Maine, Remember the Men," *AJN* 103, no. 5 (2003): 77.
5. Elizabeth Jamieson and Mary Sewall, *Trends in Nursing History*, 4th ed. (Philadelphia: W. B. Saunders, 1954): 401.
6. "Highlights in the History of the Army Nurse Corps: Chronology," www.history.army.mili tary/books/anc-highlights/chrono.htm (accessed August 7, 2015): 1–2.
7. Jamieson and Sewall, *Trends in Nursing History*, 402.
8. "The War of 1898: The Spanish American War," https://www.loc.gov (accessed January 5, 2016): 1.
9. Ann Frantz, "Clara Barton in the Spanish-American War," *AJN* 98, no. 10 (October 1998): 39–41.
10. Ibid., 41.
11. Deanne S. Nuwer, "The 1878 Yellow Fever Epidemic in Mississippi," ch. 1 in *Nurses on the Frontline: When Disaster Strikes, 1878-2010*, eds. Barb Wall and Arlene Keeling (New York: Springer Publishing, 2011): 1–15 (quote 2).
12. Ibid., 2.
13. Linda Sabin, "Sweating, Purging and a Passion for Care: The Yellow Fever Nurse in the Deep South in the Early 19th Century," in *Nursing Interventions through Time: History as Evidence*, eds. Patricia D'Antonio and Sandra Lewenson (New York: Springer Publishing, 2010). See also: Booker T. Washington, "Training Colored Nurses at Tuskegee," *AJN* 11, no. 1 (1910): 167–171.
14. Wall, "Courage to Care," 56.
15. Gertrude Fenner D.C., "The Daughters of Charity in the Spanish-American War," *Vincentian Heritage Journal* 8, no. 2 (1987): article 4.
16. Wall, "Courage to Care," 58.
17. Ibid., 59.
18. Ibid., 61.
19. Highlights in the History of the Army Nurse Corps: 1.

20. Wall, "Courage to Care," 63.

21. "A Guide to the Phillip Hench Walter Reed Yellow Fever Collection," https://www.exhibits
.hsl.virginia.edu (accessed July 25, 2016).

22. Greer Williams, *The Plague Killers* (New York: Scribner, 1969), 185–208. See also: John T.
Cunningham, *Clara Maass: A Nurse, A Hospital, A Spirit* (Belleville, NJ: Rae Books, 1968).

23. Wall, "Courage to Care," 68.

24. "Surgeon General Annual Report, 1899," in Lavinia Dock, Elizabeth G. Fox, Clara D. Noyes,
Sarah E. Pickett, Fannie F. Clement, and Anna R. Van Meter, *A History of the American Red
Cross* (New York: Macmillan, 1922).

25. Anonymous nurse, quoted in Lavinia Dock et al., *History of the American Red Cross*, 34.

26. Jamieson and Sewall, *Trends in Nursing History*, 403.

27. Kristin Rothwell, "Historical Perspective—Jane Delano: American Red Cross Nurses Continue to Walk in Her Footsteps," https://www.americanmobile.com/NurseZone (accessed
January 5, 2016): 1.

28. Doris Sterner, *In and Out of Harm's Way: A History of the Navy Nurse Corps* (Seattle, WA:
Peanut Butter Publishing, 1997).

29. "Establishment of the Nurse Corps," Act of Congress, May 13, 1908, in Lavinia Dock et al.,
A History of the American Red Cross (U.S. Congress: Washington, DC): 686.

30. Esther V. Hasson, "The Navy Nurse Corps," *AJN* 9, no. 6 (1909): 410–415 (quote 413).

31. Ethel Fenwick, quoted in Philip Kalisch and Beatrice Kalisch, *American Nursing: A History*,
4th ed. (Philadelphia: Lippincott Williams and Wilkins, 2004): 178–179.

32. Ibid., 178.

33. M. I. Feeny, "Central Directories," *AJN* 4 (1904): 797–798. See also: E. Scovil, "Openings for
Nurses," *AJN* 1(1901): 439–443.

34. Jean Whelan, "'A Necessity in the Nursing World': The Chicago Nurses Professional Registry, 1913-1950," *NHR* 13 (2005): 49–75 (quote 52).

35. Susan Reverby, *Ordered to Care: The Dilemma of American Nursing, 1850–1945* (Cambridge:
Cambridge University Press, 1987): 97.

36. Gerda Anderson, "Helps to Success in Private Duty," *AJN* 8 (1904): 11–13 (quote 11–12).

37. Mary Holleman, "The Private Duty Nurse and Her Work," *AJN* 16, no. 8 (May 1916): 708–713.

38. Whelan, "A Necessity."

39. Thelma Schorr and Maureen Kennedy, *100 Years of American Nursing: Celebrating a Century
of Caring* (Philadelphia, PA: Lippincott, 1999).

40. Nellie Miller, "The Private Duty Nurse," *AJN* 16, no. 6 (March 1916): 475–480 (quote 477).

41. Whelan, "A Necessity," 56.

42. Minnie Crawford, "Why, When and How to Bathe a Fever Patient," *AJN*, 10, no. 5 (February
1910): 314–317 (quote 316).

43. Diarmuid Jeffreys, *Aspirin: The Remarkable Story of a Wonder Drug* (New York: Bloomsbury,
2004).

44. Mary Gibson, "Care and Cure on the Hudson," paper presented at Eleanor Crowder Bjoring
Center of Nursing Historical Inquiry history forum, Charlottesville, VA, November 15, 2005.
See also: Mary Gibson, "Untiring Labor for the Suffering Child," paper presented at the South-
ern Association for the History of Medicine and Science, Atlanta, GA, March 2012, 1–12.

45. Mary Gibson, "Care and Cure," (2005): 7.

46. Barbara Brodie, "Children of the Sun: Heliotherapy and Tubercular Children," *Windows in
Time* 23, no. 2 (October 2015): 8–12 (quote 10).

47. Lina Rogers, "Some Phases of School Nursing," *AJN* 8, no. 12 (September 1909): 966–974.

48. Lillian Wald, "Medical Inspection of Public Schools," *Annals of the American Academy of Political and Social Sciences* 25 (March 1905): 91.

49. Lina Rogers, "School Nursing in New York City," *AJN* 3, no. 6 (March 1903): 448–450.

50. Arlene Keeling, "The Henry Street Settlement Visiting Nurses," ch. 1 in *Nursing and the Privilege of Prescription* (Columbus: The Ohio State University Press, 2007): 23.

51. Lavinia Dock, "School Nurse Experiment in New York," *AJN* 3, no. 2 (1902): 109.

52. Lina L. Rogers, "The Nurse in the Public School," *AJN* (1905): 764–773. See also: Lina Rogers, "Some Phases of School Nursing," *AJN* 8 (1908): 966.

53. Keeling, "Henry Street Settlement," 24.

54. Rogers, "Some Phases of School Nursing," 966.

55. Anna Kerr, "School Nursing in New York City," *AJN* 10, no. 2 (November 1909): 106–108.

56. Josephine Baker, *Fighting for Life* (New York: McMillan, 1939).

57. C. Wardell Stiles, "The Rural Health Movement," *Annals of the American Academy of Political and Social Science* 37, no. 2 (1911): 123–126; Taliaferro Clark, "The Physical Care of Rural School Children," *Public Health Reports* 38, no. 22 (June 1, 1923): 1181–1190.

58. Mary Gibson, "Hookworm, Tooth Decay, and Tonsillectomies, 1900-1925," in *Nursing Rural America: Perspectives from the Early 20th Century*, eds. John Kirchgessner and Arlene Keeling (New York: Springer Publishing, 2015): 39–52.

59. Bridget Houlahan, "A History of School Nursing" (unpublished dissertation chapters, University of Virginia, 2016).

60. Taliaferro Clark, "The Physical Care of Rural School Children," 1181.

61. Kate Hall, "Saving the Child from Hookworm," *The Public Health Nurse* 12, no. 11 (1923): 951–953 (quote 952).

62. Annie Brainard, *The Evolution of Public Health Nursing* (Philadelphia: W.B. Saunders, 1922); J. B. Gwin, "Rural Social Work," *Journal of Social Forces* 3, no. 2 (1925): 280–283.

63. Sybil Koeller, "Rural District Nursing," *American Journal of Nursing* 17, no. 4 (January 1917): 317.

64. Mary Sewell Gardner, *Public Health Nursing*, 3rd ed. (New York: Macmillan, 1936): 215.

65. Rima Apple, "Public Health Nursing in Rural Wisconsin: Stretched Beyond Health Inspection," in *Nursing Rural America*, eds. Kirchgessner and Keeling, 21–28 (quote 23).

66. Dock et al., *History of the American Red Cross*, 1227.

67. Ibid. See also: Phoebe Pollitt, *The History of Professional Nursing in North Carolina, 1902-2002* (Durham, NC: Carolina Academic Press, 2014): 60.

68. Elizabeth Turner, "One of Those Monstrosities of Nature: The Galveston Storm of 1900," *History Now: The Journal of the Gilder Lehrman Institute*, https://www.gilderlehrman.org (accessed July 21, 2016): 1.

69. Barbra Mann Wall, "The 1900 Galveston Hurricane: 'Unspeakable Calamity,'" in *Nurses on the Frontline: When Disaster Strikes, 1878-2010*, eds. B. M. Wall and A. W. Keeling (New York: Springer Publishing, 2011): 17–42 (quote 17).

70. Ibid., 17–42.

71. Ibid., 29.

72. Clyde Buckingham, *Clara Barton: A Broad Humanity* (Alexandria, VA: Mount Vernon Publishing, 1977): 298.

73. Wall, "The 1900 Galveston Hurricane," 31.

74. Barbra Mann Wall and Marie Kelly, "The San Francisco Earthquake and Fire, 1906: 'A Lifetime of Experience,'" in *Nurses on the Frontline*, eds. B. M. Wall and A. W. Keeling, 43.

75. Lucy Fisher, "A Nurse's Earthquake Experience," *AJN* 7, no. 2 (November 1906): 84–98.

76. Official reports, *AJN* 6, no. 10 (July 1906): 721–728 (quote 724).

77. "1906 Earthquake: Medical Care and Sanitation," http://nps.gov/prsf/learn/historyculture/images/EQ-field-hospitalA.jpg (accessed January 13, 2016).

78. Wall and Kelly, "The San Francisco Earthquake," in *Nurses on the Frontlines*, eds. B. M. Wall and A. W. Keeling, 49–50.

79. "Quick Facts about the 1906 Earthquake and Fires," 1906 Earthquake Resources, 2008, http://www.archives.gov/legislative/features/sf.

80. Miss Ashe, "Letter to the Editor," published in Editorial Comment, *AJN* (June 1906): 581–592 (quote 583).

81. "Letter to the Editor," *AJN* 6, no. 9 (June 1906): 581–582 (quote 583).

82. Ibid.

83. Official reports, *AJN* 6, no. 10 (July 1906): 721–728 (quote 724).

84. John Kirchgessner, "The Monongah Mine Disaster, December 1907: 'A Roar Like a Thousand Niagara's,'" in *Nurses on the Frontline*, eds. B. M. Wall and A. W. Keeling, 69–86.

85. Ibid., 72–78.

86. Ibid., 77.

87. Eugene Wolf, "December 6, 1907: No Christmas at Monongah," *Pittsburg Golden Seal Reprints* (Winter 1993): 33.

88. Michelle Hehman, "Once Seen, Never Forgotten: Nursing Ethics and Technology in Early Premature Infant Care, 1898-1943" (PhD dissertation, University of Virginia, 2016).

89. Thomas E. Cone, *History of the Care and Feeding of the Premature Infant* (Boston: Little, Brown, 1985): 25.

90. Hehman, "Once Seen."

91. "Proposal Analysis for Infant Incubator Project," report submitted February 15, 1938. Courtesy the New York World's Fair 1939-1940 records, Manuscripts and Archives Division, the New York Public Library, Series I, Box 547, Folder 3.

92. Hehman, "Once Seen."

93. A detailed photograph of a chart used to monitor temperature, growth, and weight gain can be found in James Walter Smith, "Baby Incubators," *The Strand Magazine* 12 (1896): 770–776. Similar graphs are seen on the front of individual incubators from photographs taken inside incubator exhibits, although the exact details from each record cannot be seen. These records are referenced in medical journal articles "The Victorian Era Exhibition at Earl's Court," *Lancet* 2 (1897): 161–162; "Exhibit of Infant Incubators at the Pan-American Exhibition," *Pediatrics* 12 (1901): 414–419; and "Some Medical Aspects of the Pan American Exposition: Infant Incubators," *Buffalo Medical Journal* 57 (1901): 55–56.

94. Outcome statistics quoted in "Incubator Graduates Hold a Reunion," *New York Times*, August 1, 1904; "Where Babies Are Made Strong by Artificial Means," *Washington Times*, October 2, 1904; Evelyn C. Lundeen, "History of the Hortense Schoen Joseph Premature Station," *The Voice of the Clinic* 2 (1937): 10; and Martin A. Couney, letter to J. Peter Hoguet, October 20, 1940. Courtesy the New York World's Fair 1939-1940 records, Manuscripts and Archives Division, the New York Public Library, Series I, Box 547, Folder 2.

95. Hehman, "Once Seen."

96. Ibid.

97. Julius H. Hess and Evelyn C. Lundeen, *The Premature Infant: Its Medical and Nursing Care* (Philadelphia, PA: J. B. Lippincott, 1941): 69, 82.

98. Evelyn Lundeen, "Safe Hospital Care for the Premature Baby," *Hospitals* 14 (1936): 111.

99. Julius H. Hess, "Chicago Plan for Care of Premature Infants," *Journal of the American Medical Association* 146 (1951): 891; Evelyn C. Lundeen, "History of the Hortense Schoen Joseph Premature Station," *The Voice of the Clinic* 2 (1937): 8.

100. Hess and Lundeen, *The Premature Infant*, vi.

101. Diane Hamilton, *The Metropolitan Life Insurance Company Visiting Nurse Service, 1909-1953* (PhD dissertation, University of Virginia, May 1987): 35.

102. Ibid., 68–69.

103. Ibid., 72.

104. Ibid., 74–75.

105. Lee Frankel, "Visiting Nursing from a Business Organization's Standpoint" (1913), Welfare Division files, Metropolitan Life Insurance Company archives, New York. Quoted in Hamilton dissertation, 79.

106. Ibid, 79.

107. Nellie Linsay, "Insurance Nursing in Rochester," *AJN* 11, no. 8 (May 1911): 614–616 (quote 615).

108. Cynthia Connolly, *Saving Sickly Children: The Tuberculosis Preventorium in American Life, 1909-1970* (New Brunswick, NJ: Rutgers University Press, 2008): 38.

109. Ibid., 42.

110. Cynthia Connolly, "Nurses: The Early 20th Century Tuberculosis Preventorium's 'Connecting Link,'" in *Nurses' Work: Issues across Time and Place,* eds. Patricia D'Antonio, Ellen Baer, Sylvia Rinker, and Joan Lynaugh (New York: Springer Publishing, 2007): 173–202 (quote 176).

111. Cynthia A. Connolly, "Nurses: The Early Twentieth-Century Tuberculosis Preventorium's 'Connecting Link,'" *NHR* 10 (2002): 127–157. See also: Cynthia Connolly and Mary Gibson, "The 'White Plague' and Color: Children, Race and Tuberculosis in Virginia, 1900–1935,"*Journal of Pediatric Nursing* 26 (2011): 230–238.

112. Connolly, *Saving Sickly Children.*

113. J. Palmer Quimby, "The Tuberculosis Preventorium for Children, Farmingdale, N.J." *The Modern Hospital* 8 (March 1917): 177–179 (quote 177).

114. Alfred Hess, quoted in Cynthia A. Connolly, "Nurses: The Early Twentieth-Century Tuberculosis Preventorium's 'Connecting Link," *NHR* 10 (2002): 127–157 (quote 145).

115. Connolly, "Nurses: The Early Twentieth Century," *NHR* 2002, 146.

116. Quimby, "The Tuberculosis Preventorium," 178.

117. "Farmingdale Annual Report" in Cynthia Connolly, *Saving Sickly Children,* 63.

118. "The 1911 Triangle Factory Fire," http://trianglefire.ilr.cornell.edu (accessed February 26, 2016): 1.

119. Lillian Wald Papers, Council of National Defense correspondence, Lillian Wald Papers, New York Public Library, microfilm, reel 25.

120. Sarah White Craig, "Nursing in Schoolfield Mill Village: Cotton and Welfare," in *Nursing Rural America: Perspectives from the Early 20th Century,* eds. John Kirchgessner and Arlene Keeling (New York: Springer Publishing, 2015): 53–68.

121. Ibid.

122. Ibid.

123. Deborah L. Gleason, *The Insulin Odyssey: Nursing Care of Children with Diabetes, 1915–1935* (PhD dissertation, University of Virginia, May 2012).

124. Ibid., 43.

125. Julius Freedenwall and Jon Ruhrah, *Dietetics for Nurses,* 4th ed. (Philadelphia, PA: W. B. Saunders, 1918): 333.

126. Debbie Gleason-Morgan, "A 'Cure for the Privileged': The Impact of Insulin on Nursing Care of Children with Diabetes," in *Windows in Time; The Newsletter of the Eleanor Crowder Bjoring Center for Nursing Historical Inquiry* (October 2008): 7–9.

127. Ibid.

128. "The Discovery of Insulin," http://www.nobelprize.org (accessed January 11, 2016).

129. Gleason, *The Insulin Odyssey,* 156.

130. "Lovilla Winterbottom, A Wandering Diabetes Nurse," *AJN* 31, no. 8 (August 1931): 957–958 (quote 957).

131. Ibid., 957.

132. Ibid., 958.

FURTHER READING

Apple, Rima, "Public Health Nursing in Rural Wisconsin: Stretched Beyond Health Inspection," in *Nursing Rural America: Perspectives from the Early 20th Century,* eds. John Kirchgessner and Arlene Keeling (New York: Springer Publishing, 2014): 21–28.

Baker, Josephine, *Fighting for Life* (New York: McMillan, 1939).

Brodie, Barbara, "Children of the Sun: Heliotherapy and Tubercular Children," *Windows in Time* 23, no. 2 (October 2015): 8–12.

Connolly, Cynthia, *Saving Sickly Children: The Tuberculosis Preventorium in American Life, 1909-1970* (New Brunswick, NJ: Rutgers University Press, 2008).

Connolly, Cynthia and Mary Gibson, "The 'White Plague' and Color: Children, Race and Tuberculosis in Virginia, 1900-1935," *Journal of Pediatric Nursing* 26 (2011): 230–238.

Craig, Sarah White, "Nursing in Schoolfield Mill Village: Cotton and Welfare," in *Nursing Rural America: Perspectives from the Early 20th Century,* eds. John Kirchgessner and Arlene Keeling (New York: Springer Publishing, 2014): 53–68.

D'Antonio, Patricia, *American Nursing: A History of Knowledge, Authority and the Meaning of Work* (Baltimore, MD: The Johns Hopkins Press, 2010).

D'Antonio, Patricia, *Nursing with a Message: Public Health Demonstration Projects in New York City* (New Brunswick, NJ: Rutgers University Press, 2017).

D'Antonio, Patricia, Ellen Baer, Sylvia Rinker, and Joan Lynaugheds, *Nurses' Work: Issues across Time and Place* (New York: Springer Publishing, 2007).

Editor, "Central Registries," *American Journal of Nursing* 9 (1909): 639.

Frantz, Ann, "Nursing Pride: Clara Barton in the Spanish-American War," *American Journal of Nursing* 98, no. 10 (1998): 39–41.

Gibson, Mary, "Hookworm, Tooth Decay, and Tonsillectomies, 1900-1925," in *Nursing Rural America: Perspectives from the Early 20th Century*, eds. John Kirchgessner and Arlene Keeling (New York: Springer Publishing, 2015): 39–52.

Gleason, Deborah L., *The Insulin Odyssey: Nursing Care of Children with Diabetes, 1915-1935* (PhD dissertation, University of Virginia, May 2012).

Hehman, Michelle, *Once Seen, Never Forgotten: Nursing Ethics and Technology in Early Premature Infant Care, 1898-1943* (PhD dissertation, University of Virginia, 2016).

Kirchgessner, John, "The Monongah Mine Disaster, December 1907: 'A Roar Like a Thousand Niagara's,'" in *Nurses on the Frontline: When Disaster Strikes, 1878-2010*, eds. Barbra Mann Wall and Arlene W. Keeling (New York: Springer Publishing, 2011): 69–86.

Nuwer, Deanne S., "The 1878 Yellow Fever Epidemic in Mississippi," in *Nurses on the Frontline: When Disaster Strikes, 1878-2010*, eds. Barbra Mann Wall and Arlene W. Keeling (New York: Springer Publishing, 2011): 1–15.

Sabin, Linda, "Sweating, Purging and a Passion for Care: The Yellow Fever Nurse in the Deep South in the Early 19th Century," in *Nursing Interventions through Time: History as Evidence*, eds. Patricia D'Antonio and Sandra Lewenson (New York: Springer Publishing, 2007): 49–64.

Wall, Barbra Mann, "Courage to Care: The Sisters of the Holy Cross in the Spanish American War," *NHR* 3 (1995): 55–77.

Westphal, Richard, "Remember the Maine! Remember the Men" *American Journal of Nursing* 103, no. 5 (2003): 77–78.

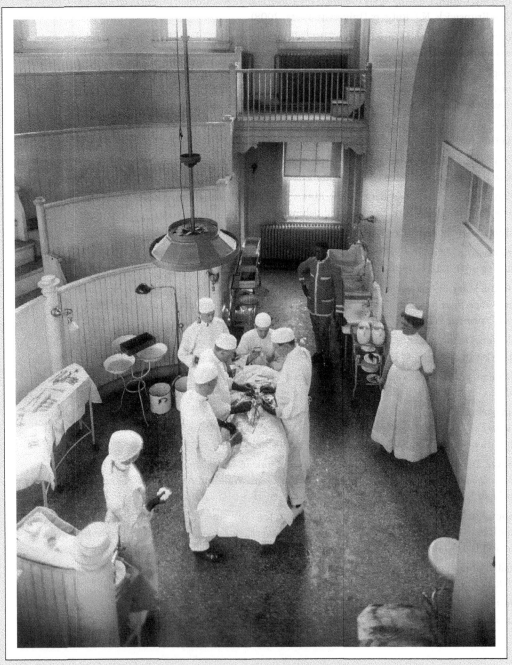

University of Virginia Hospital operating room 1913.

CHAPTER 7

Nurses, Science, and the Growth of Hospitals

1910–1930

Michelle C. Hehman

"The last thirty years have witnessed the most spectacular building of hospitals by a hopeful people that has ever taken place in the world's history. Instead of being dreaded, hospitals are now looked at with confidence and even affection as places wherein most can be done to cure disease and alleviate suffering."[1]

Writing in the *Bulletin of the American Hospital Association* in 1930, Dr. Nathaniel W. Faxon remarked on the proliferation of hospitals in the United States in the first few decades of the 20th century. Faxon concluded: "No part of medicine showed more striking advances than the development and improvement in hospitals."[3] Indeed, the total number of hospitals and hospital beds supported his assertion, growing from 4,359 hospitals with 421,065 beds in 1909 to 6,719 hospitals with 955,869 beds in 1930.[4] These increases far outpaced the growth of the population, indicating that America's image of hospital-based care had greatly improved in 20 years. During this time, the nature of hospitals changed completely. They transitioned from being charitable institutions that cared for the poor, marginalized, and chronically ill, to being institutions that embodied scientific progress and achievement, and focused on acute, specialized care for paying customers. As historian Rosemary Stevens described, hospitals are "mirrors of the culture in which we live, beaming back to us . . . the values we impute to medicine, technology, wealth, class, and social welfare."[5]

The shift from home care by family to hospital care by professionals was complex and reflected the tumultuous nature of the early 20th century. In these first few decades, U.S. citizens witnessed the social activism of the Progressive Era, the growth of mass culture and consumerism during the Roaring Twenties, and the devastating economic decline of the Great Depression. Revolutionary discoveries in science and technology changed the way people thought about and interacted with the world. Industrial growth, rapid urbanization, and large-scale immigration disrupted the traditional family system and led to new social problems, including unsafe working conditions, overcrowding, and communicable diseases.[6] Progressive reformers worked to improve individual and community health by alleviating these realities. The rising women's movement challenged traditional Victorian norms about gender roles, childbirth, and the nature of the American family. Racial tension persisted as the south remained segregated, and racially motivated violence and discrimination erupted in northern cities over housing and jobs.

> "The past thirty years in nursing show a period of intense activity, of rapid and continuous development."[2]
>
> M. Adelaide Nutting, 1923

Scientific advancement, educational reform, professional specialization, cultural changes, and racial discrimination influenced the development of the hospital industry and transformed the nurses who worked there. In turn the nursing profession influenced and transformed the nature of the hospitals and the care they provided. Virtually all aspects of the nursing profession experienced change, from education, training, and clinical skills, to practical authority and economic opportunities. But despite the upheaval and social constraints, nurses adapted to the changing circumstances and continued to combat disease and restore health in their patients.

ADVANCES IN MEDICINE, SCIENCE, AND TECHNOLOGY

Advances in medical science and technology in the early 20th century drove much of the increased demand for professional nursing care in hospitals. Discoveries by Louis Pasteur, Joseph Lister, and Robert Koch in the mid-19th century changed medical understanding of disease. Germ theory, antisepsis, and bacteriology slowly replaced the prevailing unitary and humoral theories of illness. Enthusiasm for technology also fueled improvements in laboratory analysis and medical devices in the late 19th century as physicians and inventors developed advanced diagnostic tests and instruments. They examined blood and urine to understand physiologic responses to disease. Their careful examination and tests on blood samples helped them determine hemoglobin, hematocrit, and leukocyte counts to diagnose and monitor diseases like anemia or serious infections. Blood counts became a common tool for making a prognosis. In fact, at Pennsylvania Hospital in 1900 only 5% of patients had a blood count performed; by 1920 that number increased to nearly 28%.[7]

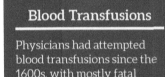

Blood Transfusions

Physicians had attempted blood transfusions since the 1600s, with mostly fatal results. In 1901 Karl Landsteiner discovered three human blood types: A, B, and C (later O); the AB blood type was discovered the following year. By 1907 cross-matching blood between the donor and the recipient led to the first successful direct blood transfusion. When long-term anticoagulants were developed in 1914 and added to blood donations, indirect transfusion and blood storage became standard.

Nurses and the New Technology

Urinalysis helped physicians diagnose and monitor kidney disease, urinary tract infections, kidney and bladder stones, and diabetes. Between 1900 and 1920 the frequency of urinalysis for inpatients at Pennsylvania Hospital increased as it had for blood counts. In 1900 a patient may have had a urinalysis performed about every 8 days, but by 1920 the test increased to one every 4 days.[8] Lab tests became common tools in a physician's diagnostic arsenal.

New medical equipment also changed physicians' understanding of physiology and broadened their diagnostic and therapeutic capabilities. As historian Joel Howell stated, "To be able to see within the human body had a profound impact on both the medical and lay communities, on medical thought, and on fundamental ideas about the human body."[9] The x-ray machine provided images that allowed physicians to accurately and less

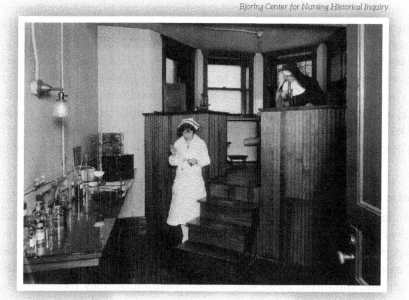

A nurse and a nun work in a laboratory.

The Electrocardiograph

In 1893, Dutch physiologist Willem Einthoven used his knowledge of the electrical activity of cardiac cells and coined the term "electrocardiogram." He also defined and identified P, Q, R, S, and T waves. By 1901 Einthoven had developed a string galvanometer to record an electrocardiograph, but the device was too heavy to be practical. After the design was improved, Mount Sinai Hospital in New York became the first hospital in 1909 to purchase an electrocardiograph for clinical use.

painfully diagnose fractures, and to improve their ability to surgically correct bony deformities. The electrocardiogram also gained popularity among the medical community, although it was a large and expensive machine. Proper use of all of these tests and technologies required extra time and specialized skills of physicians, technicians, and nurses.

Nurses were encouraged to broaden their knowledge of laboratory and x-ray science. In arguing for the addition of a laboratory course in nursing education, one scientist claimed that, "Such a course should enable them to understand the limits of their ability as well as the extent of the same. Such a course will not make pathologists or expert technicians of them; it will make their work more interesting and increase their ability."[10] Others argued that specialized knowledge and skill in these fields would make graduate nurses more marketable and expand their employment opportunities beyond private duty. Some even suggested that these specialties offered new opportunities to graduate nurses who because of their "physique or personality" might not be especially adapted to continuous bedside nursing.[11]

Nurses used all of these new technologies on a daily basis, and the amount of new information was staggering. As one physician remarked, "With the rapid advance in diagnostic methods . . . the demands on the nurses' ability are becoming more exacting."[12] To be successful, nurses needed knowledge of and familiarity with tools like thermometers and x-rays, tests like urinalysis

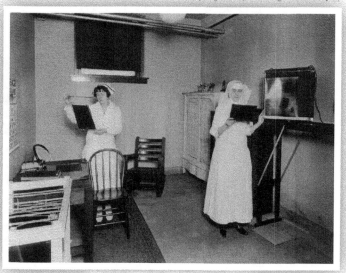

A nurse and a nun inspect x-ray films.

and blood counts, and procedures like antiseptic practices and anesthesia administration. Nursing textbooks not only described how to properly perform a task, but also the scientific reasons why it was necessary and what this meant for the patient.[13] The successful completion of a nurse's duties required intelligence, skill, and careful observation of patient responses to treatments. As nurse Mary Roberts explained, proper nursing was "not a mere series of procedures strung like beads on the wire of a doctor's orders, [but] a carefully wrought fabric in which procedures stand out like a design against the less colorful but necessary background of understanding of personal, social, and psychological factors, intelligent observation of physical and mental symptoms and conditions."[14]

Therapeutic Care

Although working with complex technology comprised an increasing part of nursing duties, much of the nurses' work still involved everyday domestic tasks, emotional support, and environmental control. Nurses still fed patients, bathed them, ensured that beds were made with fresh linens, opened windows for fresh air, and comforted those who needed reassurance. They rocked and held premature infants, and took them outside for a "sun bath."[15] Nurses continued to supervise hospitalized children as they participated in outdoor play. For many nursing leaders, these functions remained just as vital as the new technology in the process of restoring health. M. Adelaide Nutting reminded nurses, "We may have great and imposing buildings, the last word in hygienic and sanitary appliances, dazzling operation rooms and laboratories, but that stricken human being lying there has many needs that none of these can satisfy."[16]

Common domestic items like baths and beds utilized by all women in the home became therapeutic ways of healing in the hands of professional nurses. As Clara Weeks-Shaw's *A Textbook of Nursing* (1906) explained, "baths are used for remedial purposes as well as simply for cleanliness. They may be general or local, simple or medicated, cold, tepid, or hot; in the form of liquid, vapor, or air. Judiciously employed, baths are valuable therapeutic

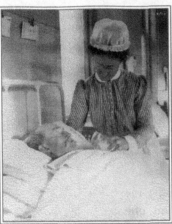

A nurse feeds a patient, which remained a core aspect of nursing duties despite technological advances.

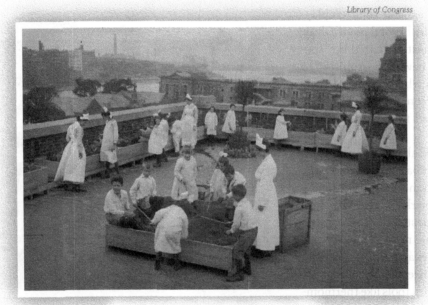

Nurses supervise children in a rooftop garden.

agents."[17] Textbooks of the time also described the different construction and use of beds. Beds could be differentiated by configuration for different patient types, for example, surgical versus obstetric; or by therapeutic purpose, as in a standard bed for resting versus a fracture bed for traction. A professional nurse was equipped with specialized knowledge and training to skillfully incorporate these devices into the patient care routine, thus distinguishing the trained nurse from the laywoman.[18]

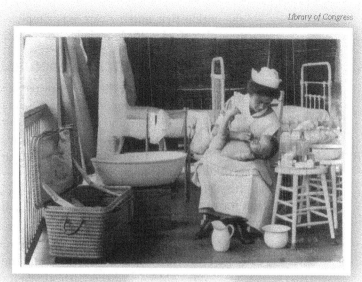

A nurse bathes a baby.

Nurses therefore occupied a unique position between laymen and physicians, sharing the use of many devices with both groups. This intermediate position, in which nurses shared use but lacked control, contributed to poor perceptions of the intrinsic value of nursing. The nursing profession failed to gain practical authority over the new medical technology and equipment; thus hypodermic syringes, stethoscopes, and incubators remained under medical control. Only physicians ordered their use; nurses simply ensured that those orders were completed. Although nurses used the new devices more often, and in some cases more efficiently than their physician colleagues, none of the instruments or tests uniquely exemplified nursing knowledge or skill. As nurse historian Margarete Sandalowski explained, "Even when nurses possessed greater knowledge than physicians, this knowledge was either not recognized or minimized, even by nurses themselves."[19] Nurses made their proficiency with new tools and procedures appear effortless; in doing so they unconsciously reinforced

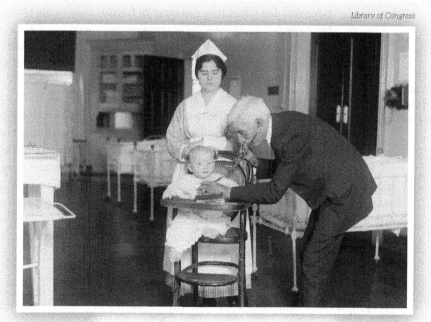

A physician examines a baby with a stethoscope as a nurse stands by.

the notion that nursing care was simply a practical ability rather than an intelligent interplay of scientific knowledge and technical proficiency.

IMPROVING MEDICAL AND NURSING EDUCATION

Medical and nursing leaders soon recognized the need to reform their educational programs to comply with contemporary scientific discovery. As one physician remarked, "The question of the proper education of the physician, as well as the proper education of the nurse, is burning hot today."[20]

"It is clear that so long as a man is to practice medicine, the public is equally concerned in his right preparation for that profession."[21]

Abraham Flexner, 1910

Until the late 19th century, American medical education lacked any sort of minimum standard or regulation. Wide variation existed among training programs, and very few states required a license to practice medicine. In response, the American Medical Association (AMA) created a Council on Medical Education in 1904 to standardize training programs for physicians. The council first created a minimum standard for physicians, calling for 4 years of medical school and the passage of a licensing exam.[23] In 1909 the AMA asked the Carnegie Foundation for the Advancement of Teaching to survey North American medical schools, with Abraham Flexner in charge of the process. Flexner's assigned duty was to assess the compliance of schools with the required minimum standards outlined by the AMA.

"Nursing is in a very special sense a national service, and the training of the nurse is a matter of vital concern."[22]

NLNE Committee on Education, 1917

The Flexner Report

Published in 1910, *Medical Education in the United States and Canada* exposed the overwhelming inadequacies of the current system of medical education and training. Remarking on the collective quality of physicians in the United States, Flexner stated, "There is probably no other country in the world in which there is so great a distance and so fatal a difference between the best, the average, and the worst."[24] Flexner also recognized a need to overhaul how medical schools taught scientific theory:

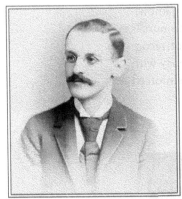

Library of Congress

Abraham Flexner, who encouraged more standardized medical education and training.

The requirements of medical education have enormously increased. The fundamental sciences upon which medicine depends have been greatly extended. The laboratory has come to furnish alike to the physician and to the surgeon a new means for diagnosing and combating disease. The education of the medical practitioner under these changed conditions makes entirely different demands in respect to both preliminary and professional training.[25]

Flexner recommended more stringent admission criteria, more qualified medical educators, and more uniform curricula that included laboratory courses and varied practical experiences. In response, American medical training became much more standardized. Numerous small medical schools were eliminated and national funding and resources were allocated to larger, professional medical schools associated with universities. Medical students began to complete a 1-year internship after they graduated from medical school, during which they focused on a chosen specialty, or experienced all areas of medicine through a rotating clerkship. By 1914 approximately 75% of all graduates finished an intern year.[26]

Nursing Education and the Goldmark Report

Nursing leaders had long lamented the character and status of American training schools. National nursing organizations had never reached consensus on admission requirements, program length, theoretical components, practice opportunities, private duty requirements, or cost; consequently, quality varied greatly across the country. State licensing laws were the first attempt to regulate the practice of graduate nurses, and nurse leaders hoped that nursing schools would adjust their curricula to ensure that students could obtain a license after graduation. But licensure exams differed from state to state, often barred African American women from taking the exam, and discriminated against students who graduated from small training schools. The National League for Nursing Education (NLNE) published the *Standard Curriculum for Schools of Nursing* in 1917 in an attempt to standardize nurse training schools, but it failed to prompt much change. The result is unsurprising given that committee members had stated that they were "not urging the unqualified adoption of this curriculum in training schools generally."[27]

Two years later, the Rockefeller Foundation financed the creation of the Committee for the Study of Nursing Education. The interprofessional group of nurses, physicians, lay individuals, and hospital industry leaders asked Josephine Goldmark to evaluate nursing education in the United States. Published in 1923, Goldmark's report, *Nursing and Nursing Education in the United States*, highlighted the limitations in nursing education and suggested the separation of training schools from the nursing service of hospitals. The report stated that the current arrangement, in which most schools lacked independent endowments and authority, demonstrated the "essential weakness of the apprentice system; [that] its first liability is service production, not education."[31] Goldmark continued, "The training of nurses is sacrificed and prolonged in deference to the needs of the hospital. . . . No actions will follow unless these facts challenge the interest of those in authority."[32]

Nursing leaders had hoped the *Standard Curriculum* and Goldmark reports would do for nursing what the Flexner report had accomplished for medical education. Unfortunately, the report received a great deal of criticism from nurses, physicians, and administrators, mainly because only 23 training schools of the highest quality had been analyzed when more than 1,700 professional nursing schools existed.[34] Hospital administrators and physicians railed against making the suggested changes, particularly granting schools complete independence from hospital service.[35] Nurses took issue with the suggestion of "a subsidiary nursing service" that would be licensed to care for patients with mild or more chronic ailments.[36]

While the Goldmark report highlighted the need to reform nursing education, it failed to create any real improvement in the system. As a profession, nursing lacked political or economic power, and fell victim to gendered stereotypes because it was overwhelmingly female. Both the Carnegie and Rockefeller Foundations had offered their money and influence to the improvement of medical education, but they did not feel the same responsibility toward the education of nurses. While the Rockefeller Foundation recognized the important role of nurses for providing public health services, it believed that nursing was ultimately an "ancillary service subordinate to physicians," and did not earnestly support the advance of nursing education.[37]

The Johns Hopkins Hospital: Model for Education

Both the Flexner and Goldmark reports praised the structure and organization of university education for medicine and nursing. The university hospital system not only offered ample and varied clinical opportunities and state-of-the-art laboratory facilities, but also allowed the schools to operate purely for educational

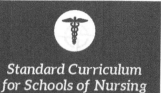

Standard Curriculum for Schools of Nursing

In the *Standard Curriculum for Schools of Nursing* (1917), committee members attempted to offer guidance rather than a "model curriculum," providing direction to schools struggling to establish their own rubric.[28] The curriculum suggested a program length of 3 years, and outlined both theoretical and practical components necessary for adequate nursing education. One nurse characterized it as a "socialized curriculum," since it emphasized preventive medicine as much as sick nursing.[29]

"The new curriculum gives us a challenge in that it stresses health not disease."[30]

Carolyn E. Gray, 1918

"The school of nursing has sought to perform two functions: to educate nurses and to supply the nursing service for the hospital. But in these two functions there lies an ever present possibility of conflict."[33]

Josephine Goldmark, 1923

"There must be wider responsibility for securing endowments for the education of women as nurses."[38]

Carrie M. Hall, 1927

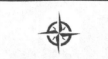

Nursing Code of Ethics

In 1926 the American Nurses Association presented a Suggested Code of Ethics at its annual convention. Nurses were to serve society as model citizens, and could achieve this by finding happiness, economic independence, and self-realization.[39] Nurses would bring their patients "all of the knowledge, skill, and devotion" required to guard their health.[40] The code emphasized good judgment rather than strict obedience, and initiated a reciprocal relationship between nursing and society.

purposes. The Goldmark report argued: "the development of the University School of Nursing has been perhaps the most notable feature in the progress of nursing education."[41] Flexner had praised the Johns Hopkins system, stating that Hopkins medical graduates were of "the highest quality the country has produced."[42] He went on to assert that the facilities "are in every respect unexcelled . . . [and] provide practically ideal opportunities."[43] The excellence established in the medical school was transferred to the Johns Hopkins Hospital School of Nursing as well. Johns Hopkins became the model that many hospitals of the time followed for both medical and nursing education and training.

The Johns Hopkins Hospital was initiated by a wealthy Baltimore merchant and financier named Johns Hopkins who had the vision and financial resources to organize a scientifically modern hospital and university system. Hopkins's interest in hospitals and nursing services originated when he contracted and nearly died of cholera during an epidemic in Baltimore in 1832. The experience left him with an appalling view of medical and nursing care available in Maryland hospitals, and he subsequently joined the governing board for Maryland Hospital.[44] An 1867 examination of the hospital's nursing services led the board to report that "the nurses did not possess either method, order, invention, or energy" and were not "sufficient in number or intelligence to discharge their duties."[45] Later that year, Hopkins secured two state bills to establish the Johns Hopkins Hospital and the Johns Hopkins University.

While the hospital and nurse training school would not open for another 22 years, Hopkins immediately created a board of trustees and began planning his new center for modern medicine. He left his entire fortune of $7 million, the largest amount any American had bequeathed for philanthropic purposes, to found the hospital and the university. His final letter of instructions to the board, written in March 1873, emphasized Hopkins's desire to establish a nurse training school associated with the Johns Hopkins Hospital to "secure the services of women competent to care for the sick" that would strengthen the community through "a class of trained and experienced nurses."[46]

Before any building projects began, Hopkins requested advice from physicians with experience in hospital construction and organization. The board appointed Dr. John S. Billings, assistant surgeon in the U.S. Army, to supervise the hospital's construction. Both Billings and Mr. Francis T. King, president of the Board of Trustees, independently travelled through Europe in the late 1870s to observe a number of hospitals, including St. Thomas Hospital in London. King even had "lengthy interviews" with Florence Nightingale, discussing the merits of the Nightingale model for the design of the hospital wards and the development of a nurse training school.[47] Nightingale heavily influenced the development of the nurse-training program at Johns Hopkins. Modeling Nightingale's school at St. Thomas, the Hopkins nursing school would be an independent women's nursing organization rather than under the medical administration, and applicants would have to be well-educated, refined gentlewomen of excellent morals and chastity.[48]

NURSING AND THE RISE OF SURGERY

Similar to other professions in the Progressive Era, American physicians joined the trend toward specialization. By 1880 specialty societies had been established for physicians practicing ophthalmology, otology, neurology, dermatology, laryngology, surgery, and gynecology. As historian Sydney Halpern notes, "specialization provided a new basis for gradients of occupational prestige because of its perceived link to progress in medical research and the growing legitimacy of the scientific method."[49] Surgery quickly claimed the top of the medical specialty hierarchy as the discovery of anesthesia and antisepsis enabled its advancement. By 1891 Dr. John Shaw Billings believed the status of surgeons was justified since "the most important improvements in practical medicine made in the United States have been chiefly in surgery."[50] As physician groups sought control over a certain disease process, organ system, or medical technology, they established different specialties that in turn contributed to a greater need for hospital-based care, particularly in the fields of surgery and obstetrics.

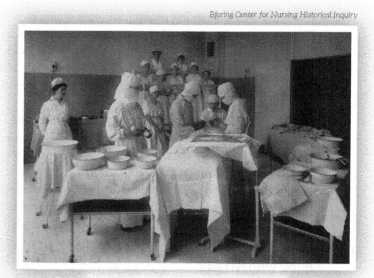

Surgery performed in the operating room at Columbia Hospital, circa 1920s.

The rise of a surgical specialty and the advances in the field fundamentally altered the practice of surgical nursing. As one nurse explained, "The rapid progress . . . has created a demand for new methods in the nursing care of surgical patients."[51] With the introduction of anesthesia, the operative process changed entirely, as surgeons found they could work meticulously and methodically without a strict time constraint. Before this surgeons were limited by their patients' tolerance for pain and suffering and operations occurred swiftly and brutally. Even if an operation was successful, postoperative complications and infections frequently resulted in death. Using anesthetics, surgeons were able to experiment with more complex and invasive procedures like hysterectomies and appendectomies, which had previously proven almost universally fatal.[52]

Once Joseph Lister's antisepsis techniques gained traction among the medical community, infection rates decreased and surgical possibilities seemed limitless. The adoption and routine use of antiseptic and aseptic techniques prompted the greatest changes

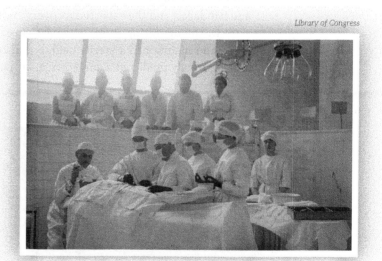

The adoption of antiseptic and aseptic techniques in the early 20th century radically changed the operating room environment.

in nursing practice. In addition to an understanding of bacteriology and "contagious nursing," nurses needed to know how to manage the surgical environment so that everyone and everything became and stayed clean. As one nurse described:

> The first requirement of a good surgical nurse is that she thoroughly understand the meaning of the word "cleanliness," and that she have the ability to carry out consistently a method by which everything unclean and unsterile is kept away

from her patient and from anything pertaining to the patient. She herself, her hair, her clothes, and particularly her hands and finger-nails, must be clean. She must have the knowledge of how to make and keep things sterile, be familiar with surgical instruments and their particular uses, and have had a training which has fitted her to care intelligently for all the different kinds of operative cases.[53]

The design of the surgical suite aided nurses in applying the new aseptic techniques. Marble walls, ventilation systems, and separate sterilization rooms all made it easier for nurses to maintain antiseptic conditions as they scrubbed walls and floors. Hospitals could easily afford the newest instruments and surgical equipment, from scalpels and clamps to rubber gloves, surgical gowns, and masks, and nurses soon became proficient in handling and sterilizing these supplies. Nurses also managed furniture, equipment, and people inside the surgical suite, and prepped and cleaned the patient's body prior to an operation. With postoperative infections posing the greatest risk to the surgical success, a great deal of the nurse's time and energy was expended to maintain antiseptic procedures.

"In the operating room, the nurse who has had contagious technic grasps more readily the methods used to obtain strict asepsis and will be less likely to contaminate articles in handling them."[54]

Ida B. Smith, 1923

New discoveries and surgical techniques occurred in rapid succession, including spinal fusions in the 1910s, joint replacement with ivory prostheses throughout the 1920s, brain tumor resection, cardiac surgery, and plastic surgery due to disfigurement of World War I veterans. This wide variety of procedures created a continuously expanding list of new operations nurses had to learn, and the effects of each on their patients. Nursing staff had to know the proper treatment of surgical patients before, during, and after each unique operation; the proper care of utensils and instruments; the different kinds of wounds and potential abnormal conditions; how to prepare different suture materials; how to make, apply, and monitor different surgical dressings and bandages; and the expected recovery trajectory for different surgeries.[55]

In the operating room, the best surgical nurses not only managed the equipment and maintained a sterile field, but also understood the entire operative process and accurately predicted a surgeon's next move. As one surgical nurse explained, "The

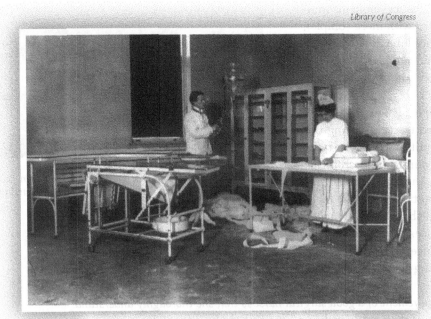

Library of Congress

An operating room between patient surgeries, where a nurse prepares bandages and a physician inspects equipment.

faculty in a nurse of anticipating the operator's wants is especially appreciated by a surgeon."[56] At Mayo Clinic, Sister Joseph Dempsey became the first surgical assistant to Dr. William Mayo, who was praised for her cooperation and quiet demeanor. Her knowledge and skill were so trusted by Dr. Mayo that "[i]t was said that if Dr. Will extended his hand and asked for instruments to begin closing the incision, and was instead handed a clamp by Sister Joseph, he automatically looked back into the incision, because it was likely that she had seen bleeding that he had missed."[57]

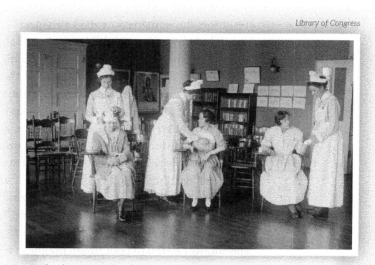

Student nurses in a bandaging lesson at Blackwell Training School.

The effect of new knowledge and surgical technique proved especially challenging for graduate nurses who did private duty nursing. Not only did they have to contend with the difficulties in keeping abreast of new methods without a guaranteed hospital affiliation, they also needed to adapt to environments that constantly changed and lacked the convenience of hospital surgical suites. When a nurse was hired for an operation performed in a private home, she was advised to start preparing the space as soon as possible, moving furniture, covering windows, scrubbing walls and floors and then draping them with sheets, gathering and sterilizing utensils, and finally setting up an operating table for the surgeon. In emergency situations, a nurse's "individual tact and executive ability" would allow him or her to prioritize and utilize the "needed safeguards" to ensure operative success.[58] Nurse educators were aware of these unique challenges in private duty surgical nursing, and attempted to prepare trainees for success in any environment. As one nursing supervisor explained, "We are preparing students to go into homes, whether as private duty nurses or public health nurses. Their experience in the hospital must not make them dependent upon fixed equipment."[59]

The organization of the hospital system and the availability of a skilled nursing staff pushed surgeons to use the hospital rather than their office or a patient's home. Having a location built specifically for surgery, fully equipped with the best tools, and surrounded by nurses, surgeons could coordinate multiple surgeries in a single day without having to worry about preparation, aftercare, or moving patients. Since hospitals were wired with electricity before the majority of private homes, some surgeons began to prefer operating in the hospital for the availability of the lights alone.[61] By 1920, surgical admissions in most hospitals had outnumbered general medical admissions. Modern aseptic surgery also offered patients a quick and effective response to illness or injury. As historian Charles Rosenberg remarked, "For the first time, patients came to their physician with the hope—and increasingly the assumption—that he might impose and not merely facilitate healing."[62] Nurses ensured that success.

> "Good aseptic technique could be carried out in a barnyard, if the brain that directs it is trained in principles and details."[60]
>
> Louella Adkins, 1903

MOVING CHILDBIRTH FROM HOME TO HOSPITAL
Toward a Safer Environment

For the overwhelming majority of human history, pregnancy, birth, and newborn care had primarily been viewed as women's work, privilege, and civic or marital duty.

Traditionally, women controlled all aspects of the birth procedure, and rules of propriety excluded men from childbirth rooms. Labor and delivery carried a high level of danger, as maternal mortality rates remained high in the 20th century, climbing as high as 92 per 10,000 live births at the height of the flu epidemic in 1918.[63] For most women, however, fears about the potential for future debility were greater than any fear of death.[64] Postpartum infections, fistulas, and poorly healed perineal tears brought constant pain and irritation to sufferers. Since women had not yet gained control over their reproductive futures, they faced the reality that multiple pregnancies and confinements would probably result in some kind of permanent physical limitation.

The location of childbirth began to change in the 19th century as a result of the increasing mobility and urbanization of families. The disruption of the traditional social networks necessary for successful home birth, as well as the shift to smaller urban dwellings, caused more women in major cities to give birth in a hospital. Lying-in hospitals specifically catered to poor urban pregnant women, acting as a replacement for postpartum home nursing care. Prior to the acceptance of germ theory and the discovery of the cause of puerperal fever, these hospitals possessed incredibly high maternal mortality rates due to postpartum sepsis.

About the time that births began occurring in hospitals, upper-class women began searching for ways to make the birth process safer and less painful. The introduction and success of new obstetrical techniques, including forceps and anesthesia, became advantageous to physicians who controlled their use.[65] Additionally, physicians carried with them the status advantages of their gender and the image of superior education.

Even so, the process of attaining professional status for obstetrics occurred slowly, as scientific medicine challenged long-held societal views of childbirth as a natural experience to be shared among women and their female attendants.

In order to have their specialty recognized and respected, obstetricians began to describe labor and delivery as potentially pathogenic and asserted that only trained physicians held the authoritative knowledge to safely guide women through birth. One of the most well-known figures in obstetric medicine, Dr. Joseph Bolivar DeLee, was "convinced that not the majority, but the minority, of labor cases is normal, and that not until the pathologic dignity of obstetrics is fully recognized may we hope for any considerable reduction of the mortality and morbidity of childbirth."[66] The high frequency of poor outcomes reinforced the new obstetric ideology that a safe labor and delivery required medical intervention.

DeLee and other prominent obstetricians recognized that the quality of obstetric care being offered to American women needed improvement. They believed that by establishing physicians as the preferred birth attendant, they would improve the quality of care. Better obstetric training for medical students became an absolute necessity, as the profession eliminated the untrained or lesser skilled midwives and general practitioners. Abraham Flexner's 1910 report, however, highlighted an appalling lack of practical obstetric experience throughout medical education, stating, "the very worst showing is made in the matter of obstetrics. Didactic lectures are utterly worthless. . . . The practice is a fine art which cannot be picked up in the exigencies of out-patient work, poorly unsupervised at that."[68]

Lay and trained midwives were pushed out of the new system almost entirely. DeLee emphatically stated that he was "opposed to any movement to perpetuate the midwife," and viewed her as "a relic of barbarism . . . a drag on the progress of the science and art of obstetrics."[70] Many obstetricians

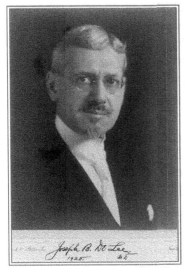

Dr. Joseph B. DeLee, an early leader in modern obstetric care.

"The nurse may smooth the path for the advance of the obstetric art. She becomes really a missionary spreading the gospel of good obstetrics."[67]

Dr. Joseph B. DeLee, 1907

shared DeLee's opinion, and viewed midwives as a barrier to the profes-sional and social advancement of obstetrics as a medical specialty. By publicly and systematically devaluing the contributions of the midwife, obstetricians were able to elevate their own status in American society as well as elimi-nate economic competitors. These efforts proved quite successful. Despite numerous studies showing significantly lower maternal mortality rates for midwife-attended births, the percentage of deliveries performed by mid-wives dropped from 50% in 1900 to only 15% in 1930.[71]

"The safety and comfort of both patients—mother and child—depend on the trained care and dexterity of the physician."[69]

Abraham Flexner, 1910

To further legitimize the specialty, obstetricians aligned themselves with surgeons, which they felt better reflected their increased tendency toward intervention and operative deliveries. As obstetrician Dr. Walter Channing stated, a physician "must do something. He cannot remain a spectator merely."[72] General practitioners were also encouraged to seek obstetric specialists for the management of birth and confinement. Hospitals emerged as the preferred location for labor and delivery, as they had immedi-ate access to the safeguards of a surgical suite. For some obstetricians, hospital deliveries became a moral obligation—the availability of the operating room, nursing staff, and the latest in medical technology made hospital birth the only safe choice for mothers and infants. As germ theory gained widespread acceptance, increased public awareness of surgical asepsis made the prospect of a sterile, scientific birth more attractive to all citizens.

But even as obstetricians supplanted midwives, wealthy women continued to deliver their children at home. It was not until the public image of hospitals shifted away from that of institutions for the poor and destitute that women began to appreciate and demand hospital childbirth. Recognizing the economic potential of paying customers, hospitals started advertising to private patients, often touting the benefits of state-of-the-art sur-gical facilities and round-the-clock nursing care. The year 1938 was a turning point in American childbirth history, as hospital births accounted for half of all births in the coun-try and would begin to supplant the home as the preferred location for confinement.

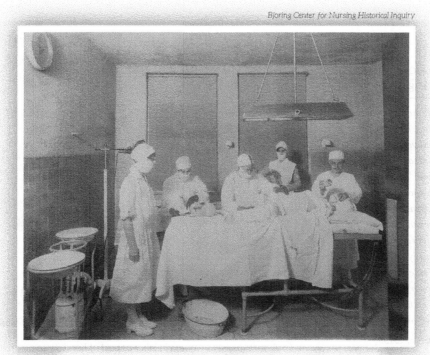

Bjoring Center for Nursing Historical Inquiry

A sterile, anesthetized hospital delivery at Columbia Women's Hospital.

Obstetricians like DeLee viewed nurses as powerful allies in promoting hospital birth, particularly private duty nurses who provided public health services and prenatal care through visiting nurse associations or settlement houses.[73] Nurses occupied a privileged position, having cultivated trusting female relationships with their pregnant patients. Obstetricians felt that the increasing acceptance of science and technology by all health professionals, plus the nurse's goal to provide the best outcome to mothers and babies, compelled nurses to advocate for hospital confinements in order to save lives.

Obstetric and Newborn Nursing Care

For both nurses and physicians, part of the appeal of hospital births over the home involved their ability to more easily control the patient and the environment. As it had for surgery, adherence to aseptic technique transformed the practice of obstetrical nursing, particularly in the hospital. A 1915 article on obstetric nursing asserted, "The duties of the nurse are manifold, but the first and foremost one is that of preventing infection by always exercising the greatest aseptic precautions in regard to the patient."[75] Hospital staff could control the cleanliness of the room, prepare the delivery bed adequately with fresh linens, wash and dress patients, and limit outside visitors, thereby "keeping the whole operating floor professionally intact."[76]

Nurses followed an extensive protocol to prepare laboring women for delivery: "The patient should have on a clean night-dress. . . . Brush the hair and braid it tightly. Give a thorough enema, and see that the bladder is emptied. It may be necessary to use the catheter. . . . You will sometimes be directed to give at this time an antiseptic douche . . . This should be done before each examination and after each micturition [urination]."[77]

Care of the parturient woman before, during, and after childbirth became much more challenging for nurses once the process was viewed as requiring medical attention. Obstetric nurses needed to know the different stages of labor and the average duration of each, normal patient responses in each stage, the best methods to assist the

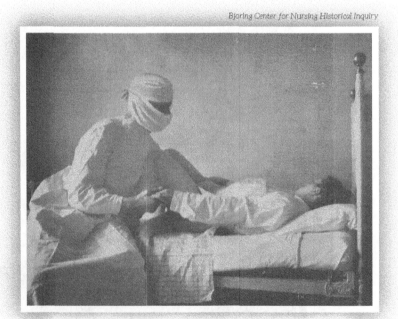

Bjoring Center for Nursing Historical Inquiry

A nurse assists a woman in labor as part of her duty to care for the mother before, during, and after childbirth.

mother and decrease her odds for perineal injury or complications, how to safely deliver the infant and tie off the umbilical cord, how to properly deliver the placenta, and methods to stimulate and stabilize the newborn. During the prescribed 10- to 14-day confinement, nurses also taught mothers how to breastfeed, and ways to manage the expected postpartum symptoms of bleeding, hemorrhoids, and fatigue.

Quality obstetric nursing in the hospital also involved an understanding of and preparation for abnormal labor progression, operative deliveries, and complications. Since obstetricians tended to follow a more interventional approach to childbirth, nurses learned about different operative techniques, the instruments involved, and how to care for the patient afterward. The increased incidence of caesarian sections, episiotomies, and use of forceps required that nurses understand the effects of these procedures on the mother and baby. Anesthesia usage also affected nursing care; obstetric nurses needed to understand how the new drugs would impact the delivery and what effects they would have on both mothers and infants. In addition, obstetric nurses had to know the causes, symptoms, and treatments for intra- and postpartum complications, including hemorrhage, eclampsia, and infection.

On the obstetric ward, nursing care both complemented and overlapped with medical practice. Describing the balance, one nursing supervisor stated that:

> In obstetrical nursing, as in all fields of nursing, the student nurse is taught to be an intelligent assistant to the physician, at the time of operation, or delivery, or dressing, or examination, to prepare for his every need and to anticipate his wants, to carry out his orders accurately and intelligently, to understand signs and symptoms and to report on them with understanding. In addition, every student nurse is taught a volume of nursing care and procedure with which the physician never concerns himself and for which he never writes orders, such as bed-making, bathing, care of body, hair, mouth, hands, and feet, and changing positions. These and many other details may be considered purely nursing procedures.[79]

Most physicians believed that a nurse's success in the hospital required that he or she understand and maintain his or her subordinate position in the organizational hierarchy.

Nursing superintendents reinforced this notion in training school lectures and ward work. However, they also prepared students for the realities of obstetric nursing, which was highly unpredictable. In her 1906 textbook, Clara Weeks-Shaw informed nurses that, "It is perhaps more often in obstetric cases than in any others that the nurse will be called upon to assume, in his absence, the responsibilities properly belonging to the physician."[80] Nurses required both the knowledge and skill necessary to appropriately and *independently* care for parturient women in the event a physician was unavailable. The time of day, particularly in the middle of the night, the availability of other support personnel, and the wide variation in the acceptable length of a woman's labor, all affected the role obstetric nurses assumed during hospital deliveries. Part of what made obstetric nurses so useful was their ability to negotiate the uncertainty and seamlessly shift between autonomous and assistant roles.[81]

In addition to caring for parturient women throughout their confinements, nurses in the hospital also tended to their newborn infants. Immediately after birth, nurses were responsible for keeping the baby warm and dry, promoting respiration, and aseptic treatment of the umbilical cord. In the event of a traumatic birth or the depressed status of the newborn, obstetricians and nurses initiated drastic resuscitation measures. They could introduce tracheal catheters to attempt manual inflation of the lungs, and administer stimulants like

"It is difficult to draw the line of demarcation between the physician's responsibilities and the nurse's duties."[82]

Carrie M. Hall, 1927

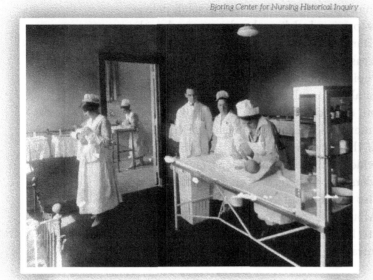

Nurses and a physician in the newborn nursery at Columbia Hospital, where nurses administered care to infants at all hours.

spirits of ammonia to treat apnea or cyanosis.[83]

Modern hospitals created well-equipped nurseries adjacent to the obstetrical wards, and nurses cared for newborn infants around the clock. Nurses placed healthy newborns in bassinets, and small, sick, or premature infants in incubators if they were available. They also made use of other equipment such as an infant scale, ceramic tubs for bathing, closed containers for clean diapers and linens, and individual thermometers.[84] Nurses frequently designed a separate room within the nursery to sterilize bottles and mix formula to ensure cleanliness.

The organization of the hospital wards and the nurses' strict adherence to aseptic principles often allowed them to exclude family members and visitors. Nursing textbooks advised that after the mother delivered, "No talking should be allowed in the room, no visitors, no excitement of any kind."[85] Nurses also followed the institutional regulation to separate mothers and their infants immediately after birth, but they provided proper identification so that infants were not accidentally mixed up. The use of the hospital completely changed the traditional childbirth experience that previously had been a family affair in the home. Families were forced into the role of outsider while nurses and physicians assumed power and authority.[86] Newborn care went from being the sole responsibility of the mother to being the exclusive responsibility of the nursery nurse.

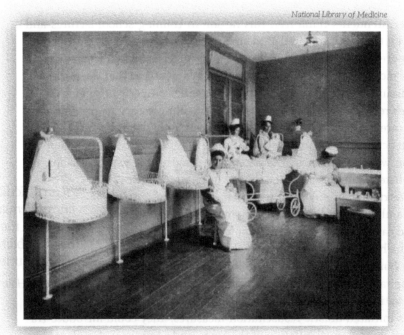

Nurses tend to their newborn patients in a hospital nursery, which was kept quiet, sterile, and separate from the infants' families.

AFRICAN AMERICAN NURSING AND SEGREGATION
Background

The passage of the 13th Amendment (abolishment of slavery) following the American Civil War and the subsequent Reconstruction years did little to improve race relations throughout the United States. Many southerners held on to long-standing prejudice against African Americans, and northern states saw increased racial tension as Black citizens moved into the cities and competed with immigrants for jobs and housing. Supreme Court decisions at the turn of the century—*Plessy v. Ferguson* in 1896 and *Cumming v. Richmond County Board of Education* in 1899—introduced the "separate but equal" doctrine and legally sanctioned institutional segregation. These Supreme Court decisions effectively "created a de facto environment of emancipation without freedom for African-Americans."[87] In addition to these legal precedents, pseudoscientific theories popularized during the Progressive Era contributed to notions of race and class hierarchies. A form of scientifically sanctioned racism occurred, using concepts like IQ testing and eugenic principles to support racial hierarchies, discrimination, and social inequality.

Even legitimate scientific concepts like germ theory were used to justify segregation. Medical and public health journals in the early 20th century argued that African Americans carried disease and posed a danger to the health of White citizens. "Germs have no color line" became the slogan of a fundraising campaign for exclusively Black hospitals, while editorials warned that "bacteria have a disconcerting fashion of ignoring segregation edicts."[91]

As hospitals increased in number and became the preferred location for health care services, two types of Black hospitals emerged—segregated and Black controlled. In the south, White philanthropists established segregated hospitals to serve Black communities. Some founders desired to provide health services for African Americans, but their creation of a separate and segregated hospital system also served another purpose—to "protect" White citizens from the illnesses of the Black patients.[92] The hospitals in northern cities that *did* offer care to all races frequently segregated patients along color lines. Wards for Black patients were often located in undesirable locations or basements. As one hospital administrator explained, "the negro department must always be as far from the white and executive as possible."[93]

Responding to discrimination in health care, African American physicians, churches, and fraternal organizations established their own hospitals. Black-controlled institutions often operated on the premise of inclusivity, refusing to discriminate against anyone needing care. African American doctors were a driving force behind the creation of Black-controlled hospitals in order to secure employment, educational opportunities, professional advancement, and future economic survival. Even as the number of African American physicians grew—increasing from 900 in 1890 to 3,500 by 1920—most Black doctors had difficulty securing a hospital appointment.[94] Their struggle mirrored that of Black women attempting to gain admittance to predominantly White nurse–training programs.

Black nurses would also benefit from the efforts of those establishing Black-controlled hospitals as they, like their physician counterparts, would need education, training, and employment. Now their own community members were willing and able to address the problem. Some of the earliest Black-controlled hospitals also established nurse training programs at the same time, knowing that the school would provide a steady supply of student

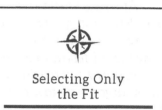

Selecting Only the Fit

The goal of eugenic philosophy in the early 20th century was to improve human heredity by eliminating all "medical and charitable activities that had artificially preserved the unfit."[88] Eugenic supporters often associated social class, race, ethnicity, and any deformity with genetic defects. In its extreme form, eugenics was used to justify forced sterilization, to restrict immigration for specific races, and to withhold treatment to newborns with certain ailments or deformities.

Supreme Court Decision

The 1927 case of *Buck v. Bell* upheld a Virginia law that forced individuals deemed "mental defectives" to be sterilized, thus highlighting the consequences of eugenic philosophy.[89] Justice Oliver Wendell Holmes Jr. proclaimed, "It is better for all the world if, instead of waiting to execute degenerate offspring for crime or to let them starve for their imbecility, society can prevent those who are manifestly unfit from continuing their kind."[90] More than 30 states enacted similar laws, causing an estimated 65,000 Americans to be sterilized without their consent.

Training School for Black Nurses

"The Problem of the Negro Nurse"

nurses to staff the hospitals. The first Black-controlled hospitals included: Provident Hospital and Nurse Training School in Chicago, established in 1891; Tuskegee Institute and Nurse Training School in Alabama, established in 1892; and Frederick Douglass Memorial Hospital and Training School in Philadelphia, established in 1895. The founding of these Black-controlled institutions resembled the efforts of women and other ethnic minority groups that created hospitals to specifically serve their own community members.

Black-controlled hospitals had done much to increase educational opportunities for African American nurses and doctors, but many programs suffered as a result of limited funding and scarce resources. Even when an assessment of the status of Black nurses was made in 1925, confirming the negative effects of racial discrimination, no improvements were ever made. The Ethel Johns report would paint a vivid picture of the marginalized status of Black nurses in the early 20th century, but its contents would remain secret for decades.

The Status of Black Nurses: The Ethel Johns Report

In 1925 the Rockefeller Foundation authorized a study of the status of Black nurses in the United States. The organization had already donated millions of dollars to urban and rural public health initiatives, and had commissioned the 1923 Goldmark report in an effort to improve nursing education and professional development. Board members of the Rockefeller Foundation noted that, "While several hospitals, both Northern and Southern, are at present giving some training to negro [sic] nurses, it is believed that there are not sufficient facilities for such instruction," and suggested funding a study to "make possible a consideration of the need and desirability of aid" for these schools.[97] Canadian nurse Ethel Johns was commissioned to examine the training conditions and practice opportunities currently available for African American nurses. The final report, *A Study of the Present Status of the Negro Woman in Nursing*, received praise from foundation officers for its depth, insight, and brilliance. John's work provided clear evidence of the struggles facing Black student and graduate nurses. While all nurses shared problems with hospital exploitation and low social standing, the educational and professional struggles of African American nurses were further exacerbated by pervasive racial discrimination and inequality.

In late 1925, Johns traveled to 16 cities in northern and southern states, visiting 23 Black hospitals and training schools to collect data. Describing the breadth of her work, Johns stated, "So far as I am able to ascertain, most of the schools with the exception of two in the far South where negro [sic] nurses are being trained in any large numbers are included in this study."[98] Johns took comprehensive field notes and recorded candid interviews from each institution. She spoke with administrators and supervisors, observed students on the wards and in the classroom, and shadowed graduate public health nurses working in the community. Overall, the study revealed the professional consequences of racism for African American nurses throughout the county. Johns concluded that Black nurses could neither train nor practice on the basis of complete equality anywhere in the United States.[99]

Johns supported improving educational standards for all training schools, and found a number of African American schools particularly lacking. Only seven out of the 23 schools in the study ranked as fairly good, with the best "barely reaching" the caliber of an average White school.[101] Most schools rated as poor or very poor. Remarking on the lectures available to students,

Johns wrote, "there is grave reason to believe that in the majority of the schools theoretical instruction is limited to just sufficient to get by the State Board of Examiners."[102] Some schools operated with "quite inadequate" curricula and equipment and "with no more than a pretense of teaching."[103]

Student nurses in segregated hospitals, which operated with very little funding, also lived and worked in deplorable conditions. Johns felt that nurse trainees bore the brunt of the economic constraints facing hospital administrators. Calling the housing facilities at most schools "abominable," Johns went on to state that "in all of these institutions money has evidently been forthcoming for good hospital equipment but the most callous disregard is shown with respect to the provisions of even the common decencies of life for the pupil nurse."[104] Like the majority of hospitals across the country associated with a nurse training school, African American hospitals exploited student nurse labor. In addition to having student nurses manage all inpatient cases, the hospitals profited by assigning students private-duty cases and pocketing the fees. Even those superintendents who opposed private duty requirements, like Martha Studley at the Dixie Hampton Training School, found themselves unable to change the system. Studley indicated to Johns that private duty would continue "because the doctors liked it very much."[105]

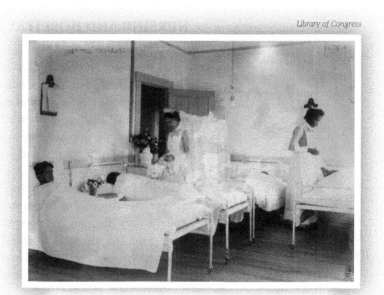

Nurses tend to patients on the boys' ward at Tuskegee Hospital, one of the first Black-controlled hospitals in the United States.

After graduation, Black professional nurses faced limited career opportunities and pay inequality. Johns tried to focus on issues other than racial discrimination, but acknowledged that "they exist and they cannot be ignored."[106] Both Black and White supervisors across the country held stereotypically racist beliefs, namely that African Americans exhibited inferior intelligence and moral character in comparison to Whites. Many of these administrators held onto prejudiced beliefs even in the face of contradictory information. For example, a public health nursing supervisor in Baltimore, Maryland, praised her Black nurses for their teaching ability and "well prepared and delivered" health talks but then she told Johns that when managing Black nurses, "you are dealing with a brain that is not the same as that of a white person."[107] Black graduate nurses also received less pay than their White counterparts in every southern state. One chief city nurse defended the disparity, claiming African American nurses were "inferior in intelligence, in judgment, and in stability."[108] Most supervisors stated that White nurses had higher living expenses than Black nurses to justify the pay inequality.

Johns's own experience and worldview undoubtedly influenced her conclusions and suggestions. She was a White woman who had been hired by the Rockefeller Foundation to develop nurse education programs in Europe. She likely had never interacted with Black nurses prior to the study, as Canadian schools of the time denied entrance to African American students. Johns stated that she had never been "brought closely into touch with any phase of the negro [sic] problem," but that "even to have touched the fringe of such an intricate and vital human problem [had] been an enriching experience."[110] By the

"No matter how high her personal and professional qualifications may be, certain doors remain closed to [the African American nurse]."[109]

Ethel Johns, 1925

report's conclusion, Johns recognized the "poignant and tragic struggle" of Black nurses, and equated their plight to the contemporary labor and women's movements.[111]

The Johns report provided firsthand experiences of Black nurses in the early 20th century. Unfortunately, the Rockefeller Foundation never released the report, leaving it buried in their archives for more than 50 years. Finally in 1982, nurse historian Darlene Clark Hine discovered and analyzed the report, stating that Johns had done her work too well, and "the deplorable conditions she described stunned the trustees of the Rockefeller Foundation and left them unable or unwilling to devise suitable strategies for redress."[113] The marginalized status and experience of Black nurses continued without published evidence of its existence, leaving Black graduate nurses without representation or a voice.

NURSING AND HOSPITAL ECONOMICS
The Modern Hospital

Changing demographics, shifts in popular culture, and the development of the middle class all helped increase the popularity of hospital-based medical care and fuel the rise in hospital systems. Large-scale immigration and urban migration had disrupted many of the traditional family ties necessary for the provision of sick nursing in the home. Crowded living spaces, lack of extended family members, and job responsibilities for nearly all members of the household forced many people to utilize medical and nursing services available in community hospitals as opposed to family care. Additionally, as everyday Americans began to accept modern scientific theory and technology, they also began to expect state-of-the-art services and advanced therapeutic techniques. Hospitals became centralized locations in which laboratory, x-ray, and surgical services were offered to every patient. As one hospital administrator remarked:

The modern hospital gives the public vastly more in the way of facilities for diagnosis, for furthering the progress of the case, with the smallest possible amount of discomfort. It provides for every form of apparatus for investigation during the entire period that the patient is confined to the institution. It provides facilities for all patients which would not have been commanded even by the very wealthiest persons only a quarter of a century ago.[114]

Finally, the creation and expansion of the American middle class also contributed to the increased popularity of hospital care. The working middle class became the target audience for hospital advertisements; they appreciated the modern convenience of a hospital and had enough income to pay for medical care.

The availability of around-the-clock, skilled nurses became a prime marketing strategy to promote hospital care. Along with technology, nursing care was presented as a life-saving service available only on the hospital ward.[117] Everything about the nursing staff reflected contemporary notions of science and modernity, from their matching clean uniforms and youthful appearances (students ranged in age from 18 to 35) to their association with an official training school and their proficiency with the latest technology. Indeed, nearly all aspects of the hospital experience were modern. Even the sounds inside a hospital reflected progress, from "the rustle of the nurse's uniform, the bell of the telegraph, the rattle of the hydraulic elevator, the hiss of steam, the murmured ritual of the operating room."[118]

The Burgess Report: *Nurses, Patients, and Pocketbooks*

In 1926, under the joint leadership of the NLNE and the AMA, the National Committee on the Grading of Nursing Schools evaluated the economic status of nursing service in the United States. The group proposed "the study of ways and means for insuring an ample supply of nursing service, of whatever type and quality is needed for adequate care of the patient, at a price within his reach."[119] Initially the goal of grading was to evaluate the quality of nurse training programs and push for higher minimum standards, but the scope of the study quickly grew. As Grading Committee Director May Ayres Burgess explained, the report would "include not only problems of grading, but problems of nursing shortage, of supply and demand, of types of service, of distribution, and of costs."[120]

Burgess, an accomplished statistician, surveyed thousands of nurses, superintendents, physicians, patients, and public health directors to present the facts surrounding the economics of nursing. Published on April 18, 1928, *Nurses, Patients, and Pocketbooks* was the Grading Committee's report that attempted to offer data without offering strict recommendations. Recognizing its lack of jurisdiction as a legislative or administrative body within the nursing profession, the committee stated, "If it has desires, it has not power to enforce them. Its function is to gather facts, make recommendations, ask questions. The answers to the questions must be found by those who have the power to act."[121] The final report included 61 diagrams, 70 statistical tables, and 819 direct quotations from survey respondents; readers were encouraged to make their own assessment based on the data.

"Not only does the educational side of the training school claim attention, but also its economics in relation to the hospital, and its responsibility to the community."[122]

E. H. Lewinsky-Corwin, 1922

The report identified the main problems affecting the economic future of the nursing profession. The Grading Committee strongly believed in reducing the overall number of nurse training schools and raising entrance requirements to bar those with "a totally inadequate social and educational background."[123] The report also recommended that hospitals replace students with graduate nurses on the wards. The committee recognized this process would be "extremely difficult," but that doing so would fulfill their social responsibility for providing high quality care to all patients.[124] Finally, the

"Awaken the public to the fact that if society wants good nursing, it must pay the cost of educating nurses."[125]

May Ayres Burgess, 1928

committee emphasized that nursing schools function strictly on an academic basis, independent of the economic and labor needs of the hospitals they were associated with.

Nursing leaders had long recognized that the relationship between a hospital and its associated training school carried high risk for mismanagement. Along with a desire to reform and standardize nurse education, the frequent and pervasive exploitation of student nurse labor by hospital trustees had provided the momentum to create national nursing organizations back in the 1890s. Although American nursing schools had been founded upon the Nightingale model, which required that the schools have independent authority over nurse training, few if any of the schools enjoyed financial and supervisory autonomy. A textbook for superintendents suggested a mutual dependence between the two entities, stating: "In large measure the existence of the hospital is quite as dependent on the training-school as the latter is upon the hospital, and both must stand or fall together."[126] In reality, the economic dependence of nursing schools upon hospital boards continued to result in the abuse of student labor.

Burgess gave two reasons why hospitals choose to associate with a training school: running a training school is cheaper than hiring graduate nurses, and student nurses are easier to control. Outlining the hypocrisy of many hospital trustees, Burgess argued:

A hospital man, be he administrator or trustee, is apt, with apparently perfect sincerity, to state that his hospital is losing money in conducting its training school; and within the next five minutes to admit that the reason the hospital wants to run the school is that graduate floor duty nurses cost too much. It is an extraordinary thing, but it seems to be a fact, that hospitals regard the suggestion that they pay for their own nursing service as unreasonable. They have been receiving free service from students for so many years that they regard it as an inalienable right.[127]

Burgess also pointed out the absurdity of training quality nurses, only to refuse to hire them at the very institutions that claim to provide excellent hospital-based care. Seventy-six percent of superintendent respondents reported that they preferred that hospital patients be cared for by their own students rather than by graduate nurses. Burgess retorted, "There would seem to be something radically wrong in the educational methods of these hospitals if, after they have had the education of a student for 3 years, they would honestly prefer to start the training process all over again with raw material, rather than to avail themselves of the services of their own product."[128] In no other business or profession would supervisors dream of continuously replacing trained staff members with a new supply of unskilled students, and yet this was precisely the model followed by hospitals of the time.

Nurses, Patients, and Pocketbooks revealed the importance of quality nursing care, and framed the education of nurses as a public service. Recognizing that the current system exploited students for purely financial reasons, the Grading Committee's report underscored the importance of demanding that society recognize the value of a well-educated and highly skilled hospital nursing staff. One hospital administrator supported the proposal, stating "Nursing education should be regarded as a public responsibility and, further, if society wants good nursing service, it must pay the cost of nursing education just as it does of educating physicians, lawyers, engineers, and other professions."[129] Many felt that they should follow the lead of the medical profession and reduce the total number of schools while increasing the educational standards of the remaining ones in order to improve the overall quality of graduate nursing care, and give the profession some economic control. A smaller number of high-quality graduate nurses would increase the value of nurses in the eyes of the consumer, thus enabling the hospitals to benefit financially.

> *"We find nursing occupying a comparatively new and rather astonishingly important place in the social and economic scheme of things."*[130]
>
> Carrie M. Hall, 1926

Burgess's report on the patient response to nursing also proved particularly insightful. She highlighted the paradox inherent in providing high-quality nursing care: "The better the nursing, the less the ordinary patient thinks about it."[131] Most of what nurses did to restore the health of their patients remained invisible to those outside the nurse–patient relationship and to the patient himself or herself. The economic value of nursing services could not be easily listed as a charge in the way a diagnostic evaluation, laboratory test, x-ray, medicine, or surgical procedure

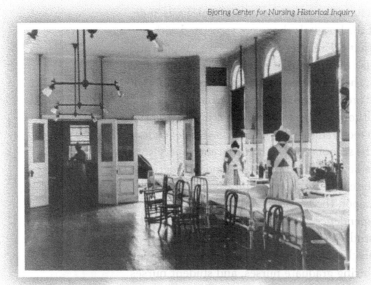

Nurses tend to patients on a ward.

could be added as a line item on a bill. Without a measurable way to show its economic worth, the value of good nursing care became difficult to communicate to hospital administrators, physicians, and patients. Since nurses at the time had no professional authority over the specific services they provided, their nursing care was rolled into the fee called "room and board rate."[132]

Advances in surgery and an elevated social status for both women and nurses gained momentum during and after World War I and the influenza pandemic of 1918. These historic events brought to the forefront the issues of nurse education and professional nursing opportunities, leading the push for an evaluation of the status of nursing across the country through the Goldmark, Johns, and Burgess reports compiled in the 1920s. The impact of many of the findings from these reports would not be fully realized until the Great Depression, when large numbers of graduate nurses ended up working in hospitals again out of economic desperation. Most nurses traded low wages for the opportunity to have consistent employment. The total number of nurse training schools also drastically decreased in the late 1920s, and the introduction of employer-sponsored health insurance changed the payment process. All of these events would have a lasting impact on the nursing profession.

> ## Collaboration in Health Care
>
> *"Nursing and medicine are, and apparently always have been, separate professions. But since they are working, even though their techniques are radically different, for exactly the same object—the health of the patient—it is essential that they work in harmony."*[133]
>
> May Ayres Burgess, 1928

For Discussion

1. How did 19th-century scientific discoveries fuel the rise in U.S. hospitals? Describe how the increased use of diagnostic test and medical devices changed the practice of nursing.
2. Describe findings from the Flexner and Goldmark reports. How did these influence the push toward university-based health care?
3. How did anesthesia and antisepsis impact surgical care? Describe the role of surgical nurses in the early 20th century.
4. What were some of the forces that compelled women to demand a hospital birth? What role did nurses play in transitioning childbirth from home to hospital?
5. Describe the findings of the Ethel Johns report. Why do you think the report was never published?
6. How did hospital economics affect the nursing profession in the early 20th century? Do these forces continue to impact the profession today? Why or why not?

NOTES

1. Nathaniel W. Faxon, "John Howard, J.R. Tenon, and Some Eighteenth-Century Hospitals," *Bulletin of the American Hospital Association* 4 (1930): 96.
2. M. Adelaide Nutting, "Thirty Years of Progress in Nursing," *American Journal of Nursing* 23 (1923): 1027.
3. Ibid., 108.
4. United States Census Bureau, *Historical Statistics of the United States: Colonial Times to 1970* (Washington, DC: U.S. Government Printing Office, 1975): 78.
5. Rosemary Stevens, *In Sickness and in Wealth: American Hospitals in the Twentieth Century* (New York: Basic Books, 1989): 15.

6. John Whiteclay Chambers II, *The Tyranny of Change: America in the Progressive Era, 1890-1920* (New York: St. Martin's Press, 2004). See also Steven J. Diner, *A Very Different Age: Americans of the Progressive Era* (New York: Hill and Wang, 1998); and Jackson Lears, *Rebirth of a Nation: The Making of Modern America, 1877-1920* (New York: Harper Perennial, 2009).

7. Joel D. Howell, *Technology in the Hospital: Transforming Patient Care in the Early Twentieth Century* (Baltimore, MD: Johns Hopkins University Press, 1996): 187.

8. Ibid., 78.

9. Ibid., 103.

10. Henry J. Goeckel, "Scientific Courses for Nurses," *American Journal of Nursing* 21 (1920): 154.

11. E. Blanche Seyfert, "Opportunities for the Nurse in the X-ray Diagnostic Laboratory," *The Trained Nurse and Hospital Review* 62 (1922): 137.

12. Goeckel, "Scientific Courses for Nurses," 152.

13. See Clara Weeks-Shaw, *A Text-book of Nursing: For the Use of Training Schools, Families, and Private Students* (New York: D. Appleton, 1906); Anna Caroline Maxwell and Amy Elizabeth Pope, *Practical Nursing: A Text-book for Nurses* (New York: G. P. Putnam's Sons, 1914).

14. Mary M. Roberts, "Modification of Nursing Procedures as Demanded by Progress in Medicine," *Hospital Progress* 12 (1931): 390.

15. Elizabeth Walker, "Saving the Babies Who Arrive Too Soon," *Ogden Standard Examiner*, September 10, 1933: 8.

16. M. Adelaide Nutting, "Apprenticeship to Duty," *American Journal of Nursing* 19 (1918): 162–163.

17. Weeks-Shaw, *A Text-book of Nursing,* 78.

18. Margarete Sandelowski, *Devices and Desires* (Chapel Hill: University of North Carolina Press, 2000): 45.

19. Ibid., 64.

20. Nathan B. Van Etten, "The Nurse Question," *American Journal of Nursing* 27 (1927): 517.

21. Abraham Flexner, *Medical Education in the United States and Canada* (Washington, DC: Science and Health Publications, 1910): viii.

22. Committee on Education of the National League of Nursing Education, *Standard Curriculum for Schools of Nursing* (New York: National League for Nursing Education, 1917): 5.

23. Paul Starr, *The Social Transformation of American Medicine: The Rise of a Sovereign Profession and the Making of a Vast Industry* (New York: Basic Books, 1983): 117–118.

24. Flexner, *Medical Education in the United States and Canada,* 20.

25. Ibid., viii.

26. Dennis Wentz and Charles Ford, "A Brief History of the Internship," *Journal of the American Medical Association* 252 (1984): 3390–3394.

27. Committee on Education, *Standard Curriculum,* 5.

28. Ibid.

29. Carolyn E. Gray, "The Standard Curriculum for Schools of Nursing," *American Journal of Nursing* 18 (1918): 792.

30. Ibid., 793.

31. Josephine Goldmark, *Nursing and Nursing Education in the United States: Report of the Committee for the Study of Nursing Education* (New York: Macmillan, 1923): 193–194.

32. Ibid., 195.

33. Ibid., 194.

34. United States Census Bureau, *Historical Statistics of the United States*, 76.

35. Susan M. Reverby, *Ordered to Care: The Dilemma of American Nursing, 1850-1945* (Cambridge, UK: Cambridge University Press, 1987): 165.

36. Goldmark, *Nursing and Nursing Education in the United States*, 15.

37. Rockefeller Foundation Archives, "Recommendations of the Conference on Nursing Education, 20 October 1925," as cited in Judith Young, "Revisiting the Ethel Johns Report on African-American Nurses," *Nursing History Review* 13 (2005): 79.

38. Carrie M. Hall, "Training the Obstetrical Nurse," *American Journal of Nursing* 27 (1927): 379.

39. "A Suggested Code: A Code of Ethics Presented for the Consideration of the American Nurses' Association," *American Journal of Nursing* 26 (1926): 600.

40. Ibid.

41. Goldmark, *Nursing and Nursing Education in the United States*, 24.

42. Flexner, *Medical Education in the United States and Canada*, 45.

43. Ibid., 235.

44. Ethel Johns and Blanche Pfefferkorn, *The Johns Hopkins Hospital School of Nursing* (Baltimore, MD: Johns Hopkins University Press, 1954): 7.

45. Ibid., 7–8.

46. Minutes of the Board of Trustees Meeting, March 11, 1873, courtesy the Alan Mason Chesney Medical Archives of the Johns Hopkins Medical Institutions.

47. Janet Wilson James, "Isabel Hampton and the Professionalization of Nursing in the 1890s," in *The Therapeutic Revolution*, eds. Morris Vogel and Charles Rosenberg (Philadelphia: University of Pennsylvania Press, 1979): 206.

48. Johns and Pfefferkorn, *The Johns Hopkins Hospital School of Nursing*, 13.

49. Sydney Halpern, *American Pediatrics: The Social Dynamics of Professionalism, 1880-1980* (Berkeley: University of California Press, 1988): 48.

50. John Shaw Billings, "Medical Progress," *The Medical News* 58 (1891): 669.

51. Anna Fuller, "New Methods in Surgical Nursing," *American Journal of Nursing* 17 (1917): 475.

52. Atul Gawande, "Two Hundred Years of Surgery," *New England Journal of Medicine* 366 (2012): 1718–1719.

53. Leila Clark Woodbury, "Surgical Nursing," *American Journal of Nursing* 3 (1903): 688–689.

54. Ida B. Smith, "Contagious Nursing Technic: Its Place in the Course of a General Hospital," *American Journal of Nursing* 24 (1923): 213.

55. See Anna Caroline Maxwell and Amy Elizabeth Pope, *A Text-Book for Nurses* (New York: G. P. Putnam's Sons, 1914); Frederick C. Warnshuis, *Principles of Surgical Nursing: A Guide to Modern Surgical Technic* (Philadelphia: W. B. Saunders, 1918).

56. Woodbury, "Surgical Nursing," 689.

57. Warren Bateman and Marilyn Bateman, "Honoring the Nurses at Mayo Clinic," Mayo Clinic Story, as quoted in Arlene Keeling, *The Nurses of Mayo Clinic: Caring Healers* (Rochester, MN: Mayo Foundation for Medical Education and Research, 2014): 19.

58. Warnshuis, *Principles of Surgical Nursing*, 24.

59. Margaret A. Tracy, "Supervision and the Teaching of Surgical Nursing," *American Journal of Nursing* 26 (1926): 797.

60. Louella Adkins, "The Care of an Obstetrical Patient," *American Journal of Nursing* 3 (1903): 710.

61. Howell, *Technology in the Hospital*, 58.

62. Charles E. Rosenberg, *The Care of Strangers: The Rise of America's Hospital System* (New York: Basic Books, 1987): 150.

63. United States National Office of Vital Statistics, *Vital Statistics—Special Reports: National Summaries Volume 35, Numbers 1 to 19, 1948* (Washington: National Office of Vital Statistics, 1951): 349–353.

64. Judith Walzer Leavitt, *Brought to Bed: Childbearing in America, 1750-1950* (New York: Oxford University Press, 1986): 28–30.

65. Ibid., 59.

66. Joseph Bolivar De Lee, *The Principles and Practice of Obstetrics* (Philadelphia: W. B. Saunders, 1913): xv.

67. Joseph B. DeLee, *Obstetrics for Nurses* (Philadelphia: W. B. Saunders, 1907): 18.

68. Flexner, *Medical Education in the United States and Canada*, 117.

69. Ibid.

70. "Society Proceedings: Progress toward Ideal Obstetrics," *Journal of the American Medical Association* 66 (1916): 56.

71. For statistics comparing maternal mortality rates of midwives versus the overall national average, see Frances Kobrin, "The American Midwife Controversy: A Crisis of Professionalization," *Bulletin of the History of Medicine* 40 (1966): 350–363; J. Clifton Edgar, "The Education, Licensing, and Supervision of the Midwife," *American Journal of Obstetrics and Diseases of Women and Children* 73 (1916): 394; and I. S. Falk, Rufus Rorem, and Martha Ring, *The Costs of Medical Care* (Chicago: University of Chicago Press, 1933): 281.

72. Walter Channing, *A Treatise on Etherization in Childbirth, Illustrated by Five-Hundred and Eighty-One Cases* (Boston: William D. Ticknow, 1848): 229.

73. Sylvia Diane Rinker, "To Spread the Gospel of Good Obstetrics: The Evolution of Obstetric Nursing," 1890-1940 (PhD dissertation, University of Virginia, 1995): 80.

74. Albert J. Ochsner, "Vast Increase in Number and Variety of Institutions is Chief Factor in Reshaping Modern Society," *Modern Hospital* 1 (1913): 2.

75. Elizabeth Burttle, "Obstetrical Nursing," *American Journal of Nursing* 16 (1915): 196.

76. Letter from Dr. J. S. to the Medical Board, January 24, 1916. Bound in *Minutes of the Medical Board 1915 to June 20, 1917*, Administrators office, Columbia Hospital, Washington, DC, as quoted in Rinker, "To Spread the Gospel of Good Obstetrics," 252.

77. Weeks-Shaw, *A Text-book of Nursing*, 275.

78. Burttle, "Obstetrical Nursing," 196.

79. Carrie M. Hall, "Training the Obstetrical Nurse," *American Journal of Nursing* 27 (1927): 373.

80. Weeks-Shaw, *A Text-book of Nursing*, 268.

81. Sylvia Rinker, "To Cultivate a Feeling of Confidence," *Nursing History Review* 8 (2000): 122.

82. Hall, "Training the Obstetrical Nurse," 373–374.

83. Julius H. Hess and Evelyn C. Lundeen, *The Premature Infant: Its Medical and Nursing Care* (Philadelphia: J.B. Lippincott, 1941): 79–81.

84. Ibid., 24.

85. Weeks-Shaw, *A Text-book of Nursing*, 281.

86. Rinker, "To Spread the Gospel of Good Obstetrics," 253.

87. W. Michael Byrd and Linda A. Clayton, *An American Health Dilemma: Race, Medicine, and Health Care in the United States 1900-2000* (New York: Routledge, 2002): 41.

88. Martin S. Pernick, *The Black Stork: Eugenics and the Death of "Defective" Babies in American Medicine and Motion Pictures Since 1915* (New York: Oxford University Press, 1996): 22.

89. *Buck v. Bell*, 274 U.S. 206 (1927).

90. Ibid.

91. Vanessa Northington Gamble, *Making a Place for Ourselves: The Black Hospital Movement, 1920-1945* (New York: Oxford University Press, 1995): 7.

92. Ibid., 7.

93. Eugene B. Elder, "The Management of the Race Question in Hospitals," *Transactions of the American Hospital Association* 12 (1907): 128.

94. Vanessa Northington Gamble, "Roots of the Black Hospital Reform Movement," in *Sickness and Health in America: Readings in the History of Medicine and Public Health*, eds. Judith Walzter Leavitt and Ronald L. Numbers (Madison: University of Wisconsin Press, 1997): 374.

95. Louise P. Nelson, "My Part," *American Journal of Nursing* 28 (1928): 355.

96. First annual report of the Frederick Douglass Memorial Hospital and Training School (Philadelphia: Frederick Douglass Memorial Hospital, 1896): 9. Courtesy the Barbara Bates Center for the Study of the History of Nursing, MC 78, box 1, folder 1.

97. "Minutes of the Rockefeller Foundation," January 15, 1924, Folder 1504, Box 121, Series 200, RG 1.1, Projects, FA 386, Rockefeller Foundation records, Rockefeller Archive Center.

98. As quoted in Darlene Clark Hine, "The Ethel Johns Report: Black Women in the Nursing Profession, 1925," *Journal of Negro History* 67 (1982): 212.

99. Ethel Johns, "A Study of the Present Status of the Negro Woman in Nursing, 1925," p. 29–41, Folder 1507, Box 122, Series 200, RG 1.1, Projects, FA 386, Rockefeller Foundation records, Rockefeller Archive Center.

100. Ibid., 6.

101. Ibid., 17.

102. Ibid., 23.

103. Johns, "A Study of the Present Status of the Negro Woman in Nursing, 1925," Exhibit J- Raleigh, North Carolina, J-5.; Hine, "The Ethel Johns Report," 216.

104. Ibid., 20–21.

105. Ibid., Exhibit H- Hampton, Virginia, H-6.

106. Ibid., 1.

107. Ibid., Exhibit F- Baltimore, Maryland, F-1.

108. Ibid., Exhibit O- Nashville, Tennessee, O-2.

109. Ibid., 6.

110. Ibid., 1.

111. Ibid.

112. Ibid., 40.

113. Hine, "The Ethel Johns Report," 221.

114. Ochsner, "Vast Increase in Number and Variety of Institutions is Chief Factor in Reshaping Modern Society," 3.

115. Charles P. Emerson, "The American Hospital Field," in *Hospital Management*, ed. Charlotte Albina Aikens (Philadelphia: W.B. Saunders, 1911): 18.

116. Henry M. Hurd, "The Hospital as a Factor in Modern Society," *Modern Hospital* 1 (1913): 33.

117. Margarete Sandelowski, *Devices & Desires: Gender, Technology, and American Nursing* (Chapel Hill: University of North Carolina Press, 2000): 3.

118. Stevens, *In Sickness and in Wealth*, 18.

119. May Ayres Burgess, *Nurses, Patients, and Pocketbooks: Report of a Study of the Economics of Nursing Conducted by the Committee on the Grading of Nursing Schools* (New York: Committee on the Grading of Nursing Schools, 1928): 17.

120. May Ayres Burgess, "Problems Involved in the Grading Program," *American Journal of Nursing* 26 (1926): 919.

121. Burgess, *Nurses, Patients, and Pocketbooks*, 23.

122. E. H. Lewinski-Corwin, "The Hospital Nursing Situation," *American Journal of Nursing* 22 (1922): 604.

123. Burgess, *Nurses, Patients, and Pocketbooks*, 448.

124. Ibid., 450.

125. May Ayres Burgess, "Nurses, Patients, and Pocketbooks': Some High Lights from Dr. Burgess' Presentation of the Book to the National Nursing Association at Louisville," *American Journal of Nursing* 28 (1928): 675.

126. Charlotte Albina Aikens, "The Training-School and Its Management," in *Hospital Management*, ed. Charlotte Albina Aikens (Philadelphia: W.B. Saunders, 1911): 334.

127. Burgess, *Nurses, Patients, and Pocketbooks*, 435.

128. Ibid., 438.

129. Robert E. Neff, "Cost of Nursing Service in the Hospital," *American Journal of Nursing* 30 (1930): 842.

130. Carrie M. Hall, "Taking Courage: The Presidential Address 1926," *American Journal of Nursing* 26 (1926): 549.

131. Burgess, *Nurses, Patients, and Pocketbooks*, 203.

132. Marcella M. Rutherford, "Nursing Is the Room Rate," *Nursing Economics* 30 (2012): 193–199.

133. Burgess, *Nurses, Patients, and Pocketbooks*, 26.

FURTHER READING

Burgess, May Ayres, *Nurses, Patients, and Pocketbooks: Report of a Study of the Economics of Nursing Conducted by the Committee on the Grading of Nursing Schools* (New York: Committee on the Grading of Nursing Schools, 1928).

Byrd, W. Michael, and Linda A. Clayton, *An American Health Dilemma: Race, Medicine, and Health Care in the United States, 1900-2000* (New York: Routledge, 2001).

Flexner, Abraham, *Medical Education in the United States and Canada* (Washington, DC: Science and Health Publications, 1910).

Gamble, Vanessa Northington, *Making a Place for Ourselves: The Black Hospital Movement, 1920-1945* (London: Oxford University Press, 1995).

Gawande, Atul, "Two Hundred Years of Surgery," *New England Journal of Medicine* 366 (2012): 1716–1723.

Goldmark, Josephine, *Nursing and Nursing Education in the United States: Report of the Committee for the Study of Nursing Education* (New York: Macmillan, 1923).

Hine, Darlene Clark, "The Ethel Johns Report: Black Women in the Nursing Profession, 1925," *Journal of Negro History* 67 (1982): 212–228.

Howell, Joel D., *Technology in the Hospital: Transforming Patient Care in the Early Twentieth Century* (Baltimore, MD: Johns Hopkins University Press, 1996).

Rinker, Sylvia, "To Cultivate a Feeling of Confidence: The Nursing of Obstetric Patients, 1890-1940," *Nursing History Review* 8 (2000): 117–142.

Rosenberg, Charles E., *The Care of Strangers: The Rise of America's Hospital System* (New York: Basic Books, 1987).

Sandelowski, Margarete, *Devices & Desires: Gender, Technology, and American Nursing* (Chapel Hill: University of North Carolina Press, 2000).

Smith, Susan L., *Sick and Tired of Being Sick and Tired: Black Women's Health Activism in America, 1890-1950* (Philadelphia: University of Pennsylvania Press, 1995).

Stevens, Rosemary, *In Sickness and in Wealth: American Hospitals in the Twentieth Century* (New York: Basic Books, 1989).

Vogel, Morris J., *The Invention of the Modern Hospital: Boston 1870-1930* (Chicago: University of Chicago Press, 1980).

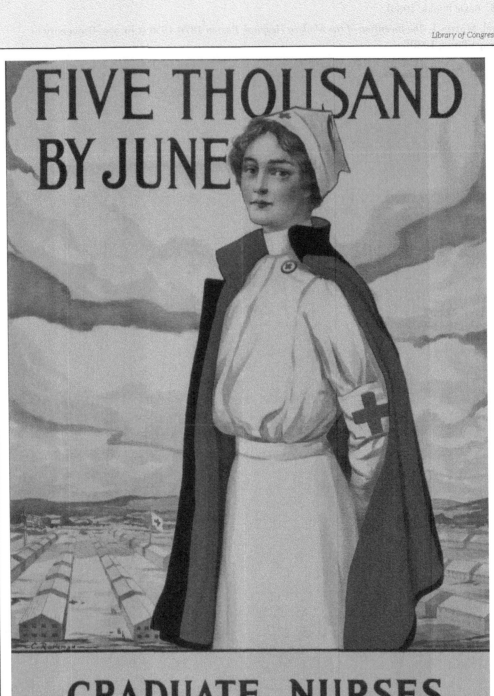

"Five Thousand by June."

CHAPTER 8

Nurses in the News: The Great War and Pandemic Influenza

1914–1919

Arlene W. Keeling

"The twentieth annual convention of the American Nurses Association, held in Philadelphia for a week covering the last days of April and the first two of May, was an unusually serious one, as such a gathering must be when the country is at war. . . . On the evening devoted to the Red Cross, the Academy of Music, which holds 3,000, was packed. . . . When the audience rose to sing the Star Spangled Banner and when it listened to the stirring addresses given by Miss Delano, [and] Miss Noyes . . . all hearts were filled with a desire to serve in this national crisis."[1]

Writing in the *American Journal Nursing* in June 1917, editor Mary Roberts recounted the stirring display of patriotism nurses demonstrated at their annual convention that spring. Just 2 months earlier, on April 6, the United States had declared war on Germany and word was spreading about the need for nurses to serve in the military.

Actually, the government had been planning for the possibility of the United States entering the war in Europe for several years, despite President Woodrow Wilson's promise that the country would remain neutral.[2] Jane Delano, chief of the Army Nurse Corps, and Clara D. Noyes, director of the Red Cross Bureau of Nursing, had themselves been involved in that process since 1916. They worked to increase the size of the Corps, to organize base hospital units, and to ensure that qualified, experienced nurses were recruited to serve. Without formal entry into the war on the part of the United States, however, those plans remained just that—plans on paper. Meanwhile, some American nurses had taken it upon themselves to support the British, French, Italian, Russian, and Belgian nurses in the war already underway against the Central Powers: Austria-Hungary, Germany, Bulgaria, and the Ottoman Empire.

U.S. NURSES IN THE GREAT WAR

U.S. nurses served in World War I, then known as the Great War, in numerous ways, not the least of which was in a voluntary capacity even before the United States entered the war in Europe in 1917. Later, after American Red Cross nurses mobilized with the Army and Navy Nurse Corps, their role became more formalized and even more important to the care of U.S. troops. By September 1917, the total number of U.S. Army nurses serving with the American Expeditionary Forces in Europe was more than 1,000. But by March 1918, that number was insufficient, and calls went out for additional nurses, including nurse anesthetists. Responding at first according to the plan for base hospitals, nursing leaders soon realized the need for special schools to train more nurses for the military. Among these were the Army School of Nursing and the Vassar Training Camp.

American Volunteer Nurses in Europe, 1914 to 1917

From 1914 to 1917, while the United States maintained its neutral stance an ocean away from the conflict, volunteer American nurses traveled to Europe to help the Allied Powers. Some worked alongside Catholic Sisters and lady volunteers in French- or Belgian-run hospitals. Others served with English Sister nurses and women of the voluntary aid detachment (VAD) units in the British Expeditionary Force. Still others worked in the Ambulance Américaine, an auxiliary hospital established in 1914 by a colony of Americans living in Paris.

During the early years of the war, Ellen La Motte, a 1902 graduate of Johns Hopkins Training School for Nurses, served as a nurse in the Ambulance Américaine. The 570-bed American-led hospital was located in the Lycée Pasteur, an unfinished school building in Neuilly-sur-Séine, just outside of Paris. Later La Motte worked at a French Army field hospital in Belgium, a few miles

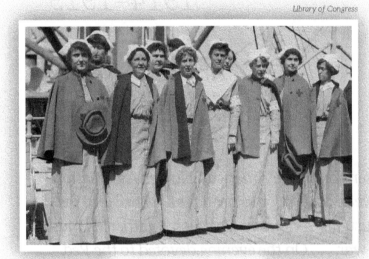

Volunteer nurses on the St. Louis.

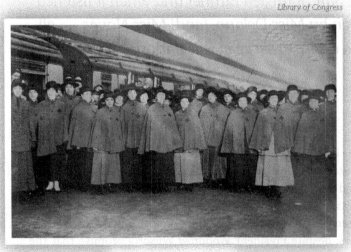

American nurses in London.

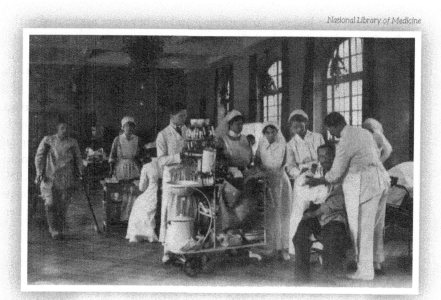

A physician and nurses in Ambulance Américaine hospital ward
attend to a soldier's amputated arm.

behind the frontlines.[3] For a young American woman who had never experienced nursing near the front lines of combat, the reality of war nursing was shocking. Day after day an endless stream of filthy men with gruesome wounds poured into the hospital.

Other American nurses also worked at the Ambulance Américaine. It was there that Dr. George W. Crile, professor of surgery at Western Reserve Medical School in Cleveland, Ohio, directed the first of several surgical teams from elite U.S. universities. Accompanying Crile was Agatha Hodgins, a nurse anesthetist who had given anesthesia to his patients in Ohio and now taught military physicians and other nurses to administer it.[5]

Day in and day out the volunteer surgical teams operated, developing new surgical techniques as soldiers with devastating war injuries presented for care. The operations provided a golden opportunity for the advancement of medical science. Moreover, Crile and his colleagues learned the importance of working with cohesive medical and nursing teams in the combat setting. Crile would return to the United States with that lesson firmly fixed in his mind.

The United States Prepares for War

In 1916, U.S. Army Surgeon General William Gorgas prepared for the possibility that the country would be drawn into the European conflict. To do so he established a General Medical Board comprised of renowned physicians from across the country. The board planned for 50 base hospitals that could be deployed to Europe should the need arise. Each base hospital would have a staff of 27 medical officers, 60 nurses, and 153 enlisted men at the least. Large U.S. hospitals and medical schools would donate staff, funds, and supplies. The plan was based on a recommendation from George Crile. Having returned from France, he argued that base hospitals should be set up by well-established universities and hospitals, reasoning that the units would be more efficient and cohesive if they were "made

"Just ambulances rolling in, and dirty, dying men, and the guns off there in the distance . . . day after day."[4]

Ellen La Motte, 1916

"The Science of Destroying"

"Richard died today . . . gas gangrene . . . the infection had developed so quickly, they could not operate as they wanted. . . . A piece of shell had broken into his brain . . . He passed a night of agony, even with many ampoules of morphia . . . the science of healing stood baffled before the science of destroying."[6]

Ellen La Motte, 1916

up of men who had similar training," and if they were associated with "a nursing staff familiar with their methods."[7]

By April 1917, 33 base hospitals were almost ready when the United States entered the war. Congress declared war on Germany shortly after German U-boats attached and sank the cargo ship, the SS *Aztec,* in British waters. As additional base hospitals were formed, chief of the Army Nurse Corps Jane Delano was struggling to recruit more nurses. Her search for qualified nurses was complicated by the gains the profession had made regarding the requirements of formal training and licensure for nurses. The patriotic spirit that spread over the nation caused thousands of women *without nurses' training* to volunteer as a nurse overseas. On April 8, 1917, the director of the Red Cross Bureau of Nursing, Clara Noyes, wrote to her colleague Adelaide Nutting, chair of the Government's Committee on Nursing, to express her concern about the volunteers:

> *There are moments when I wonder whether we can stem the tide and control the hysterical desire on the part of thousands . . . to get into nursing . . . I talk until I am hoarse, dictating letters to . . . women who want to be Red Cross nurses in a few minutes, not knowing the meaning of the word nurse or what a Red Cross Nurse is.*[8]

The issue was one that would plague the profession until the war ended. In the meantime, nursing leaders worked with the American Red Cross to enlist trained professional nurses to go abroad. On May 7, 1917, the Lakeside Unit of Cleveland (Base Hospital No. 4) sailed for Europe. The Peter Bent Brigham Unit of Boston followed on May 11, and the Presbyterian Unit of New York on May 14. Five days later, three base hospital units sailed: Base Hospital No. 21, supplied by Washington University, St. Louis, with Julia C. Stimpson as chief nurse; Chicago's Northwestern Unit with Daisy Urch as chief nurse; and Base Hospital No. 10 from the University of Pennsylvania with chief nurse Margaret Dunlop. By August 1917, Jane Delano reported that 738 Red Cross nurses were "in France or en route there," and that "the immediate need" was for 10,000 more.[9]

The Nurses Embark

"It is an inspiring picture to see the nursing personnel of a Base Hospital ready to embark. The dignified uniform of dark blue cloth, the scarlet lining of the cape giving a bit of color, the caduceus and letters U. S. on the collar . . . are impressive. . . . There are no tears. Courage is written on each countenance."[10]

Clara D. Noyes, 1917

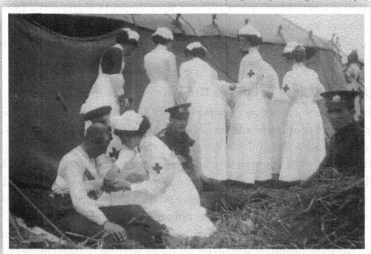

Bjoring Center for Nursing Historical Inquiry

Red Cross nurses at a field hospital tend to injured soldiers.

The Nurses of Base Hospital No. 10

The nurses of Base Hospital No. 10 from the University of Pennsylvania were among those who deployed in the spring of 1917. On arrival in Tréport, France, they reported to General Hospital No. 16 of the British Expeditionary Forces, where the British nurses welcomed them with a "cup of the inevitable tea," and showed them to bed. It was 1:00 a.m. The next day, while inspecting the hospital the nurses found that instead of the 500-bed hospital they had expected, they had 2,000 beds to staff. To make matters worse, the British nurses who had been staffing the hospital were headed home. Only a few VADs remained to help the Americans.[11]

In Tréport, the American nurses soon experienced the real nature of wartime nursing. During their first week Base Hospital No. 10 received 1,400 patients, many suffering from mustard gas attacks. According to one nurse, the summer of 1917 was a "baptism of horror and work" with patients pouring into the hospital "in great numbers, six hundred in less than 48 hours . . . their sufferings pitiful to see."[13]

In other base hospitals at the front, other American nurses also experienced the harsh reality of wartime nursing. Frances Bullard, from Mayo Clinic in Rochester, Minnesota, first worked with the Ambulance Américaines when she arrived in France in 1916. Later, she worked at a base hospital closer to the front, just miles from the front lines.[14] Describing her work in a letter home in September 1917, Bullard wrote:

> *I am at a base hospital near to the war zone; near enough so you can hear the cannon roaring all the time. . . . Tomorrow we start for the first place where it is possible to operate behind the trenches. There are sixteen surgeons . . . I am the only nurse going in this group and I am assigned to the chief surgeon. Other army nurses are coming next week . . . I realize since yesterday that this is no child's play . . . I shall have to wear a gas mask several hours a day and be in constant range of the big guns. The operating room with which I am connected is in a traveling automobile. . . . The cases are cared for a few hours and then the ambulance and stretcher-bearers carry them to the first aid hospital.*[15]

"Day after day the English nurses were transferred from the hospital until in two weeks we had but 18 VADs left. . . . A call was sent to America for a reinforcement of 30 nurses."[12]

An American Nurse From Base Hospital No. 10

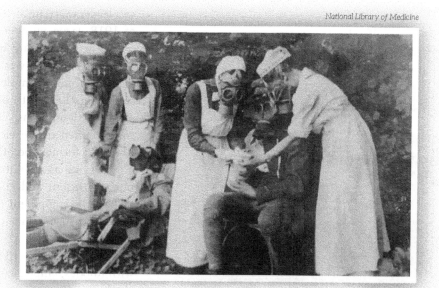

National Library of Medicine

Nurses wear gas masks to protect themselves from mustard gas attacks while they attend to wounded soldiers on the front.

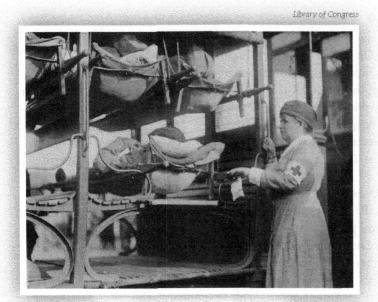

A Red Cross nurse supervises her patients.

In another letter to her colleagues at Saint Mary's Hospital in Rochester, Bullard commented on the sheer volume of injured soldiers who inundated the medical unit, noting that "all day and night," new ones arrived "as fast as others were out."[16] Working with physicians and corpsmen, Bullard and her colleagues helped stop hemorrhage, dressed and redressed wounds, and administered morphine to relieve pain. They also offered the soldiers "proper feedings" of beef tea, rice water, and milk.[17]

By September 1917, nine more base hospitals had arrived in Europe, bringing the total number of U.S. Army nurses to more than 1,000, most serving with the American Expeditionary Forces. Despite a steady increase in the size of the Army Nurse Corps over the next months, by March 1918 the shortage of military nurses at the front was a serious problem and the campaign to recruit nurses grew in importance.[18]

As more American nurses arrived in France, the need for their organization and supervision increased. In April 1918, after some confusion about appointments and lines of authority, Julia Stimpson, Matron of General Hospital No. 21 was appointed chief nurse of the American Red Cross in France.[19] (Later, in October 1918, she would become director of nursing services for the American Expeditionary Force.)

Because nursing activities of the American Red Cross and the Army Nurse Corps were "hopelessly entangled," and the nurses in the field needed both direction and supplies, Stimpson's leadership skills were soon put to the test. She performed admirably, making frequent unexpected inspection trips to the base hospitals in France to connect directly with the nurses.[20] In doing so, Stimpson gathered firsthand information about their experiences, their living conditions, and their needs. Her genius as a leader was critical. By early summer of 1918, large numbers of American nurses were arriving in Europe and Stimpson's priority was "the establishment of a more complete system" for supplying them with equipment and replacement uniforms.[21] To do so, Stimpson obtained the services of Marie B. Rhodes, a former operating room nurse now serving as a volunteer Red Cross nurse. Efficient and effective, Rhodes tackled the equipment problem immediately, ensuring that the nurses had what they needed.

One nurse described her meeting with Rhodes, emphasizing how helpful she had been to the nurses of Mobile Hospital No. 9:

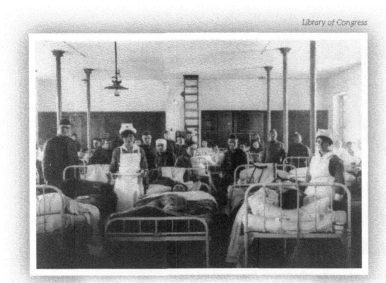

A crowded ward in an American hospital in France.

I have always believed that an efficient operating room nurse would make a good businesswoman and in the Red Cross office I found proof that I was right. The result of our conference was that each nurse was completely outfitted with a trench coat, two jersey uniforms, rain hat, rubber boots, sweater, mittens with wristlets, two suits of genuine all-woolen underwear, black jersey tights, hose, woolen kimono, . . . a set of dishes . . . a cot pillow, four blankets, bed socks, wash cloths, towels, . . . [and] a duffle bag.[22]

The Nurses of Base Hospital No. 26

On June 4, 1918, the nurses of Base Hospital No. 26 embarked on the SS *Baltic* for the transatlantic crossing to England. The group, under the charge of Chief Nurse Annie Gosman, was sponsored by Mayo Clinic and the University of Minnesota. After landing in Liverpool 12 days later, the group traveled by train to the French village of Allerey where they immediately set up camp.[23]

In Allerey, the nurses at Base Hospital No. 26 provided care to thousands of wounded soldiers, many with ragged shrapnel wounds infected from days in muddy trenches. They also cared for patients covered with burns and those whose lungs were destroyed by mustard gas. All presented challenges. Technological advances in the destructive power of weapons, including the howitzer and the machine gun, resulted in soldiers with massive injuries, internal hemorrhage, and fractured bones; all required sophisticated surgical care.[25]

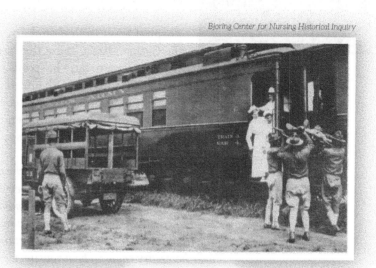

Bjoring Center for Nursing Historical Inquiry

Nurses on a troop train.

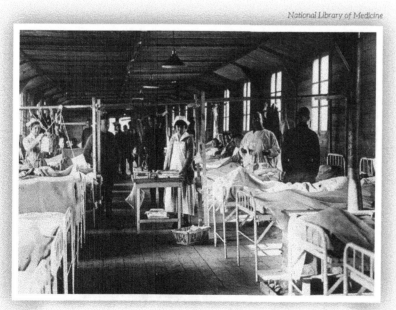

National Library of Medicine

Nurses at Base Hospital No. 26 tend to injured soldiers with infected battle wounds from trench warfare.

The Train Trip to Allerey

"The nurses were assigned six to each compartment, with knees touching. We slept as best we could—sitting up. . . . We stopped from time to time at Red Cross stations. . . . Before leaving, we were each handed a can of jam through the window. That jam, added to what we had left from our lunch box, was our food for the next three days. . . . We were three days and three nights on the way. When we arrived, we were exhausted."[24]

Mae MacGregor Given, 1918

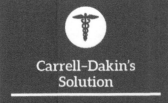
In addition to serving on surgical teams, the nurses of Base Hospital No. 26 managed wards of patients with infected wounds. As treatment they constantly irrigated the wounds with a weak bleach solution, called "Carrell–Dakin's solution." One nurse described the procedure: "several drains are inserted [into each wound] . . . and into these every two hours is pumped a dark liquid, 'Dakin,'—the idea being . . . to keep the wound in a constant bath of antiseptic."[26]

The Nurses of Mobile Hospital No. 1

During periods of intense fighting, Army nurses were sometimes dispatched to mobile hospitals closer to the front lines. At these hospitals the nurses engaged in marathon hours of duty, providing care for seriously wounded soldiers. Several Base Hospital No. 26 nurses went to Mobile Hospital No. 1 in Coulomniérs, a small village 35 miles from Paris toward the German lines. There they treated hundreds of injured soldiers before sending them to base hospitals farther from the front.[28] Nurse anesthetist Sophie Gran Jévne Winton recalled her feelings, writing: "The most pitiful thing . . . was to step outside and see hundreds of stretchers on the ground, each bearing a man who must wait hours before he could be taken care of."[29] Another nurse, Mae MacGregor Given, described the process that the nurses followed:

The seriously wounded were kept at the mobile hospital. . . . We prepared them quickly for surgery, cutting away their blood-soaked clothing. . . . As routine, we gave hypodermic injections to combat infection. . . . Everything was sacrificed to speed up the handling of the hundreds of boys lying on the ground at the front lines . . . sorting of the most urgently injured, and amputating whenever necessary came to be a routine we accomplished with speed and without words, often in near darkness, always with the noise of exploding bombs . . . in our ears.[30]

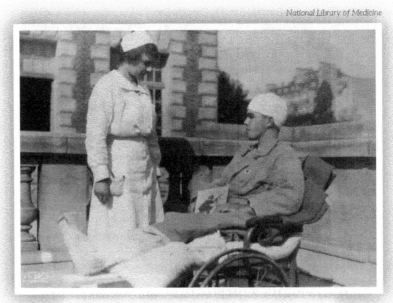

National Library of Medicine

A nurse stands by an injured soldier at Mobile Hospital No. 1.

The Nurses of Base Hospital No. 41

One hundred American nurses reported for duty to Margaret B. Cowling, superintendent of nursing for the University of Virginia's Base Hospital No. 41. The group had been organized in the spring of 1917 but was kept stateside until the summer of 1918. Finally, after months of basic training at Camp Dix, New Jersey, the nurses went to New York City to prepare for deployment. In the city, between being fitted for uniforms and taking mandatory French lessons, the nurses had time for shopping, sightseeing, and attending the theater. The war was very far away.[32]

Camilla (Katie) Louise Wills, a new graduate of the University of Virginia, deployed in July, sailing for Europe on board the USS *Cartago* with other nurses from Base Hospital No. 41.

She and her colleagues arrived at Saint Denis, France, a small town outside of Paris, on August 11, 1918.[33] The medical compound, in an 18th-century school, École de la Légion d'Honneur, accommodated as many as 2,800 patients at once, some in the historic buildings, others in a large array of tents on the enclosed grounds.[34]

Like other nurses at the front, Wills and her colleagues soon discovered the harsh reality of nursing in war. Just 1 day after their arrival in France, an onslaught of more than 100 casualties arrived at the hospital, all requiring baths, coffee, hot soup, and dressing changes before they could be admitted to the wards. In the days that followed, the nurses were overwhelmed with work. With only medical corpsmen to assist her, Wills had charge of Ward III at night, responsible for 160 patients, 144 of who required wound irrigations with the newly invented Carrell–Dakin's solution. At other times, Wills worked in the "dressing room," in charge of changing bandages.[35]

That August, after increased fighting in Marne and Amiens, more casualties flooded into Base Hospital No. 41, challenging the skills and stamina of doctors, nurses, and orderlies alike.[37]

Nurse Anesthetists

During the war, hundreds of nurses volunteered to train as nurse anesthetists. With the shortage of surgeons at the front, U.S. military leaders

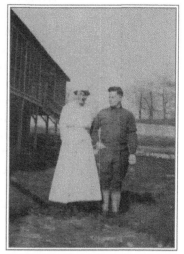

Camilla (Katie) Louise Wills, a nurse on the front at Saint Denis, France, with a soldier.

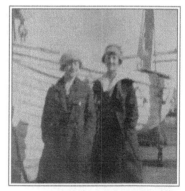

Nurses on board the USS Cartago, which set sail for Europe in July 1918.

Camilla (Katie) Louise Wills's Red Cross Card.

Base Hospital No. 41

"There are so many awfully sick boys that we don't have any hours off duty during the day and work overtime at night. I am in the dressing room at present so of course see all the wounds, a gruesome sight."[36]

Camilla (Katie) Wills, 1918

recognized that they needed more *nurse* anesthetists to free up surgeons to operate. As a result, the Army and Navy sent groups of nurses back to the United States to study the art and science of anesthesia. Many trained at the Lakeside Hospital School of Anesthesia in Cleveland, Ohio, under the supervision of nurse anesthetist Agatha Hodgins, who had returned to the States in 1915.[38] Nurses also studied at other major hospitals throughout the country, including among others the Hospital of the University of Pennsylvania, Johns Hopkins, New York Presbyterian, Mayo Clinic, and St. Vincent's Hospital in Portland, Oregon.[39]

Before the war, training for nurse anesthesia practice consisted of several months of apprenticeship in the practical and the theoretical aspects of the work.[40] Under wartime circumstances, however, the courses lasted only 6 weeks. It was important to get the new nurse anesthetists back to the front as soon as possible.[41] The goal was to have the Army nurse "administer anesthesia to fifty patients . . . on her own . . . before she left."[42]

Once trained, the military nurse anesthetists established programs for graduate nurses in military hospitals both in the United States and overseas.

The Army School of Nursing

The need for nurses extended beyond that for nurse anesthetists. In March 1918, Annie W. Goodrich and Elizabeth Burgess proposed the establishment of an Army School of Nursing. Goodrich was then president of the American Nurses Association while Burgess was assistant professor of Nursing at Teachers College and the inspector of training schools for New York; these positions had readied them for their new challenge. Their goal was to prepare thousands of new nurses for employment abroad and at home. The Army School would have central headquarters in the surgeon general's office and nursing faculty in various military hospitals. During the program students would receive room and board in addition to laundry services and textbooks.

The Army School's course of study was to be based on the standard curriculum proposed in 1917. Classes would focus on surgical nursing content, including the specialty areas of orthopedics, eye, nose, and throat—all areas of practice necessary in war. Two other priority areas were infectious disease and "mental" nursing. Considered of lesser importance for the Army School students was knowledge of specialties like pediatrics, obstetrics, and public health. For training in these areas, students would affiliate in local hospitals during the second and third years of their program.

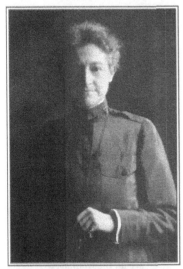

Annie W. Goodrich, who cofounded the Army School of Nursing to prepare nurses at home and abroad for war.

At their May 1918 annual convention, members of the American Nurses Association, the National League for Nursing Education, and the National Organization of Public Health Nurses vigorously debated the pros and cons of preparing full-fledged nurses versus nurses' aides for the war. They also argued over whether or not creating an Army School of Nursing was necessary in the first place. In the end, however, the three organizations voted to support the proposal for an Army School of Nursing. Their agreement did little good. Before the meeting adjourned, Goodrich received a telegram from the U.S. Surgeon General informing her that the War Department had rejected the idea.

Determined to appeal their case, Goodrich and two influential lay women, Frances P. Bolton and Florence Brewster, traveled to Washington, DC, to meet with the secretary of war. The meeting was a success. On May 25, 1918, the secretary of war approved the proposal for the Army School of Nursing. Annie Warburton Goodrich, who was then chief inspecting nurse of the Army Nurse Corps, was appointed dean.[43]

The next step was to find potential students, and during the summer of 1918 the Committee on Nursing of the Council of National Defense began a major recruitment campaign.[44]

Vassar Training Camp for Nurses

The campaign for the Army School program coincided with plans already underway at Vassar College for a rapid entry into nursing for women who already had college degrees. The Vassar plan called for a summer training camp to which college graduates could be admitted to learn "theoretical nursing."[45] That training was to be followed by a 2-year expedited clinical course in hospital nursing. In December 1917 the Emergency Committee on Nursing approved the Vassar Camp. An extensive media campaign, involving press releases and magazine advertisements, followed.

On June 24, 1918, 437 women from prestigious colleges across the nation marched into Vassar's chapel for convocation, ready to begin the program, "the first of its kind to be established in America."[47] Because each was dressed in the uniform of the school to which the applicant had been accepted for the completion of her training after the Vassar Camp, the group immediately acquired the nickname of the "Rainbow Division."[48]

Taught by a prestigious volunteer medical and nursing faculty, Vassar Camp classes included "the history of nursing, dietetics, hygiene, bacteriology, chemistry, psychology and social economics."[51] Lessons in practical nursing "took place in the college gymnasium, converted into a hospital ward with rows of beds neatly made up."[52] There students practiced giving bed baths, taking vital signs, and applying "spiral reverse bandages," among other basic nursing tasks.[53]

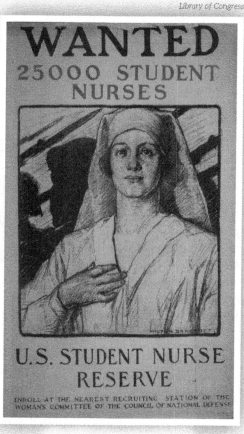

A recruitment poster for the U.S. Student Nurse Reserve.

"Among other things, we are to disprove the suspicion that a college education is in any way a disadvantage to the nursing profession."[49]

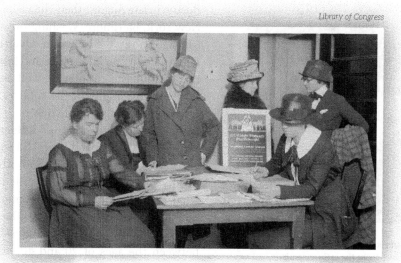

A recruitment table for Vassar College's training camp.

The Vassar Camp

"It was felt extremely important to arouse the attention and interest of young college women as it was obvious that this group could be more rapidly directed into the executive and teaching fields of nursing."[46]

Annie Goodrich, 1918

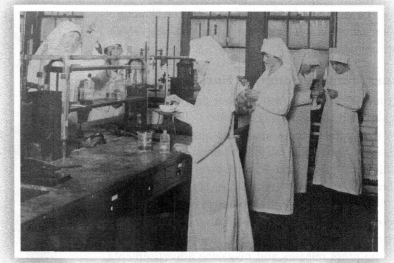

Nursing students conduct experiments in a chemistry lab as part of the Vassar Camp, starting late 1917.

That summer no one could have predicted the extent to which these young students would be needed. When the students left Vassar on September 7, 1918, to complete their education in hospital schools throughout the United States, they were hurled into an unprecedented global crisis—the worst influenza epidemic the world had ever seen. Many of the Vassar students came down with the flu themselves; seven died in the first few weeks of their probationary period. [54]

U.S. NURSES AND THE GREAT INFLUENZA PANDEMIC

In the late summer and autumn of 1918, nurses would be needed everywhere when an influenza virus that had erupted in the spring mutated and spread throughout a Kansas military camp and then throughout the world. The virus traveled across the United States with the troops, hitting Boston in late August, then Philadelphia, New York, Baltimore, Washington, and Chicago in rapid succession. Over the next weeks it spread to cities and towns throughout the country as well as to Europe, traveling with the soldiers on troop trains and ship convoys.

The mutated strain of influenza virus (now recognized as H1N1) was extremely contagious and, too often, deadly. When it was accompanied by what was thought to be pneumonia, mortality was as high as 70%. The flu was particularly lethal for young people between the ages of 20 and 40 years, and thousands of previously healthy

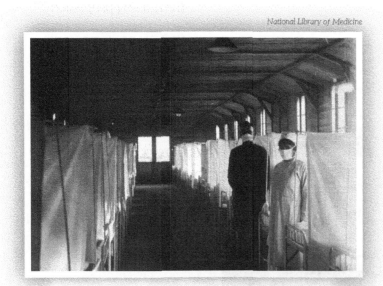

A nurse and a physician wearing masks at Base Hospital No. 26. Each bed was screened off to protect from the influenza virus, which had a mortality rate as high as 70% in some areas.

soldiers, crowded first into military camps and troop ships and then into cold and muddy trenches along the front lines, were especially susceptible.[55] To complicate matters further, the epidemic coincided with continuous air raids over Paris and with the Meuse-Argonne offensive in France and Belgium, one of the most intense and deadliest campaigns of the war.[56]

In the war zone, nurses soon became exhausted. Continuous air raids at night disrupted their sleep and now they were faced not only with an onslaught of casualties but also a deluge of soldiers with flu. The American Expeditionary Forces alone saw more than 360,000 cases.[58]

Skilled nursing care was key to surviving influenza, and the nurses fought to save lives, giving patients soup and tea, and bathing them to reduce their fevers. Nurses also dispensed Vicks vapor rub, aspirin, whiskey, and cough medicine. For the worst cases, following physician orders, nurses administered morphine, oxygen, and digitalis.[59] To control the spread of infection, doctors and nurses donned masks and isolated patients in separate wards, using screens around each bed.[60]

Despite the best efforts of the medical and nursing staff, by October 11, 1918, more than 6,000 American soldiers had already died of the flu and pneumonia in France. By the signing of the armistice on November 11 thousands more had joined them, including 127 army nurses—12 from Base Hospital No. 68 alone.[61]

Nurses on the Home Front

In the United States, both military and civilian physicians and nurses, working under the direction of Surgeon General Rupert Blue, the U.S. Public Health Service and the American Red Cross, were also trying to cope with the epidemic. Soon after the flu struck the soldiers at Camp Devens in Boston, officials had to set up an open-air tent hospital to deal with the overflow of patients.

On September 13, the Boston health department reported its first civilian case. By September 17, newspaper headlines declared that the flu was "epidemic in much of greater Boston."[62] Within the next 24 hours, health authorities recorded 41 more deaths. The next week Massachusetts Lieutenant Governor Calvin Coolidge formed an Emergency Public Health Committee to coordinate statewide efforts to curb the spread of the epidemic. The committee's first action was to telegraph the American Red Cross requesting help. Nurses were the top priority.

On September 24, the American Red Cross National Committee on Influenza assembled in Washington to discuss the epidemic. It was becoming increasingly clear that this was no ordinary flu. The new strain had devastated Boston and was now sweeping the East Coast and racing south and west. During that meeting the group drafted a decentralized plan to address the national emergency, leaving the major response to local authorities and the 3,684 local Red Cross Chapters across the country.[63] As soon as the meeting ended, director of the Red Cross Bureau of Nursing Clara Noyes

Phieffer's Bacillus

At the time of the 1918 influenza pandemic, scientists thought the flu was caused by *B. influenza*, a bacterium described by Richard Phieffer in 1892. Death was due to a complicating pneumonia or acute respiratory failure.[57]

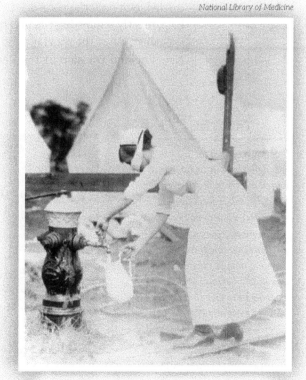

National Library of Medicine

A nurse wearing a mask draws water from a pump.

telegraphed Red Cross chapters in the 14 regional divisions wiring: "Suggest you organize Home Defense nurses . . . to meet present epidemic. . . . Provide nurses with masks."[64]

The Boston Instructive District Nurses Respond

In Boston, the Instructive District Nurses Association (classified as "home defense nurses" a year earlier) did not need to be told to organize for the epidemic: They had been seeing patients with influenza since early September. In fact, the association's newly opened headquarters on Massachusetts Avenue had been made the "administrative center for all home nursing care" related to the flu.[65] Moreover, the district's superintendent Mary Beard had been serving on the Commonwealth's Emergency Public Health Committee and was well aware of the fact that the flu was rampant in the city.

"The influenza situation overshadows everything . . . the need for nurses is tremendous."[66]

Mary Beard, 1918

In her report to a special meeting of the District's Board of Managers on September 25, Beard noted that as nurses entered homes throughout the city they found "whole families stricken. . . . In one case the father was found in bed, dead; in another room the mother lay, with two children, all very ill; and in still another, the baby, dying with pneumonia."[67] The epidemic was worse than anything the Boston nurses had experienced in the 32 years of the association's work.

Under Beard's direction, the instructive district nurses coordinated the care of "nurses of all kinds," including 15 from the Board of Health (who had volunteered under the district nurses), as well as seven tuberculosis nurses, 13 school nurses, 20 baby hygiene nurses, and the Simmons College public health nursing students. For the duration of the epidemic, the district nurses also supervised hundreds of attendants, aides, and untrained volunteers, who "poured in the Central House all day long and well into the night offering to help in any way they could."[68]

Throughout the month of September the Boston district nurses saw 4,664 new patients—more than three times the number they had seen in August.[69] Among these were 64 pregnant women with pneumonia or flu, 13 of whom died, and 11 of whom miscarried. Not only the poor needed nurses; middle- and upper-class families also sought help, mostly requesting the private duty nurses they had come to expect.

Because of the shortage and the need to make the best use of the nurses' time, the New England Division of the Red Cross declared that "an automobile and driver" be

The Crisis

"All day long and up to 11:00 at night the four telephones poured out their pitiful stories. Whole families desperately ill with no one to do the commonest things for them; patients meeting the crisis of pneumonia with no nursing care at all; distracted relatives begging us to give that which did not exist anywhere to be given—nurses to stay till the patients were better."[70]

District Nurses Report, 1918

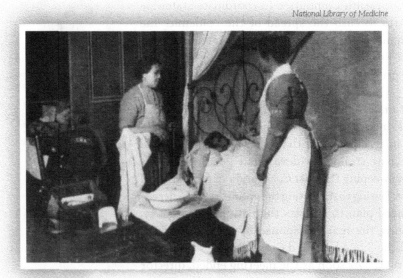

National Library of Medicine

Two district nurses attend to an influenza patient.

assigned to each nurse.[71] The directive blurred class and gender boundaries as elite White ladies, some from the district's Board of Lady Managers, worked with the local Red Cross and the Home Guard Motor Corps to transport nurses throughout the city. The plan worked: Not only did it save nurses' time, the automobile transportation allowed the nurses to carry soup, blankets, pneumonia jackets, and other necessary supplies.

By the end of September the flu situation had become increasingly serious. It was now spreading throughout the state. So, on September 26, State Commissioner of Health Eugene Kelly once again telegraphed to Washington:

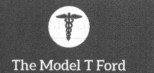

The Model T Ford

In 1908, the Ford Motor Company in Detroit, Michigan, produced America's first affordable automobile, soon known as the Model T, the "Tin Lizzie," or the "flivver." Mass-produced on an assembly line, reliable and easily maintained, the car opened road travel to the middle class.

INFLUENZA PNEUMONIA SITUATION . . . THROUGHOUT MASSA-CHUSETTS VERY SERIOUS . . . DEATHS INCREASING AT ALARMING RATE . . . MANY DOCTORS AND NURSES ILL . . . FEDERAL ASSIS-TANCE NECESSARY . . . FIVE HUNDRED DOCTORS AND ONE THOU-SAND NURSES NEEDED AT ONCE.[72]

The terse reply from Washington made it clear that no nurses were available: "Can send all the doctors you want but not one nurse."[73]

Meanwhile, although the National Red Cross had few nurses to send to Boston, several localities responded to the city's desperate appeal for help. Lieutenant Governor McCallum Grant of Nova Scotia sent nurses and doctors to Boston in appreciation of Bostonians' response to the Halifax explosion the year before. At that time the city of Baltimore had sent a "special hospital train, fully equipped with 40 beds" to East Braintree Station.[74]

On October 6, Director Beard reported that the district nurses were caring for "3,074 patients ill with influenza or pneumonia." The care that the nurses provided was basic. They put patients to bed, covered them with blankets, and opened windows for fresh air. Following medical orders, or relying on their own nursing expertise and making do with what they had on hand, the nurses bathed patients, changed bed linens, and administered such treatments as ice packs and aspirin to reduce fever, Listerine gargles for sore throats, and mustard plasters and cough syrups to alleviate lung congestion.[75] They also provided nourishment, giving patients "gruels, cereals, milk toast, eggs, and milk."[76]

Following directions from the National Red Cross, the nurses wore masks as they cared for flu victims.[77] It was a mandate created with the hope of protecting nurses and others from "the bacteria that were floating in the air around each patient." The demand for masks was enormous. In Boston, Red Cross volunteers worked 7 days a week to produce 83,606 gauze masks during the last week of September and the first weeks of October.[78]

Philadelphia Visiting Nurses Society Response

From Boston the epidemic spread to Philadelphia. On September 19, hundreds of sailors on the naval base became sick and over the next 10 days civilians also succumbed. After September 28, when the city held its scheduled Liberty Loan parade to raise money for the war effort, the epidemic exploded.[79] Hospitals soon reached capacity and the city set up emergency facilities in warehouses, churches, and schools. Given the nursing shortage because of the war, officials turned to pupil nurses, medical students, and Red Cross volunteers to help. They worked under the direction of retired physicians who had returned to practice.

With hospitals overflowing, patients were advised to stay home. As a result, the demands for nurses increased. In response Health Commissioner William Kreusen

"If you would ask me the three things Philadelphia most needs to conquer the epidemic, I would tell you 'Nurses, more nurses, and yet more nurses.'"[83]

William Kreusen, Health Commissioner, 1918

placed his entire staff of 120 nurses at the disposal of the Visiting Nurse Society. They worked under the direction of Superintendent Katherine Tucker and Assistant Director Elizabeth Scarborough.[80]

Even with more help, however, the nurses were stretched to their limits. In many families, more than one member was ill—and when both parents succumbed to the flu, the nurses not only had to care for the sick, but they also had to supply food for the entire family. To do so, the nurses turned to the soup kitchens set up by churches, synagogues, and the Junior League. When the parents in a family died, the nurses' work got even more complicated. Now they had to find placement for the orphans left behind.

As family after family succumbed to the flu, Philadelphia's social infrastructure crumbled. There was no one to drive streetcars, operate telephones, collect garbage, or bury the dead. By October 15, Philadelphia had reported 10,046 deaths, and the newspapers reported: "Bodies were being brought to the cemeteries faster than they could be buried.[82] When the nurses also became sick, the need for help became critical. Newspapers not only advertised for help, but also reported on the participation of society's elite women, local college girls, and members of the Junior League.

Before nurses could be obtained, however, the epidemic peaked and then began to subside. By late November, the epidemic was over. In December, the district nurses began to focus on cases "needing aftercare."[84] The December 1918 minutes from the children's ward of the Hospital of the University of Pennsylvania reflect the pressing need for follow-up care:

Several children who were admitted during the epidemic . . . are still with us and others still need care at home. . . . Clifton, an influenza-pneumonia patient, is beginning to come back to life after having been ill in the ward since October. Application has been made to have him admitted to the Children's Seashore Home."[85]

Lillian Wald and the Henry Street Visiting Nurses Respond

In New York City, Lillian Wald, director of the Henry Street Settlement Visiting Nurses, was all too aware of the alarming rapidity with which the flu was affecting the city's residents. Since 1893 the Henry Street nurses had been responding to calls from the Lower East Side where epidemics were commonplace. In September 1918, it seemed this was just another bad flu epidemic.

This time, however, the intensity of the disease and the devastation it caused was remarkable. While making their rounds, nurses found "households where whole families were ill . . . without anyone to give them the simplest nursing care."[86] As in other cities, hospitals overflowed and patients had to be cared for at home. As one student nurse recounted: "Almost overnight the hospital was inundated. Wards were emptied hastily of patients convalescing from other ailments . . . only emergency operations were performed. Cots appeared down the center of wards."[87]

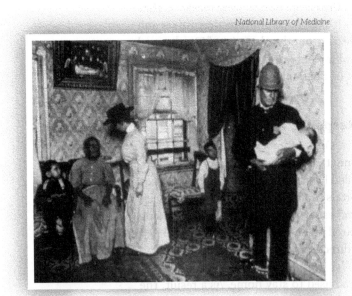

National Library of Medicine

A visiting nurse visits a family with a policeman.

On October 10, the New York nurses met and voted unanimously to organize the Nurses' Emergency Council to coordinate nursing activities throughout the city. Lillian Wald was elected chair.[89] Wald's leadership skills were needed; all over the city people were succumbing to the deadly virus. Lillian Wald described the problem, writing:

> *The home is in upper Harlem; the family consists of seven—a father, mother and five children. The mother lies ill with influenza, the father has lobar pneumonia, two children have measles and bronchopneumonia and one child is only four weeks old. . . . The family had been without care of any kind until the case was reported to the visiting nurse. This is a situation duplicated in hundreds of homes.*[90]

The Nursing Situation in Chicago

Conditions in Chicago, the location of the nation's largest railroad hub, were much the same as those in New York and Philadelphia. Reports of flu at the Great Lakes Training Station surfaced in Chicago as early as September 9, by September 22, 100 sailors had died and 4,500 were ill.[91] On October 1, Cook County Hospital reported 260 cases, 60 of which had arrived that day.[92] That same day, Commissioner of Health Dr. John Dill Robertson ordered "virtual quarantine for every case of influenza" in the city, commanding "every victim . . . to go to his home and stay there."[93] By October 2 the city reported that

National Library of Medicine

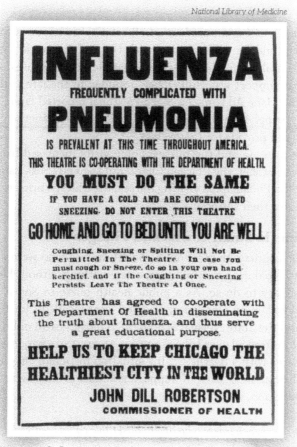

Chicago's West Side

"We were very hard hit on the west side of Chicago. . . . Dirty streets, dirty alleys and just as dirty houses, and lack of proper sleeping quarters have made our work more than usually difficult."[96]

Mary Westphal, assistant superintendent

"The Ghetto was a hotbed of influenza and pneumonia."[97]

Mary Westphal, 1918

Influenza poster advising readers in Chicago to stay at home if they were ill.

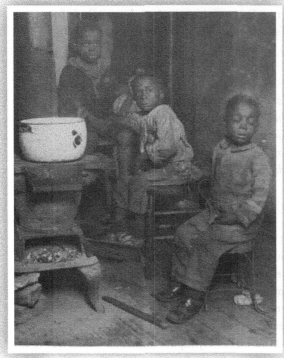

Three children in a Chicago tenement room.

hospitals across the city had reached capacity.[94] By October 10 Chicago was reporting "1,421 cases of flu and 340 of pneumonia, with 72 deaths from pneumonia and 55 from influenza."[95] During that month, the rise in cases of flu, the overcrowded hospitals, and the "virtual quarantine" in the city all served to increase the work of the Chicago Visiting Nurse Association.

Assistant Superintendent Mary Westphal described a nurse's typical day during the epidemic, writing:

The houses in this area are very close together and many families live under one roof. The people watched at their doors and windows, beckoning for the nurses to come in. One day a nurse, who started out with 15 patients to see, saw nearly fifty before night. . . . Sometimes, before getting out of her first case, the nurse was surrounded by people asking her to go with them to see other patients. Physicians could not get around to all of the people needing them, it was impossible to get orders, and consequently the nurse had to try to be many things to all people."[98]

Fortunately, the Chicago visiting nurses had a well-established network to whom they could turn for support, and, in collaboration with the Red Cross, decided that they would try to "cover all families for whom it was impossible to get private duty nurses or aides."[99] Critical to that support was Hull House, founded in the late 19th century by Progressive Era reformer Jane Addams. As Mary Westphal reported later: "Hull House helped us wonderfully, supplying warm gowns, baby clothes, bed linens . . . [and] soup for families that could not provide for themselves."[100]

As the epidemic wore on and the nurses' home visits increased from 12,000 to 25,750 in the month of October, the Chicago Chapter of the Red Cross issued an appeal for volunteers.[101] Like the Philadelphia visiting nurses, the Chicago nurses could no longer meet the demands for their services.

Nursing Flu Victims in Small Towns and Villages

In remote areas of the country, the few public health nurses who were available also responded to calls for help during the epidemic, often working without help and without the supplies necessary to do so. As a public health nurse in South Dakota who worked as superintendent in an emergency hospital later recalled: "for five weeks we used the dormitory and the State Normal School, then moved to an old residence. The patients were brought in from all over Lake County . . . many farm hands with pneumonia. We treated 175 cases with 4 deaths."[102] The situation in Denio, Oregon, was much the same. In isolated rural areas, lack of supplies and lack of help were typical. One nurse described her situation, writing:

Our patients are . . . sheepherders who live in miserable cabins scattered in most inaccessible places. . . . There is no food, no bedding and absolutely no conception of the first principles of hygiene and sanitation, or of nursing care. I have taken over the hotel as a hospital and the Big Boss, who employs the sheep-herders, is having all who are not too ill to be moved, brought in here."[103]

In coal-mining communities and small towns in Kentucky, West Virginia, and Alabama, Red Cross nurses cared for hundreds of miners who had come down with influenza. By November 1 conditions were so serious in certain mountain communities that the Red Cross begged for extra help. Twenty-four graduate nurses, 45 practical nurses, and 83 Catholic Sisters responded. In another Kentucky town where almost half of the 2,500 inhabitants were ill, one nurse cared for the sickest patients in an emergency hospital set up in the Young Men's Christian Association (YMCA); she visited others in their homes. Neighbors helped whenever possible.[104]

In the Black Belt in the Deep South, where racial segregation, geographic isolation, and poverty made conditions even worse for African Americans, the nursing shortage was extreme. In the segregated town of Greenville, Mississippi, where more than 1,800 African Americans succumbed to the flu during the month of October, the local Red Cross society opened an emergency hospital and put out a special call for Black nurses. In Montgomery, Alabama, African American nurse Euphemia Davis recalled a similar situation, noting how she was "on duty four weeks in succession during the influenza" at the St. Bernard Mining Company Hospital. And in the backwoods of Talladega, Alabama, nurse Betsy Hawse reported her determination to do whatever she had to do to help those who were sick, writing:

> *Eight miles from Talladega in the back woods, a colored [sic] family of ten was in bed and dying for the want of attention. No one would come near. I was asked . . . if I would go. I was glad of the opportunity. As I entered the little country cabin I found the mother dead in bed. Three children buried the week before; the father and remainder of the family running a temperature of 102–104. Some had influenza; others had pneumonia . . . I milked the cow, gave medicine, and did everything I could to help . . . I didn't realize how tired I was until I got home."*[105]

> *"I rolled up my sleeves and killed chickens and began to cook. I forgot I was not a cook, but I only thought of saving lives."*[106]
>
> Betsy Hawse, 1918

African American Nurses in Camp Sherman and Camp Grant

As the epidemic raged in military camps throughout the United States, the Army made exceptions to its policy of denying the enlistment of African American nurses. It sent Black nurses to Camp Sherman, one of the military camps with the highest mortality rate from influenza, and to Camp Grant in Illinois, where physicians, nurses, and orderlies were collapsing from overwork.[107] Clinical expertise mattered more than color and in both camps Black nurses cared for both Black and White soldiers. Nonetheless, some prejudice remained; the Black nurses lived in segregated quarters.

The Aftermath

By November 1918 nurses in cities throughout the country were trying to recuperate

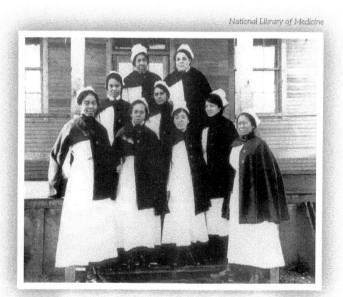

Nurses at Camp Sherman, where they cared for Black and White soldiers.

themselves, treat patients who were recovering, and help address "the social wreckage" left in the wake of the epidemic. In Boston, the strain on the Instructive District Nurses Association was serious. Sixty-six percent of the staff, and some of the students, had been ill "at one time or another" during the 8 weeks of the epidemic.[108] Indeed, every department of the service had been "stressed to the utmost."[109] Now they had to follow those who had lingering effects of the illness. The flu caused serious complications, including "ear troubles" in children, pneumonia, debilitating muscle weakness, and hair loss in adults.[110] As for the social devastation, some families were left fatherless. In other cases, when both parents died, children were orphaned. Getting back to normal would take a coordinated effort. The visiting nurses turned to affluent citizens for financial support and to social workers for their skills in placing orphaned children and helping families find work, food, and medicines.

Red Cross Nurses in Alaska

While nurses in the lower 48 states were dealing with the aftermath of the epidemic, Alaskan Red Cross nurses, teachers, and salmon packers were just beginning to confront the deadly flu. The flu had arrived in Alaska on October 20, 1918, when the steamship *Victoria* docked at Nome, a small town on the coast of the Seward Peninsula.

Alaska's governor Thomas Riggs had imposed a marine quarantine of 14 days after the arrival of the ship, and had stationed U.S. marshals at all ports, trail heads, and the mouths of Alaska's rivers to ensure that travelers did not bring the disease into any of the territory's remote communities. Despite those precautions, however, the flu spread to small villages and towns. By the end of November, 35% to 40% of the native population in villages from Nome to Shishmarez was dead. In the tiny village of Brevig Mission, 72 of the 120 Inuits died in less than 10 days.

Within weeks, the epidemic spread from the Seward Peninsula all along the Alaskan coasts, attacking Juneau, Anchorage, Homer, Cordova, Kodiak, and small settlements on the Aleutian Islands. On November 7, with many dead and the risk of more deaths from flu increasing, Governor Riggs issued a special directive to all

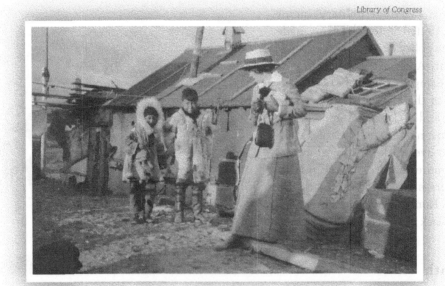

A nurse with native Alaskans, whose population was ravaged by influenza throughout the fall and winter of 1918.

Alaskan natives, urging them to stay at home and avoid public gatherings. It was an order in direct opposition to the Inuits' traditional value of the importance of community. As a result, many ignored the directive, continuing to gather in public places. Others, fearful of hospitals, too sick to move from their homes, or too sick to make a fire, froze to death. Some, too weak to bait their traps or hunt for reindeer, died of starvation. When most of the village members were sick, they could not care for each other. As a result, entire communities were devastated. And when the adults died, children were orphaned. Meanwhile, their parents' bodies were left to freeze or be ravaged by wild dogs. Throughout the territory, medical and nursing personnel were desperately needed.

In December 1918, 10 physicians and 10 nurses, "together with medical supplies furnished by the Northwest Division of the Red Cross," left Seattle for a relief expedition to Alaska. They sailed under the command of Dr. Emil Kurlish, captain of the U.S. Public Health Service. The expedition members spent a month in Alaska, tending to natives and others on Prince of Wales Island, Juneau, Cordova, and Kodiak. Meanwhile, Alaskan Red Cross chapters were active throughout the epidemic, not only in cooperating with Kurlish's expedition but also providing assistance "on their own account."[111] In the meantime, Governor Riggs traveled to Washington, DC, to appeal to Congress for funds, noting that the alarming situation was "beyond" his "control."[112]

> "There have been deaths all over the Territory, 90 percent of which have been among the Eskimos . . . and the epidemic is still raging."[113]
>
> Governor Riggs, 1919

Appearing before a congressional subcommittee to make his case, Riggs asked the federal government to appropriate $200,000 to help Alaska respond to the flu, noting that the territory's entire medical relief fund was only $75,000—an amount that was already budgeted to maintain its five to six hospitals and the few physicians and nurses they employed. The subcommittee asked questions and debated the role of local versus federal government and their respective responsibilities during a major epidemic. Finally, in recognition that the Bureau of Indian Affairs had been granted funds to support other native populations, the federal government provided Riggs with $100,000. What he needed, however, were nurses.

During the winter, with waterways frozen, Alaskans were left to battle the epidemic on their own. In one case, when no nurses could be found, a local schoolteacher volunteered to work in the temporary hospital in Ketchikan. At Brevig Mission, where there were hundreds of children left on their own, the church was used as an orphanage. Meanwhile, hundreds of Inuits died, their bodies frozen in place in their huts.

Finally on June 3, 1919, 12 American Red Cross nurses and six doctors left San Francisco for Alaska, sailing on the steamship *Unalga*. After a stormy voyage, the party landed in the Aleutian Islands where the group divided into smaller teams to visit villages along the coast. There, they found deplorable conditions with "heaps of dead bodies on the shelves and floors of the huts."[115]

After visiting several other small villages, where more orphans were found, the Red Cross relief parties returned to their ship on June 29, 1919, for the voyage back to Seattle. The epidemic was over; the dead had been buried, and the orphans taken into missions. There was little more that the teams of volunteer nurses and physicians could do. Alaskan's native population had been decimated.[116]

Nursing in Kanakanak

"ursinurses, Miss Mary Conley and Miss Rhoda Ray . . . had been working practically night and day for weeks on end doing all the janitor's work, the cooking for the entire hospital, all the nursing and caring for a number of children and babies whose parents were either dead or dying."[114]

American Red Cross Report, July 1919

With the end of the Great War and the end of the flu epidemic, U.S. nurses turned their attention to "maternity and other preventive work."[117] In 1919, maternal and infant mortality were at all-time highs and the country needed to find ways to address these issues. Nurses, working in public health departments in cities and towns across the country, in demonstration projects in Appalachia, and on assignment with the Bureau of Indian Affairs, would be essential players in that process. In doing so, they would find their work extending beyond individual care to families and communities. The health of the nation was at stake.

For Discussion

1. What was the reasoning for sending fully developed base hospitals to Europe?
2. Discuss the role of nurse anesthetists in World War I.
3. How did racial prejudice affect enlistment in the U.S. Army and Navy Nurse Corps in World War I?
4. Why did so much responsibility fall to American Red Cross nurses and visiting nurses during the influenza epidemic of 1918?
5. Discuss the challenges of nursing in the territory of Alaska and in rural states during the influenza epidemic.

NOTES

1. "Editorial Comment," *American Journal of Nursing* 17, no. 9 (June 1917): 761–765 (quote 761).
2. Mary Sarnecky, "The Army Nurse Corps in World War I," in *A History of the U.S. Army Nurse Corps*, ed. Mary T. Sarnecky (Philadelphia: University of Pennsylvania Press, 1999): 80–132.
3. http://www.medicalarchives.jhmi.edu/papers/LaMotte (accessed May 3, 2016).
4. Ellen LaMotte, *The Backwash of War: The Human Wreckage of the Battlefield as Witnessed by an American Nurse* (New York: G. P. Putnam's Sons, 1916): 115–116.
5. Virginia Gaffey, "Agatha Cobourg Hodgins: She Only Counted Shining Hours," *American Association of Nurse Anesthetists Journal* 75, no. 2 (April 2007): 97.
6. La Motte, *The Backwash of War*, 24–26.
7. Sarnecky, *A History of the U.S. Army Nurse Corps*, 81.
8. Clara Noyes, correspondence to Adelaide Nutting, April 8, 1917, as quoted in Philip Kalisch and Beatrice Kalisch, *American Nursing: A History*, 4th ed. (Philadelphia: Lippincott Williams and Wilkins, 2004): 199.
9. Jane Delano, "The Need for Increased Enrollment, "*American Journal of Nursing* 17, no. 11 (August 1917): 1092–1097 (quote 1092).
10. Clara Noyes, quoted in Lavinia Dock, Sarah Pickett, Clara Noyes, Fannie Clement, Elizabeth Fox, and Anna Meter, *A History of American Red Cross Nursing* (New York: McMillan, 1922): 575–576.
11. "Pennsylvania Base Hospital No. 10," 82–83. https://archives.org/details/historyofpennsyl 00unit_10.
12. Ibid.
13. Sarnecky, *A History of the U.S. Army Nurse Corps*, 96
14. Lawrence Gooley, "Florence Bullard: Local Nurse, World War One Hero" (June 27, 2011), http://www.adirondackalmanack.com/2011/06/florence-bullard-local-nurse-world-war -one-hero.html.

15. Frances Bullard, correspondence, September 26, 1917, *St. Marys Alumnae Quarterly* (November 1917), Mayo Historical Unit.

16. Gooley, "Florence Bullard."

17. Christine Hallet, *Containing Trauma: Nursing Work in the First World War* (Manchester, UK: Manchester University Press, 2009): 107.

18. Sarnecky, *A History of the U.S. Army Nurse Corps*, 98.

19. Christine Hallet, *Veiled Warriors: Allied Nurses of the First World War* (Oxford, UK: Oxford University Press, 2014): 221.

20. Sarnecky, *A History of the U.S. Army Nurse Corps*, 99–101.

21. Dock et al., *A History of American Red Cross Nursing*, 575–576.

22. Ibid., 288.

23. "Hospital Center in France," Saint Marys School of Nursing, 1919 annual report, reprint, Mayo History Unit, 1–2.

24. May MacGregor Given, quoted in Arlene Keeling, *The Nurses of Mayo Clinic: Caring Healers* (Rochester, MN: Mayo Clinic, 2012): 39.

25. I. M. Rutkow, "History of Surgery," in *Sabiston Textbook of Surgery: The Biological Basis of Modern Surgical Practice*, 17th ed., eds. C. M. Townsend, B. M. Evers, and K. L. Mattos (Philadelphia: Saunders, 2004): 3–19.

26. "Mademoiselle Miss," quoted in Arlene Keeling, "Historical Research and WOC Nursing: A Strange and Wonderful Relationship," *Journal of Wound, Ostomy and Continence Nursing* 29 (2002): 180–183 (quote 181).

27. Army Medical Services, "Carrel-Dakin Treatment of Wounds," *British Medical Journal* 2, 2966 (November 3, 1917): 597–599 (quote 597).

28. May MacGregor Given, quoted in Arlene Keeling, *The Nurses of Mayo Clinic*, 38–39.

29. Lorrie Bennett and Barbara Jerabek, "Sophie Gran Jévne Winton: A Woman and Nurse Anesthetist before Her Time: April 24, 1887-April 24, 1989" (master's thesis, Mayo School of Health Related Sciences, Rochester, MN, 1999), Archives of the American Association of Nurse Anesthetists.

30. Keeling, *The Nurses of Mayo Clinic*, 38–39.

31. Ibid.

32. Hallet, *Veiled Warriors*, 220.

33. Camilla Louise Wills Collection, Eleanor C. Bjoring Center for Nursing Historical Inquiry, University of Virginia.

34. Ibid.

35. Hallet, *Veiled Warriors*, 241.

36. Jennifer Cassavant, *American Red Cross Nursing during World War I: Opportunities and Obstacles* (PhD dissertation, University of Virginia, 2007): 138.

37. Hallet, *Veiled Warriors*, 242.

38. Gaffey, "Agatha Cobourg Hodgins," 1.

39. Ira Gunn, "The History of Nurse Anesthesia Education: Highlights and Influences," *American Association of Nurse Anesthetists Journal* 59, no. 1 (1991): 53–61 (quote 55).

40. Hallet, *Veiled Warriors*, 949.

41. Sarnecky, *A History of the U.S. Army Nurse Corps*, 130.

42. Ibid., 131.

43. Kalisch and Kalisch, *American Nursing*, 208–210.

44. Dock et al., *A History of American Red Cross Nursing*, 288.

45. Katherine Smith, *Both a College Woman and a Professional Nurse: College Educated Women Who Became Professional Nurses, 1890-1920* (publicly accessible Penn dissertations, 2015): Paper 1139, 43.

46. Annie Goodrich, in Annie Goodrich Collection MC4, Series I, folder 4. The Barbara Bates Center for the Study of the History of Nursing (hereafter BBCSHN), University of Pennsylvania (hereafter UPENN).

47. Gladys Bonner Clappison, *Vassar's Rainbow Division: The Training Camp for Nurses at Vassar College* (Huntsville, AL: Graphic Publishing, 1964): 30.

48. Smith, *Both a College Woman*, 34.

49. Clappison, *Vassar's Rainbow Division*, 40.

50. Ibid.

51. Smith, *Both a College Woman*, 49.

52. Clappison, *Vassar's Rainbow Division*, 81.

53. Ibid., 81.

54. Ibid., 90.

55. Carol Byerly, *Fever of War: The Influenza Epidemic in the U.S. Army during World War I* (New York: New York University Press, 2005).

56. Ibid.

57. Jeffrey Taubenberger, Johan Huilton, and David Morens, "Discovery and Characterization of the 1918 Pandemic Influenza Virus in Historical Context," *Antiviral Therapeutics* 12, no. 4 (2007): 581–591.

58. Hallet, *Veiled Warriors*, 229.

59. Arlene W. Keeling, "Alert to the Necessities of the Emergency: U.S. Nursing during the 1918 Influenza Pandemic," *Public Health Reports: Special Supplement on Pandemic Influenza* 125, supplement 3 (April 2010): 105–112.

60. Byerly, *Fever of War*, 75.

61. Sarnecky, *A History of the U.S. Army Nurse Corps*, 121.

62. "Grippe Making Great Headway," *Boston Daily Globe*, September 17, 1918, 1.

63. Marian Moser Jones, "'The Greatest Mother' and the Great Pandemic" (unpublished manuscript, April 10, 2009), paper presented at the National Influenza History Seminar, the University of Michigan, Ann Arbor, Michigan.

64. Clara Noyes, "Memo to All Division Directors," September 25, 1918, National Archives and Records Administration, College Park (hereafter NARA, CP), box 689, 803.11.

65. Minutes of the Instructive District Nurse Association (hereafter IDNA) Board of Managers Meeting (October 23, 1918): 1. IDNA Collection, Howard Gotlieb (hereafter HG) Archives, Boston University (hereafter BU) N34, box 11.

66. Minutes of the IDNA Board of Managers Meeting (September 25, 1918): 2, HG Archives, BU, N34, box 11.

67. IDNA, *Emergency Bulletin 1918*, HG Archives, BU, N34, box 11.

68. IDNA Board of Managers' Minutes, September 25, 1918, HG Archives, BU, N34, box 11.

69. Ibid.

70. Report of the Director, IDNA Annual Report, 1918, HG Archives, BU, N34, box 11, folder 5, p. 34.

71. American Red Cross New England Division, "Memo, October 3, 1918," NARA, CP, box 689, 803.11 Epidemic, Flu, Massachusetts.

72. Eugene Kelly, *Telegram to Congressman George H. Tinkham*, September 26, 1918, NARA, CP, box 689, 803.11.

73. Alfred W. Crosby, *America's Forgotten Pandemic* (New York: Cambridge University Press, 2003): 51.

74. IDNA Minutes, October 23, 1918, HG Archives, BU, box N34.

75. "What the Boston Metropolitan Chapter of the Red Cross Accomplished during the Epidemic," November 18, 1918, NARA, CP, box 689, 803.11 Epidemic, Flu, Massachusetts, 2–3.

76. "How to Care for Influenza and Pneumonia Patients," *The Public Health Nurse*, 10, no. 7 (November 1918): 238–245 (quote 244).

77. Ibid.

78. "What the Boston Metropolitan Chapter of the Red Cross Accomplished," 2–3.

79. John Barry, *The Great Influenza* (New York: Penguin Book Group, 2003): 208.

80. "Influenza Kills 143 in this City," Visiting Nurse Society (hereafter VNS) Scrapbook, BBCSHN, UPENN.

81. "Volunteer Nurses Care for 1200 Grip Patients," unidentified newspaper clipping, VNS Scrapbook, BBCSHN, UPENN.

82. "Influenza Increases the Country Over," *New York Times* (October 19, 1918).

83. "No Increase Reported in Influenza Deaths," unidentified newspaper clipping, VNS Scrapbook, BBCSHN, UPENN.

84. "Report of Work in Ward G for December 1918," MC 166 Women's Auxiliary of the Hospital of the University of Pennsylvania's Ward G (Children's Ward). Minutes, 1917–1927, box 1, folder 1, BBCSHN, UPENN.

85. Ibid.

86. Pamela Doty, "A Retrospect," *The Public Health Nurse* 11, no. 12 (1919): 949–957 (quote 954).

87. Dorothy Deming, "Influenza, 1918: Reliving the Great Epidemic," *American Journal of Nursing* 10 (1957): 1308–1309 (quote 1308).

88. Ibid., 1308.

89. Doty, "A Retrospect."

90. Keeling, "Alert to the Necessities of the Emergency," 105–112.

91. "100 Sailors at Great Lakes Die of Influenza," *Chicago Daily Tribune* (September 22, 1918).

92. "All Flu Cases Quarantined by Order of City," *Chicago Daily Tribune* (October 1, 1918).

93. Ibid.

94. "Influenza Cases Overtax Nurses and Physicians," *Chicago Daily Tribune* (October 2, 1918).

95. "Society Women Work as Nurses in Flu Hospital," *Chicago Daily Tribune* (October 10, 1918).

96. Mary Westphal, *Report*, November 8, 1918, Chicago Visiting Nurse Association (hereafter VNA) papers, Chicago Historical Society.

97. Ibid.

98. Ibid.

99. "The VNA in Epidemics," Chicago VNA Collection, Chicago History Museum, box 16, folder 1-1, 9.

100. Westphal, *Report*.

101. "The VNA in Epidemics."

102. Keeling, "Alert to the Necessities of the Emergency," 105–112.

103. Ibid.

104. Ibid.

105. Darlene C. Hine, *Black Women in the Nursing Profession: A Documentary History* (New York: Garland Publishing, 1992): 18.

106. Ibid.

107. John Barry, *The Great Influenza* (New York: Penguin Book Group, 2003): 210–219.

108. 1918 Annual Report IDNA, box 13, N34, folder 11, p. 32, HG Archives, BU.

109. Ibid.

110. IDNA Board of Managers Minutes, December 4, 1918, HG Archives, BU, N34, box 11, folder 5.

111. "Alaska Handled Flu with Efficiency and Dispatch," *Report of the Northwest Division of the American Red Cross,* January 18, 1919, NARA, CP, box 689, 803.11 Epidemic Flu.

112. Thomas Riggs, "Influenza in Alaska and Puerto Rico," hearings before the Subcommittee of House Committee on Appropriations, 65th Congress (Washington: Government Printing Services, 1919): 3–18 (quote 4).

113. Ibid.

114. Ibid., 3.

115. American Red Cross Report, "Alaska, Flu," July 1919, NARA, CP, 803.11 Epidemic, Flu.

116. Arlene W. Keeling, "A Most Alarming Situation: Responding to the 1918 Influenza Epidemic in Alaska," *Windows in Time: The Newsletter of the Eleanor Crowder Bjoring Center for Nursing Historical Inquiry* 21, no. 1 (October 2013): 8–11.

117. Westphal, *Report*.

FURTHER READING

Byerly, Carol, *Fever of War: The Influenza Epidemic in the U.S. Army during World War I* (New York: New York University Press, 2005).

Casavant, Jennifer, *American Red Cross Nursing during World War I: Opportunities and Obstacles* (PhD dissertation, University of Virginia, 2007).

Crosby, Alfred, *America's Forgotten Pandemic: Influenza 1918*, 2nd ed. (Boston: Cambridge University Press, 2003).

DeValpine, Maria, and Arlene Keeling, "The Alaskan Influenza Epidemic, 1918-1919," in *Nurses and Disasters: Global Historical Case Studies*, eds. Arlene Keeling and Barbra Mann Wall (New York: Springer Publishing, 2015): 91–113.

Doty, Pamela, "A Retrospect of the Influenza Epidemic," *The Public Health Nurse* 11, no. 12 (1919): 949–957.

Geister, Janet, "The Flu Epidemic of 1918," *Nursing Outlook* 5, no. 10 (October 1957): 582–584.

Hallet, Christine, *Containing Trauma: Nursing Work in the First World War* (Manchester, UK: Manchester University Press, 2009).

Hallet, Christine, *Veiled Warriors: Allied Nurses of the First World War* (Oxford, UK: Oxford University Press, 2014).

Hallet, Christine, *Nurse Writers of the Great War* (Manchester, UK: Manchester University Press, 2016).

Hine, Darlene C., *Black Women in the Nursing Profession: A Documentary History* (New York: Garland Publishing, 1992).

Keeling, Arlene, "'The Ghetto was a Hotbed of Influenza and Pneumonia': District Nursing during the Influenza Epidemic, 1918-1919," in *Everyday Nursing Life, Past and Present*, ed. Sylvelyn Hahner-Romback (Stuttgart, Germany: Franz Steiner Verlag Publishers, August 2009): 63–80.

Keeling, Arlene, "'When the City Is a Great Field Hospital': The Influenza Pandemic of 1918 and the New York City Nursing Response," *Journal of Clinical Nursing* 18 (September 2009): 2732–2738.

Keeling, Arlene, "Alert to the Necessities of the Emergency: U.S. Nursing during the 1918 Influenza Pandemic," *Public Health Reports: Special Supplement on Pandemic Influenza* 125, supplement 3 (April 2010): 105–112.

Keeling, Arlene, *The Nurses of Mayo Clinic: Caring Healers* (Rochester, MN: Mayo Clinic, 2012).

Keen-Payne, Rhonda, "'We Must Have Nurses': Spanish Influenza in America, 1918-1919," *Nursing History Review* 8 (2000): 143–156.

LaMotte, Ellen, *The Backwash of War: The Human Wreckage of the Battlefield as Witnessed by an American Nurse* (New York: G. P. Putnam's Sons, 1916): 115–116.

Noyes, Roger, "Clara D. Noyes, RN: Life of a Global Nursing Leader" (Manchester Center, VT: Shires Press, 2017).

Rockefeller, Nancy, "In Gauze We Trust: Public Health and Spanish Influenza on the Home Front, Seattle, 1918-1919," *Pacific Northwest Quarterly* 77, no. 3 (1986): 104–113.

Sarnecky, Mary, "The Army Nurse Corps in World War I," in *A History of the U.S. Army Nurse Corps*, ed. Mary T. Sarnecky (Philadelphia: University of Pennsylvania Press, 1999).

Toman, Cynthia, "Sister Soldiers of the Great War: The Nurses of the Canadian Army Medical Corps" (Toronto, CA: UBC Press, 2017).

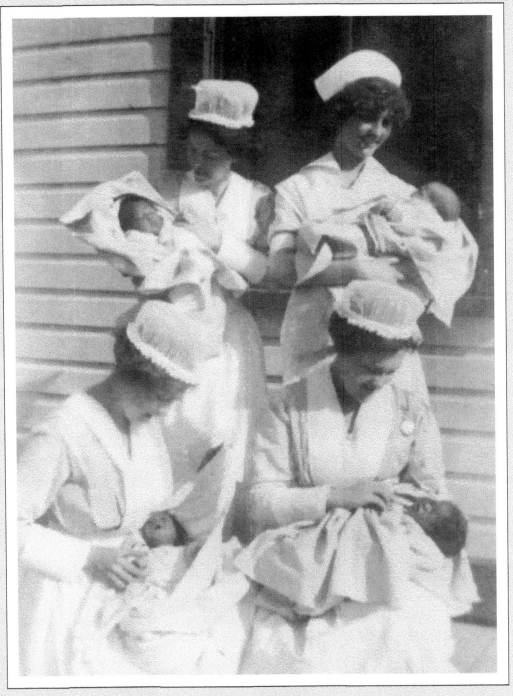

Nurses with babies.

CHAPTER 9

Nurses, Babies, and Public Health

1920s

Arlene W. Keeling

"Whereas, the National Organization for Public Health Nursing, believing that protection of maternity and infancy is of vital importance to the welfare of the country, finds itself in full sympathy with the provisions incorporated in Senate Bill 3259 [Sheppard–Towner Bill], therefore be it resolved: That the National Organization for Public Health Nursing express its approval of this bill. Be it further resolved, that a copy of this resolution be sent to Julia C. Lathrop, Chief of the Federal Children's Bureau . . . under whose auspices the bill was drafted, and also to Honorable Mr. Sheppard of the United States Senate." [1]

Writing in the *American Journal of Nursing* in June 1920, Stella Fuller reported on the events of the nursing convention held that spring. The three national nursing organizations—the American Nurses Association, the National Organization of Public Health Nurses, and the National League for Nursing Education—had met in Atlanta to consider their agenda for the future. In particular, Fuller noted that public health nurses supported the Sheppard–Towner legislation being proposed to Congress. Its purpose was to promote the "welfare and hygiene of maternity and infancy." [2]

For decades, maternal and infant mortality in the United States had been higher than that of other developed countries, including England and Denmark. [3] Finally, the issue was coming to the forefront of the nation's concern, and nurses, long interested in promoting maternal and infant health, were eager to endorse legislation that addressed it. As Harriet Leete, director of Field Work for the American Child Hygiene Association, wrote just 2 years later: "This twentieth century does belong to the child, and unless we as nurses—not just public health nurses, but *all* nurses—meet this challenge . . . we shall be liable to the reproach of those who follow us."[4]

Nurses were not alone in their concern for promoting the health of mothers and infants. The poor health status of many army recruits in World War I brought attention to the fact that something needed to be done to prepare a healthier nation. Even Congress was interested in ensuring that each generation had a healthy cohort of men able to serve the country in the future.

By 1921, members of both the House and the Senate were well aware that women had just received the vote and were now a group they had to appease. In fact, as the *Ladies' Home Journal* reported it: "If the members [of Congress] could have voted secretly in their cloak rooms," the bill "would have been killed as emphatically as it was passed in the open under the pressure of the Joint Congressional Committee of Women."[6]

However, since the men of Congress were in fact eager to please the new constituency of women, Congress passed the Sheppard–Towner Act in October 1921 by an overwhelming majority (House 279 to 39; Senate 63 to 7). President Warren G. Harding signed the act into law in November.[7] A separate division of the Children's Bureau, the "Division of Maternity and Infancy," would administer Sheppard–Towner funds from its headquarters in Washington, DC.

Although many pediatricians supported the bill, both anti-suffragists and the American Medical Association opposed it. Anti-suffragists denounced it as a "feminist plot," while the American Medical Association feared government control of medical practice. Once enacted, however, the Sheppard–Towner legislation had a major impact on public health nurses' work over the next 9 years.[8] The law allocated $1,240,000 annually for both maternal and child hygiene, granting $5,000 to states outright and then on a matching basis. States used the money for various projects, including "conferences" [clinics] in which physicians and nurses examined pregnant women and children, health promotion demonstrations, and the production of printed materials containing information about maternal and child health care.[9]

THE PROBLEM OF MATERNAL/INFANT MORTALITY

The enactment of the Sheppard–Towner bill was timely; the problem of maternal and infant mortality was not going away on its own. During the opening decades of the 20th century, concern for safe deliveries and the public's growing acceptance of hospitals had already led many upper- and middle-class urban White women to turn to delivery of their babies in a hospital under the care of obstetricians[10] rather than at home. In contrast, poor urban European immigrants, like those on the Lower East Side of New York City, continued to use lay midwives to deliver their babies at home, while others turned to general practitioners with little experience in obstetrics. Meanwhile, in rural areas of Mississippi, Alabama, and North Carolina, a significant portion of the population was Black and infant mortality was twice that for Whites. In these southern states, women turned to African American "granny midwives" to deliver their babies.[11] Similarly, in remote mountainous areas like Leslie County, Kentucky, poor White women relied on untrained and illiterate White granny midwives to attend their babies' births. Now, the availability of Sheppard–Towner funds would support nurses' and physicians' efforts to provide for *all* American women to have access to safe maternity care. Throughout the country, state boards of health soon

"It may seem like a cold-blooded thing to say, but . . . the world war was a backhanded break for children."[5]

Josephine Baker, 1919

The Sheppard–Towner Act, 1921

The Sheppard–Towner Act authorized more than $1 million in federal funds for maternal and infant health. It would have a major impact on maternal and child health care in the 1920s.

Library of Congress

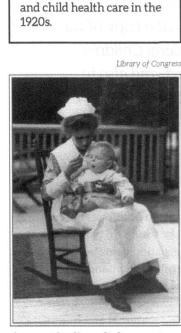

A nurse feeding a baby.

developed plans to provide care for women in every region; public health nurses would be the central players.

Margaret Sanger and Birth Control

Long before the passage of the Sheppard–Towner Act, nurses were aware of the critical problem of maternal and infant mortality. In fact, trained nurses in urban areas had been caring for mothers and their newborns through the services of visiting nurse associations, parish nurses, and missions since the late 19th century. They had seen for themselves the need for basic instruction on prenatal care, the exhaustion mothers suffered after multiple unwanted or unplanned pregnancies, and the reality of infants dying in their first years of life. Some nurses, aware that women had little if any control of their pregnancies, wanted to address that issue.

Margaret Higgins Sanger, a mother and nurse, frequently accepted maternity cases in New York City in 1912. On her calls she came face to face with women's problems on a daily basis. In July of that year, a physician asked Sanger to visit Sadie Sachs, a young mother who was deathly ill from a self-induced abortion. With the physician's direction and under Sanger's care for 3 weeks, the woman survived. When Sanger was about to leave for the last time, Sachs asked her for help to prevent another pregnancy. Not knowing the answer, Sanger left the home. Just 3 months later, Sanger again was directed to care for Sadie Sachs, but this time she watched helplessly as Sadie died from yet another pregnancy. For Sanger the incident was a turning point; she resolved to help women plan their pregnancies.[12] As she noted later: "Pregnancy was a chronic condition" for women—especially for the very poor, many of whom lived in the tenement district.[13]

Sanger had witnessed many women suffering from poverty and the problems of having too many unwanted pregnancies, especially when she worked in the immigrant neighborhoods on the Lower East Side. The women were desperate for information about spacing their pregnancies. Sanger recalled what happened when she went to visit one mother:

> As soon as the neighbors learned that a nurse was in the building they came in a friendly way to visit, often carrying fruit, jellies or "gëfullter fish" made after a cherished recipe. . . . Always back of the gift was the question. . . . "Tell me something to keep from having another baby."[15]

Other evidence of the problem was all too apparent. On Saturday nights, Sanger frequently saw "from 50–100 women with their shawls over their heads waiting outside the office of a $5.00 abortionist." Realizing someone had to give voice to these women, Sanger read the existing literature on birth control and traveled to Europe to learn more. She then conceived the idea of a magazine to be called *The Woman Rebel*, "dedicated to the interests of the working woman."[16]

However, Sanger's plan was short-lived. The distribution of the magazine was in direct violation of the 1873 Comstock Act, which considered any information about contraception "obscene." Arrested for distributing "lewd" information and "unprepared to defend herself," Sanger fled to Canada and later to England where she investigated various means of birth control.[17] Returning to the United States in 1916, she and her sister opened a birth control clinic in a predominantly Jewish neighborhood at 46 Amboy Street,

Margaret Sanger, birth control advocate.

"I knew something must be done to rescue these women."[14]

Margaret Sanger, 1938

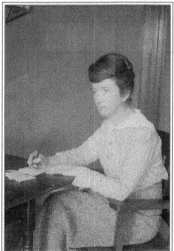

Margaret Sanger.

"46 Amboy Street... All Mothers Welcome"

On October 16, 1916, Margaret Sanger opened a birth control clinic in Brownsville, Brooklyn. For 10 cents, clients received instructions on the use of contraceptive devices and a free copy of *What Every Girl Should Know*, a pamphlet discussing female growth and development, sexuality, and reproduction. In violation of the Comstock Act of 1873, Sanger was arrested and the clinic shut down on October 26.

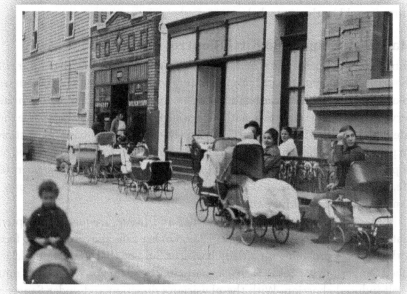

The street outside Margaret Sanger's birth control clinic in Brownsville, Brooklyn.

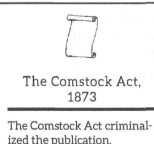

The Comstock Act, 1873

The Comstock Act criminalized the publication, distribution, or possession of any information about unlawful abortion or contraception. It was named for Anthony Comstock, a zealous crusader who was against what he considered to be obscene.

Brooklyn. It was the first birth control clinic in the nation. To Sanger, prevention of an unwanted pregnancy seemed to be the perfect solution to a complicated problem; the 100 women who lined up at the clinic on the first day agreed.

Within 2 weeks of the clinic's opening, Sanger was arrested a second time. Several weeks after her arrest, Sanger appeared in a crowded courtroom and faced a judge who sentenced her to 30 days in a workhouse. After serving her time, Sanger resumed her crusade for women's health, serving as president of the American Birth Control League until 1928.[18] For her, the answer to the problem of too many unwanted pregnancies was "knowledge and health care" for *all* women, not just the fortunate few who could obtain information from their private physicians.[19]

IMPACT OF THE SHEPPARD–TOWNER ACT

The passage of the Sheppard–Towner Act would affect nursing throughout the country. For some organizations, it would provide funding to offset costs they had already incurred as they had tried to implement measures to decrease maternal/infant mortality earlier in the century. For others, it would mean the expansion of care to citizens in rural areas of the country, particularly in the southeast and southwest, but also in remote regions like Alaska. One of the first to be affected was the Maternity Center Association, an organization whose roots were established even before the Sheppard–Towner Act took effect.

Maternity Center Association

Approaching the issue of pregnancy from the perspective of promoting the health of the mother and baby regardless of whether the pregnancy was wanted, a group of obstetricians, social reformers, and public health nurses established the Maternity Center Association in New York City. They did so in 1918, just a few years before Congress passed the Sheppard–Towner legislation. The Association's major goal was to ensure that every pregnant woman saw a physician during her pregnancy. To achieve that goal, the Association offered "complete maternity care to poor women in a small demonstration area of Manhattan." They divided the city into 10 zones, each with a nurse who would attempt to reach every pregnant woman. Philanthropic groups, including among others, the New York Milk Committee and the Women's City Club, funded the nurses.[20]

The first major hurdle the nurses had to overcome was gaining the women's trust in the nurses' expertise and in "American ways" of care. They tried to establish trust by providing free classes on childbirth and the care of the newborn, and giving demonstrations on how to prepare safe infant formula. The nurses also made "friendly visits" to women's homes during their pregnancies, following the instructions of a manual:

> *The nurses may find it necessary to make many friendly visits before even mentioning a doctor's examination or any real nursing care. She may find inviting the patient to see the demonstration at the Center, or to come in and get help making baby clothes, the best way to gain her confidence.*[21]

The work was challenging. Nurses had to deal with immigrant women who held longstanding and often inaccurate beliefs about pregnancy and childbirth, and had cultural preferences about the care of the newborn. Some new mothers, for example, would not open a window near the baby's crib; others refused to bathe the infant with soap and water. The nurses, working in the context of Western medicine and with a goal of assimilating immigrants into American culture, attempted to convert young mothers to modern childcare methods. At the same time, some nurses supported cultural differences, allowing immigrant mothers to use childcare traditions advocated by their mothers and grandmothers. Sometimes they allowed the mother to clean a newborn's skin with olive oil instead of washing with soap and water, or to use lard for the baby's first bath. In all cases, however, nurses promoted the airing of the room in which the baby slept, serving as the messenger for the advice of American physicians.[24]

At first nurses who worked for the Maternity Center Association visited women on the "margins of New York City area." But in 1922, the Association expanded its reach "to include middle-class women" throughout the city by developing pamphlets and other educational materials on pregnancy and childbirth.[26] Educational material hung in the Maternity Association's clinic on West 34th Street provided instructions for prenatal care. Exhibit 4, "Advice for Mothers," stated:

Diet: Eat the food you are used to. Do not eat what you know gives you indigestion . . . Drink eight glasses of water every day. Drink all the milk you can . . . Do NOT drink any beer, whiskey, wine, or other alcohol. These hurt the kidneys and thus may poison the baby.

Sleep: At least eight hours every night with windows open.

Exercise: Do your regular housework, but lie down several times a day if only for five minutes. If possible take a walk out of doors.

Constipation: . . . drink a cup of coffee before breakfast . . . During the day eat stewed fruit . . . all the water you can . . . and four to six prunes.

Telephone the Maternity Center if you need a nurse.[27]

By 1926, the Maternity Center Association expanded to reach upper-class, private patients as well. The goal of the Association was to have a physician, preferably an obstetrician and not a general practitioner, attend *each and*

"We learned . . . that finding mothers and teaching them the need for care during pregnancy was no easy task."[22]

Hazel Corbin, 1928 Report

Advertising the Maternity Center Association

"We tried everything— Posters on large billboards giving locations of the Center. . . . Small posters in shop windows . . . smaller cards in mailboxes . . . [and] newspaper stories."[23]

Hazel Corbin, 1928

Airing the American Baby

"The nursery should be aired at least twice a day—in the morning after the child's bath, and again in the evening before the child is put to bed for the night. Airing may begin with a healthy child, even in cold weather, when he is one month old, at first for only 15 to 20 minutes at a time."[25]

Dr. L. Emmett Holt, 1920

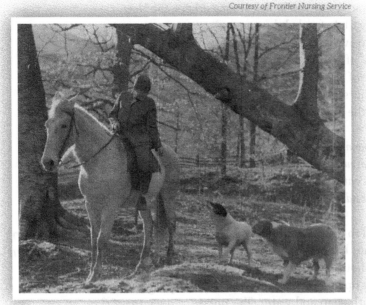

Mary Breckinridge, founder of the Kentucky Committee for Mothers and Babies that provided midwives for rural populations.

every birth.[28] To overcome "American prudishness" about any discussion of the delicate topic of pregnancy, the Association launched several innovative public relations campaigns in the 1920s and 1930s "making full use of modern advertising methods." Among these efforts was the "16,000 White Carnations" campaign, with each flower standing for one of the 16,000 American women who died annually due to inadequate prenatal care. The campaign, launched on Mother's Day, generated a great deal of publicity for the cause of safe maternity care.[29]

Realizing that safe maternity care was dependent on having properly trained nurse-midwives at deliveries, the Maternity Center Association opened an educational program in 1931, called the Lobenstine Clinic and Midwifery School. It was the first school for nurse-midwives in the United States. Two of its graduates, Sisters M. Helen and M. Theophane, later opened the Catholic Maternity Institute in Santa Fe, New Mexico, in 1944.

The Frontier Nursing Service

In remote areas of the country, connecting pregnant women with physicians was even more complicated than in large cities like New York. Leslie County, one of the poorest counties in the Appalachian Mountains of Eastern Kentucky, presented various challenges for accessing care. In the remote region, the external conditions—particularly the shortage of physicians, the lack of telephone service, the mountainous terrain, and few roads—made access to medical care a challenge. Leslie County, for example, had only five state-registered physicians who could see patients. According to one report:

> *In most instances, there is no telephone service available, someone must ride the entire distance, varying from 4 to 20 miles, to summon the doctor, who usually lives in some small village or town where he maintains a practice. It is often impossible for him to leave his patients for the length of time necessary to make a trip into the mountains. . . . In winter, when snow covers the ground and the creek beds are frozen, it is difficult if not impossible for the mountaineer to go for the doctor and equally out of the question for the doctor to come to the patient.*[30]

The extreme poverty of the citizens of Leslie County only compounded the problem of access to physicians for prenatal care and delivery. A family's average income was $183.53 a year, hardly enough for food and housing, and not nearly enough to pay a physician who charged "$1.00 per mile for every mile spent in travel to the case, as well as an additional basic charge of $5.00."[31] Given these circumstances, most mountain women relied on untrained granny midwives to attend their births.[32] However, the midwives' care centered only on the birth itself and did not include care during the pregnancy or follow-up care for the mother and newborn after delivery.

Mindful of these problems and eager to apply for Sheppard–Towner funds, the Kentucky State Board of Health not only formed the Bureau of Maternal and Child Health in 1922 but also mandated that the Bureau protect

"The granny woman just came and done what she could—and she hardly ever come back."[33]

Della Gay, 1923

and promote the health of mothers and children in the state. Their work soon coincided with a program of privately funded nursing services started by Mary Breckinridge. Breckinridge, an upper-class woman who had both family and political connections in Kentucky, had lost her two small children to disease and was determined to save other families from a similar fate. She chose the familiar territory of Leslie County, Kentucky, to achieve her goal. Her decision to set up a nursing service in the remote mountainous area was based in part on her awareness that rural children were often worse off than those in cities.

During the summer of 1923, Breckinridge rode through the mountains of Eastern Kentucky to survey the existing state of midwifery there. Her findings supported what she already knew to be true: most women used granny midwives to deliver them and the area needed professional nurse-midwives. Knowing that the British prototype of *nurse-midwives* might be an effective program to replicate in the United States, Breckinridge first traveled to England and Scotland to see how district nursing was implemented. She also trained as a midwife herself. Breckinridge then returned to Kentucky, and in 1925 formed the Kentucky Committee for Mothers and Babies, introduced the idea of a nurse-midwifery service in Leslie County, and gained the support of local physicians.[35]

Working closely with local doctors, Breckinridge arranged for a medical committee in Lexington to write standing orders—*Medical Routines*—for the nurses to follow in the absence of a physician. She also agreed to pay half the salary for the county health officer to serve as "general consultant" to the nurses and treat any patients admitted to the small hospital in Hyden, only a few miles from her headquarters at Wendover.[37]

In May 1925, members of the Kentucky Committee for Mothers and Babies met and approved Breckinridge's plan. By September, Breckinridge had hired two nurses and opened a clinic in her log cabin headquarters. In that first month, she and two other nurses saw 233 patients in the clinic and visited 46 homes.

Originally, Breckinridge staffed the service with British nurse-midwives. Later she added American public health nurses whom she had sent to England for midwifery training.[38] Initially, these few nurse-midwives worked out of Wendover, traveling by horseback

> "While much has been done for city children, remotely rural children have been neglected."[34]
>
> Mary Breckinridge

> "Midwives are essential here. I wish they might be nurses as well."[36]
>
> Kentucky Physician, 1924

Courtesy of Frontier Nursing Service

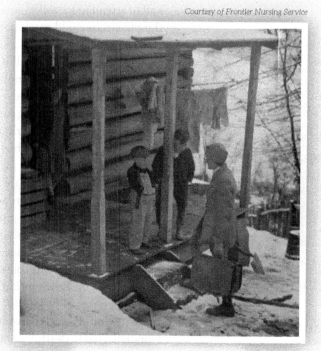

A Frontier nurse visiting her patients.

"Catching Babies"

> "The whole of the district work . . . is done with the aid of two pairs of saddlebags . . . In these we have everything needed for a home delivery . . . In one of the pockets we carry our Medical Routines."[39]
>
> Frontier Nurse Vanda Summers, 1938

Red Bird Clinic

"The center at Red Bird is perfectly exquisite—a log building with a big veranda, a living room with an open stone fire, two bedrooms . . . a large waiting room. . . . The barn has stalls for visiting horses . . . a feed room screened against rats. . . . The whole property is the gift of Mrs. Henry Ford."[43]

Mary Breckinridge, 1929

along creek beds and mountain trails to the remote cabins where their patients lived. They attended births and cared for the sick, using supplies and medicines that they carried in their saddlebags.

Gradually, more nurses joined the staff and Breckinridge added more clinics, spaced throughout the county, to decrease the nurses' travel time to and from remote areas. All of the clinics were funded with private donations raised by Breckinridge herself on her extensive lecture tours. By 1929, the Frontier Nursing Service had six clinics in which the nurses both lived and worked.[40] Operating out of these decentralized locations, the Frontier nurses covered a total of approximately 700 square miles and delivered care to nearly 10,000 people.[41]

While mothers and babies were their primary concern, the Frontier nurses soon realized that they had to address the health needs of the entire community. Thus, nurses who were not midwives soon joined the service. One of their first priorities was to administer hundreds of typhoid and diphtheria inoculations. Both diseases were prevalent in the Kentucky mountains, and the Frontier nurses traveled the territory to "inoculate the whole creek," riding horseback nearly an entire day to visit everyone.[44] At other times, they held vaccination days in one or more of the clinics, immunizing hundreds of citizens in a day.

Besides preventing or treating typhoid and diphtheria, Frontier nurses treated patients for a host of other diseases and injuries that occurred in the mountain community. Without adequate nutrition and housing, and without electricity and sanitation, people suffered from vitamin deficiencies, colds, and dysentery, along with infectious diseases such as measles, scarlet fever, whooping cough, tuberculosis, influenza, and pneumonia. Barefoot children contracted hookworm; pregnant women had anemia and hypertension. Accidents and injuries were commonplace among men in the coal-mining or lumber industries; family feuds left others with gunshot wounds.

Given the setting and the physician shortage, Frontier nurses often cared for their patients on their own, relying only on the written *Medical Routines* to guide them.[45]

Sometimes, the Frontier nurse-midwife had to attend to a medical situation *until* the physician could reach her; at other times, she might have to assume complete responsibility for a life, knowing that the physician could not reach her in time to help. This was especially true when the nurse was caring for a woman with postpartum hemorrhage, a life-threatening situation in which a woman began to bleed before the placenta was delivered. In this situation, the nurse had to respond quickly and in accordance with her training and the guidelines in the *Medical Routines*. "Slipping on a fresh glove," the nurse would have to insert her hand into the uterus to remove the placenta. Following that intervention with doses of Ergotrate, the nurse-midwife could save the mother from hemorrhaging to death.[46] At other times,

Courtesy of Frontier Nursing Service

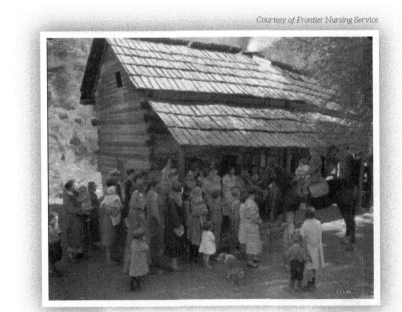

A crowd of rural patients gathering in front of a Frontier nurse clinic on Clinic Day.

the Frontier nurses performed external rotations of babies in the womb, administered sedation and anesthesia to the mothers, and performed other life-saving measures.[47]

Working to the limits of their knowledge, authority, intuition, and skills, Frontier nurse-midwives provided safe care for thousands of citizens in Leslie County during the 1920s and 1930s. In their first 1,000 deliveries, the Frontier nurses had only two maternal deaths, both caused by chronic heart conditions. In the second 1,000 deliveries, they had no maternal death from any cause.[48] The nurses' impact went beyond a decrease in maternal and infant mortality, however. By 1934, the Frontier nurses were caring for "1,146 families, including 256 babies, 1,139 preschool children, and 2,243 school-aged children," as they provided primary and preventive services to the entire mountain community.[49]

Nurses and Black Midwives in the Southeast

While Mary Breckinridge was addressing the lay-midwife problem with the development of a privately funded nurse-midwife service, other states took a different approach. They focused on educating the lay-midwives already in practice instead of replacing them. In Mississippi, White public health nurse Laurie Reid traveled through the state in 1921 "tracking down the names of midwives and registering the women county by county." Discovering more than 4,000 midwives in the state, she concluded that the high maternal–infant mortality in Mississippi was most likely due to "poor health care for pregnant women from 'careless physicians' and illiterate, ignorant midwives."[50] Indeed, during the 1920s in the state of Mississippi, "half the population was black" and the "vast majority of midwives were black women." Lay-midwives delivered 80% of African American babies and 8% of the White babies.[51]

Given the shortage of physicians and the absence of trained nurse-midwives in Mississippi, the plan to target the education of lay-midwives was a logical solution. Over the decade of the 1920s, the Mississippi Board of Health hired 125 White and six Black public health nurses to train the lay-midwives. The nurses instructed the midwives to wash their hands, deliver women in bed rather than on the floor, maintain clean delivery bags and equipment, and wear clean white gowns when they assisted in childbirth. They also required the midwives to attend monthly club meetings in which they heard lectures on the "proper" care of pregnant women, the baby, and their equipment. Sometimes, the midwives received the instruction readily; at other times, they balked at the nurses' interference, especially if the nurse suspended a midwife's license for an infraction of the rules.

One reason for suspending a midwife's license was for her breaking the rule that forbade her conducting an internal examination on a woman during childbirth. Another was for the midwife testing positive for syphilis, or refusing to be vaccinated for typhoid and smallpox.

Most public health nurses in Mississippi worked closely with the midwives rather than against them, realizing that "midwives were assets" to their community work, rather than detriments to the health of mothers and babies. In fact, the nurses relied on the midwives to connect them to the community. Lay-midwives provided health instruction to adults and children through churches and schools, encouraged people to be vaccinated, and worked on various health promotion activities, including the "annual May Day child health program."[53] As historian Susan Smith has argued: In southern rural areas in the early 20th century, "black midwives were important health workers beyond their midwifery role . . . [proving] to be a vital link between poor African Americans and health departments."[54]

Like state officials in Mississippi, public health leaders in other southern states used Sheppard–Towner funds to help mothers and babies. As early as 1917, the North Carolina Bureau of Infant Hygiene had been advocating for women to see their physicians early in their pregnancies and to breastfeed their infants to save them from "diarrheal diseases."

When Sheppard–Towner monies became available to support their ongoing efforts, North Carolina reorganized the Bureau of Infant Hygiene into the Bureau of Maternity and Infancy in 1922 to better align with the funding opportunity. That bureau began a program using public health nurses to educate and supervise the "approximately 5,000 midwives in active practice" in the state. As was true in Mississippi, the North Carolina legislature passed "Model County Midwife Regulations" requiring that lay-midwives "have a physical examination and instruction and demonstrations given by doctors and nurses in the procedures of a normal delivery." Over the course of the 1920s, public health nurses conducted midwife classes in 30 counties throughout North Carolina.[56]

White nurses frequently taught and supervised African American midwives. However, in the racially segregated South, Black nurses were occasionally hired to teach Black midwives. In Alabama, where officials were particularly concerned about maternal and infant mortality among African Americans, the state paid for Eunice Rivers, a graduate of Tuskegee Institute, to join a three-member team of Macon County's "Movable School." Traveling the state with a carpenter and a teacher in 1923, Rivers had wide-ranging responsibilities to teach families how to improve their homes and health. For Rivers, that meant teaching them the "rudiments of home nursing, including training lay-midwives how to safely deliver a baby, how to wash their hands and cut their fingernails, and how to prepare a bed for delivery."[57]

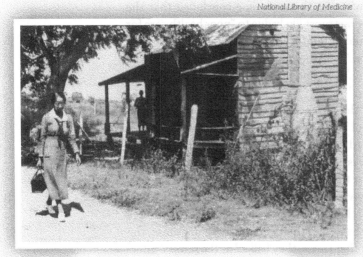

National Library of Medicine

A Black public health nurse making home visits.

"We had an awful time trying to train the mothers to use the bed instead of the floor [for delivery]."[58]

Eunice Rivers, 1923

Nurses in other southern states also benefited from Sheppard–Towner funds. In Florida, larger problems, including the eradication of mosquitoes, the destruction caused by hurricanes, and the prevalence of hookworm, vied for public health officials' attention. With state funds allocated for these other projects, the federal Sheppard–Towner funds were essential for promoting the health of women and children. In the 1920s, Ruth E. Mettinger became one of the first Sheppard–Towner nurses to assist with child welfare. In 1924, the funding allowed nurses to make 4,033 prenatal visits to Black women and 2,406 visits to White women.[59] Later, Rosa Brown, an African American nurse, joined the crusade for child health, covering approximately 2,500 square miles in Palm Beach County by "adapting her work to fit the community."[60]

In Georgia, where public health nursing was "small, underdeveloped, and underfunded" and the state had "a long tradition of refusing to acknowledge . . . maternal morbidity," Sheppard–Towner monies provided a critical infusion of support to public health.[62] In 1925, the State Board of Health hired 18 "itinerant nurses," assigning them the responsibility to supervise 5,000 midwives across the state.[63]

A Red Cross Nurse in Alaska

While many of the lower 48 states used Sheppard–Towner funds to employ public health nurses, the territory of Alaska relied on the Red Cross nurses for help. On October 1, 1922, Stella Fuller was appointed as a Red Cross nurse to the islands off Alaska, where living conditions were "appalling" and health conditions among the natives "deplorable," due to the absence of doctors, dentists, clinics, and dispensaries. In Unalaska, Fuller worked on her own, acting as nurse, midwife, physician, and health educator. One day she "attended one woman in childbirth, took care of mother and baby, sterilized and demonstrated the arrangement of the delivery room in the homes of three prenatal cases . . . called on a chronic case, and answered one emergency request."[64] It would be years before medical services in the remote northern territory would change for the better.

Public Health Nurses in the West and Southwest

During the 1920s, some states utilized "Home Hygiene" nurses from the American Red Cross program to provide instruction to lay women in rural areas. The program, started as a "tangible memorial" to Red Cross leader Jane A. Delano after her death, honored Delano's vision for the Town and Country Nursing Service to "offer all women and girls fifteen lessons in Home Hygiene and Care of the Sick."[65]

Camilla Wills, who had returned from France in 1919 after her work with Base Hospital No. 41 in World War I, was one of the nurses who responded to the call for instructors. An active member of the National Organization of Public Health Nurses in 1920, Wills participated in the Home Hygiene and Care of the Sick program for the Bureau of Public Health in Clovis, New Mexico. Working in that program from 1920 to 1922, she taught home nursing courses. Later Wills did the same in Las Vegas, Nevada, followed by a stint on the staff of the Cragmore Sanatorium in Colorado Springs, Colorado. To reach patients and her students, Wills drove across the desert in her car, which she affectionately called "Elizabeth."[66]

In Montana, the State Board of Health hired four field nurses in an attempt to decrease maternal and infant mortality. In 1925, nurse Henrietta Crocket conducted an infant health clinic on a Montana Indian reservation, engaging tribal members in her public health campaign. That year, public health nurse Margaret Thomas traveled throughout western Montana "organizing well-baby clinics, [and] lecturing on nutrition and the care of the sick."[67]

Nurses and the Indian Health Service

In addition to funding from the Sheppard–Towner Act and the American Red Cross, the 1921 Snyder Act supported the employment of public health nurses. Specifically, the Snyder Act funded nurses who would work "for

Bjoring Center for Nursing Historical Inquiry

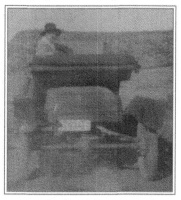

Camilla (Katie) Louise Wills in "Elizabeth," which she used to visit her patients isolated by desert.

Bjoring Center for Nursing Historical Inquiry

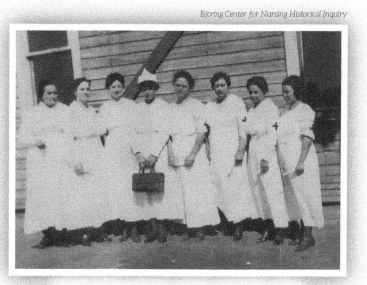

Wills's first Home Hygiene and Care of the Sick nursing class for the Red Cross.

"I didn't have a horse or a wagon back then . . . so I had to make my calls on foot."[70]

Lula Owl Gloyne, 1920s

the benefit, care and assistance" of Indian tribes. Using these funds, North Carolina hired Lula Owl Gloyne, a Cherokee Indian of the North Carolina Eastern Cherokee Band, to work among her people. After obtaining her degree in 1916 from Pennsylvania's Chestnut Hill Hospital School of Nursing, Lula Owl had married and worked as a missionary school nurse on the Standing Rock Sioux Reservation in South Dakota. In 1921, the couple returned to North Carolina, where Mrs. Gloyne assisted a physician in a small clinic on the Cherokee reservation.

Sometimes she left the clinic and traveled to isolated areas of the reservation to reach her patients. Far from the clinic and a doctor, she worked on her own, relying on her training and experience to direct the care she provided. Recalling those days, Gloyne said: "I got caught in places [too far from the clinic] where I'd just have to do what had to be done. Men got cut up and I'd have to sew them up. Women would call on me to deliver their babies . . . there was no one else."[69]

As a Native American Indian herself, Lula Owl Gloyne was an exception to the stereotypical public health nurse who worked for the Bureau of Indian Affairs (later called the Indian Health Service) during the 1920s and 1930s. The majority of nurses who accepted jobs in the government's experimental program on Indian reservations were middle-class White women, in part because they reflected the general population of nurses in the United States at the time, but also because the Bureau discriminated against nurses of color. Some of these White nurses sought adventure and travel after returning from World War I; others wanted freedom from the constraints of hospital nursing they had known as students.[71] The majority were single women, free of family responsibilities. Most were middle class, as they all had to have sufficient funds to pay for their own uniforms and to travel by train, sometimes across the entire country, to reach distant Indian reservations.

As was true of nurses supported by the Sheppard–Towner Act, as well as those who worked for the American Red Cross, nurses who worked for the Bureau of Indian Affairs were hired to promote the health of the communities in which they worked. In particular, they focused on the health of women and children. They were also expected to assist physicians in specialty clinics. The nurses who worked with the Navajo held clinics to treat tuberculosis and trachoma, two diseases most prevalent on the reservation. Other responsibilities included participating in the prevention of disease by administering vaccines and educating the Indians about diet and sanitation. The nurses' work often exceeded the areas of health promotion and disease prevention, however. Since most reservations were short of physicians, nurses were frequently on their own to treat patients.

Public health nurse Elizabeth Forster, who first joined the Bureau of Indian Affairs in 1924, was assigned to the Navajo Reservation in the Four Corners region, where Colorado, New Mexico, Utah, and Arizona meet. The isolated reservation, sparsely dotted with buttes and rocks, pinon trees, and

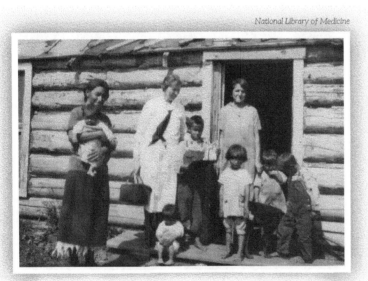

National Library of Medicine

A nurse visiting a family on the White Earth Indian Reservation.

desert grasses, was home to more than 100,000 nomadic sheep-herding Navajo who had been forced to settle the region in the late 19th century.

The initiative to provide civilian medical services to the Indians had begun in 1849 when the government transferred the oversight of the Bureau of Indian Affairs from the War Department to the Department of the Interior. The government's transfer of services was intended to show a desire to create a less hostile environment for working with Native Americans. The initiative, however, had been under-resourced. The reality was that there was little funding, few physicians to do the work, and no nurses available until the 1890s, when the Bureau hired several nurses to work in Indian boarding schools.[73] In fact, it was not until 1911 that Congress allocated $40,000 for general health services to Indians, the first significant funding it had ever provided.

Finally, in 1913, Congress ordered a survey to identify the Indians' health care problems. According to their findings, the most pressing need was for better sanitation. The report also recommended that more hospitals and better qualified and better paid physicians be provided, and field nurses (registered nurses with public health training) be hired to provide care for patients outside the hospitals. The major emphasis, however, was on preventing trachoma and tuberculosis from spreading to White Americans.[74] Despite the report's recommendations, the Bureau continued to hire minimally qualified field matrons rather than public health nurses to care for patients in the community.

Finally, in 1922, the use of matrons was challenged after the American Red Cross conducted a survey of health needs on the reservations. Based on the survey results, the Red Cross recommended "the immediate establishment of an organized public health nursing service as part of the Indian health program."[75] As a result, three trained Red Cross nurses were assigned to be visiting nurses on the Navajo reservation.

Shortly after the Red Cross survey, a prestigious staff of scientists and physicians, under the leadership of Lewis Meriam, investigated the reservations. In 1928, they published the results in *The Problem of Indian Administration*, soon widely known as the *Meriam Report*. The report recommended a plan "to replace field matrons with public health nurses as rapidly as possible."[76] The plan was implemented. Between 1924 and 1934, the number of field nurses working on reservations grew from three to 98. Among them was a young nurse, Elizabeth Forster.

Upon arriving in Arizona, Forster found herself alone in Red Rock, a small remote trading post, doing the best she could to care for patients who came to her dispensary, some with minor conditions, others seriously ill.

Sometimes, Forster worked from her little clinic, using hot soup and coffee to lure in patients. Other times, she traveled the length and breadth of the reservation to see patients in their homes (hogans).[77] That travel, often up to 2,500 miles a month, had its difficulties. In the monsoon season, unexpected torrential downpours caused flash floods over the "wash" (wide dry riverbeds capable of carrying raging torrents of water).[78] In summer, sandstorms, high winds, and searing heat could make any trip miserable; in winter, snow could block roads for days.[79] Automobiles that broke down and the occasional absence of an Indian guide complicated Forster's ability to get where she needed to be.

Frequently the Indian Health Service nurses worked with doctors in specialty clinics. One clinic was set up to diagnose and treat trachoma, an

"I was forever trying to teach my people that . . . I was there to . . . prevent illness, not to treat it."[72]

Dorothy Loope, circa 1930

A Letter Home

Dear Emily,
A typical day's work in my dispensary:
Man—with trachoma— eyes treated
Baby—diarrhea, diet and treatment outlined to mother
Woman —ear irrigated to remove louse
Child—extensive impetigo . . . Allowed the removal of scabs and the application of ointment without a murmur.
Old man—Chill last night, pain in chest, general aching, headache, and temperature 101. Refuses to be taken to hospital.

Elizabeth Forster, 1932

Travel on the Reservation

"The sun blazes and no tree offers shade, the dust flies in smothering clouds, and yet we dread the coming of the seasonal rains which either cause us to stick in the mud or wait for hours on the bank of a wash while the water goes down."[80]

Elizabeth Forster, 1932

infectious eye disease that affected the conjunctiva and then the cornea. Aggravated by the hot dry climate, as well as the dust and winds of the desert, trachoma caused granular bumps to form on the inside of a patient's eyelids that scratched the cornea, causing excruciating pain. The only treatment available until years later was the daily application of painful eye drops. The discovery in 1937 that sulfa drugs could cure the disease changed the treatment to the simple and painless application of an antibiotic ointment.[81]

The field nurses also worked with the reservation's contract doctors in general clinics. There they treated patients with a wide variety of problems, including colds, ear infections, pneumonia, venereal disease, burns, spider bites, diabetes, meningitis, appendicitis, breast abscesses, or infectious diseases such as whooping cough, measles, chicken pox, and polio.[82]

Working on their own, nurses held "conferences" to instruct the Navajo women about infant and child care, sanitation, nutrition, and the importance of prenatal care. The conferences were held to make baby clothes, give immunizations, weigh and measure babies and children, and check their overall health status.[83] Often, however, these conferences turned into "nurse-run clinics," as the Navajo mothers arrived with sick infants and children. In the clinics, nurses treated babies for conditions such as diaper rash and infantile diarrhea. The field nurses worked as public health nurses, teaching the expectant and new mothers how to sew layettes for their infants, how to bathe their babies with "green soap," how to prevent infantile diarrhea, and how to provide a more nutritious diet for their children.[84] The nurse's teaching often included her recommendation to the mother to supplement the child's diet of "coffee and Navajo bread" with cod liver oil.[85]

The nurses' major goal was to improve health through educational activities. Nonetheless, when the nurses' skills were required and they had no other options, they provided treatment themselves. They treated both babies and children for a wide variety of problems, including colds, sore throats, ear infections, measles, mumps, and impetigo.

The public health nurses who worked for the Indian Health Service were not certified nurse-midwives and were careful to work within their professional boundaries. Rather than delivering infants themselves, the field nurses transported expectant mothers to hospitals. Mollie Reebel reported one case in which she went to extremes to get the patient to the hospital rather than deliver her at home:

One of the most difficult trips I have ever made was in response to a call about two o'clock one afternoon to go out and see a lady reported as having been in labor for three days with no result. The man who came for me had started before daylight on foot and after reaching the highway had caught a ride. I inquired how far the Hogan was, and was assured that it was not very far. Maybe six miles off the highway, and about twelve miles up the highway. . . . With the Indian man as guide, we started out. After we left the highway we went sixteen miles over places where there was not even a wagon road. Found the patient in terrible condition, put her in the car and headed for Ship Rock where we arrived at 7 PM having covered sixty-four miles. The patient was given immediate attention and is now recovering.[88]

Saving Mothers and Babies in the 1920s

By the late 1920s, a majority of states and the territory of Hawaii had nurses involved in health promotion activities for expectant mothers and their

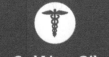

Cod Liver Oil

"Cod Liver Oil Squibb is very rich in those health giving vitamins—A and D. . . One teaspoonful . . . is approximately equal to a pound of the best butter in vitamin value!"[86]

Squibb Advertisement, 1924

Field Nurse's Report

"Five clinics held this week, three general and two baby clinics. Mothers bathed their babies and were given material to cut out and make gowns for baby. Preschool children were weighted, inspected, and mothers advised about diets for underweights [sic]."[87]

Dorothy Williams, 1931

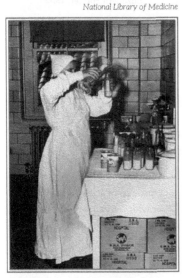

A nurse preparing safe baby formula.

children. According to the Children's Bureau statistics for 1927, nurses in these areas had held at least "21,347 child health conferences and 3,231 pre-natal conferences," resulting in a gradual decrease in maternal and infant mortality.[89] By 1929, 45 states and Hawaii had child health agencies, 33 more than in 1921. Moreover, "during the last four years of the funding alone," public health nurses reached "more than four million infants and children and about 700,000 pregnant women."[90] Overall, according to one research analysis, Sheppard–Towner activities accounted for an 11% to 12% decline in infant mortality over the decade. Not all activities had equal impact, however; interventions based on one-to-one contact between a nurse and a mother proved more beneficial

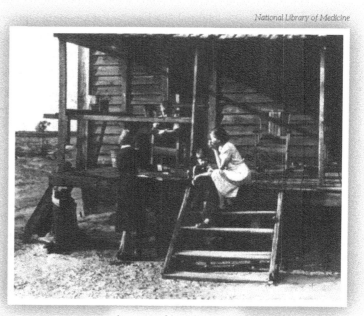

A nurse making a home visit.

than classes and demonstrations. In addition, building clinics and providing public health nurse visits to the home lowered mortality—especially for non-White populations.[91] Key to the nurses' success was their promotion of mothers breastfeeding their infants during the first year of life.

Sheppard–Towner funding came to an end in 1929, the same year that the U.S. stock market crashed. Both events would have an impact on the nursing profession, as unemployed private duty nurses would seek jobs in hospitals, in public health departments, and in numerous other areas. During the 1930s, the decade that would later be labeled "The Great Depression," Congress would pass legislation that established the Civil Works Administration, the Works Progress Administration, and the Social Security Act. Specific to nursing, these acts would provide new opportunities for employment, both inside hospitals and in public health.

"It is now almost universally recognized that breast milk is the best food for infants."[92]

Edna Foley, Public Health Nurse, 1924

For Discussion

1. Discuss the importance of the 1921 Sheppard–Towner Act. What was its impact on nursing and the public?
2. Describe Margaret Sanger's contributions to maternal–child health. What are the ethical issues related to her work?
3. What factors led Mary Breckinridge to establish the Frontier Nursing Service in Leslie County, Kentucky, in 1925?
4. Compare and contrast the work of the Maternity Center Association with that of the Frontier Nursing Service.
5. What issues of the 1920s are still concerns in the United States today?

NOTES

1. Stella Fuller, "The Atlanta Convention," *American Journal of Nursing* (hereafter *AJN*) 20, no. 9 (June 1920): 720–722 (quote 721).
2. Ibid.

3. Editorial, "Lack of Care of American Mothers," *AJN* 26, no. 4 (April 1926): 297–299.

4. Harriet Leete, "The Maternity and Infancy Law and State Nurse Directors," *AJN* 22, no. 6 (March 1922): 453–457 (quote 453).

5. Josephine Baker, *Fighting for Life* (New York: New York Review Books, 1919): 165.

6. Carolyn Mochling and Melissa Thomasson, "'Saving Babies,' the Contribution of Sheppard-Towner to the Decline in Infant Mortality in the 1920s," http://www.colorado.edu (accessed August 12, 2016): 1–24 (quote 7).

7. Ibid., 7.

8. Ibid.

9. Editorial, "Lack of Care," 297.

10. Sylvia Rinker, "To Cultivate a Feeling of Confidence: The Nursing of Obstetric Patients, 1890-1940," *Nursing History Review* (hereafter *NHR*) 8 (2000): 117–142. See also Sylvia Rinker, "The Real Challenge: Lessons from Obstetric Nursing History," *Journal of Obstetric, Gynecologic, and Neonatal Nursing* 29, no. 1 (2000): 100–106.

11. Susan Smith, "White Nurses, Black Midwives, and Public Health," *NHR* 2 (1994): 30–31.

12. Joan Lynaugh, "The Death of Sadie Sachs," *Nursing Research* 40, no. 2 (March–April 1991): 124–125.

13. Margaret Sanger, *Margaret Sanger: An Autobiography* (New York: W. W. Norton, 1938): 88.

14. Ibid., 106.

15. Ibid., 87.

16. Ibid., 88–106 (quote 106).

17. Lynaugh, "The Death of Sadie Sachs," 124.

18. Sanger, *Margaret Sanger.*

19. Lynaugh, "The Death of Sadie Sachs," 125.

20. Laura Ettinger, "Nurse-Midwives, the Mass Media and the Politics of Maternal Health Care in the United States, 1925-1955," *NHR* 7 (1999): 47–66 (quote 55).

21. Anne Steven, "The Work of the Maternity Center Association," November 1919, womhist .alexanderstreet.com (accessed July 26, 2016).

22. Ettinger, "Nurse-Midwives," 56.

23. Ibid.

24. Barbara Brodie, "Snippets from the Past," *Windows in Time: The Newsletter of the Eleanor C. Bjoring Center for Nursing Historical Inquiry,* University of Virginia 24, no. 1 (2016).

25. L. Emmett Holt, *The Care and Feeding of Children: A Catechism for the Use of Mothers and Children's Nurses* (New York: D. Appleton, 1910): 27–30.

26. Ettinger, "Nurse-Midwives," 55.

27. Anne Stevens, "The Work of the Maternity Center Association," reprinted from the *Transactions, 10th Annual Meeting, American Child Hygiene Association,* November 11–13, 1919, Asheville, NC, Women's City Club of New York Papers, Archives and Special Collections, Hunter College, New York, microfilm, reel 20, frames 209–231.

28. Ettinger, "Nurse-Midwives," 55–56.

29. Maternity Center Association Finding Aid, http://library-archives.cumc.columbia.edu (accessed September 11, 2016): 1.

30. Ettinger, "Nurse-Midwives," 55–56.

31. Mary Willeford, *Income and Health in Remote Rural Areas: A Study of 400 Families in Leslie County Kentucky* (New York: Frontier Nursing Service, 1932): 38–39.

32. Laura Ettinger, *Nurse-Midwifery: The Birth of a New American Profession* (Columbus: The Ohio State University Press, 2006): 36.

33. Della Gay, interview by Dale Deaton, September 8, 1978, interview #79OH19, transcript p. 8 and 15, Frontier Nursing Service Collection, University of Kentucky, Special Collections

(FNSC, UK-SC). Della Gay, a young woman in the 1920s, described the work of granny women.

34. Mary Breckinridge, *Wide Neighborhoods* (Lexington: University Press of Kentucky, 1952): 111.

35. Carol Crowe-Carraco, "Mary Breckinridge and the Frontier Nursing Service," *Register of the Kentucky Historical Society* 76, no. 3 (July 1978): 181.

36. Breckinridge, *Wide Neighborhoods,* 229.

37. Edwin Harper, "Then and Now," *FNS Quarterly Bulletin* 64, no. 3 (1969): 6.

38. Anne Cockerham, "Mary Breckinridge and the Frontier Nursing Service: Saddlebags and Swinging Bridges," ch. 6 in *Nursing Rural America,* eds. John Kirchgessner and Arlene Keeling (New York: Springer Publishing, 2015): 83–102.

39. Vanda Summers, "Saddlebag and Log Cabin Technic," *AJN* 38, no. 11 (1938): 1183–1184 (quote 1184).

40. Cockerham, "Mary Breckinridge."

41. Breckinridge, *Wide Neighborhoods,* 228.

42. Ibid.

43. "Rounds," *Quarterly Bulletin* 5, no. 2 (September 1929): 5–6, cited in Cockerham, "Mary Breckinridge."

44. Breckinridge, *Wide Neighborhoods,* 190.

45. Arlene W. Keeling, "Providing Care in the Hoot Owl Hollers," ch. 3 in *Nursing and the Privilege of Prescription, 1893-2000* (Columbus: The Ohio State University Press, 2007).

46. Breckinridge, *Wide Neighborhoods,* 308.

47. Donna Schminkey and Arlene Keeling, "Frontier Nurse-Midwives and Antepartum Emergencies, 1925 to 1939," *Journal of Midwifery and Women's Health* 60, no. 1 (2015): 48–55.

48. Keeling, "Providing Care," 67.

49. Ibid., 68.

50. Smith, "White Nurses, Black Midwives," 32.

51. Ibid., 30–31.

52. Mary Osborne, quoting a nurse in Washington County (Report, May 1924), cited in Smith, "White Nurses, Black Midwives," 36.

53. Smith, "White Nurses, Black Midwives," 37.

54. Ibid., 29.

55. North Carolina Bureau of Infant Hygiene, *Biennial Report of North Carolina State Board of Health* 17 (1917–1918), University of North Carolina Health Sciences Library, http://archives .hsl.unc.edu/nchh/nchh-02/nchh-02-017.pdf (accessed August 12, 2016): 1.

56. "History of Public Health Nursing in North Carolina," nursinghistory.appstate.edu/NC -public-health-nursing (accessed August 5, 2016).

57. Darlene C. Hine, *Black Women in White: Racial Conflict and Cooperation in the Nursing Profession, 1890–1950* (Indianapolis: Indiana University Press, 1989): 154–156.

58. Ibid., 155.

59. Mochling and Thomasson, "Saving Babies," 11.

60. Christine Ardalan, *Forging Professional Public Health Nursing in a Southern State: Florida's Public Health Nursing, 1889-1934* (dissertation, Florida International University, 2012): 306.

61. Rosa Brown, quoted in Ardalan, "Forging Professional Public Health," 306.

62. Patricia D'Antonio, *American Nursing: A History of Knowledge, Authority, and the Meaning of Work* (Baltimore, MD: Johns Hopkins University Press, 2010): 119.

63. Mary Hall, "The Second Twenty-Five Years," https://dph.georgia.gov/sites/.../HistoryofPublic HealthNursinginGeorgia (accessed August 12, 2016): 11.

64. Clara Noyes, "The Delano Red Cross Nurses," *AJN* 11 (November 1924): 1113–1115 (quotes 1114–1115).

65. Lillian White, "Home Hygiene and Care of the Sick," *AJN* 22, no. 4 (January 1922): 266–269.

66. Camilla Wills Collection, boxes 1–4, Eleanor Crowder Bjoring Center for Nursing Historical Inquiry, University of Virginia.

67. "Expanding Their Sphere: Montana Women in Education Administration and Public Health," montanawomenshistory.org (accessed August 13, 2016): 1.

68. Lula Owl Gloyne, quoted in Phoebe Pollitt, *The History of Public Health Nursing in North Carolina, 1902–2002* (Durham, NC: Carolina Academic Press, 2014): 66.

69. Lula Owl Gloyne, quoted in *History of Public Health Nursing in North Carolina*, nursinghistory .appstate.edu/NC-public-health-nursing (accessed August 5, 2016): 1–4.

70. Ibid.

71. Both Mary Zillitas and Delores Young wrote of this desire for adventure in their responses to the Indian Health Service Nursing Questionnaires (hereafter IHSNQs) in the Northern Arizona University-Cline Library (hereafter cited as NAU-CL), Virginia Brown, Ida Bahl, and Lillian Watson Collection (hereafter: BBWC), MS 269, box 1.

72. Dorothy Loope, IHSNQ to Ida Bahl, 1974. NAU-CL, BBWC, MS 269, box 1, folder 1.4.

73. Mary Breckinridge, "Yarb Lore in the Kentucky Mountains," *FNS Quarterly Bulletin* 35, 2 (1959): 3–17 (quote 3).

74. United States Public Health Service (USPHS), *Contagious and Infectious Diseases among the Indians*, Senate Document #1083, 62nd Congress, 3rd Session (Washington DC: Government Printing Office, 1913): 1–85.

75. Lewis Meriam, *The Problem of Indian Administration* (hereafter *The Meriam Report*) (Baltimore, MD: Johns Hopkins University Press, 1928): 20.

76. Ibid., 16.

77. "Field Nurses' Narrative Reports," National Archives Records Administration, Washington, DC (hereafter NARA), Bureau of Indian Affairs Record Group (hereafter RG75), E779, box 9 [no folders].

78. Laura Gilpin, *The Enduring Navaho* (Austin: University of Texas Press, 1974): 19.

79. Mollie Reebel, "Field Nurse's Narrative Report, April 1933," NARA, RG75, E779, box 9, [no folders], 1–4.

80. Elizabeth Forster to Laura Gilpin, August 1, 1932, in Martha Sandweiss, *Denizens of the Desert: A Tale in Word and Picture of Life among the Navajo Indians, the Letters of Elizabeth Forster* (Albuquerque: University of New Mexico, 1998): 102.

81. Katherine Schlosser, "Trachoma through History," https://www.nps.gov/elis/learn/educa tional/upload/Trachoma-Through-History-2.pdf (accessed August 6, 2016): 1–13 (quote 9).

82. Field Nurses' Narrative Reports, NARA, RG75, E779, box 9 [no folders].

83. Lillian G. Watson, "Annual Narrative Report, March 1955 to July 1956," original manuscript, NAU-BBWC, MS 269, box 1, folder 1.3.

84. Nena Seymour, "Field Nurse's Narrative Report, August 1935," NARA, RG75, E779, box 9 [no folders].

85. Arlene Keeling, "My Treatment Was Castor Oil and Aspirin": Field Nursing among the Navajo People in the Four Corners Region, 1925-1955," ch. 4 in *Nursing and the Privilege of Prescription, 1893–2000* (Columbus: The Ohio State University Press, 2007): 86.

86. Squibb Advertisement, "Cod Liver Oil," *AJN* 24, no. 13 (October 1924): inside cover.

87. Dorothy Williams, quoted in Keeling, "My Treatment Was Castor Oil," 84.

88. Reebel, "Field Nurse's Narrative Report, April 1933," 2.

89. Grace Abbot, "Children's Bureau Report," *AJN* 28, no. 2 (1928): 142.

90. Mochling and Thomasson, "Saving Babies," 8.

91. Ibid., 1.

92. Edna Foley, "Breast Feeding," *AJN* 24, no. 9 (September 1924): 751–757 (quote 753).

FURTHER READING

Abel, Emily, "We Are Left So Much Alone to Workout Our Own Problems," *Nursing History Review* 4 (1996): 43–64.

Ardalan, Christine, *Forging Professional Public Health Nursing in a Southern State: Florida's Public Health Nursing, 1889–1934* (dissertation, Florida International University, 2012).

Breckinridge, Mary, *Wide Neighborhoods* (Lexington: University Press of Kentucky, 1952).

Cockerham, Anne, "Mary Breckinridge and the Frontier Nursing Service: Saddlebags and Swinging Bridges," ch. 6 in *Nursing Rural America*, eds. John Kirchgessner and Arlene Keeling (New York: Springer Publishing, 2015).

Cockerham, Anne, and Keeling, Arlene, *Rooted in the Mountains, Reaching to the World: Stories of Nursing and Midwifery at Kentucky's Frontier School, 1939–1989* (Louisville, KY: Butler Books, 2012).

Ettinger, Laura, "Nurse-Midwives, the Mass Media and the Politics of Maternal Health Care in the United States, 1925-1955," *Nursing History Review* 7 (1999): 47–66.

Ettinger, Laura, *Nurse-Midwifery: The Birth of a New American Profession* (Columbus: The Ohio State University Press, 2006).

Hine, Darlene C., *Black Women in White: Racial Conflict and Cooperation in the Nursing Profession, 1890–1950* (Indianapolis: Indiana University Press, 1989).

Keeling, Arlene, "Providing Care in the Hoot Owl Hollers," ch. 3; and "My Treatment Was Castor Oil and Aspirin: Field Nursing among the Navajo in the Four Corners Region, 1925–1955," ch. 4 in *Nursing and the Privilege of Prescription: 1893–2000*, ed. Arlene Keeling (Columbus: The Ohio State University Press, 2007).

Lynaugh, Joan, "The Death of Sadie Sachs," *Nursing Research* 40, no. 2 (March–April 1991): 124–125.

Meckel, Richard, *Save the Babies: American Public Health Reform and the Prevention of Infant Mortality, 1850–1929* (Baltimore, MD: Johns Hopkins University Press, 1990).

Pollitt, Phoebe, *African American and Cherokee Nurses in Appalachia: A History 1900–1965* (Jefferson, NC: McFarland, 2016).

Ruffing-Rahal, Mary Ann, "The Navajo Experience of Elizabeth Forster, Public Health Nurse," *Nursing History Review* 3 (1995): 173–178.

Schminkey, Donna, and Keeling, Arlene, "Frontier Nurse-Midwives and Antepartum Emergencies, 1925 to 1939," *Journal of Midwifery and Women's Health* 60, no. 1 (2015): 48–55.

Smith, Susan, "White Nurses, Black Midwives, and Public Health in Mississippi, 1920–1950," *Nursing History Review* 2 (1994): 29–49.

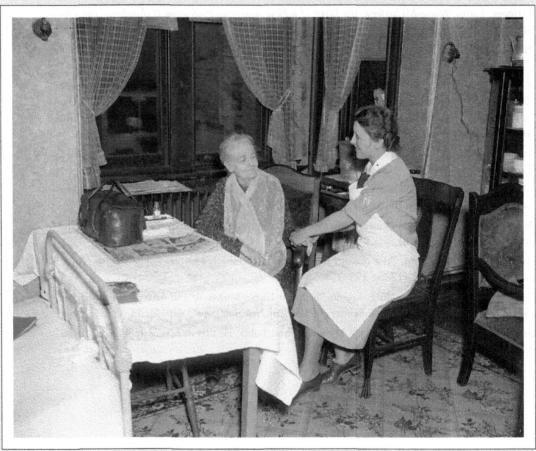

A home visit.

CHAPTER 10

Nursing in the Great Depression

1930–1940

Arlene W. Keeling

"The influence on nursing of the turbulence and tragic economic uncertainty of the world in the past year is too far-reaching to be completely evaluated in the close range. But it is possible that we may, in years to come—look back on this year of black depression as that in which powerful forces converged [so that nursing could] turn towards true professional status." [1]

Writing in January of 1933, Mary Roberts, the editor of the *American Journal of Nursing*, was optimistic about the nursing profession's ability to weather the storm of the Great Depression (1930–1940) and emerge with "true professional status." Only a few years before Roberts wrote this, in 1929 the stock market had crashed, the U.S. economy had collapsed, and millions of Americans lost their jobs. In fact, when President Franklin Delano Roosevelt took office in January 1933, manufacturing had "all but ground to a halt," and 15 million Americans were unemployed. [2] Among them were thousands of nurses.

During the Depression, the nursing profession faced several problems: (a) many private-duty nurses were unemployed, as few people had money to hire them; (b) public health nurses were in short supply when the demand for their services was increasing; and (c) the medical profession was rapidly developing the field of anesthesia, and as more physicians began to practice this specialty, they not only competed with nurse anesthetists for jobs, but also began to challenge the legality of nurse anesthesia practice.

Describing the conditions nurses faced in "the richest country in the world," Roberts wrote about the difficult experiences of visiting nurses. She told of those who entered tenement homes where entire families were suffering because the "heat had been cut off." She described how families from "proud homes" in farming communities only called for a nurse "in the gravest emergencies because of lack of money to pay." She also noted that payment, "if it was made at all," was made in "butter, eggs and other products of the land."[3]

THE CRISIS IN PRIVATE-DUTY NURSING

Patients and their families were not the only ones reeling from the economic crisis. Private-duty nurses were desperate for work. Nursing schools in the 1920s had proliferated, doubling the number of graduates seeking work and saturating the field of private-duty nursing. The over supply of nurses converged with the economic disaster of the Depression to cause a critical shortage in opportunities for those nurses seeking work in private homes. Hiring a private-duty nurse at $6.00 to $7.00 for a 12-hour shift was simply too expensive for most Americans at a time when they could hardly afford medical care. Now too many nurses were vying for too few positions.[4]

> "The tragic unemployment among private duty nurses has sent many . . . back to their homes."[7]
>
> Editor, American Journal of Nursing, 1933

In 1932, at the height of the Depression, between 8,000 and 10,000 U.S. nurses were searching for work.[5] One nurse wrote to the *American Journal of Nursing* describing the nurses' predicament, noting that many private-duty nurses were "seeking help from home, borrowing on insurance, using up savings and investments." Others supplemented their incomes by "gardening, raising poultry, doing sewing, [and] even resorting to domestic work."[6]

Some states, short of positions for their own residents, took out ads in the *American Journal of Nursing*, warning nurses from other areas of the country not to come. The ad that Florida nurses posted was typical:

> To nurses contemplating coming to Miami we wish to present the following facts: There are several hundred nurses out of employment in Miami at the present time. There is less work here now than there has been at any time during the past eleven years. Florida has passed a state law that all nurses practicing their profession in this state pay a tax of $15.00, this being county and state tax. This, added to the state registration fee, makes a total of $25 that has to be put out in order to nurse in the State of Florida.[8]

As a result of the shortage of work, during the 1930s graduate nurses increasingly turned to hospitals for employment. Hospitals were the ones that benefited. Hospital administrators found that "employing private duty nurses who could be hired and dismissed as patient occupancy rates rose and fell, was an easy way to temporarily supplement short staffs and save the expense of permanent employees."[10] The former private-duty nurses would work as "general duty" nurses even if that meant they could only work on a per diem basis at a lower rate of pay (sometimes $3.00–$5.00 a shift) or for room and board.[11] The nurses had little choice. Meanwhile, hospitals acquired experienced graduate nurses who could manage the care of several patients, serve as head nurses on the wards, or care for the most seriously ill patients.

> "Nurses are advised not to come to Oklahoma for work, as the private duty field is more than full."[9]
>
> American Journal of Nursing, 1930

In 1933, congressional approval of the Federal Emergency Relief Act and the establishment of the Civil Works Administration provided hope. The American Nurses Association could now work with the Women's Division of the Federal Emergency Relief Administration to help unemployed nurses. According to the American Nurses Association's report: "In the interests of safeguarding the health and welfare of every community in the United States, it is advised that relief nurses be assigned to some already existing organization such as a hospital, institution, nurses' association, public health organization et cetera; also that no nurse be assigned to work as a nurse, excepting under paid, qualified, nurse supervision." Their goal was to remedy "the tragic unemployment of nurses without affecting quality of care."[12]

Francis Helen Zeigler, a nurse at the Medical College of Virginia, explained how this new policy helped both White and Black nurses, writing: "We, in the hospital division . . . had no difficulty in creating jobs. The census had been steadily increasing. Had we not had the increase in personnel through our Civil Works Administration projects, I hardly know what we would have done. As it was, we added . . . seven white and three Negro graduate nurses for general staff nursing."[13]

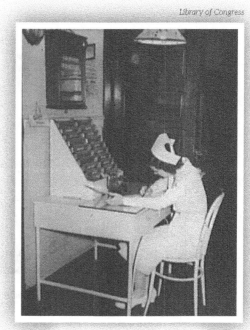

A graduate nurse completing her notes on patients.

NEW OPPORTUNITIES OUTSIDE THE HOSPITAL

In addition to opportunities inside hospitals, new jobs were created in the community. Under the Civil Works Administration (later called the Works Progress Administration), the U.S. Public Health Service initiated community-based services in which nurses "in financial need" could be employed.[14]

By 1936, approximately 6,000 graduate nurses worked in the New Deal programs initiated by President Roosevelt when he took office in 1933. Funded by the Federal Emergency Relief Act and the Works Progress Administration, some of these nurses worked in public health departments, others in school hygiene, in tuberculosis and orthopedic clinics, or as assistants to county health officers. A few conducted tuberculosis surveys. According to a 1937 editorial in the *American Journal of Nursing,* "the Works Progress Administration nursing programs (1) gave employment to nurses who had no other means of support; (2) provided much-needed assistance to health departments and hospitals which were very much understaffed; and (3) introduced many recent graduates . . . to the field of public health."[15]

"Since the beginning of the fiscal year 1936, 75 projects which provide for the employment of graduate nurses in 16 different states have been approved by the Works Progress Administration."[16]

American Journal of Nursing, 1937

Public Health Nursing in Gees Bend, Alabama

No one needed a competent public health nurse more than the geographically isolated, poor Black community of Gees Bend, Alabama. The 5-mile long and 8-mile wide bend of land in the Alabama River was seven miles away by foot from the nearest town, and accessible by ferry only when it was running. The only "nurse" was an African American midwife named Sally.[17] Gees Bend was home to a group of Black sharecroppers who even before the Depression had been living hand to mouth, making do with what they had. With only wood stoves to heat their tumbledown shacks, the women of Gees Bend made quilts to keep their families warm, piecing together scraps of cotton, corduroy, and feed sacks to do so. Living on credit from the local merchant in hopes of a "better crop next season," the sharecropper families were always in debt. With the drop in cotton prices from 13¢ to 5¢ a pound in the early 1930s, that debt only got worse. The benevolent merchant who had always extended them credit died suddenly and the merchant's family demanded payment of their notes. Within a short time, the people of Gees Bend were in crisis as they watched their food, animals, tools, and seed confiscated as debt repayment. Most were left destitute. They had lived on cornbread and molasses in good times; now, with nothing to trade and not a penny to their name, the sharecroppers ate whatever they could forage off the land. Paying for medical or nursing care was simply out of the question.

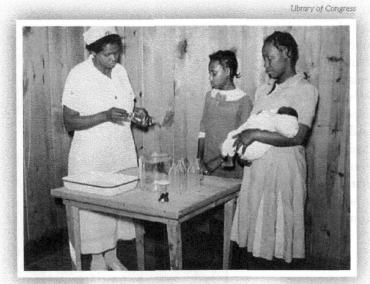

Nurse Shamburg with Gees Bend residents.

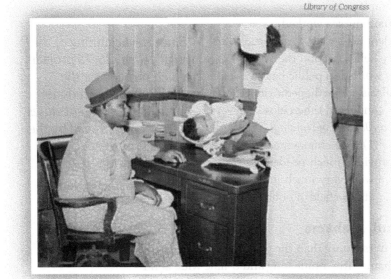

Nurse Shamburg weighing a baby.

Two groups stepped in to respond to the community's desperate situation: the American Red Cross and the Farm Security Administration. The American Red Cross provided immediate help, arriving with truckloads of flour, meat, cornmeal, used clothing, and shoes. In an attempt to provide a longer term solution, the Farm Security Administration purchased land in Gees Bend and established Gees Bend Farms, Inc., a pilot project that included "Roosevelt" houses, a schoolhouse, and a clinic. Federal funds paid the salaries of Miss Shamburg, a nurse, and Dr. R. E. Dixon who staffed the clinic. In addition to assisting Dr. Dixon with medical procedures and immunizations, Miss Shamburg held well-baby clinics, taught nutrition classes, and made home visits to the sick. For the first time, the Gees Bend community had access to professional nursing care.

Nursing in West Coast Migrant Camps

Shamburg was not the only nurse to be hired by the government to help those in need. Other nurses worked for health departments, some in routine jobs and others in federally funded migrant camps established throughout the nation. A small number of graduate nurses found jobs in California in migrant workers' camps, some of the first to be built. Employed first by state public health departments and later under the Farm Security Administration's Federal Emergency Relief Act, the camp nurses collaborated with physicians and social workers to provide care to the thousands of destitute U.S. farmers.[18]

With the collapse of the U.S. economy, farmers had been particularly devastated when farm income plummeted from $6.7 billion in 1929 to $2.3 billion in 1932. At the same time, tractors were replacing manual labor, and farmers in the Plains states plowed thousands of acres of prairie grasses in their desire to increase crop production. However, when a devastating drought and subsequent dust storms hit the plains in 1933, choking the farms with black sand, the crops did not grow.[19] Unable to pay their mortgages, the farmers were eventually evicted from their homes. More than 250,000 farmers and their families left the "Dust Bowl" states and migrated to the West Coast to harvest fruits and vegetables.[20] Traveling in rickety automobiles packed with "tents, bedding, and a few household items," the "baked out and broke" families headed to California on Route 66.[21]

Arriving in the towns of California's Imperial and San Joaquin Valleys, the migrants concentrated in appalling numbers, only to discover that work was scarce, pay was little, and living conditions in the squatter camps were horrid. In California, "there were two and three men for every job." As a result, wages were low. With little cash left after the long trip, the migrants accepted whatever pay was offered, forcing earnings even lower.[22] Homeless, the migrants lived in rickety cabins owned by their employers or in makeshift "squatter camps" hastily erected along irrigation ditches and dirt roads close to the fields.[23] Without indoor plumbing, families used ditch water for bathing, drinking, and toileting.

Poor living conditions combined with the migrants' inadequate diet decreased their ability to fight infection and many succumbed to communicable diseases. Inevitably dysentery, diarrhea, and other diseases broke out.[24] Tuberculosis was endemic. Other prevalent diseases included conjunctivitis, colds, whooping cough, strep throat, scarlet fever, mumps, and measles.[25] "In one camp 26 cases of small pox developed before the outbreak was even documented."[26]

Soon Californians saw the filthy tent cities and the Dust Bowl refugees with their "grimy, coughing children" as menaces to their own health.[28] Under pressure from local citizens, the State Department of Health was asked to intervene—the migrants had no money for medical care. However, the displaced migrant families were not considered residents in their states of destination, and therefore did not qualify for state relief. As a result, the states soon sought help from the federal government. In response, the federally funded Agriculture Workers Health and Medical Association set up clinics near the ditch camps and employed local public health nurses and part-time physicians to care for the migrants.[29]

The care provided to the migrants was multifaceted, involving not only treatment with medicines, vitamins, and supplements, but also paying attention to housing and sanitary conditions, and providing health education. The nurses had to stop epidemics, give first aid, help families cope with floods, keep the community well, and provide prenatal and postpartum care for mothers and babies. While visiting the families in their ramshackle tents and shacks, the nurses taught hygiene and proper diet—or simply provided the destitute families with food and housing. One nurse documented her visit to a

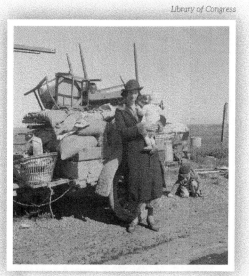

Migrant family in front of their loaded car after leaving the Dust Bowl.

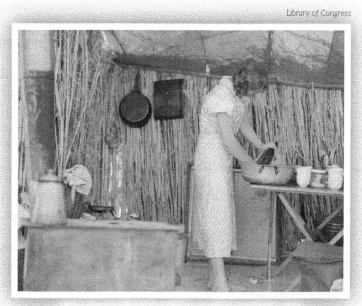

A woman working in a ditch camp in Imperial County, California, in 1937.

"There is a continual epidemic of measles, mumps, whooping cough, scarlet fever and pneumonia."[27]

Journalist Sanora Babb, 1935

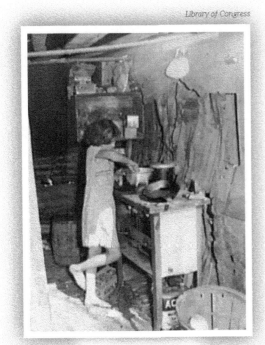

*A child preparing a meal in
a migrant camp in 1939.*

family of six, living in a makeshift structure in the corner of a pea field, writing:

The parents were away working . . . the four children were all sick. The baby was wracked with whooping cough. . . . I left a note for the parents—where to come for a tent and for surplus foods. . . . The family received a new tent, bedding, clothing, and rations . . . [including] prescriptions from the grocery store for three high-caloric diets.[30]

Malnutrition was more common than any other problem the nurses encountered. Food was scarce and most migrant families subsisted on a diet of salt pork, boiled beans, cornbread, potatoes, and baking powder biscuits with gravy.[31] As one nurse described it: "During potato-picking season, the children might have potato sandwiches for lunch—sliced raw potatoes between two slices of bread."[32] Health problems followed. One mother who had been living for weeks on a diet of hotcakes cooked in fatback arrived at the clinic with "the skin of her hands and wrists cracking and becoming infected."[33] According to the Farm Security Administration's chief medical officer Ralph Williams, "most every child in camp" suffered from "nutritional defects"; many had pellagra, a preventable disease caused by lack of niacin.[34]

In addition to treating nutritional deficiencies with vitamins and food, camp nurses had to educate young mothers about food preparation. In one case, even though the family had powdered milk given to them "off relief from the government," the mother did not use it, explaining to the nurse: "I don't guess I know how to mix it up." The nurse responded by demonstrating its preparation. She also recorded the outcome, noting: "the two children devoured it voraciously."[35]

In the ditch camps, the lack of proper kitchens, indoor plumbing, refrigeration, and household goods added to the nurses' challenges. Nurses had to make do with what the family had on hand, teaching the mother to prepare baby formula using a "saucepan, an empty flask, and a tin spoon"—or how to make a baby crib from an "orange crate and an old quilt."[36]

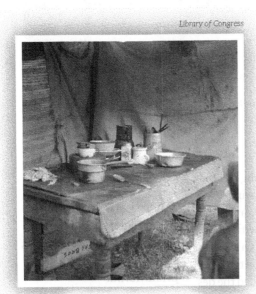

A sparse migrant food table.

Health teaching about the importance of hygiene was another aspect of the nurses' role. Teaching new mothers how to care for their infants took up much of the nurses' time, especially because the migrant mothers were young and living away from their mothers and grandmothers who might have helped. One nurse documented her interaction with a new mother, writing that on making a postpartum visit she found the mother bathing the new baby by "dabbing about his head" with a cloth. After asking why the mother did not place the baby in a tub on such a hot day, the mother replied: "Well, I ain't never, reckon I might—but no notion as how [sic]." According to the nurse, this called for a "demonstration baby bath," followed by further instruction on washing baby bottles, keeping them refrigerated and away from flies.[37]

Because the migrants moved frequently to new fields as they followed the crops from harvest to harvest, locating pregnant women for pre- and postnatal care was difficult. In an attempt to solve this problem, the nurses distributed "change of address" postcards to the women, encouraging them to keep in touch. Finding their patients was still not easy, however, as nurses had to decipher the new addresses from an often vague set of instructions. One woman wrote:

> "Dear Nurse: We moved Sunday from Doran's to the Ballard Ranch. Turn south where Hanford road turns north from Corcoran go south and turn west at first road west . . . pass highline . . . about one mile north you can see the camp. . . . We are in a tent."[39]

Given directions like these, the nurses spent an inordinate amount of time searching for their patients.

The severe floods in March 1938 aroused Californians to the tragedy of the Dust Bowl migrants.[40] Speaking to the Bakersfield Rotary Club a few months after the floods, the assistant regional director of California's migrant camps recounted what had happened:

> The rain kept pouring down and pea pickers kept pouring in, stretching leaking tents over muddy puddles. A week later more than 3,000 people were picking peas . . . scattered over 10 more or less disreputable campsites. At the end of the first week, the nurse had found 151 cases of illness, among them 27 cases of whooping cough, 23 cases of measles, 21 cases of chickenpox, and 14 cases of mumps. But there was no opportunity for medical care as the Board of Supervisors of that county had voted to hospitalize "extreme emergency cases only."[41]

Kings County suffered the worst. Much of the cotton, grain, and beets were in the old Tulare Lake Basin, and as it filled up with water, camp after camp washed way. Now nurses had to deal with the flood emergency in addition to their usual work.

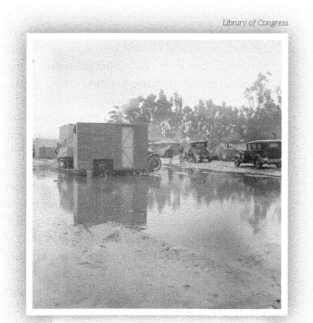

Aftermath of the floods in 1938, which washed away entire migrant camps.

Preventing the Spread of Disease

"One mother had to be made to understand that by bathing four small children with one basin of water using the same towel, she spread impetigo and pink eye among them. It might almost have been better not to have bathed them at all."[38]

Camp Nurse, 1937

The Floods

"March 3, 1938—This morning I started to Moore's camp to make a survey for the well-baby conference. When I came to St. John's River . . . I found the concrete bridge completely under water . . . I contacted the Red Cross. Together the worker from the Red Cross and I made a survey of the conditions of all camps bordering rivers and creeks and advised the campers that the auditorium in Visalia was to be opened with beds and food."[42]

Faverman Report, 1938

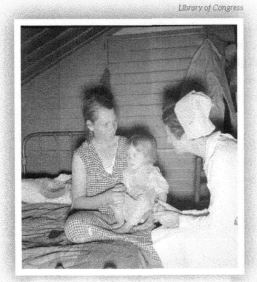

A nurse visiting a migrant mother and child
in their shelter in Tulare Camp in 1939.

*"They have a deep sense of
what living in America
should mean."⁴⁵*

Journalist Sanora Babb, 1936

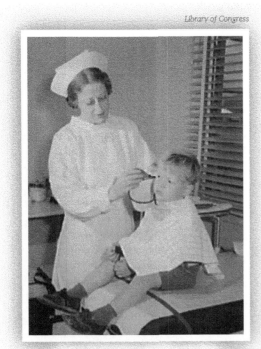

A nurse irrigating a child's ear at the
Tulare migrant camp, 1940.

Nurses would soon receive help from the federal government. They convinced state officials that something had to be done to help the migrants who had lived so much better before the economic collapse and the drought. As a result, the Farm Security Administration established its first structured federal camps. The camps, called "Farm Workers Communities," were set up in areas where the migrants concentrated.⁴³ The new camps had wooden platforms on which families could pitch tents. They also had showers, toilets, and laundry facilities, as well as a community hall in which the families could gather for social events, council meetings, and elections. In addition, the typical camp had a clinic with a nurse, a first aid room, and nursery where children could be cared for while their parents worked in the fields.

Public health nurse Mary Sears was assigned to Brawley, one of the first Farm Worker camps to be established. She recalled that when the camp first opened, "migrants came pouring in, their jalopies crammed with their worldly goods and their ragged children. They were coming to a place where they were able to wash their rags, sleep off the ground, and live more like human beings."⁴⁴

Full-time public health nurses, chosen for their "experience, personality . . . and ability to obtain the confidence and cooperation of poor people," were "instrumental in the organization and operation of the migrant health program" in the camps.⁴⁶ In addition to screening all family members on arrival, the nurse would also provide immunizations, give first aid, and teach the migrant mothers how to care for "cuts, abscesses, sore eyes and rashes."⁴⁷

Although physicians were in attendance a few days a week, often working well beyond their set hours on any given day, camp nurses accepted a "striking degree of responsibility" when there was no physician available. The nurses assessed patients, treated them according to standing order sets, and triaged them according to severity of illness.⁴⁸ More complicated cases were "referred to specialists, dentists, x-ray and clinical laboratories."⁴⁹ In these camps, nurses merged their traditional role with an expanded one, diagnosing and treating patients using physician-written protocols and standing orders.⁵⁰

The nurses' role in the camps was not without controversy, particularly related to their scope of practice. Nursing supervisors themselves were concerned. The director of the Division of Public Health Nursing for the Oregon State Board of Health, Olive Whitlock, expressed her worry in a letter to her supervisor, writing: "It seems the nurse is to see all patients requiring medical care, and refer them to the contract physician if she is unable to give the necessary care herself . . . My chief concern is over the amount of responsibility placed upon the nurses."⁵¹

Officials in the Farm Security Administration were quick to defend the camp nurses, however. Responding to a letter criticizing the nurses' work, Dr. Ralph Williams wrote:

We are thoroughly aware of the dangers of permitting any nurse to assume too much responsibility in connection with the treatment of disease. We have been punctilious in this respect relative to the nurses employed in the Migrant Labor Camps . . . Dr. R. G. Leland of the American Medical Association recently spent two weeks in visiting the labor camps. . . . He had no criticism of the work of the nurses in any way."[52]

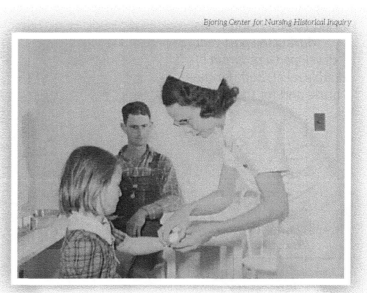

A nurse tending to a child in the Shafter Migratory Camp, 1940.

The camp nurse's role was not always questioned, especially if she spent most of her time performing traditional nursing activities, providing a listening ear, and offering comfort and support. Even the camp newspaper editors supported that role. For example, a 1939 article in the Indio Camp newsletter announced the arrival of a new camp nurse, Lena Pimentol, and followed with: "Do come in and meet her, and bring all your troubles along."[53]

The same held true when the nurse worked within her traditional public health role—case finding, visiting the sick, and teaching the principles of disease prevention and health promotion. Eventually, the editors of the camp newspapers allotted the nurses space for a column giving health advice. They also advertised the information about nursing clinics. In the Shafter Migratory Camp, Mrs. Crain, the nurse, wrote an educational column in the *Covered Wagon News* from time to time. In one letter, she urged families to "put forth a definite effort to keep the babies well by washing all fruits and vegetables" and to make sure that children were not allowed to drop fruit on the ground and then pick it up and eat it.[54] In other camp newsletter columns, the clinic nurses provided information on what mothers should do about contagious diseases. Sometimes translating the advice into Spanish for their "Mexican friends," the nurses also encouraged mothers to attend vaccination and well-baby clinics.[55]

Since the camp nurse's role was to focus on the prevention of illness, the nurses organized "Mothers' Health Clubs" and camp health committees to "generate interest" in the health education programs they offered. As camp nurse Pauline Koplan remarked: "Every day was different. One day might be set up for well-baby clinics . . . another time it was immunization day."[57]

By the end of the decade, nurses were working in migrant camps scattered throughout the San Joaquin and Imperial Valleys. By May 31, 1939, the Agriculture Workers Health and Medical Association not only employed 10 registered nurses in California, but also had seven in Arizona, and others in Texas, Oregon, Utah, Washington State, and Florida.[59]

Public Health and Migrant Nursing in Florida

In 1933, after the Florida State Nurses Association discovered that 200 nurses had been unemployed for at least 6 months, the association worked with the State Board of Health to hire nurses under the Federal Emergency

---

"What to Remember About Whooping Cough"

It is a highly contagious disease and is especially dangerous for babies and young children . . . It is spread by discharges from the nose and throat . . . Keep the child completely away from other people. All discharges should be burned . . . Have special dishes . . . and wash separately with soap and hot water."[56]

Indio Camp Nurse, *The Migratory Clipper*, 1939

"The first Well-Baby Clinic of the new year will be held on Friday, January 27, from 1-3 PM. Diphtheria and small pox [vaccinations] will be given."[58]

Clinic Nurse, The Weedpatch Cultivator, 1939

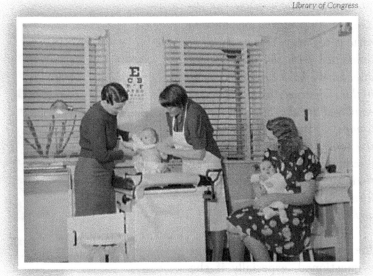

Nurses tending to a baby in the well-baby clinic in the Tulare migrant camp, 1940.

> "Florida, as other states, has during the past year developed a program of double relief; both for the nurse and for the sick."[60]

Preparation for New Recruits

"Before assigning a nurse to a county, she is placed for a period of three weeks on the Visiting Nurse Staff in Jacksonville or Tampa where she receives lectures in public health nursing . . . experience in home visiting [and] rural school nursing."[62]

Ruth Mettinger, 1934

Relief Association Nursing Project. In that project, 286 newly recruited nurses worked under 15 experienced public health nurse district supervisors at different locations throughout the state. At the Florida State Nurses Association in 1935, Ruth Mettinger, director of Florida's Public Health Nursing Department, reported that the 300 nurses employed with federal funds were mostly "out of work private duty nurses."[61]

The new public health nurses also worked with local physicians as well as with Black Red Cross nurses and local midwives—both Black and White—directing their efforts toward health promotion and disease prevention. Under the State Nursing Project, the nurses completed "physical inspections of children in families receiving relief," screened those in need of medical care, arranged for the "correction of defects" as ordered by physicians, provided nutrition counseling, "distributed prenatal literature," ensured that pregnant women received "an obstetrical pack" with necessary supplies for delivery, and cooperated with the county medical societies to provide immunizations.[63]

The nurses employed under the federal programs did not always work in traditional public health settings, however. With the migration of tens of thousands of dispossessed sharecroppers to Florida after they were evicted from farms in Tennessee, North and South Carolina, Alabama, and Georgia, squatter camps were springing up near orchards and fields throughout the state. And, like those in California, Oregon, and Washington, the disenfranchised migrants in the Florida camps needed nurses.

The nurses employed in Florida's squatter camps faced problems similar to those facing the nurses on the West Coast; however, East Coast nurses cared for many more African American workers. Both Black and White sharecroppers migrated to Florida in search of work. Both groups needed help, but the Black workers and their families were near desperate, living at the bottom of the social ladder in the segregated Jim Crow South. As one Black family member

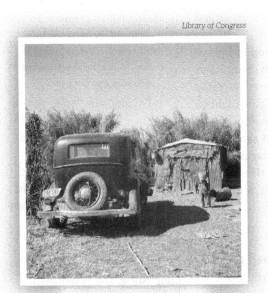

House in Belle Glade made of tin and burlap, 1939.

put it: "We ain't lived like hogs before, but we sure does now!"[64]

Some displaced sharecroppers migrated to Winter Haven and the newly opened Belle Glade-Pahokee region, an area on the southern shore of Lake Okeechobee, where workers harvested vegetables. There they lived in tin shacks in segregated camps near bean and potato packing plants. Living conditions were abysmal, particularly for African Americans. In 1933, John P. Ingle, president of the Statewide Health Committee, deemed the living conditions as the "filthiest, most insanitary conditions" he had "ever seen."[65] Some families lived in windowless wooden shacks near irrigation ditches; others in tents with their car serving as one side of the shelter. None had electricity or indoor plumbing. Drinking water came from ditches; city water could be purchased at 1¢ a bucket. Working with families living in these conditions, nurses not only cared for the sick but also taught basic hygiene, nutrition, first aid, and well-baby care.[66]

After reports of the shocking living conditions of the migrant workers in Belle Glade, the Farm Security Administration opened Osceola in 1933, a segregated "army-like camp for 533 black and white migrant farm families." In addition to providing families with access to clean water, bathtubs for the children, and a place to hang out the laundry, the camp had a clinic building where 2 to 3 days a week a local physician and the camp nurse would see patients.

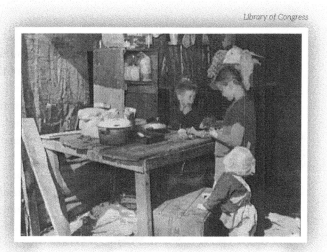

Migrant children in Belle Glade amuse themselves while their parents worked all day and far into the night, 1939.

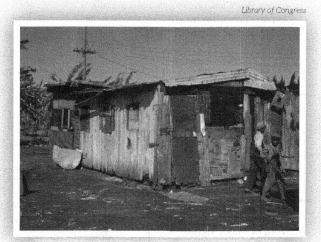

The African American section of the Belle Glade camp in 1941, where the conditions were even worse—no electricity or indoor plumbing, and little access to clean water.

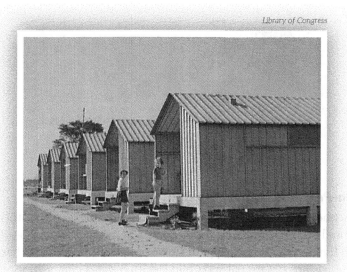

Osceola camp in 1941, which had access to clean water for all residents and a clinic building for a part-time local physician and a camp nurse.

"In Hector Quarter at Belle Glade . . . four tumbledown privies serve the entire community."[67]

James Snyder, 2004

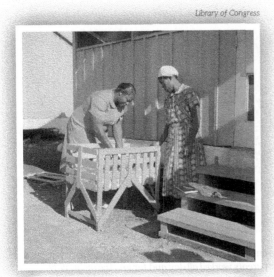

A camp nurse at Okeechobee migratory labor camp, Belle Glade, in 1940, examining a baby as part of camp nurses' efforts to decrease the high maternal death rate in Florida.

As was true in the migrant camps on the West Coast, on days that a physician was not in camp the nurse would care for patients with minor problems, treating sore throats, fevers, and colds. She also immunized both adults and children. Because the maternal death rate in Florida was "extremely high," camp nurses placed special emphasis on prenatal care, preparation for delivery, and post-partum care.[68]

Essential players in the government camps, nurses worked with physicians and African American aides to promote the health of the community, insisting that *all* Americans live in decent environments with access to clean water, education for their children, and the right to obtain medical and nursing care for themselves and their families. As the social service director for the Federal Emergency Relief Act put it: "Health is both a necessity and a luxury for the enjoyment of life. There is an increasing recognition that adequate health and medical care is a social necessity, in fact, a social right for those who cannot provide it for themselves. The question is how and by whom this medical care is provided."[69]

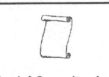

Social Security Act, 1935

The Social Security Act was an event of major significance to the people of the United States. The legislation not only provided assistance to crippled children and funding for maternal–child health, but also encouraged "cooperative efforts between official and voluntary nursing agencies." In addition, the act provided scholarships for nurses and federal funding to the states to establish public health services.[70]

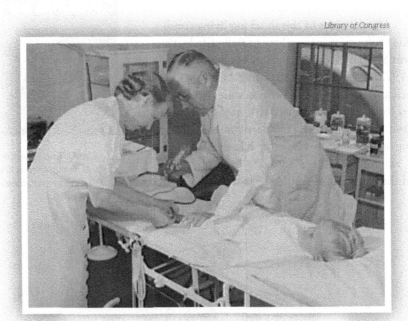

Physician and nurse tending to a child in a migrant camp, 1940.

The *Curandera-Parteras* in New Mexico

In 1935, the enactment of the Social Security Act gave New Mexico, like other states, funds to expand and improve programs for mothers and infants that had been started in the 1920s with funding from the Sheppard–Towner Act. With the use of these funds, officials from the Division of Maternal and Child Health began a demonstration project in San Miguel County in 1936. The project had two purposes—to enhance maternal and child public health nursing and to provide "field training" for public health nursing students. Both were needed.

In the early 20th century, more than 800 *curandera-parteras* (traditional Hispanic midwives) were working in New Mexico. Most of them were located in the rural, isolated, Hispanic villages in the northern part of the state that was culturally isolated from the rest of the United States. Typically, the *curandera-parteras* were middle-aged or older Hispanic women who had learned midwifery practices from their mothers and grandmothers and held key positions in the community. Often they relied on herbal treatments and attributed some of the complications of labor and delivery to superstition. But in the 1930s, New Mexico's maternal mortality rate (8.9 per 1,000 live births) was 20% higher than the U.S. average.[71] Officials knew they had to do something. Their goal now was to improve standards for the *curandera-parteras'* performance by supervising them with individual education.

The project began first in the county of San Miguel but soon encompassed the entire state. With a staff of 11 nurses—one supervisor, eight public health nurses, one nurse-midwife, and one nurse for venereal disease work—the nurses established clinics, *La Clinica*, in all the counties of New Mexico. In remote areas, they used an automobile as the clinic. Jean Egbert, the nurse-midwife, worked with the *curandera-parteras*, teaching them and providing direct supervision for their work.

Later, in 1938, the county added a Midwifery Consultant Program, employing two more nurse-midwives, Eva Borden and Frances Fell. Both saw patients in prenatal clinics and provided classes for the *curandera-parteras*. By 1938, the public health and nurse-midwives had taught almost all of the *curandera-parteras* in the state. Those who completed the course received a midwifery certificate and a regulation bag and equipment.[72]

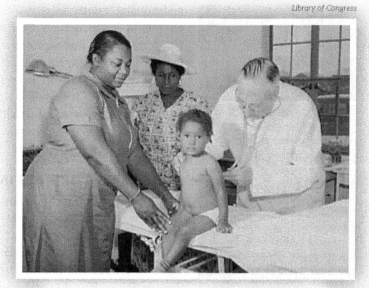

Physician and nurse tending to a child in a migrant camp, 1940.

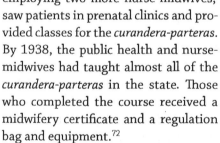

"They taught us to do everything—how to take care of the lady, how to take care of the baby, and when to ask a doctor for help."[73]

Dona J. Aragon,
Curandera-Parteras

NURSES AND ANTIBIOTICS

By the mid-1930s, nurses and doctors began to change the treatment of patients with infectious diseases from simply relieving symptoms to curing the disease. To do so they used a new type of drug: the antibiotic. In 1932, scientists discovered a new drug to treat commonly occurring streptococcus infections. The first in its class of sulfonamides, Prontosil would lead to a new era in medicine

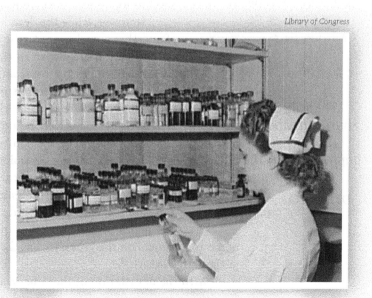

A nurse inspecting medications, which took on greater significance as antibiotics were discovered.

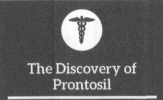

The Discovery of Prontosil

In 1932, German scientist Gerhard Domagak, working with his colleague Josef Karere at Bayer Pharmaceuticals, experimented with chemical dyes, testing them for their effect on streptococcus, the bacteria responsible for diseases such as scarlet fever, rheumatic fever, pneumonia, and strep throat. In 1936, the drug gained widespread recognition after it was used to cure a throat infection in President Franklin D. Roosevelt's son.

Courses for Nurses

"Charity Hospital of Louisiana in New Orleans offers a post-graduate course of eight months in Anesthesia and Gas Therapy. The course includes all types of anesthetic agents and practice in the use of modern equipment. Write Director, School of Anesthesia, Charity Hospital."[77]

Advertisement, *American Journal of Nursing*, 1939

"The skillful, well-trained nurse anesthetist has been responsible for the great improvement in the practice of anesthesia."[80]

Dr. Evarts Graham, Washington University, 1933

and nursing.[74] Sulfa drugs could be used to cure patients with "streptococcus meningitis, puerperal fever, gonococcal infections, erysipelas, pneumonia, scarlet fever, and septic sore throat (strep throat)."[75] The drug was not without side effects, however. Writing in the *American Journal of Nursing* about the administration of Prontosil solution, which contained a red dye, one nurse noted: "It is well to remember several symptoms will occur. The patient's skin takes on a pinkish hue and the . . . urine becomes highly colored with red dye. These symptoms should be expected and should cause no alarm."[76]

NURSE ANESTHETISTS IN THE 1930S

Hard-pressed to find work of any kind during the Depression, some nurses left their home states to seek further training in public health, surgical nursing, or anesthesia.

For those who turned to training as a nurse anesthetist, the time was right. In 1931, nurse anesthetist Agatha Hodgins established the National Association of Nurse Anesthetists (later to become the American Association of Nurse Anesthetists) and the specialty, with support from the American Hospital Association, was gaining in strength and recognition. In fact, by the 1930s nurses were giving anesthesia in more than 2,000 hospitals across the country.[78] Since the late 19th century, nurse anesthetists had been giving safe and economical care. Now, "many of the best surgeons" in hospitals throughout the United States were employing them.[79]

The practice of nurse-delivered anesthesia had started first in the Civil War, when Catholic Sisters assisted physicians during surgery. After that war, nurse anesthetists flourished at Mayo and Cleveland Clinics. In 1917 to 1918, with the shortage of anesthetists in World War I, the nurses' role developed even further. By the 1930s, there were more than 20 schools for nurse anesthesia across the country, each offering 6 months to a year of postgraduate nursing training in the specialty. Included among these were the Lakeside Hospital in Cleveland, Mayo Clinic in Rochester, Johns Hopkins Hospital in Baltimore, Barnes Hospital in Saint Louis, New York Hospital in New York, St. Joseph's in Milwaukee, Emory in Atlanta, Yale in New Haven, and Presbyterian in Chicago.[81]

However, while the decade of the 1920s had seen a growth in schools of anesthesia, resistance to the practice of nurse anesthesia was beginning as more physicians began to choose anesthesia as their medical specialty. The situation was further complicated by the discovery of new types of anesthesia and new methods of delivery. In short, giving anesthesia was beginning to require increasingly complex scientific knowledge and clinical skill, and physicians were becoming interested in the specialized field.

Since the 1910s, the number of physician anesthesia training programs had increased and the possibilities for research in the field had expanded. Professional groups of medical anesthetists started to form and tensions between physician anesthetists and nurse anesthetists escalated. As early as 1928, the California Board of Medical Examiners adopted a resolution and mailed it to all hospitals in California—requesting the termination of nurse anesthetists on the grounds that they were practicing in violation of the state's medical practice act.[83]

With the devastation of the American economy in the 1930s, tensions between physician anesthetists and nurse anesthetists increased even further. Hopeful that organization, standardization, and unity in nurse anesthesia practice would help, the National Association of Nurse Anesthetists voted to affiliate with the American Nurses Association. However, the American Nurses Association was hesitant to assume legal responsibility for a group that could be charged with practicing medicine without a license and refused to accept the nurse anesthetists' request to affiliate.[84] As it turned out, the American Nurses Association's fears were not unfounded. In 1934, the Los Angeles County Medical Association, represented by William V. Chalmers-Francis, sued nurse anesthetist Dagmar A. Nelson for "the illegal practice of medicine."[85] The trial began on July 12, 1934, and lasted 12 days. In the end, the judge decided in Nelson's favor, concluding that:

> *The administration of general anesthetics by the defendant Dagmar A. Nelson, pursuant to the directions and supervision of duly licensed physicians and surgeons, as shown by the evidence in this case, does not constitute the practice of medicine or surgery . . . and . . . constitutes the practice of nursing within the meaning of the laws of the State of California.*[86]

In response, Dr. Chalmers-Francis filed another suit against Nelson in 1936, which again resulted in a ruling *for* nurse anesthetists.[87] In 1938, the physicians appealed the case to the California *Supreme* Court. When the case was heard, the amicus curiae [letters that supported the nurses] submitted by the National Association of Nurse Anesthetists argued that the reason for this lawsuit was primarily that nurse anesthetists were taking work away from physicians during a time of national economic hardship.

The National Association of Nurse Anesthetists also noted that they believed "that safety of the patient is the most important thing to be considered in determining whether nurse anesthetists ought to be permitted to administer anesthetics." Relying on their positive relationships with surgeons and the American Hospital Association, they further explained: "the nurse anesthetist is content to rest her case with surgeons and laymen alike on that single proposition."[89]

Upholding the decisions of the lower courts, the California Supreme Court ruled in favor of Nelson, stating that she was not practicing medicine because she was "under the immediate direction and supervision of the operating surgeon."[90] Thus, in 1938 legal precedent was established: the administration of anesthesia by a nurse was *within* the scope of nursing practice and *not* the practice of medicine. The landmark decision soon became known as "The Captain of the Ship Doctrine," referring to the fact that the operating surgeon was "captain of his ship" and responsible for everything that happened in the operating room, including the nurse anesthetist's practice. The ruling would have lasting implications for nurse anesthetists' practice for years to follow.[91] In the short term, the decision was timely; nurse anesthetists would be in demand in civilian hospitals and in the military just a few years later when the United States entered World War II.

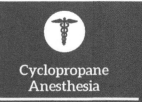

Cyclopropane Anesthesia

"Introduced by Ralph Waters in 1934, cyclopropane offered the advantage of decreased pulmonary irritation for inhalation anesthesia and less agitation during induction."[82]

Nurse Anesthetists: An Economic Threat to Medicine

"Since the onset of the economic disturbance of the past few years, agitation has sprung up in certain quarters to restrict the right to administer anesthetics to . . . licensed physicians, thus eliminating nurse anesthetists from the field of anesthesia. We believe that the aforesaid economic disturbance and the agitation against the nurse anesthetist bear a direct relationship."[88]

National Association of Nurse Anesthetists, 1938

NURSES IN OFFICES, ON AIRPLANES, AND ON PASSENGER TRAINS

A far cry from delivering anesthesia in the operating room, some nurses turned to new venues for work. Some accepted employment in industrial plants and private medical offices, where duties varied according to the job setting. Writing in the *American Journal of Nursing* in 1935, Mabel Detmold described some of the challenges of office nursing, including the variation in skills needed and the challenges of dealing with the telephone:

> *The kind of office assistance required by a doctor will vary according to the branch of medicine or surgery practiced. A nurse in the office of a neurologist will find that her duties differ greatly from those for a dermatologist. . . . To preside over the telephone is fast becoming an art.*[92]

While office nurses mastered the telephone, a handful of nurses who found work as nurse-stewardesses on airplanes and passenger trains faced other challenges. The nurse-stewardesses' purpose was to ensure the safety and comfort of the American public as they traveled. Airlines first employed nurses; railroads followed within a few years. There were never enough positions open, however; most nurses who applied for the jobs were turned away. According to one note in a 1938 edition of the *American Journal of Nursing*, there were "relatively few openings for nurses in the transportation lines at the present time."[93]

For "the young, attractive, single nurse" who did manage to get a job as a nurse-stewardess on a passenger plane, it was a unique and rare opportunity, provided she did "not mind hours in the air, temporary lodging in distant hotels, and long flights back and forth between major U.S. cities." On May 15, 1930, Boeing Air Transport (the predecessor to United Airlines) hired registered nurse Ellen Church as head stewardess on the Boeing 80A from Oakland/San Francisco to Chicago. Making the "20-hour journey with 13 stops," Church's role was to keep the 14 passengers calm, comfortable, and safe during the flight.[94] Over the next 8 years, other airlines followed suit. By 1938, five airlines employed a total of 326 nurses.[95]

The role of the nurse on a passenger train was similar to that of the nurse in the air: she was to ensure the safety and comfort of the travelers. In August 1935, officials of the Union Pacific Railroad "selected seven graduate nurses . . . to serve on the popular tourist deluxe coach train, the *Challenger*."[96] Similar to the requirements for the airlines, any nurse applying for a job on a passenger train had to be young and present "an attractive personality and appearance." Physical requirements included: "age 25 to 28, height 5' 3" to 5' 7", and corresponding weight of 125 to 145 pounds." In addition, each nurse had to be "registered and a member of the American Nurses Association." It was also essential that the nurse demonstrate "adaptability in understanding situations confronting her."[97]

The nurse's "adaptability" was particularly important. Eunice Hoevet described the role in the *American Journal of Nursing*, noting:

> *The first duty of the stewardess was to assist mothers in the care of their children. With fifty children under the age of five on one train, one nurse found plenty to keep her busy—bottles to be sterilized, formulas to prepare, and vegetable and cereal feedings to be served. Each nurse learns to know the different types of formulas prescribed by pediatricians from every section of the country.*[98]

THE RISE OF HOSPITAL NURSING

During the late 1920s and 1930s, nurse leaders were advocating for changes in nursing education, particularly regarding the practice of staffing hospitals with student nurses. In their final report, the Grading Committee "strongly urged the increased employment of graduate nurses for bedside nursing," and by 1938, the National League for Nursing Education emphasized the

Nursing on the Union Pacific

"Diabetic, chronic cardiac and asthmatic patients are frequent travelers. They are usually educated to their symptoms . . . but at the same time . . . grateful for the attention of the nurse on board. . . . The young mother traveling to California with three children and suffering from asthma could not administer her own hypodermic injections of adrenalin when her attacks became severe. The nurse remained with her until she was relieved."

Eunice Hoevet, 1937

"A physician may be secured at any time en route."[99]

Eunice Hoevet, 1937

need "for larger numbers of general staff nurses in hospitals that had training schools . . . to safeguard the care of patients . . . and to stabilize the nursing service."[100]

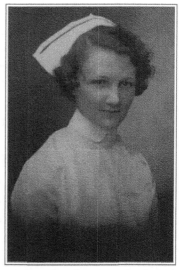

At the same time, nurse leaders stressed the importance of raising standards in nurse training schools and closing those of poor quality—those whose directors would "barter professional standards for a mess of pottage."[101] In addition, some nurse leaders advocated for the 8-hour workday for special duty nurses. As nurse leader Stella Goostray wrote:

> There are still employable nurses who are not employed sufficiently to provide [them with] basic economic security. Yet we still have nurses working twenty-four hours, twenty hours, and twelve hours. We must not turn back in our effort until the eight-hour working day for graduate nurses is universally accepted.[102]

Theodora Wynbeek, RN.

Meanwhile, new graduates continued to flood the market, many looking for work in hospitals. With the beginning of Blue Cross and Blue Shield health insurance, patients could afford to go to the hospital and hospitals needed nurses to care for them. With increasing numbers of surgeries and hospital deliveries, as well as developments in technology and science, hospitals needed graduate nurses who could assume leadership and clinical positions, and could supervise students.[103] Writing to the *American Journal of Nursing* in 1935, Sophie Nelson stated her thoughts on the matter, noting that, "The day of freelance nursing is over, and because of the tendency to have health services paid for in hospitals under some group insurance plan, . . . nurses will be employed under the auspices of some agency."[104]

As the 1940s approached, Sophie Nelson's prediction became a reality. Hospital administrators employed 5,700 more general staff nurses in 1937 than they had in 1935.[105] By 1941, 100,000 nurses were working in general duty positions in hospitals. They would be needed. The entry of the United States into World War II would create an unprecedented demand for nurses at home and abroad.

For Discussion

1. What factors converged to change opportunities for nurses in the Great Depression?
2. In the migrant camps, how did nurses combine their role as agents of the government with the traditional nursing values of caring and social justice?
3. What challenges did nurse anesthetists face during the Great Depression?
4. What is the significance of the California Supreme Court decision in *Chalmers-Francis v. Nelson* for nurse anesthetists today?
5. Discuss transitions in nursing during the Great Depression. Do you think nurses gained or lost professional autonomy during the 1930s?

NOTES

1. Editorial, "In 1932," *American Journal of Nursing* (hereafter *AJN*) 33, no. 1 (January 1933): 1–4 (quote 1).

2. Adam Cohen, *Nothing to Fear: FDR's Inner Circle and the Hundred Days that Created Modern America* (New York: Penguin Books, 2009): 14.

3. "Editorial," *AJN* 33, no. 5 (May 1933): 469–472 (quote 469).

4. Jean Whelan, "'A Necessity in the Nursing World': The Chicago Nurses Professional Registry, 1913-1950," *Nursing History Review* 13 (2005): 49–75 (quote 55).

5. Barbara Brodie, "Nurses' Struggles during the Great Depression: Prelude to Professional Status," *Windows in Time: The Newsletter of the UVA School of Nursing Center for Nursing Historical Inquiry* 20, 1 (April 2012): 8–12.

6. Francis Helen Zeigler, "Relief Employment," *AJN* 34, no. 8 (1934): 760–763 (quote 760).

7. "Editorial," (May 1933), 469.

8. "The Open Forum," *AJN* 3 (March, 1930): 343–244 (quote 344).

9. Ibid., 344.

10. Whelan, "A Necessity," 62.

11. Ibid., 61.

12. Editorial, "Private Duty and Unemployment," *AJN* 33, no. 12 (December 1933): 1177–1179 (quote p. 1178).

13. Zeigler, "Relief Employment," 761.

14. M. Louise Fitzpatrick, "Nursing in the Great Depression," *AJN* 75, no. 12 (December 1975): 2188–2190 (quote 2190).

15. "WPA Projects for Registered Nurses," *AJN* 37, no. 1 (January 1937): 35–37 (quote 37).

16. Ibid.

17. "History of Gee's Bend," https://www.prairiebluff.com (accessed September 1, 2016): 1.

18. Sanora Babb, "Research Notes," Sanora Babb Collection, file 19.2: "Migrant Labor," Special Collections, Harry Ransom Archives, University of Texas, Austin.

19. Timothy Eagan, *The Worst Hard Time: The Untold Story of Those Who Survived the Great American Dust Bowl* (New York: Harcourt Publishing, 2006).

20. Michael R. Grey, "Dustbowls, Disease, and the New Deal: The Farm Security Administration Migrant Health Programs, 1935-1947," *Journal of the History of Medicine and Allied Sciences* 48 (1993): 3–39 (quote 3).

21. Russell Freedman, *Children of the Great Depression* (New York: Clarion Books, 2005): 65.

22. Case History, Louis Family, Hollenberg Collection, Bancroft Library (hereafter HC-BL), carton 2, folder 25, 1–5 (quote p. 3).

23. Grey, "Dustbowls, Disease," 10.

24. Ralph Williams, "Nursing Care for Migrant Families," *AJN* 41, no. 9 (1941): 1028–1032 (quote 1030).

25. Mary Sears, "The Nurse and the Migrant," *Pacific Coast Journal of Nursing* 37, no. 3 (March 1941): 144–146.

26. "The FSA's Low Cost Medical Program," HC-BL, Farm Security Administration, carton 2, folder 2, 1.

27. Sanora Babb, "Report," Sanora Babb Collection, Special Collections, Harry Ransom Archives, University of Texas, Austin.

28. Freedman, *Children of the Great Depression*, 13.

29. Sears, "The Nurse and the Migrant," 144–145.

30. Mary Sears, "The Flat-Tired, Flat-Tired People," "Voices from the Past," in *The Californians*, ed. Anne Loftis (March–August 1989): 14–17, 58 (quote 15).

31. Laura Bolt, "Nutritionist's Report," in Anita Faverman, Edna Rockstroh, Freda Whyte, and Laura Bolt, *Report of the Second Year of the Migratory Demonstration Project, July 1937—June 1938*, HC-BL, carton 2, folder 2:11, 1, 28–38.

32. Arlene Keeling, "Nursing the Migrants in the Great Depression: Floods, Flies and the Farm Security Administration," ch. 7 in *Nursing Rural America*, eds. John Kirchgessner and Arlene Keeling (New York: Springer Publishing, 2015): 103–119 (quote 107).

33. Farm Security Administration Case Report (1938), HC-BL, carton 2, folder 2–11, 1.

34. Williams, "Nursing Care," 103.

35. Anita Faverman, Edna Rockstroh, and Freda Whyte, "Trailing Child and Maternal Health," *Report of the Second Year,* HC-BL, University of California (hereafter UC)-Berkeley (1937–1938): 38.

36. Ibid., 32.

37. Quoted in Keeling, "Nursing the Migrants," 109.

38. Faverman et al., "Report of the Second Year," 32.

39. Ibid., 29.

40. Agricultural Workers Health and Medical Association (hereafter AWHMA), HC-BL, UC-Berkeley, container 2, folder 2:1, 1.

41. Eric Thomsen, "Migratory Labor—Asset or Liability," speech to the Bakersfield Rotary Club (July 29, 1938): 1–14 (quote 5), HC-BL, UC-Berkeley. Thomsen was the assistant regional director in charge of California Migrant Labor Camps.

42. Faverman et al., "Report," 34–35.

43. Wanda Mann, "Migrant Nursing," *Pacific Coast Journal of Nursing* 37, no. 11 (November 1941): 658–660 (quote, 658).

44. Sears, "The Flat-Tired, Flat-Tired-People," 14–17, 58.

45. Sanora Babb, "Research Materials, Farm Security Administration Work, 1936-1940," file 18.8, Sanora Babb Collection, Special Collections, Harry Ransom Archives, University of Texas Austin.

46. Grey, "Dustbowls, Disease," 18.

47. Faverman et al., "Report," 32.

48. Grey, "Dustbowls, Disease," 18.

49. Sears, "The Nurse and the Migrant," 145.

50. Michael R. Grey, *New Deal Medicine: The Rural Health Programs of the Farm Security Administration* (Baltimore, MD: Johns Hopkins University Press, 1999): 94.

51. Ibid., 97.

52. Ralph C. Williams to Coffey (October 1939), Region XI, United States Department of Agriculture (hereafter USDA), Farm Security Administration (hereafter FSA), General Correspondence files, 1935–1942. RG 96, National Archives and Record Administration (hereafter NARA), Federal Records Center, Seattle, p. 1.

53. "Announcement," *Indio Camp Newsletter* (September 16, 1939), NARA, San Bruno, Record Group (hereafter RG) 96, Regional Guides and Research Aids (hereafter RR) Case Files (hereafter CF) 32-163-01.

54. Mrs. Crain, "Camp Nurse," letter in *Covered Wagon News* (July 19, 1941), Shafter Migratory Camp, NARA, San Bruno, RG96, FSA, box 2, RR CF27-163-01.

55. "Health News," *Indio Camp Newsletter* (August 12, 1939), NARA, San Bruno, RG96, FSA, RR CF32-163-01.

56. Indio Camp Nurse, "What to Remember about Whooping Cough," *The Migratory Clipper Newsletter,* Indio Camp (December 9, 1939), NARA, San Bruno, RG96, RR CF32-163-01.

57. Pauline Koplan, quoted in Grey, "Dustbowls, Disease," 19.

58. *The Weedpatch Cultivator* (January 1939), NARA Archives, San Bruno, RG96, RR CF32-163-01.

59. AWHMA, HC-BL, UC-Berkeley, (carton) container 2, folder 2:1, 7.

60. Mabel Berry, "Florida ERA Social Service and Public Health Program," speech to the Sixth Annual Meeting of the Florida Public Health Association, Inc., Jacksonville, Florida (December 3–5, 1934), Florida State Archives, RG810 S899, box 1, folder 1, 1–6 (quote 4).

61. Christine Ardalan, *Warm Hearts and Caring Hands* (Miami, FL: Centennial Press, 2005): 70.

62. Ruth Mettinger, "Public Health Talk," speech to the Sixth Annual Meeting of the Florida Public Health Association, Inc., Jacksonville, Florida (December 4, 1934), Florida State Archives, RG810 S899, box 1, folder 1, 4.

63. Ruth Nulting, "Public Health Talk," speech to the Sixth Annual Meeting of the Florida Public Health Association, Inc., Jacksonville, Florida (December 4, 1934), Florida State Archives, RG810 S899, box 1, folder 1, 2.

64. James Snyder, *Black Gold and Silver Sands: A Pictorial History of Agriculture in Palm Beach County* (Palm Beach, FL: Historical Society of Palm Beach County, 2004): 100.

65. Ibid.

66. Ibid.

67. Ibid.

68. Mettinger, "Public Health Talk," 3–4.

69. Berry, "Florida ERA," 2.

70. Fitzpatrick, "Nursing in the Great Depression," 2188–2190.

71. Felina M. Ortiz, "History of Midwifery in New Mexico: Partnership between Curandera-Parteras and the New Mexico Department of Health," *Journal of Midwifery and Women's Health* 50, no. 5 (October 2005): 411–417 (quote 411).

72. Ibid., 415.

73. Ortiz, "History of Midwifery in New Mexico," 415.

74. John E. Lesch, "Prontosil," ch. 3 in *The First Miracle Drugs: How the Sulfa Drugs Transformed Medicine* (New York: Oxford University Press, 2007).

75. Dorothy Best, "Sulphanilamide and Nursing Care," *AJN* 37, no. 9 (September 1937): 950–952 (quote 950).

76. Ibid., 951.

77. Advertisement, *AJN* 39, no. 12 (1939): 36.

78. Arlene Keeling, "Nurse Anesthetists, 1900-1938," ch. 2 in *Nursing and the Privilege of Prescription* (Columbus: The Ohio State University Press, 2007): 28–48.

79. Marianne Bankert, *Watchful Care: A History of America's Nurse Anesthetists* (New York: Continuum Publishing, 1989): 79.

80. Ibid.

81. "AANA Timeline, created for 75th anniversary," http://www.aana.com/resources2/archives-library/Pages/Timeline-of-AANA-History.aspx (accessed January 16, 2005): 1.

82. Rebekah Carmel, *Over the Drape: Olive Berger and Blue Baby Anesthesia, 1944–1954* (PhD dissertation, University of Virginia, 2015): 129.

83. Ibid.

84. Virginia Thatcher, *History of Anesthesia with Emphasis on the Nurse Specialist* (New York: Lippincott, 1953).

85. Agnes McGarrell, Official Reporter, Superior Court California, July 1934. *Transcript on Appeal, Volume I, in the Supreme Court of the State of California,* William V. Chalmers-Francis, William Dewey Wightmann, George P. Waller, Jr., and Anesthesia Section of the Los Angeles County Medical Association (Plaintiffs) v. Dagmar A. Nelson and St. Vincent's Hospital (Defendants). L.A. SC of Appeals No. 364130, RG08113, American Association of Nurse Anesthetist's Executive Office, Historical Files (hereafter AANA HF), Chicago, Illinois (1934), 95–345.

86. "Findings of Fact and Conclusion of Law in Recent Nurse-anesthetist Decision," *Western Hospital Review* 41, 3 (September 1934): 11.

87. *Chalmers-Francis v. Nelson,* cited in Arlene Keeling, "Nurse Anesthetists: Practicing Medicine without a License?" ch. 2 in *Nursing and the Privilege of Prescription* (Columbus: The Ohio State University Press, 2007): 45–58.

88. Brief of National Association of Nurse Anesthetists, Amicus Curiae, in the Supreme Court of the State of California, L.A. No. 15162. 1–2, AANA, HF, Chicago.

89. Ibid., 2.

90. *Chalmers-Francis v. Nelson,* cited in Keeling, "Nurse Anesthetists," 45–58.

91. Keeling, "Nurse Anesthetists," 47.

92. Mabel Detmold, "The Office Nurse," *AJN* 35, no. 8 (August 1935): 725–727.

93. "Planes, Trains, Ships and Nurses," *AJN* 38, no. 11 (November 1938): 1199–1201 (quote 1201).

94. Shane Nolan, "United Airlines Celebrates 80 Years of the Flight Attendant Profession," avstop.com/.../united_arilines_celebrates_80_years_of_the_flight_attendant_profession (accessed August 26, 2016): 1.

95. "Planes, Trains, Ships and Nurses," 1199–1201.

96. Eunice Hoevet, "Nurse Stewardesses, Nursing Takes to the Railroad," *AJN* 37, no. 1 (January 1937): 18–20 (quote 18).

97. Ibid., 18.

98. Ibid., 18.

99. Ibid., 19.

100. "More General Staff Nurses," *AJN* 38, no. 2 (1938): 186–190 (quote 186).

101. Stella Goostray, "What Lies Ahead for the Nursing Profession?" *AJN* 35, no. 8 (August 1935): 765–771 (quote 769).

102. Ibid., 769–770.

103. Brodie, "Nurses' Struggles," 9.

104. Sophie Nelson, "Social and Economic Factors as They Affect Nursing Services to the Public," *AJN* 35, no. 10 (October 1935): 943–946 (quote 945).

105. "More General Staff Nurses," 186.

FURTHER READING

Bankert, Marianne, *Watchful Care: A History of America's Nurse Anesthetists* (New York: Continuum Publishing, 1989).

Brodie, Barbara, "Nurses' Struggles during the Great Depression: Prelude to Professional Status," *Windows in Time: The Newsletter of the UVA School of Nursing Center for Nursing Historical Inquiry* 20, no. 1 (April 2012): 8–9.

Brown, Rosa, "A Negro Nurse in the 'Glades'," *Opportunity: Journal of Negro Life* XV, no. 11 (November 1937): 336–338.

Fitzpatrick, M. Louise, "Nursing in the Great Depression," *American Journal of Nursing* 75, no. 12 (December 1975): 188–190.

Grey, Michael R., "Dustbowls, Disease, and the New Deal: The Farm Security Administration Migrant Health Programs, 1935-1947," *Journal of the History of Medicine and Allied Sciences* 48 (1993): 3–39 (quote 3).

Grey, Michael R., *New Deal Medicine: The Rural Health Programs of the Farm Security Administration* (Baltimore, MD: Johns Hopkins University Press, 1999).

Keeling, Arlene, "Nurse Anesthetists, 1900-1938," ch. 2 in *Nursing and the Privilege of Prescription* (Columbus: The Ohio State University Press, 2007): 28–48.

Keeling, Arlene, "Nursing the Migrants in the Great Depression: Floods, Flies and the Farm Security Administration," ch. 7 in *Nursing Rural America*, eds. John Kirchgessner and Arlene Keeling (New York: Springer Publishing, 2015):103–119.

Mann, Wanda D., "Migrant Nursing," *Pacific Coast Journal of Nursing* 37, no. 11 (November, 1941): 658–660.

Ortiz, Felina M., "History of Midwifery in New Mexico: Partnership between Curandera-Parteras and the New Mexico Department of Health," *Journal of Midwifery and Women's Health* 50, no. 5 (October 2005): 411–417.

Sears, Mary, "The Nurse and the Migrant," *Pacific Coast Journal of Nursing* 37, no. 3 (March 1941): 144–146.

Whelan, Jean, "'A Necessity in the Nursing World': The Chicago Nurses Professional Registry, 1913-1950," *Nursing History Review* 13 (2005): 49–75.

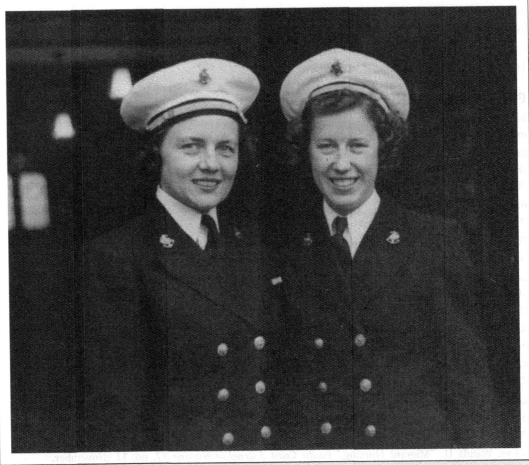

Navy nurses.

CHAPTER 11

Nursing in World War II: Overseas and at Home

1940–1945

Arlene W. Keeling

"American nurses are needed now in great numbers to care for the armed forces and to relieve the suffering of helpless people in our hospitals, in air raid shelters, and in the evacuation line of 'target' cities. All American men and women will be listed for service to our country. Many thousands more nurses are needed to perform services which only the professional nurse can give. . . . If you are a graduate of a school meeting Red Cross requirements, if your health is good, if you are not over fifty years of age, apply today for enrollment in the national nursing reserve of the Red Cross."[1]

Writing in the January 1942 issue of the *American Journal of Nursing (AJN)*, director of the American Red Cross Nursing Service, Mary Beard, made this urgent appeal for nurses to serve in the military. The need was acute; only weeks before, with the December 7, 1941, Japanese attack on U.S. battleships anchored in Pearl Harbor, war had become a grim reality.[2] Since 1939, the Red Cross Nursing Service had been working to build up an enrollment of nurses for the possibility of the United States' entry into the war in Europe, but, as *AJN* editor Mary Roberts noted: "the emergency lacked drama," and nursing recruitment efforts "fell on deaf ears."[3] Nursing leaders had made some efforts toward recruitment. In July 1940, with Germany's Adolf Hitler controlling much of Western Europe, representatives of national nursing organizations, several federal agencies, and the Army and Navy Nurse Corps had formed the Nursing Council on National Defense to plan for war.[4] However, in December 1941, fewer than 1,000 nurses were on active duty with the military. Now that would change as the U.S. declaration of war on Japan, Germany, and Italy provided American nurses "a new and powerful unity of purpose."[5]

In the months that followed the attack on Pearl Harbor, thousands of nurses enlisted in the military, volunteering to care for soldiers overseas and in military camps throughout the United States. Others cared for civilians on the home front, working in organizations like the U.S. Public Health Service, the Indian Health Service, the Frontier Nursing Service in Appalachia, or in local hospitals, schools, and industrial plants.

NURSING OVERSEAS

Not all American nurses waited for the United States to enter the war before they volunteered their services. By the late 1930s, some American nurses were serving with the British and French in Europe; others were in "Zone of the Interior" in existing army hospitals within the continental United States and its outlying territories.

Mayo Clinic nurse Martha Thevoz was one of those serving in Europe. She had volunteered to help the Allies and was working in the American Hospital in Paris when the Germans attacked the city in 1940. She and others like her were in the thick of the battle in Europe.

Meanwhile, other military nurses were working within the United States and its outlying territories, far from the scenes of battle. About 50 Army nurses were stationed in four military hospitals in isolated areas of Alaska.[7] Lucille Carter recalled the routine nature of their work there: "No one was often sick and there were no battles. The nurses spent most of the day trying to make life easier for the soldiers and officers—dancing with the officers nightly and [making cookies] for the soldiers."[8] For the nurses, the real challenges were in dealing with loneliness, boredom, slow mail service, and the harsh realities of the weather—the "grey wet blanket" of the Aleutian fog in summer and the frigid wind and snow of winter.[9]

Letter From Martha Thevoz, 1940

"*War is more or less at Paris' gates. Yesterday, June 34rd, there was heavy bombing of the city . . . we are at our post near our wounded soldiers during the bombardment. Our first duties on the floors are: Close the shutters and windows, draw the curtains, close the gas and stay with the patients. These men, during an air raid, get very nervous because they have just come from the battlefields where they were so heavily bombarded. Now, there are over 100 men here—mostly head or spinal cases . . . these men are desperately ill and have suffered such a great shock. Every nurse is doing her utmost.*"[6]

Martha Thevoz, 1940

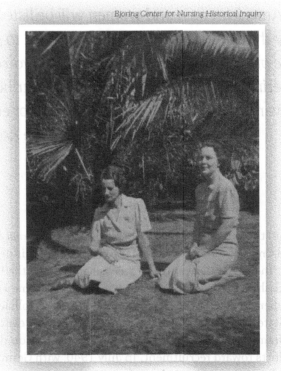

Bjoring Center for Nursing Historical Inquiry

Navy nurses relaxing.

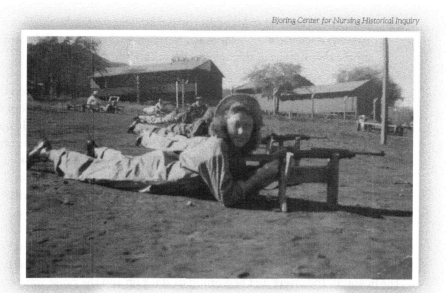

Nurses were instructed how to shoot properly in field training in Ie Shima.

By the fall of 1941, some Army and Navy Nurse Corps volunteers were stationed on the Hawaiian Islands; others on islands scattered throughout the South Pacific, including Ie Shima and islands in the Philippines. The majority of the nurses were young women eager to serve their country, eager for adventure and travel, and thrilled to be assigned to a "charmed life" in a tropical paradise.[10] All had no idea of what would happen if the United States actually entered the war.

The Nurses of Pearl Harbor

Fewer than 100 military nurses were in Pearl Harbor, Hawaii, in early December 1941, some in the Navy and others in the Army Nurse Corps. Among them was Ruth Erickson, who had joined the Navy Nurse Corps in 1936. She had served on the USS *Relief* from November 1938 until April 1940 when she was transferred to the U.S. Naval Hospital in Pearl Harbor. Erickson was there, "talking over coffee," on Sunday morning, December 7, 1941, when the Japanese launched their surprise attack on the harbor, sinking five battleships and severely damaging several others. As she later recalled:

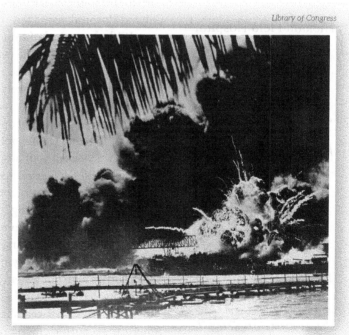

> *My heart was racing, the telephone was ringing, the chief nurse . . . saying, "Girls, get into your uniforms at once! This is the real thing!" I was in my room by that time; changing into uniform. . . . Smoke was rising from the burning ships . . . I ran to the orthopedic dressing room, drew water into every container, and set up the instrument boiler. The first patient came at 8:25 a.m.*

Immediately after the Japanese attack on December 7, 1941, the nurses stationed at Pearl Harbor attended to the thousands of wounded soldiers and base personnel.

with a large opening in his abdomen and bleeding profusely. . . . Then the burned patients streamed in. . . . There was heavy oil on the water and the men had dived off the ship and swum through it to Hospital Point.[11]

On that "day that would live in infamy," 76 Army nurses were serving in two Army medical facilities: Tripler General Hospital, and Schofield Hospital, both in Oahu.[12] Six others were stationed at the newly opened, 30-bed Hickam Field Hospital, located on Hospital Point in Pearl Harbor. Among them was Monica Conter, a second lieutenant in the Army Nurse Corps, who had arrived in Hawaii only a few months earlier.

Conter was on duty at Hickam when the bombing began. She flew into action, evacuating patients from the hospital's third floor to the first floor where they would be safer. Suddenly the power went out; all of the clocks stopped at 7:55 a.m.[13] Within minutes, casualties started to arrive. Meanwhile, the bombing continued. Conter recalled the chaos: "All of these patients were coming in, and we were putting them all out on the porch. There were some who were killed, and we were putting them out in the back yard behind the hospital. They were just beginning to stack up and the noise was terrible."[14]

The scene in front of the hospital was sheer chaos. Conter recalled the nurses' efforts at treatment while patients waited for surgery or transfer:

In the meantime, we were giving morphine. . . . They gave us 10cc syringes. We would fill those . . . and go down that porch giving shots . . . trying to stop the hemorrhaging and the pain . . . we would give it just as fast as we could. . . . We told them not to let anyone give them another shot. . . . We went in to fill up and came back out where we left off and gave more. . . . That was the only thing we knew to do in the middle of all of this.[15]

The wounded and those carrying them swarmed Hickam's front lawn; trucks and ambulances filled the driveway. In less than an hour the 30-bed hospital had exceeded capacity. The team refocused their efforts, converting Hickam into an evacuation hospital. All critical cases were sent to Tripler General Hospital, just a few miles away.

With the arrival of hundreds of casualties, nurses at Tripler were also overwhelmed. Nurse Nellie Osterlund, who had been awakened by the bombing, was so terrified by the radio broadcast ordering all personnel to the hospital that she could barely control her shaking fingers to button her uniform. By the time she reported for duty, the injured were already pouring in. Shifts were unending; eight operating teams worked continuously for 11-hour stretches.[18] Second Lieutenant Elma Asson, an operating room nurse, worked around the clock without stopping until she was finally ordered off duty.[19]

The nurses' experience at Schofield Barracks mirrored that at Hickam Field and Tripler. Army doctors, nurses, and volunteers worked continuously throughout the day and night to provide care to the deluge of casualties. As Army nurse Myrtle Watson recounted: "the three days following the attack were a blur of activity," during which time the staff survived on chocolate bars and coffee while "nursing dying men, giving morphine and whiskey, filling old vodka bottles with hot water to serve as hot water bottles, checking vital signs and placing basins under the thin mattresses to catch the leaking blood."[20]

Casualties on December 7 included 2,403 dead and 1,178 wounded Americans—both civilian and military.[21] By sunset that day, the influx of patients into Hawaii's military hospitals had decreased; now hospital per-

"We hoped we were saving their lives, keeping them from pain, and maybe stopping some of the hemorrhaging.[16]

Monica Conter, 1941

Hickam Field Hospital on December 7, 1941

"Inside the hospital, doctors, staff, and volunteers were overwhelmed by the ferocity of the attack and the number of wounded flooding the facility. There were only six of us nurses, and we couldn't possibly begin to take care of all the wounded and dying men. The decision was made to treat patients with first-aid-type care and send them to Tripler General Hospital in ambulances. Soon there weren't enough ambulances so the local people drove patients in their cars."[17]

Sara (Sally) Entrikin, 1941

sonnel had to deal with the difficulties of fear of another attack and caring for the wounded in total blackout conditions.

That same day (already December 8 in the Philippines), the Japanese also attacked the Army and Navy bases in the Philippines, targeting Camp John Hay and then Clark Air Field. The attacks killed 100 soldiers and wounded 93 others. Over the next weeks repeated bombings caused more casualties and the staff of 14 Army and three Filipino nurses at Fort Stotsenberg Station Hospital struggled to care for the critically injured soldiers. By Christmas 1941, all of the nurses of Fort Stotsenberg had to be evacuated to Manila, as attacks continued; however, on December 26, 1941, General Douglas MacArthur, the commander of the U.S. Army in the Far East, ordered the nurses' evacuation to Bataan. There they worked in General Hospital 1 on Manila Bay and General Hospital 2, located further inland in the jungle.[22]

Under continuous Japanese attacks, General Hospital 1 was soon forced to evacuate, while the numbers of patients at General Hospital 2 mushroomed. In that makeshift jungle hospital, the nurses worked in open-air wards under the trees; they placed their patients in old iron beds on mattresses stuffed with rice straw. Food and supplies were scarce or nonexistent, flies swarmed, and water had to be obtained from the Real River nearby.[23] Making do with what they could find, the nurses did their best to provide their patients with food and fluids.

Only months later, after continuous enemy attacks, on April 8, 1942, the 88 nurses of General Hospital 2 were ordered to retreat from Bataan and go to Corregidor. For the next months, they lived and worked underground in the Malinta Tunnel until they were forced to surrender to the Japanese.[25]

On July 2, 1942, the Army nurses from Bataan and Corregidor became Japanese prisoners of war, joining 11 navy nurses who had been forced to surrender earlier. Both groups would spend the next several years in Japanese internment camps, suffering from severe malnutrition, but continuing to nurse others in the camp.[27]

While the war raged in the Pacific in the opening months of 1942, millions of U.S. citizens mobilized for war. Young men from every state enlisted in the military or were drafted into service. With the increase in military personnel came the ever-increasing demand for nurses.

A National Campaign for Nurses

The sudden demand for nurses after the United States entered the war was immediately manifested in a national campaign to recruit them. Recruitment posters appeared on billboards, in magazines, in trains and buses, all speaking to the need. Within 6 months, the number of military nurses increased from 1,000 to 12,000. Both Black and White nurses responded to the calls, but only White nurses were accepted. Racial prejudice and the widely accepted social norm of segregation presented a significant barrier; military officials and nurse leaders could not fathom an integrated nurse corps. In fact, the war was close to ending before the military accepted African American nurses.

Meanwhile, White Army nurses received only "relative rank" and Navy nurses received "officer's privileges." Both of these designations amounted to "an officers' uniform and title without an officer's commission, retirement privileges, dependents' allowances, or pay."[29]

Male nurses were also underutilized—not only because very few men were nurses but also because the Army refused to commission them as officers, a designation that

"Food was so scarce, the last ration we received in the camp was two bags of moldy rice for over 4,000 people."[28]

Madeline Ullom, 1942

"I was in charge of feeding 90 people from a 12 quart bucket . . . a kind of Bataan stew with maybe mule or horsemeat . . . even monkey . . . with rice and a few green weeds."[24]

Hortense McKay, 1942

In the Malinta Tunnel

"I wish I could forget those endless, harrowing hours. Hours of giving injections, anesthetizing, ripping off clothes, stitching gaping wounds . . . sterilizing instruments, bandaging . . . covering the wounded we could not save. . . . While it's happening there's a sort of blessed numbness that keeps you going, keeps you making the right moves, finding the right things to do."[26]

Juanita Redmond, 1942

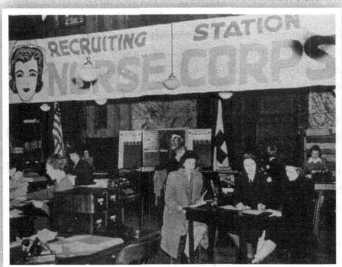

Nurse recruiting stations helped swell the numbers of enlisted nurses from 1,000 to 12,000 in the 6 months after Pearl Harbor.

"The troops moved fast and we hardly stayed in one place more than a few days. There were so many casualties as we followed the battles, working steadily, then moving on, setting up and working again."[31]

Esther Edwards, 10th Field Hospital, 1942

would identify them in rank and privilege as separate from medical corpsmen. The Army Medical Department eventually allowed men to join the Red Cross Reserve, but never let them work as nurses under military command during World War II.

Nurses in the European Theater

With America's declaration of war in 1941, the military mobilized teams of medical and nursing personnel, sending some to Europe and others to the Pacific. Some worked in field hospitals, close to the front lines. Others staffed general hospitals in towns and cities farther away. In a middle zone were the evacuation hospitals.

The mobile evacuation hospitals were particularly needed in Europe where U.S. General George S. Patton used rapid maneuvers of the Third Army to attack the enemy. He expected supplies, equipment, and medical support to keep pace with him. Thus, numerous field and evacuation hospitals followed battles from North Africa into Italy, France, Belgium, and Germany. These units provided emergency treatment to the wounded, after which the men were sent farther back from the front lines to general hospitals in cities and towns near the battle zones. The Eighth Evacuation Hospital kept pace with the fighting in North Africa and Italy from 1942 to 1945, its staff packing up repeatedly to move from one battle to another, contending with mud and snow as the seasons changed.[30]

The typical 750-bed evacuation hospital was mobile, constructed of canvas tents that could be disassembled easily and moved along with the army. When possible, it might be situated near buildings that could also be used. Specifications mandated that an evacuation hospital have a total of at least 417 personnel with 47 commissioned officers, 52 commissioned nurses, and 328 soldiers.[32]

Nurses in the Eighth Evacuation Hospital

The Eighth Evacuation Hospital, organized by the University of Virginia hospital, was typical of hundreds of other military evacuation units sponsored by major U.S. hospitals during the war.[33] On February 27, 1942, the secretary of war approved the formation of the Eighth Evacuation Hospital, one of 23

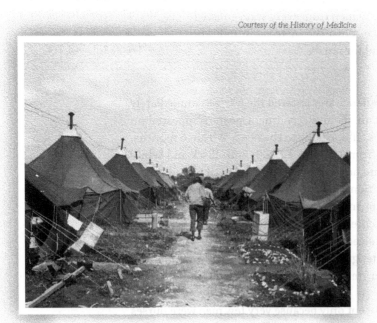

Ambulance turn around area, 8th Evacuation Hospital, Italy.

that would be mobilized by March 1943.[34] University of Virginia's Dr. Staige Blackford and Chief of Surgery E. Cato Drash had responsibility for recruiting all personnel. Blackford immediately recognized the need to have an experienced nurse as supervisor. Professional nursing leadership would be critical to the effective and efficient running of an evacuation hospital. Years earlier, Blackford had met Ruth Beery when she was a science instructor in the University of Virginia's School of Nursing. Writing to her at the University of Minnesota where she was employed, Blackford convinced Beery to return to Virginia and accept the job of chief nurse. She was a perfect choice for the leadership position: she had a calm temperament, remained composed under pressure, and focused on the welfare of her staff and patients.[35]

> "If American boys are going into danger, it is up to America's nurses to care for them. That is our duty and we cannot escape it."
>
> Ruth Beery, 1942

Ruth Beery first had to recruit nurses—a task more difficult than she had imagined, and she spent a great deal of time on correspondence and travel to do so. The newly commissioned First Lieutenant Beery spoke to nursing groups in cities and towns throughout Virginia in an effort to procure enough nurses.[36]

Gradually, the Eighth Evacuation Hospital's roster grew as nurses responded to Beery's call. In early spring 1942, the unit was completely staffed; its personnel ready for training and deployment. After basic training at Camp Kilmer, New Jersey, the Eighth Evac received orders to deploy. On November 1, 1942, the unit traveled to New York City where unit personnel boarded a troop transport ship, the *Santa Paula*. The next day the ship set sail, crossing the Atlantic in a convoy of 35 to 40 ships. The Eighth Evac was headed for North Africa, to take part in Operation TORCH, the first large-scale offensive military operation the Allies executed. Securing North Africa would give the Allies a staging platform from which to launch an invasion of Sicily and Italy, in the hope of defeating the German forces who occupied that territory.[37]

Operation TORCH provided the Eighth Evacuation Hospital nurses with their first experience in the combat theatre. During this extensive campaign, mobile field hospitals and evacuation hospitals played a critical role. Once stable enough to move from the front, a wounded soldier was evacuated to a field hospital where he received emergency care. From there he was transferred to an evacuation hospital 3 to 30 miles from the front lines, where nurses would perform triage, sending the soldier who was sick to a medical tent, and the one who was injured to a surgical tent. If seriously injured and needing intensive nursing care, the patient would be admitted to a shock ward.

Arrival in North Africa

"There were pools of blood beneath some of them [soldiers], where dressings had not been changed since the first shock dressing was applied in the field. I don't know how the other girls felt, but I experienced at once a violent anger—bitter, surging anger—against the people that out of greed and power and lust would cause such things to happen to young manhood."[38]

Ruth Haskell, 1942

Nurses in the shock ward worked 12-hour shifts—longer when heavy fighting caused increased casualties. In this setting, the boundaries between medicine and nursing blurred as nurses took on tasks that were customarily performed by physicians. In addition to their usual tasks of monitoring vital signs and administering antibiotics, morphine, tetanus toxoid, and other medications, the nurses started blood transfusions, performed phlebotomy to collect blood samples, gave oxygen, and changed bandages.[39]

Bjoring Center for Nursing Historical Inquiry

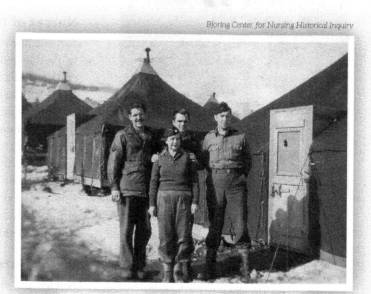

Ruth Beery, chief nurse at Eighth Evacuation Hospital.

Once stabilized, patients were sent to the operating room where circulating and scrub nurses worked as part of the surgical team. In the case of the Eighth Evacuation Hospital, the operating room was housed in a cramped embassy building where doctors and nurses operated "in the face of swarms of flies . . . falling plaster, and a failing sewage system."[41]

When casualties poured in after a battle, the teams worked round the clock. Modern warfare often caused severe chest wounds from high-velocity bullets and shrapnel. Wounds that prevented adequate ventilation, such as sucking chest wounds and hemothorax, required urgent thoracotomy. Chest wall debridement, placement of chest tubes, and thoracentesis were all commonplace, and nurses assisted physicians in an efficient and coordinated effort to complete the procedures.

With a shortage of physician anesthetists during the war, nurses were also asked to give anesthesia. Dorothy Sandridge, a 21-year-old nurse with the Eighth Evacuation Hospital, was one of many nurses who responded to an advertisement to do so.

After only a few weeks of training in the art and science of anesthesia administration, Sandridge and the other nurse anesthetists worked side-by-side with the surgeons for 16-hour shifts, collaborating in a united effort to save the injured soldiers. Recalling her work in Italy with Dr. Prentice Kinser, Jr., Dorothy Sandridge stated: "I think he knew, instinctively, that I was having kind of a difficult time being so young and so new at everything and he just couldn't have been nicer to me . . . He taught me to do IVs and all that, because in those days nurses didn't learn how to do IVs when they were in school."[42]

During the time spent in Italy, the Eighth Evacuation Hospital admitted 6,597 patients and had only 33 deaths—in part because the critically injured died before they reached the evacuation hospital, and in part because of two advances in medicine: the widespread use of penicillin and the establishment of a hospital-based blood bank. Interprofessional collaboration was also a key to success. By 1945, the nurses, physicians, and enlisted men of the Eighth Evacuation Hospital had provided care for more than 70,000 patients. As Sandridge later recalled, "we [were] all in it together."[44]

Nurses of the 26th General Hospital

Not all nurses worked in evacuation hospitals. Some worked in general hospitals further from the front. General hospitals were the more permanent structures, sometimes built as one-story wooden buildings with a capacity of 1,000 beds, and in other instances established in confiscated buildings. From December 7, 1941 to July 1, 1942, 15 General Hospitals were sent to theaters of war around the world. Among these was the 26th General Hospital sponsored by the University of Minnesota, sent first to England and then to North Africa. Arriving without supplies, the unit had to "make do" for several weeks, with the nurses outfitted in oversized men's uniforms.[45]

Flight Nursing

Nurses and physicians were "all in it together"—on land, on the sea, and in the sky. Flight nursing, originating as

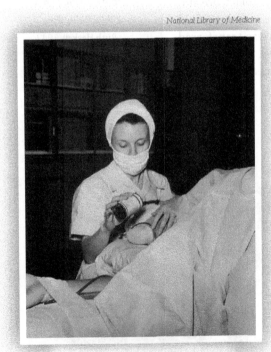

National Library of Medicine

A nurse anesthetist whose training was reduced from months to weeks due to the anesthetist shortage during the war.

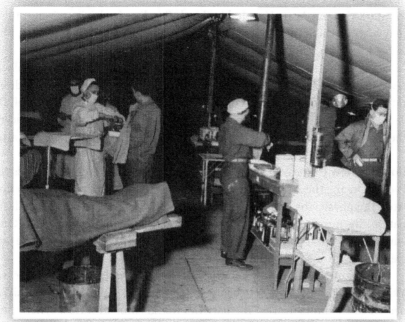

Operating tent in the 94th Evacuation Hospital, where patients were cared for at all hours immediately after a battle.

the Aerial Nurse Corps of America in the 1930s, rapidly developed into a division of the Army Air Force in June 1942. With the deployment of American servicemen to Europe and North Africa, "evacuation of the sick and wounded by air became a medical and military necessity."[47] According to Colonel Wood S. Woolford, evacuation by air required female flight nurses—the most highly trained medical personnel available for these missions. In November 1942, Air Surgeon Brigadier General David N. W. Grant issued a call for nurses, particularly those with "experience as stewardesses or pilots" to join the Army Nurse Corps for assignment as air evacuation nurses.

The nurses who responded received a month of intensive training at Bowman Field, Kentucky—the center of Air Force operations. Training for flight nursing included hands-on practice in loading and unloading air ambulances, as well as formal classroom instruction on military customs and the special ways of treating patients in the air. Among the topics were how to administer intravenous medications and oxygen at high altitudes, and what procedures to follow if the plane was shot down.

The training was important. No physician would be present on the medical evacuation planes and the nurses would be on their own. They would also be, according to General Grant, air surgeon of the Army Air Force, "closer to the front lines than any other group of women personnel" and could "expect . . . to be the target of enemy aircraft."[48] On Christmas day, December 1942, the newly trained flight nurses left Bowman Field. They were part of the 802nd Aeromedical Evacuation Squadron headed for North Africa.[49]

"We were trained to load the patients on litters with just the help of our corpsmen. . . . The plane was refitted to hold 18 litters; nine on each side, three tiers high. There was a small area for walking wounded and room for our rather large, very heavy medical kit."[50]

Nurse Margaret C. Hofschneider

Nurses in the Pacific Theater

While the war was raging in Europe, some medical units remained stateside, awaiting orders. The 71st General Hospital, organized by Mayo Clinic, was one of those, and included more than 50 nurses. Finally, after months of meetings and drills in Rochester,

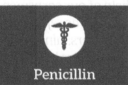

Minnesota, in December 1942 the nurses of the 71st General Hospital left for Stark General Army Hospital in South Carolina for basic training. There they learned the basics of life in the military, including how to salute, how to fire a weapon, and how to use a gas mask.[52]

In August 1943, new orders arrived and the 71st General Hospital was divided into two equal-sized Station Hospitals: the 233rd under the direction of Dr. Charles W. Mayo and the 237th under the leadership of Dr. James T. Priestley.[53] Accompanied by physicians, enlisted men, and officers, the nurses journeyed by train to Camp Stoneman, California. Soon after New Year's Day, 1944, they boarded the *New Amsterdam,* a troopship destined for New Guinea. After 14 days at sea, zigzagging their way across the Pacific Ocean, the hospital units arrived in Sydney, Australia.[54] A month later, the physicians, officers, and enlisted men set sail for their final destination. The nurses, under orders from Dr. Mayo, remained in Australia. Only when the hospital buildings and nurses' barracks had been built in the jungles of New Guinea were they allowed to set sail.[55]

Once in New Guinea, the nurses worked with physicians to treat casualties evacuated by air from the campaign against Japan.[56] One physician described the units' work: "The patients would come in waves. When there was action going on up north, there would be a lot of casualties," and the nurses, like everyone else on the medical teams, would be busy "around the clock."[57] Given the complications of wound infections during war, almost every casualty received penicillin—the new miracle drug.

When they were not caring for the wounded, the teams turned their attention to patients with infectious diseases. In the rain forest, "dysentery . . . malaria and scrub typhus" were common."[60] Mosquito-borne malaria was a particularly vexing problem and the staff members themselves were not immune. One of the nurses working with the 233rd Hospital developed cerebral malaria. According to Dr. Delmar Gillespie: "Everyone knew her and we were all concerned. . . . We gave her massive doses of intravenous Atabrine, and, by gad, she survived! And she wouldn't go home; she stayed there with us!"[61]

Living in open barracks "divided into individual cubicles," with "latrines, showers, and laundry facilities all within their stockade," the nurses considered themselves pretty lucky. Nonetheless, they were still at war and far from home. To cope with their homesickness and the boredom that set in during the slow days, the nurses turned to gardening, movies, dances, and music.

Nurses in the Normandy Invasion

On June 6, 1944 more than 150,000 Allied forces landed on five beaches along a 50-mile stretch of France's Normandy region. Thousands were killed or injured. No nurses were allowed to participate in the invasion but within a week Army officials decided that nurses were essential for the field hospitals to function. They ordered the nurses to cross the English Channel to France immediately. On June 10, the first nurses arrived in Normandy, some from the 51st Field Hospital, others from the 45th Field Hospital and the 128th Evacuation Hospital. Nurses from the 91st Evacuation Hospital and the 42nd Field Hospital soon joined them.[63] All worked with thousands of casualties over the following days; most of whom required surgery.

NURSING AT HOME

The departure of large numbers of nurses to serve in the military during the war left a shortage of nurses for civilians on the home front. Nurses were needed in traditional roles in public health departments, schools, clinics, and hospitals to replace those who had left to serve in the military. In addition, new federal programs for maternal–child health, an increase in manufacturing for the war effort, the creation of Japanese American internment camps, federal initiatives to increase the number of students in nursing schools, and restrictions on world travel for American missionaries all served to generate new opportunities for nurses.

Refresher Courses for Nurses

Responding to the increased demand for nurses in civilian hospitals and public health departments, hospitals throughout the country offered refresher courses for nurses who had earlier left the profession to become full-time

Library of Congress

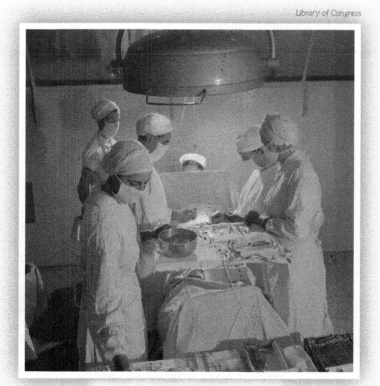

Nurses in the operating room attending to a patient in surgery.

Nurse Rivers and the Tuskegee Experiment, 1932–1972

Among those who did not receive penicillin were 399 poor, rural, African American men who were being studied for the long-term effects of untreated syphilis. Eunice Rivers, a trusted Black nurse in Macon County, Alabama, worked to keep them enrolled in the study, giving them vitamins, aspirin, and rides to the clinic. The study went on for 40 years, with publications in respected medical journals. "In a setting where there was neither racial, gender, nor class justice," Rivers was caught between keeping her job, supporting the White physicians who were conducting the study, and doing what was best for the men. Keeping silent, she may have found "the only solution she thought possible."[59]

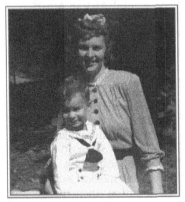

Charlotte Wynbeek traveled to Memphis, Tennessee, to join her husband on the naval base.

wives and mothers. Those who attended the refresher courses in hospital nursing or public health could return to active work in the profession—even if it was only on a part-time basis. The state of Ohio was typical of this trend, reporting that "687 graduate nurses enrolled for refresher courses" in that state in 1942, and 184 were "doing at least some part time work in hospitals."[65]

Other states, including Michigan and New Jersey, offered refresher courses for public health nursing and industrial nursing. One letter to the editor in the *AJN* was typical:

Public health nurses in Michigan who have been inactive during the past few years now have an opportunity to take a short, intensive refresher course arranged by the Michigan Department of Health. The course . . . includes a two-week period of lectures . . . on communicable disease control, maternal and child health, school nursing . . . and field practice.[66]

Nurses and the Emergency Maternal and Infant Care Program

Nurses were also needed to care for women and children in cities and towns surrounding military bases as thousands of women followed their enlisted husbands. Tacoma, Washington, located near the Fort Lewis army base, was one of the first military boomtowns flooded with "suitcase wives and 'storkers'"[68] (newlyweds and pregnant wives). In Tacoma, two problems became apparent almost immediately: a shortage of medical facilities for women and children, and the soldiers' inadequate income to pay for their families' care. Base hospitals were prepared for war, not women, and were ill-equipped to deal with the needs of new mothers, infants, and children. Moreover, private medical care was too expensive for most soldiers' families. The $28.00-per-month dependent allotment that the soldiers received was hardly enough to cover rent and other essentials—much less "the $50.00 fee charged by most physicians for a hospital delivery."[69]

National Library of Medicine

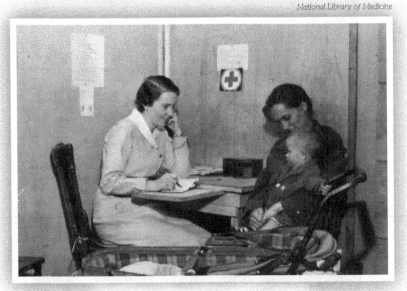

Providing care for a mother and child under the Emergency Maternal and Infant Care program.

In Fort Lewis, as local hospital obstetrical wards filled to capacity and nurses were stretched thin, military authorities and Washington State Health Department officials appealed to the U.S. Government's Children's Bureau for help. They needed to fund a program that would include obstetrical deliveries, prenatal and postpartum care, and infant follow-up care. The request was granted. The program—Maternal and Child Hygiene Medical Care Program for Servicemen's Wives—provided maternal and infant medical care to military dependents in the Fort Lewis area. By July 1942, almost 677 women had registered for care under the program that would "protect mothers and babies" and "promote the best interest of the soldier."[70] The demand for this type of assistance spread: all over the United States military wives and their children needed care. As a result, on March 18, 1943, Congress passed the Emergency Maternal and Infant Care program.

The Emergency Maternal and Infant Care Act not only provided military families with care, but also opened up job opportunities for nurses. In civilian hospitals near military bases, local area nurses found jobs in obstetrical wards and newborn nurseries. Others found employment in public health departments. Additional public health nurses were needed to make antenatal visits and later follow patients after they gave birth, teaching young mothers how to care for their infants.[72]

Nurse Anesthetists and the Blue Baby Surgeries

While other nurses were being "refreshed" and retooled for work, nurse anesthetists continued to work in hospitals throughout the United States, giving anesthesia to thousands of patients. Their role was especially important during the war, as increasing numbers of physician anesthetists left for the military.

At the Johns Hopkins University Hospital in Baltimore, one nurse anesthetist would soon be involved in the cutting-edge "blue baby" surgeries performed by Drs. Alfred Blalock and Helen Taussig. The innovative surgery, called the Blalock–Taussig shunt, first done in 1944, repaired the cardiac anomaly, Tetralogy of Fallot, also known as the "blue baby syndrome." The repair allowed more of the baby's blood to return to the lungs for oxygenation, thereby reducing the cyanosis that babies with this condition experienced. Present at the first operation, nurse anesthetist Olive Berger administered the anesthesia. After that, Blalock requested her presence for the majority of his surgical procedures. In fact, Berger kept a detailed notebook of the first 100 cases, as well as the 475 succeeding cases. Recognized for her expertise and skill, Berger was appointed an instructor in anesthesia at the Johns Hopkins School of Medicine.[74]

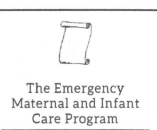

The Emergency Maternal and Infant Care Program

In 1943, Congress passed the Emergency Maternal and Infant Care Act, funding it with special appropriations. The new program provided free maternal care to thousands of pregnant women as well as care to the infants of military personnel until 1949.[71]

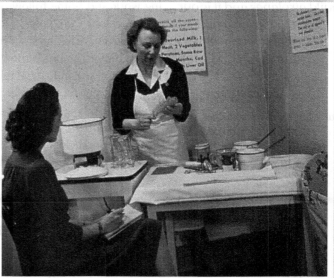

National Library of Medicine

A nurse teaching a patient as part of the Emergency Maternal and Infant Care Act, passed by Congress in early 1943 and designed to give free care to pregnant women and infants.

"Lots of places had nurse anesthetists but also had a physician anesthetist in charge . . . but we didn't. Dr. Blalock did not want it, and Dr. Blalock had great faith in us."[73]

Olive Berger, Nurse Anesthetist, 1946

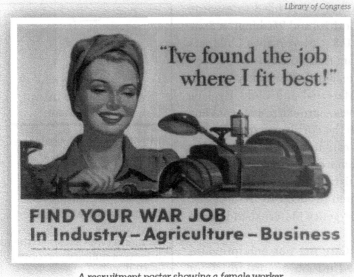

"I've found the job where I fit best!"

FIND YOUR WAR JOB
In Industry – Agriculture – Business

A recruitment poster showing a female worker.

Nurses in Industry

The exponential increase in manufacturing for the war effort also provided new employment opportunities for nurses. Manufacturing plants, particularly those that produced airplane parts, textiles for soldiers' uniforms, parachutes, and ammunition, could not afford any production slowdowns due to employee injuries or illness. Keeping both male and female workers healthy and on the job was a priority, and having nurses on site in the factories could help companies meet this goal. The increase in the number of nurses employed at Lockheed Aircraft Corporation was typical of other manufacturing plants. Lockheed had initiated a visiting nurse department in 1939, and by 1942 the department had nine visiting nurses on staff, covering work and home follow-up care at both Lockheed and its affiliate, the Vega Airplane Company.[75]

"Sick or injured men cannot build airplanes and it is our job to help get a patient back on the job with as little delay as his health and general condition will permit."[76]

Nurse Louise Davidson, Lockheed
Aircraft Corporation, 1942

In industrial nursing, much of the nurses' work was dedicated either to first aid or the prevention of injury. According to a report by Lockheed's chief nurse, the industrial nurses dealt with eye injuries, tuberculosis, first aid, sore throats, and infections. They also kept a list of possible blood donors and advised workers on "the use of dust respirators."[77]

In addition, nurses ensured that safety precautions were taken, insisting on such modifications as adequate lighting in hallways, safety shoes for ladders, and the use of facemasks for personal protection.[78]

Nurses' work in large plants could be intense. Nurse Leona D. McConnell worked for the McNeil Construction Company in Las Vegas, Nevada, and wrote of her experience there:

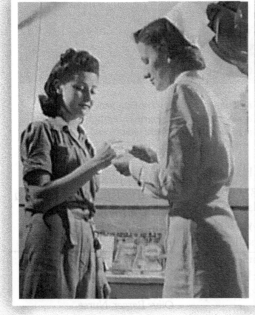

Our company is doing all the construction for basic magnesium, which you no doubt have read a lot about. It is a big defense plant and hazards are many, although our department has been given many compliments on our work in handling chlorine gas patients and hot magnesium metal burns.[80]

A full-time plant nurse attending to a worker's injured finger so she can return to making dive bombers, 1943.

Opportunities in industrial nursing grew as the war continued and more and more women joined the production lines. In 1941, there were 5,512 nurses in factories throughout the United States; by 1943 that number had more than doubled, reaching 11,220. Nonetheless, these numbers represented only 6% of nurses in active duty in the United States. Hospitals and schools of nursing employed 39%, while the U.S. Public Health Service employed 10%.[81]

A poster encouraging chest x-rays to detect
tuberculosis and keeping sick workers at home.

Experience of an Industrial Nurse

"The work is mainly first aid,
with much clerical work
included. We have a main
First Aid station with several
sub-stations out on the area.
The 15-bed hospital, which is
to serve as an emergency
hospital only, will soon be
ready and we're anxious to get
settled there. Patients needing
indefinite hospitalization are
taken to Baraboo or Madison.
With about 9,000 employees
here, we are kept busy and
have about 200–250 cases
each day. The plant itself is
immense, covering an area of
ten square miles."[79]

Ann Eubank, 1942

Nurses in Japanese American Internment Camps

During World War II, the U.S. Public Health Service also needed additional nurses, not only for the usual public health nurse jobs but also to care for those held in the newly built Japanese American internment camps. Immediately after the attack on Pearl Harbor, U.S. government authorities began a program in which they arrested Japanese Americans, who lived on the west coast of the United States, seizing their assets, closing Japanese banks, and revoking Japanese business licenses. It was a regrettable plan of action begun in hatred for the Japanese and fear that Japanese Americans would aid the enemy. It only got worse. On February 19, 1942, President Franklin Roosevelt signed Executive Order 9066, authorizing the identification of military areas from which any or all persons of Japanese descent, even if they were Americans, could be denied their freedom. The order denied Japanese Americans their civil liberties. A series of

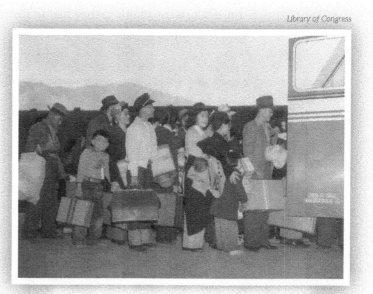

Japanese Americans waiting to board a bus to landlocked
internment camps established as part of Executive Order 9066,
leaving their belongings, businesses, and lives behind in 1942.

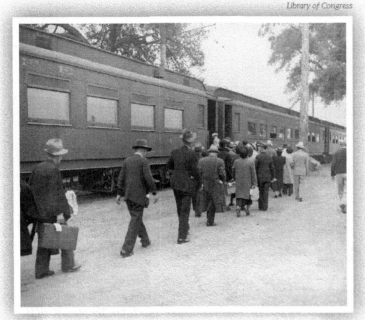

Japanese Americans boarding a relocation train at Santa Anita, California, destined for an internment camp.

public proclamations and orders came in quick succession and Japanese Americans from the coasts were sent first to staging areas (often in unused barns and storage sheds on fairgrounds) and later to 10 relocation camps in areas of the interior of the country.

The areas of the interior had been designated because of the availability of water, nearby railroads, and space for growing food. However, geographic isolation, extreme environmental temperatures, and sudden dust storms often defined the camp locations.[82] The camps included Manzanar and Tule Lake in California, Colorado River (Poston) and Gila River in Arizona, Topaz in Utah, Minidoka in Idaho, Heart Mountain in Wyoming, Granada in Colorado, and Jerome and Rohwer in Arkansas. Enclosed with barbed wire and surrounded by military outlook towers, the camps were designed to keep Japanese Americans isolated from American society and away from any possibility of helping the enemy.

The camps, modeled after military bases, needed doctors and nurses. Each camp had a group of hospital buildings: administration, doctors' and nurses' quarters, general patient wards, outpatient clinics, obstetrical areas, surgery, pediatrics, isolation, and a morgue. Standard wooden barracks wrapped in black tar paper served as housing; common buildings housed mess halls, laundry rooms, and latrines. Entire families crammed into tiny spaces partitioned by walls that did not reach the ceilings. In summer, the uninsulated barracks were stifling; in winter, snow sifted in. In such conditions, infections spread rapidly. Nurses had to deal with epidemics of measles, colds, chickenpox, and tuberculosis. In addition, they had to institute public health measures to prevent the epidemics in the first place.

Both the U.S. Public Health Service and the Bureau of Indian Affairs assigned physicians and nurses to the camps. However, both medical and nursing personnel were in short supply. While some were recruited from the civilian sector, for the most part Japanese American doctors and nurses who had already been evacuated to the camps staffed the hospitals and clinics themselves.[83]

Camps also relied on young Nisei (second-generation Japanese American) women who were trained to work as nurse aides. These young women provided most of the direct patient care, including bathing and feeding patients. They also assisted in orphanages. Training as a nurses' aide did provide the

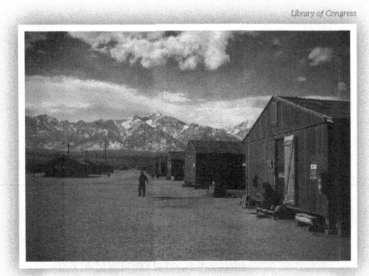

Camp Manzanar in California, which processed 11,070 Japanese Americans from 1942 to 1944.

young Nisei with opportunities, however. Having been introduced to nursing in the camps, many young Nisei aides were eager to become nurses. When the U.S. Cadet Corps program began in 1943, providing free training for thousands of student nurses without racial and ethnic discriminatory policies, almost 200 young Nisei women enrolled.[84]

Due to the severe shortage of nurses, in some camps authorities resorted to hiring Black nurses—despite the prevalent racial prejudice in America and the existing segregation laws. The African American nurses proved themselves to be a valuable asset. Discussing Black nurses, Elizabeth Vickers, the supervisor nurse at Poston camp, noted:

> *Their total contribution to the nursing service surpasses that of both the white nurses and the evacuee nurses . . . they are the only ones who have been ready and willing to do everything requested of them within their range of ability, such as operating room and delivery room duty, classroom teaching for nurses aides and supervision of nurses aides on the wards, night duty as well as day duty, outpatient service as needed, all of which they have done with efficiency and ease.*"[85]

The American Red Cross Volunteers and the Cadet Nurse Corps

To meet the increased demands for nurses on the home front and to prepare new nurses for the military, the federal government created two new programs: the American Red Cross Volunteer Nurse's Aide Program in 1941 and the Cadet Nurse Corps in 1943.[86] One would provide immediate help for nurses in civilian hospitals at home; the other would prepare a new generation of registered nurses for the future.

The American Red Cross volunteer program, begun early in 1941, grew in popularity after the United States entered World War II. Citizens wanted to help and hospitals across the nation opened their doors to American Red Cross volunteers. Saint Marys Hospital, part of Mayo Clinic in Rochester, Minnesota, did so early in 1942. Women volunteers, called "Grey Ladies," prepared surgical dressings, delivered reports from the clinical laboratories to the

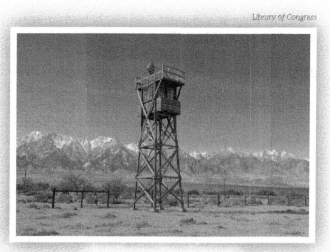

Watchtower at Camp Manzanar.

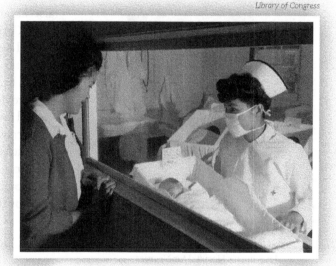

A Japanese American nurse showing a baby in an internment camp nursery.

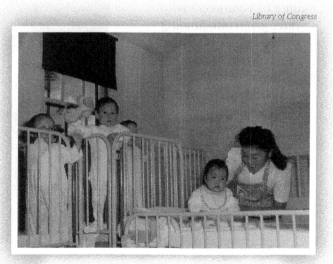

A nurses' aide playing with children in an orphanage at Camp Manzanar, 1943.

wards, helped in nursery schools for the nurses' children, and supplied patients with magazines. They also organized linen closets, changed babies' diapers, transported patients in wheelchairs, answered call-lights, made beds, filled water pitchers, and put away supplies. In short, they did everything the nurses asked them to.[88]

The Grey Ladies at Saint Marys were not the only women who volunteered. By 1945, more than 165,000 lay women in the United States had taken the Red Cross volunteer nurses' aide course and were serving more than "a million hours a month" in hospitals and other nursing agencies across the country.[89]

The wartime nursing shortage, however, could not be met with Red Cross volunteers alone; nursing schools would have to graduate more nurses and would have to do so quickly. To do that, schools needed money, faculty, and students who had full scholarships. Congresswoman Frances Payne Bolton (Ohio) sponsored federal legislation in 1942 to establish the Cadet Nurse Corps. Congress passed the bill (also known as the Nurse Training Act) creating the Cadet Nurse Corps of the Public Health Service on June 15, 1943. The bill subsidized the education of students who agreed that after they graduated, they would serve in military or civilian health agencies for the duration of the war. Students were provided tuition, fees, and books, along with a monthly stipend for the length of their training. Participating schools also received funds for instructional facilities and postgraduate education for their nursing faculty.

To administer the program, the U.S. Public Health Service established the Division of Nurse Education within the Office of the Surgeon General with Lucile Petry (later Petry Leone) as director. Because the Bolton Act stipulated that

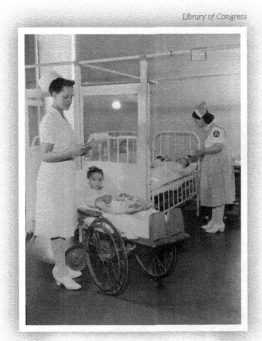

Red Cross volunteer nurses' aides at Freedmen's Hospital for Negroes tending to patients.

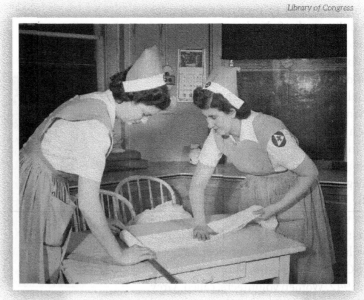

Red Cross volunteer nurses' aides rolling bandages.

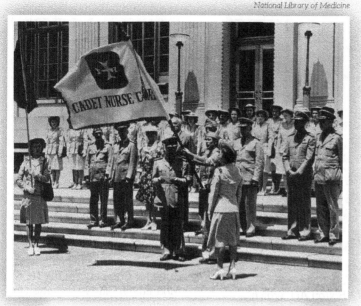

Cadet nurses standing behind the Cadet Nurse Corps flag.

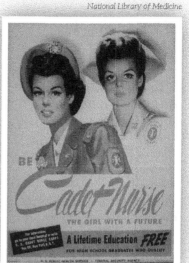

A recruitment poster for the Cadet Nurse Corps, which subsidized students' education if they worked in civilian or military health agencies for the remainder of World War II.

there "shall be no discrimination . . . on account of race, creed, or color," nursing schools throughout the United States immediately opened their doors to applicants from diverse backgrounds and from all races, including African Americans and Japanese Americans.[91] Saint Marys School of Nursing and the Kahler School of Nursing, both associated with Mayo Clinic in Rochester Minnesota, admitted Japanese American women, some directly from the internment camps. Fumiye Yoshida Lee arrived at Mayo Clinic from the Minidoka Relocation Camp. According to Lee: "It was a fantastic opportunity to be accepted at one of the best hospitals in the United States . . . [The program] opened doors to us when we were facing discrimination."[92]

One of the requirements of the cadets in training was that in the last 6 months of their educational program, the seniors would cover shortage areas, filling in for nurses who had gone to war. Cadet nurse Florence Nudelman, who joined the Corps in 1943 in her second year of nursing school at Hahnemann Hospital in Pittsburg, was sent to Turtle Mountain Indian Reservation in North Dakota, where she worked with two physicians. In a small clinic, caring for the Chippewa, she took on the new responsibilities of taking blood pressures and attending births after one of the physicians had a heart attack. She called the one remaining clinic physician only when absolutely necessary.[94]

The Bolton Act set minimum educational standards for schools that trained cadet nurses and required the schools to have separate budgets from the hospitals with which they were affiliated. These policies, combined with federal money to the schools, had a significant impact on nursing education after the war, promoting the break from the hospital-based apprenticeship model of education to a university model. By the end of the war, the cadet nurse program had subsidized the education of nearly 179,000 nursing students in more than 1,125 schools.

Medical Mission Sisters in New Mexico

The war affected all nurses in the United States, regardless of their place of practice or their specialty. New opportunities arose due to various circumstances. In one case,

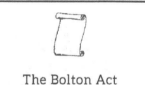

The Bolton Act

On June 15, 1943, Congress passed a bill introduced by Frances P. Bolton of Ohio, establishing the Cadet Nurse Corps. The bill had a major impact on the integration of nursing schools, as it stipulated that any nursing school receiving federal funds could not discriminate "on account of race, creed, or color."

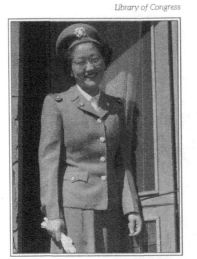

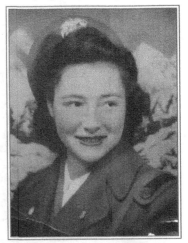

On Leaving an Internment Camp

"For three years I had lived with my family of seven members in one little room in a city of barracks. Leaving for the outside world, alone, was a little frightening. Arriving in Rochester, I was overwhelmed . . . St. Marys seemed enormous! . . . The standard of education [there] was the highest, the instructors were excellent, and the medical care, the finest!"[93]

Teruko Yamashita Okimoto, Cadet Nurse, 1945

Cadet Kay Fakudo, who served with the Cadet Nurse Corps under the Bolton Act, which forbid discrimination based on "race, creed, or color."

Cadet Florence Nudelman, who cared for Chippewa at the Turtle Mountain Indian Reservation in North Dakota.

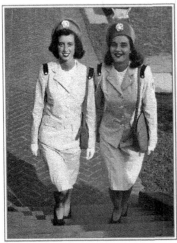

Cadets from the University of Virginia.

international travel restrictions coupled with medical and nursing shortages in all areas of the country provided a unique opportunity for a group of missionary nurses. The Medical Mission Sisters, a community of Catholic sisters founded in 1925 by Dr. Anna Dengel, usually worked in India. The travel restrictions, however, made them search for locations within the continental United States where they might be needed. They found a new place to serve in Santa Fe, New Mexico, where the shortage of physicians and nurses was severe, and maternal–infant death rates were "devastatingly high" among the predominantly Catholic, Spanish American population.[95]

Responding to this situation in 1944, the Medical Mission Sisters opened the Catholic Maternity Institute in Santa Fe, where they offered nurse-midwifery care to local Spanish American women. Originally, the Maternity Institute had two registered sister-nurse-midwives on staff: Sister Theophane Shoemaker and Sister Helen Herb, both graduates of the Lobenstine School for Nurse Midwifery in New York City.

At first, the Sisters attended births in their patients' homes. However, because many of the women lived long distances from the mission, in "unsuitable" conditions for birth in the home, the Mission Sisters soon opened "La Casita"—a tiny two-room adobe structure where they could attend maternity cases. La Casita's close proximity to Santa Fe's only hospital, St. Vincent's, facilitated rapid transfer of mothers and babies who experienced complications. A delivery at La Casita was safer, especially for high-risk mothers who needed careful monitoring.[97]

Advertisements highlighted that births at La Casita were "set up as nearly like a home as possible." One nurse-midwifery school alumna recalled:

The concept and actual functioning of La Casita was very unique, providing such a wonderful homelike atmosphere for the patient. It was a big factor in helping all of us, including the mother and husband, realize how normal and natural the experience of giving birth is meant to be.[98]

Thus, the care at the Maternity Institute emerged as a new solution to maternity care problems in Santa Fe in 1944 while providing the Medical Mission Sisters a new location in which to practice during the war.

The Frontier Nursing Service and War Shortages

Among those also affected by the war were the nurses of the Frontier Nursing Service in the mountains of Kentucky. For years, the Frontier nurse-midwives had prided themselves on their services to families living in Leslie County, Kentucky. They visited pregnant mothers, assisted with home births, and cared for their newborns. From the establishment of the organization in 1925 until 1939, the Frontier Nursing Service recruited experienced midwives from Great Britain to provide care to the people of Leslie County. Thus, the staff was decimated when Great Britain declared war on Germany in 1939, and 18 of 22 nurse-midwives from England decided to return to their own country. To replace them, Director Mary Breckinridge opened her own midwifery education school, admitting two students to the 4-month-long program on November 1, 1939. In the absence of midwives from England, Breckinridge trained *American* midwives.[99]

The shortage of midwives was not the only problem facing the Frontier Nursing Service. When the United States entered the war, the government directed all resources of iron and cotton toward military production, creating critical shortages of horseshoes and diapers throughout the country. The shortages nearly crippled the Service. In the remote Kentucky backwoods, horses provided the only transportation through creek beds, over rugged terrain, and up steep mountain paths to reach the families. Without horses, the midwives had to hike for days to an outlying cabin. Clearly, the nurses needed the horses and the horses needed shoes. Moreover, the Frontier nurses needed a steady supply of cotton diapers if they were going to help the impoverished Appalachian mothers. Frequently nurses not only offered nursing and medical care, but also gave basic necessities such as shoes, coats, diapers, and baby clothes to their patients' families. For newborns, the most important of these supplies were diapers.[100]

Breckinridge tackled the problem of the horseshoe shortage first, taking the issue to legislators in Washington, DC, but finding it "hard to convince officials that horseshoes were essential to childbirth."[101] Undaunted, Breckinridge argued that horseshoes were absolutely essential to the work of the Frontier nurses. In 1943, horseshoes were removed from the government's priority list for the war effort.[102]

Diapers were even more important to the nurses' work than horseshoes. Now, with the country's textile looms dedicated to making cotton for military uniforms, diapers were low on the manufacturing priority list and were in short supply nationwide. The shortage was so noteworthy, in fact, that Congresswoman Frances P. Bolton, a longtime Frontier nurse

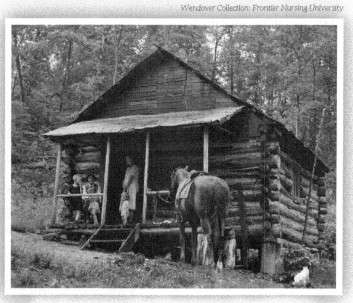

Wendover Collection: Frontier Nursing University

Frontier nurse at a cabin with a pregnant mother and children in the rural United States, where the shortage of nurses and nursing supplies was severe during the war.

supporter, referred to it as "the national problem of diapers," when she advocated that Congress address the issue. Meanwhile, to address the local problem of diapers for babies in Kentucky, Breckinridge appealed to her circle of wealthy friends around the country to send diapers. Even with this assistance, the diaper supply barely kept up with the demand.

Race and Gender Issues in the Military

Throughout the war, the Army Nurse Corps maintained restrictive racial quotas, and the Navy Nurse Corps excluded all African Americans. These restrictions, combined with the willingness of Congress to consider drafting nurses in 1944, turned public opinion against the armed services' discriminatory policies. As a result, in January 1945, both corps lifted their racial restrictions and accepted African American female nurses. Male nurses, however, faced a more entrenched form of military discrimination than their Black female nurse counterparts. Tradition and sentiment had long dictated that nursing was a woman's field, and Congress, in establishing the nurse corps, ruled that only women could be appointed as military nurses. Male nursing students and graduates were subject to the Selective Service Act draft, and most volunteered for military service rather than waiting to be drafted.

NEW DEVELOPMENTS

On February 3, 1945, the U.S. military rescued the nurses from the Santo Thomas internment camp. Later they welcomed them to Hawaii to recuperate and gain strength before going back to the mainland.

On May 8, 1945, Nazi Germany unconditionally surrendered to the Allied Forces, ending the war in Europe. On August 13, 1945, Japan also surrendered. More than 59,000 American nurses served in the Army Nurse Corps during World War II and over 201 Army nurses died while in service to their country.

After the war, the profession made further progress in its own war against discrimination on the basis of race and gender. In 1947, military nurses were awarded full

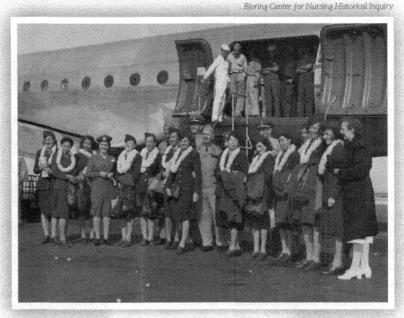

Bjoring Center for Nursing Historical Inquiry

Rescued nurses from the Santo Thomas internment camp in the Philippines.

commissioned status. Concurrent with the new policy came the end of racial segregation in the military and an end to discrimination toward male nurses.

When World War II came to an end, the presence of many more African American registered nurses, many of whom were graduates of the Cadet Nurse Corps, caused state nurses associations to remove racial barriers of membership. General integration into the American Nurses Association was hastened in 1948, when its House of Delegates called for racial integration at district and state levels and granted individual membership to African American nurses barred from their state associations. In 1950, only two state associations still had discriminatory racial practices and the National Association of Colored Graduate Nurses announced its dissolution. By 1952, all state nurses associations had removed racial restrictions for membership in the American Nurses Association.

Unfortunately, the end of overt professional discrimination against African American nurses and male nurses did not eradicate the more subtle and entrenched forms of prejudice. For Black nurses, the struggle to be fully accepted as professionals by patients, hospitals, and fellow heath care colleagues continued to be a problem.[106] The postwar years would see many changes: a rise in the growth of hospitals through funding from the Hill Burton Act, nursing shortages as more women chose to leave the workplace and return home, and an increase in obstetric care as birth rates boomed. Other changes would include the introduction of recovery rooms and intensive care units, a vaccine for polio, innovations in emergency care through MASH (Mobile Army Surgical Hospital) units during the war in Korea, and new opportunities for nurses in remote areas like West Texas, where drillers had just struck oil!

> ## Victory in Japan
>
> "After leaving the hospital ship Refuge, I was stationed at the Brooklyn Navy Hospital in New York. On V-J Day, four of us girls went to Times Square in our uniforms. What bedlam! It was a mass of people, and the sailors were going around kissing and hugging everyone. There is this famous photograph that is printed year after years as they commemorate the end of World War II. In it a sailor has a nurse in a big clinch and is kissing her, and I always look to see if we are in the picture."[105]
>
> Helen Wentz Miller,
> U.S. Navy, 1945

For Discussion

1. What was the impact of World War II on the nursing profession in the United States?
2. How did the Bolton Act, forming the Cadet Nurse Corps, affect nursing schools?
3. What changes occurred in the profession on the U.S. home front during World War II?
4. Discuss the impact of the Emergency Maternal and Infant Care Act on nursing and access to care.
5. Discuss the ethical and professional dilemmas facing nurses as they worked in Japanese internment camps in the United States during the war.

NOTES

1. Mary Beard, "A State of War Exists," *American Journal of Nursing* (hereafter *AJN*) 42, no. 1 (1942): 1.

2. Patricia Ballard, *Angels of the Mercy Fleet: Nursing the Ill and Wounded Aboard the U.S. Navy Hospital Ships in the Pacific during World War II* (PhD dissertation, University of Virginia [hereafter UVA], May 2000).

3. Mary Roberts, "We See the Face of Danger" (editorial), *AJN* 1 (January 1942): 62.

4. Judith Bellafaire, "The Army Nurse Corps: A Commemoration of World War II Service" (Washington, DC: U.S. Army Center of Military History). Last modified October 3, 2003, http://www.history.army.mil/books/wwii/72-14/72-14.HTM.

5. Mary Roberts, "We See the Face," 62.

6. Arlene Keeling, "Mayo Influences, Nursing Transitions, 1940-1970," ch. 3 in *The Nurses of Mayo Clinic: Caring Healers,* ed. Arlene Keeling (Rochester, MN: Mayo Clinic, 2012): 59–85 (quote 60).

7. Barbara Tomblin, *GI Nightingales: The Army Nurse Corps in WWII* (Lexington: University Press of Kentucky, 1996): 183.

8. Ibid., 185.

9. Ibid.

10. Elizabeth Norman and Sharon Elfried, "How Did They All Survive?" *Nursing History Review* no. 3 (1995): 105–107 (quote 105). See also: Elizabeth Norman, *We Band of Angels: The Untold Story of American Nurses Trapped on Bataan by the Japanese* (New York: Pocket Books, 1999).

11. "Oral History of the Pearl Harbor Attack, 7 December 1941, Lieutenant Ruth Erickson, NC, USN," https://ehistory.osu.edu/oral-histories/RuthErickson (accessed June 6, 2012).

12. Bellafaire, "Army Nurse Corps."

13. Gwyneth Milbrath, "The Bombing of Pearl Harbor, Hawaii, December 7, 1941," ch. 6 in *Nurses and Disasters: Global Historical Case Studies,* eds. Arlene Keeling and Barbra Mann Wall (New York: Springer Publishing, 2015): 145–167.

14. Ibid.

15. Ibid.

16. Ibid.

17. Gwyneth Milbrath, "We Just Had to Line Them Up," *Windows in Time: Newsletter of the Eleanor Crowder Bjoring Center for Nursing Historical Inquiry* (hereafter *ECBCNHI*) 22, no. 2 (October 2014): 9–11 (quote 10).

18. Tomblin, *GI Nightingales,* 15–16.

19. Mary Sarnecky, *A History of the U.S. Army Nurse Corps* (Philadelphia: University of Pennsylvania Press, 1999): 185.

20. Myrtle Watson, quoted in Tomblin, *GI Nightingales,* 15.

21. Milbrath, "We Just Had to Line Them Up," 11.

22. Sarnecky, *A History,* 187.

23. Norman, *We Band of Angels,* 43.

24. Sarnecky, *A History,* 189.

25. Ibid., 189.

26. Ibid., 190–191.

27. Norman and Elfried, "How Did They All Survive?" 105–107.

28. Madeline Ullom in Diane Fessler, *No Time for Fear: Voices of American Military Nurses in World War II* (East Lansing: Michigan State University Press, 1996): 92.

29. Philip A. Kalisch and Beatrice J. Kalisch, *American Nursing: A History,* 4th ed. (Philadelphia: Lippincott Williams & Wilkins): 302.

30. Patricia Kinser, "'We Were All in It Together': Medicine and Nursing in the 8th Evacuation Hospital, 1942-1945," *Windows in Time: Newsletter of the ECBCNHI* 19, no. 2 (November 2011): 7–11.

31. Fessler, *No Time for Fear,* 131.

32. "Capturing, Preserving and Interpreting U.S. Army Medical History," http://history.amedd .army.mil (accessed January 3, 2016): 1.

33. Teresa Opheim, "Mayo in the Pacific," Reprint, *Mayo Alumnus* (Spring, 1990): 3–14. Mayo Historical Unit (hereafter MHU), Mayo Clinic, Rochester, Minnesota.

34. "Capturing," http://history.amedd.army.mil.

35. Bill Brown, "Nursing in the 8th Evacuation Hospital, WWII," class Project (unpublished manuscript, UVA, 2009).

36. Ibid.

37. "Operation Torch: Allied Invasion of North Africa," http://www.historynet.com/operation-torch-allied-invasion-of-north-africa.htm (accessed December 20, 2015).

38. Tomblin, *GI Nightingales*, 71.

39. Brown, "Nursing in the 8th Evacuation Hospital."

40. Raymond Scott, "Eleventh Evacuation Hospital in Sicily," *AJN* 43, no. 10 (October 1943): 925–926 (quote 926).

41. Kinser, "We Were All in It Together," 10.

42. Ibid.

43. Ibid.

44. Ibid.

45. "26th General Hospital: Unit History," https://www.med-dept.com/unit-histories/26th-general-hospital (accessed June 20, 2016).

46. Keeling, "Mayo Influences," 64.

47. Judith Barger, "Origin of Flight Nursing in the US Army Air Force," *Aviation, Space and Environmental Medicine* 50, no. 11 (November 1979): 1176–1178.

48. Ruth White, "Army Nurses—in the Air," *AJN* 43, no. 4 (April 1943): 342–344 (quote 344).

49. Barger, "Origin of Flight Nursing," 1178.

50. Tomblin, *GI Nightingales*, 62.

51. The Kahler School of Nursing, "Alumnae," *The Link* (March 1944): 8.

52. Keeling, "Mayo Influences."

53. Mayo Vignette, "World War II: Mayo Goes to New Guinea," *Mayo Alumnus* 23, no. 2 (Spring 1987): 1–2.

54. Keeling, "Mayo Influences," 64–65.

55. "Historical Data," MHU: Station Hospital 233 and 237.

56. John Henderson, *A Brief History of the Army of the United States 71st General Hospital* (Rochester, MN: MHU, Mayo Clinic, September 1996): 1–3.

57. Opheim, "Mayo in the Pacific," 7.

58. Milton Wainwright, *Miracle Cure* (Cambridge, UK: Basil Blackwell, 1990): 6. See also: Barbara Brodie, "The Search for Penicillin," *Windows in Time: Newsletter of the ECBCNHI* 12, no. 2 (November 2004): 6–8, 11.

59. Susan Reverby, "Rethinking the Tuskegee Syphilis Study: Nurse Rivers, Silence and the Meaning of Treatment," *Nursing History Review* 7 (1999): 3–28.

60. Opheim, "Mayo in the Pacific," 7.

61. Ibid., 8.

62. Ibid., 9.

63. Tomblin, *GI Nightingales*, 127.

64. Ibid., 128.

65. "Refreshers Help Stretch Nursing Service," *AJN* 43, no. 1 (January 1943): 51.

66. "News about Nursing," *AJN* 43, no. 2 (February 1943): 214–231 (quote 216).

67. Matilda Davis, "Fiftyish and Refreshed," *AJN* 43, no. 5 (May 1943): 434–435 (quote 434).

68. Elizabeth Temkin, "Driving through: Postpartum Care during World War II," *American Journal of Public Health* 89 (1999): 587–595 (quote 588).

69. Vivian Pessin, Leona Baumgartner, and Helen M. Wallace, "Distribution of Costs under the Emergency Maternity and Infant Care Program," *American Journal of Public Health* 41 (April, 1951): 410–416.

70. Nena Patterson, *Protecting America's Future Citizens: An Historical Analysis of Nursing Roles in the Emergency Maternal and Infant Care Program* (PhD dissertation, UVA, 2011).

71. Ibid.

72. Anna Moore and Marie Chard, "Private Don Jones' Baby," *AJN* 43, no. 1 (January 1943): 46–50.

73. Olive Berger interview, cited in Rebekah Carmel, *Over the Drape: Olive Berger and Blue Baby Anesthesia, 1944–1954* (PhD dissertation, UVA, June 2015): 65.

74. Ibid.

75. Louise Davidson, "Rescuing Man Hours for Production," *AJN* 42, no. 2 (1942): 168–172 (quote 168). Davidson was chief nurse of Lockheed Aircraft Corporation, Burbank, California.

76. Ibid., 168.

77. Ibid.

78. Ibid.

79. Ann Eubank, "Letter to the Editor," *Saint Marys Alumnae Quarterly* (October 1942): 12, Saint Marys Hospital Archives, Mayo Clinic, Rochester, Minnesota.

80. Leona Dale McConnell, "Letter to the Kahler School of Nursing Alumnae News," *The Link* (June 1943): 10.

81. "Wartime Nursing is Different," *AJN* 43, no. 9 (September 1943): 835–838.

82. Susan Smith, "Women Health Workers and the Color Line in the Japanese American 'Relocation Centers' of World War II," *Bulletin of the History of Medicine* 73, no. 4 (1999): 590.

83. Rebecca Coffin, *Nursing in the Japanese American Incarceration Camps, 1942–1945* (PhD dissertation, UVA, 2015).

84. Smith, "Women Health Workers," 589.

85. Ibid., 594.

86. Susan Winters, *Enlightened Citizen: Frances Payne Bolton and the Nursing Profession* (PhD dissertation, UVA, 1997).

87. "Training Program Announced for 100,000 Nurses' Aides," *Hospital Management* 52 (September 1941): 44–45 (quote 44).

88. Elizabeth Wilson, "Alleviate Your Nursing Shortage with Aides," *AJN* 43, no. 3 (March 1943): 184–188.

89. Elizabeth Bell, quoted in Editorial, "A Nursing Service Adjusts to Wartime Pressures," *AJN* 44, no. 6 (June 1944): 537–540 (quote 540).

90. Ibid., 540.

91. "Cadet Nurse Corps," https://en.wikipedia.org/wiki/Cadet_Nurse_Corps (accessed May 29, 2017).

92. Fumiye Yoshida Lee, cited in Keeling, "Mayo Influences," 63.

93. Ibid.

94. Arlene Keeling, personal communication with Florence Nudelman Kornblat, RN, April 23, 2016.

95. Anne Cockerham and Arlene Keeling, "Finance and Faith at the Catholic Maternity Institute, New Mexico, 1944-1969," *Nursing History Review* 18 (2010): 151–166 (quote 153).

96. Catherine Shean, cited in Anne Z. Cockerham and Arlene W. Keeling, *Rooted in the Mountains, Reaching to the World: Stories of Nursing and Midwifery at Kentucky's Frontier School, 1939-1989* (Lexington: Frontier Nursing University, 2012): 156–157.

97. Ibid., 156.

98. Sister M. Paula D'Errico, in *CMI Graduates and Faculty Remember Nurse-Midwifery in Santa Fe, New Mexico*, eds. Rita Kroska and Catherine Shean (Tucson, AZ: Medical Mission Sisters/Catholic Maternity Institute Historical Project, 1996): 38.

99. Cockerham and Keeling, *Rooted in the Mountains*.

100. Ibid., 32.

101. Mary Breckinridge, *Wide Neighborhoods* (Lexington: University Press of Kentucky, 1952): 330.

102. Cockerham and Keeling, *Rooted in the Mountains*, 32–33.

103. Ibid.

104. Madeline Ullom, in Fessler, *No Time for Fear*, 93.

105. Fessler, *No Time for Fear*, 255.

106. Ibid.

FURTHER READING

Ballard, Patricia, *Angels of the Mercy Fleet: Nursing the Ill and Wounded Aboard the U.S. Navy Hospital Ships in the Pacific during World War II* (PhD dissertation, University of Virginia, May 2000).

Carmel, Rebekah, *Over the Drape: Olive Berger and Blue Baby Anesthesia, 1944–1954* (PhD dissertation, University of Virginia, June 2015).

Cockerham, Anne, and Keeling, Arlene, "Finance and Faith at the Catholic Maternity Institute, New Mexico, 1944–1969," *Nursing History Review* 18 (2010): 151–166.

Fessler, Diane, *No Time for Fear: Voices of American Military Nurses in World War II* (East Lansing: Michigan State University Press, 1996).

Milbrath, Gwyneth, "We Just Had to Line Them Up," *Windows in Time* 22, no. 2 (October 2014): 9–11.

Milbrath, Gwyneth, "The Bombing of Pearl Harbor, Hawaii, December 7, 1941," ch. 6 in *Nurses and Disasters: Global Historical Case Studies*, eds. Arlene Keeling and Barbra Mann Wall (New York: Springer Publishing, 2015): 145–167.

Norman, Elizabeth, *We Band of Angels: The Untold Story of American Nurses Trapped on Bataan by the Japanese* (New York: Pocket Books, 1999).

Reverby, Susan, "Rethinking the Tuskegee Syphilis Study: Nurse Rivers, Silence and the Meaning of Treatment," *Nursing History Review* 7 (1999): 3–28.

Robinson, Thelma, *Nisei Cadet Nurse in World War II: Patriotism in Spite of Prejudice* (Black Swan Mill Press, 2005).

Sarnecky, Mary, *A History of the U.S. Army Nurse Corps* (Philadelphia: University of Pennsylvania Press, 1999).

Smith, Susan, "Women Health Workers and the Color Line in the Japanese American 'Relocation Centers' of World War II," *Bulletin of the History of Medicine* 73, no. 4 (1999).

Temkin, Elizabeth, "Driving through: Postpartum Care during World War II," *American Journal of Public Health* 89 (1999): 587–595.

Tomblin, Barbara B., *GI Nightingales: The Army Nurse Corps in World War II* (Lexington: University Press of Kentucky, 1996).

Winters, Susan C., *Enlightened Citizen: Frances Payne Bolton and the Nursing Profession* (PhD dissertation, University of Virginia, 1997).

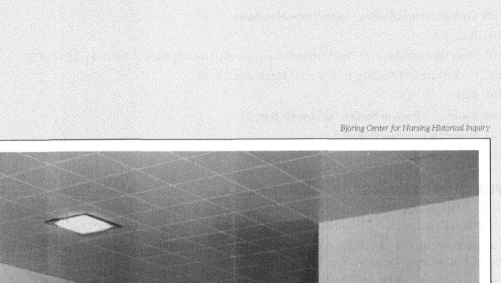

Nurses station.

CHAPTER 12

Mid-Century Transitions and Shortages

1945–1960

John C. Kirchgessner

"That the Call System is abused, I heartily agree; but, to ask a Director of a Nursing Service to be responsible for [the] functioning [of the hospital] . . . without permitting the Departmental Supervisors to be paged is difficult to understand. . . . To function adequately for the safety of the patient with the present conditions in the nursing world is a herculean task; we have exerted every effort to safeguard the patient through holding the Departmental Supervisor responsible for the young inexperienced graduate Charge Nurse and the student nurse alone on wards at periods of the day." [1]

Virginia H. Walker, January 14, 1946

In 1946, the director of nurses at the University of Virginia Hospital wrote these words to the hospital administrator, Dr. Carlisle S. Lentz, expressing her concern over a new rule regarding the paging system. Since the hospital's Executive Committee had not consulted with Walker, they had passed a rule that would ultimately hinder communication between the nurses and their supervisors, thus putting patient care in jeopardy. The new rule prohibited student nurses and new graduate nurses from paging their supervisor. Walker went on to note that the hospital now had a higher percentage of acutely ill patients than in previous decades and fewer private-duty nurses to care for them. [2] Under the new rule, nursing supervisors could not be paged over the intercom, making it impossible for them to know who needed them. They simply could not be everywhere, and new graduate nurses and student nurses covering wards at night often needed advice.

POSTWAR TRANSITIONS

Even without the new "paging" issue, Walker's problems were typical of what other nursing directors faced during the years after World War II. The nursing profession in the mid-20th century was in a period of transitions and shortages. Several factors were causing increased demands on nursing services: the increase in the number of patients admitted to hospitals, the rise in patient illness acuity, and the shortage of registered nurses. These problems would continue to plague nurse leaders for the next two decades.

Other factors would also affect the profession during the postwar era. Hospital construction and renovation, emerging ideas about patient care delivery, medical specialization, and advances in science would transform nursing practice; so would a polio epidemic. Meanwhile, women were being pushed out of the workforce due to the prevailing social norm that "a woman's place was in the home," coupled with a postwar "Baby Boom," and World War II veterans returning to their prewar job. Put simply, more women chose to stay home to care for their families. This reality, combined with an increase in the demand for more nurses in hospitals, resulted in a critical shortage of staff for the nursing profession.

The Baby Boom

As the war came to an end, and military personnel returned home, dramatic societal and cultural changes occurred in the United States. One of the greatest changes was an increase in the birth rate. In the decade prior to the World War II, the birth rate in the United States had declined as families struggled to survive the Great Depression. However, during World War II the birth rate began to increase dramatically, partly due to the improved economy and partly due to peoples' uncertainty about the future, loving goodbyes, and eager reunions. In 1940, the birth rate was just under 23 births per 1,000 people in the population. In 1947, the rate increased to 26.5 births per 1,000. The National Center for Health Statistics reported that in 1925 there were 2.9 million births in the United States; in 1946 the number increased by 20% to 3.4 million births; it peaked in 1957 when 4.3 million babies were born. In fact, the increase in numbers of births during this period was unprecedented. The infants who were born from mid-1946 to mid-1964 became known as the "baby boomers." Because of their sheer numbers, the group would have a profound effect on society in the postwar period and for years to come.

Development of the Modern Hospital

As the profession of medicine advanced, so too did the need for more modern hospitals. In 1946 the 79th U.S. Congress passed The Hospital Survey and

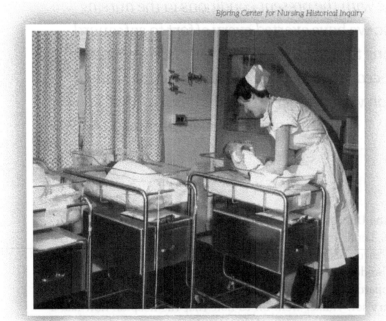

Nurse tending to a newborn, part of the rapidly expanding baby boomer generation after the war.

Construction Act to promote the expansion and construction of nonfederal hospitals. The Act, more commonly known as the Hill–Burton Act, resulted in a rapid expansion in a number of hospital beds. This increase in beds, along with an increase in the overall number of hospitals, resulted in a severe shortage of nurses throughout the country.

POLIO: THE PARALYZING FEVER

At no time was the post–World War II nursing shortage felt more acutely than during the poliomyelitis epidemics of the 1940s. Epidemics in the summers of 1946, 1949, and 1950 spurred fear throughout the nation. Intensive, time-consuming nursing care was required for patients in the initial phases of the illness, and total care for those confined to iron lungs. Scientists worked to find a cure or a vaccine to prevent the deadly disease and finally in the early 1950s hope for prevention was discovered in the form of a vaccine to prevent the poliovirus.

Polio and Its Epidemics

Poliomyelitis was nothing new; it had plagued civilizations for millennia. Ancient Greek physicians Hippocrates and Galen had described patients with polio-like symptoms; 18th-century medical literature described illnesses that presented as a fever followed by muscle weakness of the limbs.[3] Polio was caused by the poliovirus that spread in fecal material. Although the disease could present in a variety of ways at its onset, fever was often the only initial symptom. Muscle weakness in the arms and legs occurred, and in some cases, paralysis followed. When the virus attacked the central nervous system, the diaphragm and other respiratory muscles became paralyzed, making the patients unable to breathe and often causing death. Polio was also called "infantile paralysis," as infants and children were usually the victims of the paralyzing disease. In fact, during the major polio epidemic of 1916, 95% of those infected were children less than 9 years old.[4] That summer 6,000 children, adolescents, and young adults died and at least 27,000 were left permanently crippled.[5]

In the 1940s, outbreaks of the disease occurred mostly in the summer months. Entire communities curtailed summer activities, including swimming in lakes and pools and attending movies, all in the hope of preventing the contagious disease from spreading. Sometimes whole households were quarantined. Nurses and doctors made house calls and families were educated in the proper techniques for preparing food, washing laundry, and disposing of body waste.[6] The summer of 1946 was especially difficult as the epidemic leapfrogged unpredictably across the United States. But the polio outbreak of 1946 was not the last of the summertime epidemics. A second major epidemic in 1949 and a third in the summer of 1950 left thousands of individuals ill and spurred fear throughout the country.

Nursing Care and Polio Treatments

Nursing care during the active phases of the illness was intensive. Patients required continuous monitoring and in many cases complete and total patient care. The National Foundation for Infantile Paralysis and the American Red Cross established training sessions for registered nurses to better prepare them in the complex care of polio victims, especially those who required respiratory support from the iron lung. These specially trained nurses became known as polio nurses; many of them traveled the nation from epidemic to epidemic using their expert knowledge and experience to train others and to care for the victims.[7]

Sister Elizabeth Kenny, a self-taught Australian nurse, perfected a method she began in the early 20th century to care for victims of polio who suffered from paralysis of the limbs. Kenny maintained that patients' affected muscles and limbs should be wrapped in hot packs and exercised—not immobilized, as was the customary medical treatment. Kenny's method was most successful on early cases *before* deformities and paralysis occurred. The treatment was done in three stages. In the first stage, hot moist packs were applied to the patients' muscles; this helped to relax both the muscle and the pain. Next, gentle manipulation of the affected limb and muscles was performed. As treatments continued, the patients were allowed to move their own limbs with assistance until they were able to independently do so.[8]

Despite her successes, Kenny's ideas met with resistance and caused controversy in the medical community. Many physicians continued to advocate for immobilization and splinting of affected limbs. In 1940, Sister Kenny traveled to the United States to present her controversial method to American physicians and nurses in major cities, including (among others) Chicago, New York, Minneapolis, and Rochester, Minnesota. In Minnesota, Kenny received support. By 1943, the "Kenny Method" had become the standard treatment for polio at Mayo Clinic and Mayo-affiliated hospitals.

> *"Every available wool or cotton blanket was run under hot water and wrung out, then wrapped around the legs of the patients with polio."*[9]
>
> Saint Marys Hospital, Mayo Clinic, 1940s

When the "epidemics raged," Saint Marys Hospital in Rochester, Minnesota, "swarmed with polio patients," as it was the "only hospital in the region with facilities capable of dealing with major outbreaks of contagious diseases."[10] Between July 5 and October 11, 1946, Saint Marys Hospital admitted "110 patients for the treatment of polio. . . . Frequently there were three patients in respirators, requiring the services of nine nurses in a 24-hour period."[11] In 1949, the epidemic was even worse. On August 9, 1949, Sister Domitilla reported on the "Polio Situation." There were "21 patients in isolation—18 of them with polio."[12] September 5, the polio "situation" had changed to the "polio problem" at Saint Marys with "13 patients in the Isolation Department . . . and 35 post polios on first floor."[13] Since the first of June, 108 patients had been admitted to the hospital for poliomyelitis.[14]

The nurses needed help. Providing care for polio patients was both physically and emotionally exhausting. Care of patients with polio involved time-consuming treatments consisting of hot packs and splints. Nurses were also responsible for monitoring patients for complications related to immobility, including pneumonia, urinary tract infections, and pressure ulcers. Some patients were sedated to help control the pain of the severe cramps that also attacked the muscles.[15] For those victims who required mechanical respiratory assistance, the negative pressure ventilators (iron lungs) allowed patients to breathe despite their paralyzed chest muscles. The patients confined in the machines were completely dependent on nurses to provide all of their care. Part of that care involved intensive monitoring of the patients for aspiration, cyanosis, and skin breakdown.[16]

> *"Any graduate nurse who can give a few hours a day for a period of a week to two months is urged to contact the nursing department or the personnel department . . . immediately."*[17]
>
> Newspaper Ad, 1949

Because of the intensive nature of care needed for polio victims and the sheer numbers of patients requiring that care during epidemics, hospital administrators established respiratory centers—forerunners of the intensive care unit (ICU)—to group patients requiring respirators. Teamwork was essential. Moving patients in and out of the iron lungs required up to four nurses at a time. One nurse described her experience, writing:

> We always had fifteen to twenty respirators in service. Tracheotomies were done right in the unit . . . almost every patient in the unit was receiving oxygen; almost every patient had to be suctioned and each one had to have his own set up for this care. Most patients on this unit were unable to swallow properly, so most of them had feeding tubes or were being nourished intravenously or by clysis. The number

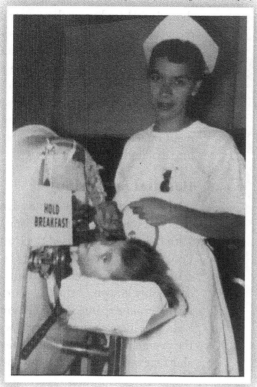

Eleanor Crowder, RN, caring for a patient in an iron lung

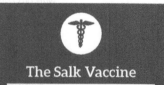

The Salk Vaccine

On March 26, 1953, American medical researcher Dr. Jonas Salk announced his discovery on a national radio show. He had found a way to prevent polio. Tests confirmed the success of a vaccine against poliomyelitis, the virus that caused the crippling disease. In 1954, a large-scale field test of the vaccine was conducted, involving more than 1,600,000 school-age children across the United States.[21] Considered one of the greatest scientific breakthroughs of the century, the Salk vaccine began to eradicate polio and its devastating paralysis. By 1955, the vaccine was distributed throughout the United States.

of nurses available for this unit was not sufficient so each nurse had to be assigned as many as four patients daily. (Teamwork on this unit was a reality not a thesis!).[18]

When there were power failures, the work that was required of nurses to maintain the patients' respirations became even more arduous. According to one nurse: "Once the current on three of the respirators failed. Until maintenance could restore it we had to man the respirator bellow by hand. This is extremely hard to do, the person pumping tiring within a minute or two."[19]

Hope for Polio Prevention

Some of the help nurses needed came from the National Foundation for Infantile Paralysis. The Foundation not only supplied funds to train nurses, physicians, and physical therapists in the new polio techniques but also provided monies for research to find a vaccine or a cure for the deadly disease. Discovery of a vaccination, however, would take time. And with each year as spring turned to summer, parents and medical personnel alike feared the possibility of another epidemic. Finally, in the early 1950s Dr. Jonas Salk discovered a vaccine to prevent the virus.

CHANGES IN HOSPITALS, MEDICINE, AND TECHNOLOGY

During the 1940s and 1950s, dramatic advances in medicine and surgery changed the hospital industry, medical practice, and nurses' work. Throughout this period, new discoveries occurred that led to advances in the care of the mentally ill, new cancer treatments,

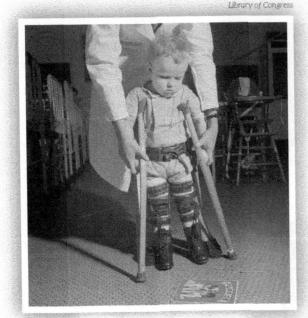

A child paralyzed by polio learning to walk on crutches.

peritoneal and hemodialysis, and more advanced thoracic and cardiovascular surgeries. Postoperative recovery rooms and surgical ICUs were established and reflected the increased demand for acute care. Societal changes throughout the postwar era and increased consumerism changed how care was delivered. In less than 10 years, as hospitals across the nation became centers for the diagnosis and treatment of acutely ill patients, hospital services grew into a billion-dollar industry.

Hospital Expansion

As the profession of medicine advanced, so too did the need for more modern hospitals. In 1946, the 79th U.S. Congress passed the Hospital Survey and Construction Act to promote the expansion and construction of nonfederal hospitals. The Act, more commonly known as the Hill–Burton Act, resulted in the rapid expansion in the number of hospital beds. This increase in beds, along with an increase in the overall number of hospitals, resulted in a severe shortage of nurses throughout the country.

Advances in Surgery and Specialized Care

Beginning in the 1940s, new discoveries occurred in renal therapy, cancer treatments, and cardiovascular surgery in particular. The new treatments of peritoneal and then hemodialysis revolutionized the care of patients with chronic renal failure. Nurses' involvement became highly specialized as they learned to manage complex machines, adjust fluids pouring into and out of patients' abdomens, and cope with emergency situations related to the patient's response to treatments.

Meanwhile, new techniques in thoracic and cardiovascular surgery greatly increased the demand for surgical and perioperative nurses and the demand for postanesthesia care units and ICUs in hospitals. At Mayo Clinic

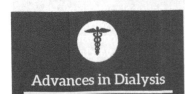

Advances in Dialysis

In 1943, Dr. Willem Kolff, a young Dutch physician, constructed the first artificial kidney, a mechanical "drum dialyzer," after watching a young man die slowly of kidney failure. During the next 2 years, he treated 16 patients with little success. In the 1950s, University of Washington's Dr. Belding Scribner used a new material called "Teflon" to develop the "Scribner Shunt" —dialysis tubing that could be kept in place longer. The invention provided new hope for patients requiring long-term care.

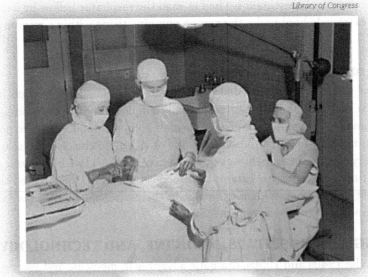

An operating room in 1943.

in Rochester, Minnesota, the demand for nurses increased when thoracic surgeon Dr. O. T. Clagett began to perform life-saving chest surgeries on hundreds of adults and children.[22] Nurses were essential members of Clagett's team; some prepared patients for surgery, others circulated and scrubbed during the complicated thoracic surgeries, and still others cared for and observed patients after the procedure. In this era before ICUs, many hospitals were just beginning to introduce the recovery room to care for critically ill patients. The nurses who cared for the postoperative patients needed to be adept at using such equipment as oxygen tents, suction catheters, and chest tubes. Such was the case at the Johns Hopkins Hospital in Baltimore, Maryland. There the rise in Drs. Blalock and Taussig's "blue baby" surgeries increased the need for physician and nurse anesthetists, surgical nurses, and nurses for the intensive postoperative care unit. As chest surgeries moved from "blue babies" to the general population in need of cardiac bypass surgeries across the nation, hospitals and nursing services were once again transformed.

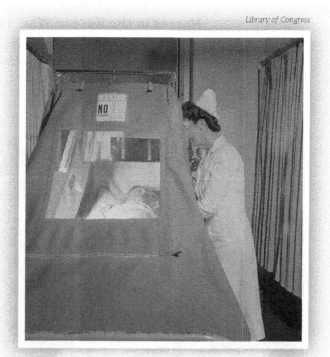

A nurse tending to a patient in an oxygen tent in 1942.

Beyond the walls of the Johns Hopkins Hospital, other hospitals throughout the United States also became centers for the diagnosis and treatment of acutely ill patients. Many hospitals established postoperative recovery rooms and surgical ICUs, basing their innovations on the increasing demand for acute care. The new medical centers were larger than hospitals of previous decades and far more complex.

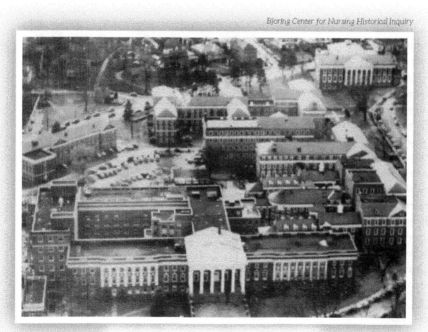

University of Virginia Hospital, circa late 1950s.

Nurses in the Korean War, 1950–1953

As in previous wars in other decades, nurses played an important role in the military conflict in Korea. In fact, when President Harry S. Truman ordered troops into South Korea in 1950 just after the North Korean People's Army invaded, nurses joined the incursion just days later. By the end of that year, 200 army nurses were in South Korea. On September 15, General Douglas MacArthur and his troops landed at Inchon; army nurses of the First Mobile Army Surgical Hospital (MASH) and the Fourth Field Hospital accompanied them. Just a few weeks later, in October 1950 as the nurses were on the move to Pusan, they hurriedly took cover in roadside ditches when the enemy attacked their convoy.

Anna Mae Hays was among those who served in the Korean War. She was assigned to the Fourth Field Hospital, a unit that cared for more than 25,000 patients over a 10-month span in 1950. Working in MASH near the front lines, Hays and other army nurses assisted military surgeons and worked with enlisted men to treat the onslaught of casualties that arrived in the unit for care. Some casualties came by helicopter, cared for by medical staff who used the new aeromedical evacuation procedures. Others came in trucks. Sometimes the nurses treated more than 400 patients in 1 day in a unit set up for 200. Nurses provided state-of-the-art care,

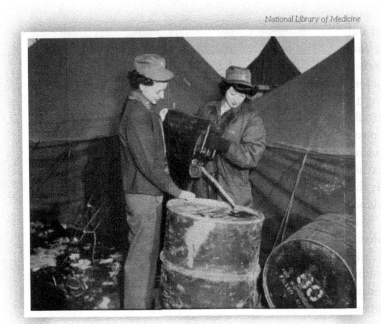

Members of a First Mobile Army Surgical Hospital (MASH) unit filling an oil drum.

Nursing in Korea

"I learned a lot from other people. I think that one of the things about us being in the service, is that you are exposed to so many different people from so many different places. If you're wise, you can pick up a lot of good information from them. If you're not wise, then you become very regimented in your own thinking and you just never progress very far . . . I grew from that experience, both as a nurse and as a person."[23]

First Lieutenant
Mary C. Quinn, 1952

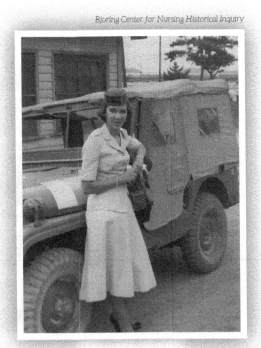

Eleanor Crowder, RN.

including trauma surgery, blood transfusions, and fluid resuscitation for shock.[24] During the conflict, 17 nurses died; for the most part their deaths were due to aircraft crashes.[25]

In fact, the use of helicopters and medevac airplanes grew exponentially in the Korean War. Early treatment saved lives, and flight nurses played a significant role in the evacuation of casualties. Captain Lillian Kinkela Keil, a member of the Air Force Nurse Corps and one of the most decorated women in the U.S. military, flew several hundred missions as a flight nurse in Korea. Among numerous other medals, she received the Korean Service Medal with Seven Battle Stars, and the Presidential Citation, Republic of Korea.[26]

By July 29, 1953, when the war ended, thousands of military nurses had served. These included more than 700 Army nurses, more than 4,000 Navy nurses, and dozens of Air Force nurses.[27]

Hospital Expansion and Blue Cross Insurance

Back at home, Congress continued its commitment to the nation's hospitals and continued to increase Hill–Burton funding for improving existing hospitals and constructing new ones. In 1959, congressional funding for hospitals totaled $186.2 million; by 1962, it had grown to $226.2 million. The number of new hospital beds rose in direct portion to the Act's funding. In 1957, there were 253,000 hospital beds in the nation; by 1963, America had a total of 1,700,000 hospital beds. This transformation led hospital administrators across the nation to be confronted by issues that other businesses had faced for a long time: concern for their product, the cost, and the need for a competent workforce.[28] The most important issue for hospitals was finding and retaining a competent workforce of registered nurses. The problem with this issue was there simply were not enough nurses to meet the increased demand.

Both the medical profession and the American Hospital Association wholeheartedly supported hospital expansion.[29] However, nursing leaders were less enthusiastic, as they predicted a crisis in the making. In addition to the increase in the number of patients in the hospital, new technologies, new surgeries, and more complex procedures placed increased demands on the nurses who were already employed. In addition, the physical expansion of the nation's hospitals not only increased the number of hospital beds, but also changed the architecture of hospitals. Semiprivate and private patient rooms soon replaced the large patient wards. These new spaces, along with rising acuity of illness, changed the way in which nurses worked.[30]

Prepaid health insurance coverage funded by companies such as Blue Cross and Blue Shield also changed hospital care. In the immediate postwar years, medical insurance became part of employee benefits; in fact, fringe benefits were used in place of employee raises. By 1950, there were 90 Blue Cross plans and 79 Blue Shield plans (physician payment plans) in the United States and Canada, covering 50% of the civilian population's medical expenses. By 1960, 75% of the population was

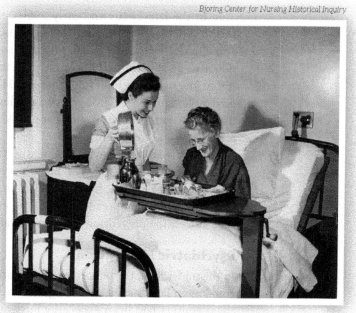

Bjoring Center for Nursing Historical Inquiry

A student nurse caring for a patient in a private room, often funded by insurance companies, which covered 50% of the civilian population's medical expenses.

covered by some form of private hospital insurance.[31] Insurance companies paid for semiprivate and private rooms for their subscribers, and more and more patients began to demand rooms that provided privacy and comfort. They no longer wanted to stay in large open wards that afforded little privacy.[32]

While changes in hospital architecture and the flexibility in the choice of rooms benefited the patients and their privacy, the use of semiprivate and private rooms increased the need for more nurses at a time when the profession was already not meeting the demand. Open hospital wards had provided nurses with the ability to see large numbers of patients at once. Now patients were isolated in semiprivate and private rooms, and the nurses' ability to monitor and assess their patients was diminished.[33] In the past, two nurses could care for all the patients in one open ward. Now, with patients ensconced in their private and semiprivate rooms, more nurses were needed.[34]

The growing number of patients in hospitals during the postwar years reflected the public's demand for service. In 1941, just more than 10,000 patients were admitted to hospitals each year; by 1946, the number had increased to more than 14,000.[35] By 1953, more than 19,000 patients received hospital care each year, bringing the average daily hospital census to 1,335,673.[36] As patient admissions continued to climb, the quest for hospital personnel intensified. Nurses were in high demand.

Medical Research, Science, and Technology

Medical science grew rapidly during the post–World War II era. At the center of the expansion was medical research. Funded by the federal government, new research findings directly influenced the physicians' income, their power, and how they practiced. New discoveries in biomedical research served to enhance physicians' abilities to diagnose and treat disease. Findings also improved their understanding of disease prevention.

Discoveries in antibiotic therapies also changed medical care. The widespread use of penicillin and sulfa drugs in the 1940s led to the control of infectious and communicable diseases. A decade earlier, infectious diseases had caused more than two thirds of all deaths in the United States. By 1945, two thirds of all deaths were caused by chronic illnesses.[37] Now scientists and physicians could turn their attention to finding cures for cancer, obesity, heart disease, and mental illness.[38]

In the late 1940s and early 1950s, the expansion of the National Institutes of Health (NIH) and the establishment of a Communicable Disease Center (CDC) would also impact health care. Besides expanding the physical size of the NIH, the organization also demonstrated impressive growth in its grants program and overall budget. "From just over four million dollars in 1947, the program grew to more than one hundred million in 1957."[39] Congress was willing to spend money for researchers and scientists to prevent illness and cure disease. With this knowledge came advances in medical technology and treatments.

The CDC did not have as impressive financial support as the NIH; however, it was established to initially focus on malaria, typhus, and other infectious diseases. Malaria continued to be a public health problem in the southern United States. The Center continued to expand its breadth of focus to eventually include all infectious diseases and also address the prevention of communicable diseases and chronic illnesses.

Psychiatric Medications

In the mid-1950s, the majority of psychiatric patients were housed in large state-sponsored psychiatric facilities throughout the United States. Prior to this time, nurses in these centers had been especially busy and involved in the care of their psychiatric patients. They had been responsible for preparing, monitoring, and sometimes even administering nursing-intensive treatments such as hydrotherapy, fever therapy, shock therapy, and lobotomies. In contrast to that care, by the mid-1950s as new drugs were introduced, nurses were only responsible for the safety and hygiene of the patients, and supervised the staff; in many cases, they were faced with patients who were docile. The introduction of new medications changed the nurses' role to a certain degree as they now prepared and administered the medication and monitored the patients for side effects.[40]

The following description of one nurse's daily routine in a state psychiatric hospital illustrates the shift in nursing responsibilities after the introduction of the antipsychotic medications. "Ms. Shelton described the period between 1958 and 1961 when the Thorazine pills arrived in barrels and had to be counted. Ms. Shelton recalled when the nurse functioned 'like the pharmacist and refilled the individual stock bottles for each ward.' Ms. Coltrane remembered that frequent blood pressures were needed and stated, '[taking vital signs] was all you would get done,' before more nursing staff were hired to assist."[41]

As government funding fueled medical research and medical science, new diagnostic tests and equipment were developed to assist physicians in the diagnosis and management of their patients' health problems. A logical place to house this new technology was in the nation's hospitals. In fact, hospitals soon became technologic centers capable of providing patients with the latest in modern services and equipment.[42] During the 1950s, physicians took full advantage of modern hospital equipment and technology, increasing the number of patients they hospitalized.[43] As historian Rosemary Stevens notes, the health insurance industry's willingness to pay for technology further exaggerated modern medicine's high-technology emphasis and encouraged the public to seek admission to hospitals for diagnostic work-ups.[44]

Starting in the 1950s, researchers focused on America's top three causes of mortality: heart disease, cancer, and stroke.[47] Unprecedented federal funding allowed scientists to make great strides in the discovery of the cause of diseases and the development of new therapies to treat them. Hyperbaric chambers improved wound healing; hemodialysis provided a new treatment for renal failure, and internal pacemakers saved lives for patients with heart block. Advances in medical research and technology radically modified surgical techniques, as reflected by lifesaving transplantation of kidneys and livers.[48]

The very success of medical science and technology directly affected the severity of the nursing shortage and the demands made on the profession. As patient admissions increased and patient care grew more complicated, directors of nursing faced the problem of finding more nurses. Just as important was the intellectual demand that was placed on nurses. Nurses were continually pressed to learn how to use new technology, dispense new medications, and care for patients whose needs were far more complex than in previous times.

The entire situation was made more complex by the fact that physicians and nurses had to address the health care needs of the elderly. The nation's population was aging. In 1950, 12.3 million Americans were older than 65 years of age; by 1960, that number had risen to 16.6 million.[49] Moreover, many of the elderly suffered from multiple chronic illnesses such as diabetes, heart disease, and arthritis, thus adding to the complexity of their medical care needs. An aging population required more frequent hospitalizations,

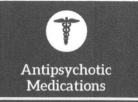

Antipsychotic Medications

In the mid-1950s, new medications were introduced to better manage psychiatric disorders. First called major tranquilizers, later neuroleptics, and then antipsychotic medications (Thorazine and Stelazine), these medications not only changed how psychiatric nurses cared for their patients, but also changed the lives of psychiatric patients themselves. Eventually, these drugs were prescribed to existing and newly diagnosed psychiatric patients, allowing them to remain in their communities rather than in an institution.

"The Thorazine pills arrived in barrels and had to be counted."[45]

Ms. Shelton

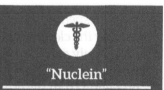

"Nuclein"

In 1953, scientists James Watson and Francis Crick suggested what is now accepted as the first correct double-helix model of DNA structure in the journal *Nature*. Identifying the double-helix model was perhaps one of the greatest biomedical discoveries in the immediate postwar period. It would provide further clarity into heredity and contribute to a better understanding of the intricate relationships between genes and disease.[46]

more complicated medical procedures, and increasingly complex nursing care—all of which increased the demand for professional nurses.

Advances in medical science and technology also led to the rapid proliferation of medical subspecialties after World War II. As the 1950s dawned, new areas of medical care emerged, including oncology, cardiology, endocrinology, and nephrology. Directly related to this increase was the greater complexity within hospitals. During the 1950s, hospital organization changed as more clinical departments were established.[50]

With the rise of subspecialties came an increased demand for additional nursing personnel, space, and equipment. Soon, whole hospital floors were designated for patients with cardiac disease, metabolic disorders, orthopedic surgery, plastic surgery, and ophthalmology. Moreover, it was expected that nurses working in these specialties would have adequate knowledge specific to their patients' individual care.

NURSING EDUCATION, NURSING PRACTICE, AND WORKFORCE REALITY

After World War II, the changes that occurred in science, medicine, and the hospital industry contributed to the nationwide shortage of nurses. Without nurses hospitals could not function. As the shortage continued to escalate and with little end in sight, dramatic changes in how nurses practiced and were educated occurred. Changes in nursing service administration, the increased use of licensed practical nurses, and the establishment of associate degree programs in nursing reflect an attempt to meet the needs of society and provide safe, quality care.

The Nursing Shortage

The nationwide shortage of nurses led some hospitals to eliminate the number of beds, just as they had done during the war. In 1947, an American Hospital Association survey revealed that in 3,219 of its member hospitals, 494 were forced to close a total of 17,524 beds.[51] The study further revealed that the closing of general hospitals depended on the region of the country in which the hospital was located, and the population of the area. In the eastern United States, 30 of every 1,000 beds closed; in the western states, only 20 of every 1,000 beds closed. Administrators soon realized that while closing beds was a necessary solution to the lack of nurses, it was a temporary solution at best and did not address the escalating nursing shortage.

"The desperate need for opening the closed wards is certainly evident to all concerned. It can be done by taking from the other floors sufficient number of nurses."[52]

Virginia Walker, 1945

Among those most actively engaged in trying to resolve the nursing shortage were the profession's leaders and educators. The post–World War II nursing shortage served as a powerful stimulus for dramatic changes in how nurses practiced and how they were educated. Professional nurses were challenged to provide uncompromised advanced patient care in a time of inadequate nursing manpower. As patient care became more advanced and greater demands were placed on nurses, the profession's leaders, clinicians, and educators were forced to examine the essentials of nursing care, the utilization of registered nurses, and nursing education. For almost 75 years, hospitals had relied on student nurses as their major workforce. In the 1940s, major changes to nursing education would change that practice. As the education of nurses moved from an apprenticeship form of training to a collegiate model, students could no longer be the major patient care providers in hospitals.

Nursing Education and the Brown Report

By the late-1940s, the National League for Nursing Education was well aware that nursing educators faced many critical issues. Not only were schools of nursing hard-pressed to recruit students, they also faced the reality that the structure of nursing education needed to undergo radical changes. As social anthropologist Esther Lucile Brown noted:

"Almost without a dissenting voice" those who were familiar with trends in professional education in the United States agreed that preparation of nurses belonged "squarely within the institution of higher learning."[53] "Training" in skill sets was no longer adequate; education that encompassed a full breadth of the sciences and humanities was necessary to prepare nurses for their work in the second half of the 20th century.

To address the issue, in 1946 the National Nursing Council commissioned Esther Lucile Brown to study professional nursing education in the United States. After an extensive study, Brown made recommendations that would allow nursing to keep pace with advances in health care. One of Brown's most significant recommendations was to move nursing education out of hospital-based schools and into colleges and universities. Although baccalaureate programs had existed since 1909, 3-year nursing diploma programs still provided training for the majority of the nation's nurses.

The profession responded. During the 1950s, the movement to increase the number of generic baccalaureate nursing programs and baccalaureate-prepared nurses gathered momentum. In an increasingly high-tech and complex medical environment, the value of higher education was clear to nursing leaders and educators. However, the more pressing issue was how to prepare adequate numbers of nurses to meet the rising demands for more nurses in the shortest time possible.

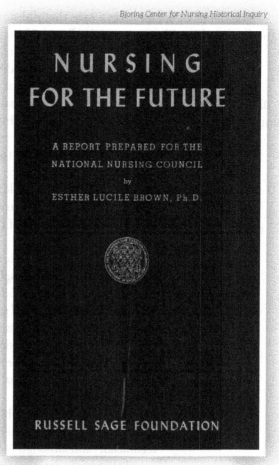

The Brown report, which emphasized that nursing education should primarily take place in universities rather than hospital-based training programs.

Nursing leaders and educators saw the Brown report as a blueprint for the profession's future, while physicians and hospital administrators criticized it for being unrealistic. They were concerned that the proposed education changes would lead to the closure of large numbers of hospital-based "diploma" nursing schools, and in turn, further deplete the number of nurses.[56] Despite the controversy, after 1955 diploma programs continued to decrease in number while the number of baccalaureate and associate degree nursing programs increased. By 1962, 30 baccalaureate nursing education programs and 50 new associate degree programs existed in the country.[57]

Associate Degree Programs

Responding to the changes in health care and the Brown report in 1951, nurse educator Mildred Montag proposed that nursing education programs be located in the nation's ever-increasing number of community colleges. The basis for Montag's proposal was the recognition that contemporary patient care required varying levels of skills and knowledge. Nurses' aides, whose numbers were increasing to fill gaps in care that resulted from the nursing shortage, were educated in brief programs and sometimes on the job. They were not trained to perform independent care, but rather to work under the supervision of a registered nurse. Aides provided basic nursing

"With the maintenance of health . . . as the future goal of medicine . . . it is obvious that greatly increased nursing competence will be demanded."[54]

Esther L. Brown, 1947

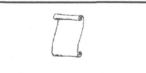

Nursing for the Future

The Brown report, released in 1948, urged that only college graduates be regarded as truly professional nurses and that "technical" nurses be prepared in associate degree programs.[55]

care that did not require the knowledge and skills of a registered nurse: feeding, bathing, and ambulating patients.[59] Meanwhile, registered nurses provided more complex, high-tech care to acutely ill patients. These responsibilities involved in-depth preparation in the sciences and humanities—the preparation that Esther Lucile Brown had discussed in her report insisting that professional education should take place in a collegiate setting.

Recognizing that the skills for some nursing tasks resided somewhere between those of aides and those of professionally educated nurses, Montag referred to them as "intermediate functions." These were more technical in nature but nevertheless required a certain level of skill. Moreover, these skills could be learned in a technical training program. In order to describe what she meant, Montag used the provision of fluids for patients to illustrate the function of the various levels of the nursing care:

> The aide may be instructed to fill the water containers for these patients and to keep them filled throughout the day. The nurse with technical training may be assigned the responsibility for keeping the fluid intake of these patients within the amount prescribed for the day. This would entail spacing the fluids allowed so the patient experiences a minimum of discomfort from the restriction of fluids. The nurse with professional preparation would assume the responsibility for the giving of fluids to those patients whose fluid intake must be adjusted according to fluid loss and a given ratio between the two maintained.[60]

Montag also noted that while the boundaries between the three roles were not fixed, they demonstrated that there were limits to each role. The new role was titled "nursing technician" and although Montag admitted that it would "not satisfy forever," she proposed that it was one that indicated "more accurately" the person who had semiprofessional preparation—those whose functions were "predominantly technical."[61]

The decision about which educational institution should house these programs also had to be considered. Montag knew that students needed both a general education and technical or vocational education in order to have the necessary knowledge and skills required for nursing. She noted: "The preparation which the nursing technician requires is what is usually called terminal-technical, dual in character and including vocational and general. This kind of preparation is in keeping with the trend in other professional areas as is indicated by the number of junior colleges and technical institutes now in existence offering many different curricula."[62] Divided into regular college courses and courses in nursing, these programs were usually 2 years in length. Thus, junior and community colleges seemed to be the logical places for technical nursing programs. Community colleges were actually the preferred location, as they offered a variety of curricula and they were available locally. It was hoped that they would prepare nurses who would then remain and work in the local community.

The first of the associate degree programs for nursing began in 1952. By the mid-1960s, associate degree programs were the fastest growing nursing programs in the United States; in 1955, 19 schools offered associate degree programs; by 1962, 84 schools existed.[63] As historians Joan Lynaugh and Barbara Brush note, by the 1970s the associate degree movement in nursing education was "booming."[64] While the associate degree programs provided a means of educating more nurses more quickly, this entry level for registered nurses would remain a controversial issue within the profession for decades to come.

Meanwhile, moving nursing education into colleges and universities proved to be a double-edged sword for hospital nursing directors. The closing of hospital diploma programs meant that fewer students were available to give care to hospital patients. Although baccalaureate and associate degree students continued to use hospital wards for their clinical experiences, nursing directors no longer had control over the students' clinical assignments. Nor did they have the responsibility to choose the shift the students would work, or the length of time they would work on any given day. Nursing instructors were now responsible for students' assignments. Students were in the hospital to learn, not to staff units.

The Retention of Nurses

As the nursing shortage persisted, nurses became dissatisfied with their working conditions and the lack of any improvement. Many nurses perceived the failure to improve working conditions as the hospital administrators' lack of effort to make them better. The reality was, however, that administrators were all too aware of the nurses' dissatisfaction and knew that changes needed to occur if they were to retain the nurses they already had and recruit new ones.

In 1955, Northwestern Hospital in Minneapolis, Minnesota, conducted a survey about nurses' resignations. The survey revealed that the 165 registered nurses who resigned from the hospital that year cost the hospital $552.67 in personnel staff time per resignation. The study concluded that there were two categories of the reasons nurses left: unavoidable and avoidable. Unavoidable reasons included marriage, moving out of the area, or pregnancy. "Avoidable" reasons for staff turnover were low morale, poor working conditions, inadequate pay, and poor employee–management relations.[65]

Licensed Practical Nurses and Auxiliary Personnel

Forced to develop strategies to provide nursing care with fewer professional nurses, administrators and nursing directors began to examine the specific types of care patients needed. From their experiences with a shortage of nurses during the war, nursing directors knew that nonprofessionals could do many of the tasks usually performed by registered nurses. The use of more licensed professional nurses (LPNs) and nurses' aides appeared to be a logical solution. Supervised by registered nurses, LPNs were capable of performing such nursing tasks as wound dressings, while nurses' aides could assume the responsibility to make beds, bathe, and ambulate patients. The increased use of these auxiliary personnel would allow more efficient use of registered nurses' time. In 1950, there were more than 144,000 LPNs providing patient care in America's hospitals.[66] By 1953, the number of LPNs had risen dramatically to 370,819 nationally.[67] Hospital administrators and nursing directors clearly viewed the use of LPNs and aides as one solution to their nursing service woes.

Although the use of LPNs and auxiliary nursing personnel did help to provide more bedside patient care, it unexpectedly became a source of dissatisfaction for registered nurses. As nurse historian Barbara Brush has noted, the strategy not only diluted the role of the registered nurse, but also resulted in changing registered nurses from care providers to managers of LPNs and aides.[68] In doing so, the change in role contributed to a decrease in registered nurses' pride in their profession. While the strategy provided help, it also had a negative impact on a hospital's ability to retain and recruit registered nurses.

Nursing Practice in the 1950s

During the 1950s, directors of nursing who were besieged by multiple demands attempted to respond to the nursing shortage while simultaneously improving the quality of care for their patients. The movement away from student-nurse labor to an all-graduate

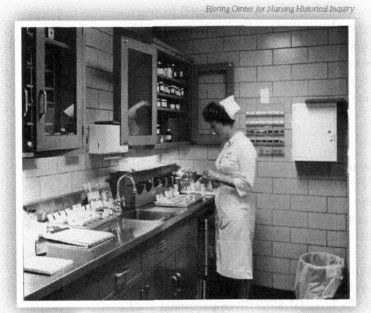

A nurse organizing medications, which became a primary task of registered nurses as ancillary staff took over the tasks of bedside care.

nursing staff that had begun in the 1930s intensified in the early 1950s as more registered nurses left private-duty nursing to become hospital employees. As a result, the graduate nurses assumed a greater percentage of patient care than they had in the past. As hospitals employed more graduate nurses in "general duty" positions, nursing service departments became more complex. In fact, it was soon necessary to employ associate and assistant directors of nursing in addition to nursing supervisors for all three shifts. Specific clinical services, including obstetrics, psychiatry, and operating rooms, needed to have supervisors as well as a head nurse and an assistant head nurse. Some of these positions were created and others were redefined.

In addition to changes in nursing service administration, changes also occurred in the delivery of patient care. With fewer nurses and more ancillary staff, a system to provide safe, efficient care was needed. Soon labeled "team nursing," the new system relied on registered nurses to serve as "team leaders," managing auxiliary staff. Teams consisting of registered nurses, licensed practical nurses, nurses' aides, and orderlies provided complete care to a certain number of patients on a unit or ward. The team took vital signs, changed bedding, bathed and ambulated patients all under the supervision of the registered nurse. While the ancillary staff focused on the bedside care, the registered nurses administered medications and treatments.

Head nurses and nurses in charge of the shift made rounds with the physicians, reviewed physicians' written orders, and communicated any changes in care to the teams. Although the introduction of more ancillary staff to assist with patient care helped to alleviate the burden of care in light of the nursing shortage, many registered nurses found it difficult to adjust to the lack of time they had to deliver direct patient care, caused by an increase in their administrative tasks.

Working Conditions, Hours, Wages, and Nurses' Dissatisfaction

Poor working conditions and low wages proved to be two of the greatest reasons that registered nurses left the profession. Although the 40-hour workweek was the norm for most of America's workforce, in 1950 registered nurses were still required to work more hours. By the mid-1950s, the major reasons nurses cited for leaving their jobs were: they were required to perform non-nursing tasks, they had to work between 44 to 48 hours per week, and they had less time for direct patient care.[69]

While nurses were dealing with low wages, long hours, and increased responsibilities in an increasingly high-tech hospital environment, leaders of the profession were struggling to identify what was unique about professional nursing: what separated it from the medical profession, and what separated it from pharmacy, physical therapy, occupational therapy, and other allied health professionals. In an attempt to carve out nursing's scope of practice, in 1955 the American Nurses Association published the "Model Definition of Nursing":

The practice of professional nursing means the performance for compensation of any act in the observation, care and counsel of the ill . . . or in the maintenance of health or prevention of illness . . . or the administration of medications and treatments as prescribed by a licensed physician . . . The foregoing shall not be deemed to included acts of diagnosis or prescription of therapeutic or corrective measures.[71]

The definition, soon adopted by the majority of state legislatures, would have a profound impact on the future of the profession: the Association's exclusion of the acts of diagnosis and prescription would undermine nurses' autonomy in rural and urban underserved areas where they provided care to the poor and disenfranchised. The definitions also set the stage for conflicts about the role of nurse practitioners when the idea was introduced in the 1960s.[72]

Progressive Patient Care

In the late 1950s, hospitals established special units to care for patients who were gravely ill. The idea came from Faye Abdellah and her colleague Josephine Starchan, both nurses at Manchester Memorial Hospital in Connecticut. Together they proposed a system of "Progressive Patient Care," defining it as "the organization of facilities, services, and staff around the medical and nursing needs of the patient."[73] In this system, patients would progress from special care units where they received care when they were critically ill, to "step-down units," and on to "home care."[74]

Across the nation, nurses, hospital administrators, and physicians eagerly accepted Abdellah and Starchan's plan. Of particular interest was the concept of intensive care, the most exciting and innovative aspect, and the one that would generate the most hospital income. Grouping critically ill patients in one area—with nurses who specialized in their treatment—made sense. It would also decrease the demand for private-duty nurses to "special" critically ill patients in private rooms.

Among the first units to be established were postsurgical recovery rooms and ICUs. Although not equipped with the advanced technology that was present in later recovery rooms and ICUs, these units had experienced and vigilant nurses.[75] In fact, physicians often demanded that nursing supervisors only place the most experienced nurses in the ICU. Those nurses began to specialize in their chosen field, often acquiring advanced medical knowledge and new nursing skills. Soon these nurses, seeking new opportunities to expand their clinical expertise, began to develop specialized nursing organizations.

ICUs also offered nurses an improved work environment. In the ICUs, they could provide direct care for one or two patients, they gained respect for their increased specialty knowledge, and they developed an esprit de corps with their colleagues. Saving patients in dramatic situations, they received thanks for their work. A sense of pride in their accomplishments helped to retain experienced, highly qualified nurses to work in these units.

The Nursing Shortage and Public Health

The postwar nursing shortage also affected the nation's public health system. Fewer and fewer nurses were available to care for patients in their homes, in clinics, and in rural areas. This was especially true in the far western regions of the United States, areas that were remote from most conveniences, including health care. In west Texas, for example, ranchers, oilmen, and their families had to rely on their own knowledge and experience

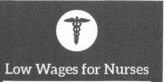

Low Wages for Nurses

In 1946, the starting gross monthly salary for general duty registered nurses averaged $172; by 1950, their average monthly gross income averaged $253. At the same time, the 1955 gross monthly salaries for secretaries and factory workers averaged approximately $315 and $323 more per month, respectively.[70]

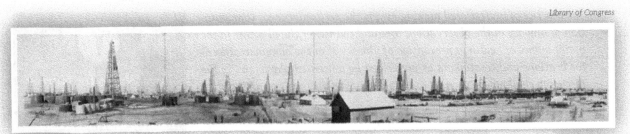

Oil wells in Texas, where workers and community members often needed to travel hours to receive health care.

when dealing with minor illnesses and injuries. When they were seriously ill or injured, they often had to travel hours to get to the nearest hospital, clinic, or physician.

Oil prospecting began in Pecos County in 1900. When oil was discovered, an instant boomtown developed as workers arrived from around the country. Iraan, Texas, was one of the boomtowns. In an effort to move workers and their families to the new town, oil companies rushed to build company houses and drill water wells. In 1927, they built a school and hired teachers; a year later the town opened a post office. By 1930, Iraan had 60 businesses and an estimated population of 1,600.[76] However, access to health care remained a challenge for the citizens of this remote corner of Texas. There was one doctor for the area and only a few nurses. The closest hospital was in Fort Stockton, 65 miles away. Roads were often in poor condition and the lack of transportation presented a challenge when acutely ill or injured citizens needed medical services. In addition, the few health care resources that existed were strained by the lack of state funding and services.[77]

In the 1950s, the county hired Dr. Alan Sherrod to help them. He, in turn, asked his wife, Judy, a registered nurse, to assist him in providing services for the new town. Together they would be the sole source of medical and nursing support in the town.

The first day Dr. Sherrod's office opened in September 1949, there were 95 people in line for care. Mrs. Sherrod, a registered nurse, remembered looking out the door wondering what they were going to do for all of them. Each day continued to be the same as citizens of the town and surrounding county sought health care.

Much of the care the doctor/nurse team delivered occurred on ranches or on drilling sites, on roadways, or in fields. There was no easy access. When Dr. Sherrod was traveling from ranch to ranch seeing families and their ranch hands, Mrs. Sherrod was in the office, suturing lacerations, giving injections, writing prescriptions, and bandaging open wounds. When asked if she was concerned that some would think she was practicing medicine, Mrs. Sherrod responded: "No, of course not. I knew what Dr. Sherrod would have done and what he would want me to do. I was trained in the OR and he showed me how to suture, set broken bones, and debride wounds. I was just doing what he would want me to do."[78]

In the late 1940s, the community of Iraan was in dire need of health promotion and prevention programs, and when Mrs. Sherrod was not in the office, she set up immunization clinics and classes for mothers of infants and small children. The goal of these clinics was to protect the health of the public, while also improving hygiene in the home and a higher level of infant care.

The clinic's success did not go unnoticed by the community leaders; nor did it go unnoticed by the state when several years later, a representative from the Texas State Health Department came to Pecos County to help immunize the children in the region.[80] Town leaders told the representative that

Practicing Medicine Without a License?

"You know, I wasn't prescribing medicine for people. I had a prescription pad that was stamped with his name on it, and I knew what to give the patients. I was very aware of what they needed and what Alan would want me to give them. Besides, I was knowledgeable about pharmacology as a nurse. I was just doing what I had to do under the circumstances. There was no one else to do it."[79]

Judy Sherrod, 1948

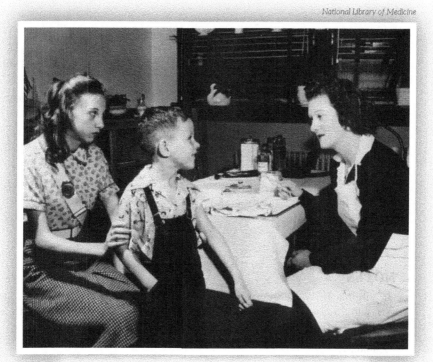

A nurse preparing to administer an immunization to a young patient.

the state's help was not needed: Dr. Sherrod and his nurse had immunized all the children.[81]

Judy Sherrod's venture into medical territory was not the first, nor would it be the last. During the first half of the 20th century, other nurses had provided care in remote rural areas in the absence of physicians, using "standing orders" to cover them legally. Among these were the Frontier nurses in Appalachia and the nurses working with the Indian Health Service on reservations and in Alaska. At the same time, in busy hospitals and medical centers physicians had been increasing the number of procedures they delegated to nurses. By the 1950s, nurses were taking blood pressures and using stethoscopes to listen to patient's heart and lungs—tasks that in the past only physicians had done. With increased specialization, nurses were also accepting other new responsibilities. In renal units, nurses were hanging bottles of solution for peritoneal dialysis; in surgical ICUs, they were managing patients on respirators, suctioning tracheostomy tubes, regulating intravenous medications, and hanging blood. Over the next two decades, nurses' responsibilities would only continue to increase as care became increasingly dependent on new machines and new technology. The line between medicine and nursing was blurring.

For Discussion

1. Describe the role of nurses in the polio epidemics of the 1940s and 1950s. How did their role change with the introduction of the Salk vaccine?
2. Compare and contrast the conventional medical therapy used to treat polio victims and Sister Kenny's method of treatment.

(continued)

NOTES

1. Virginia H. Walker. Correspondence Virginia H. Walker to Carlisle S. Lentz, January 14, 1946. University of Virginia Health Science Center Special Collections: University of Virginia Hospital Director's Office Collection, 1.
2. Ibid., 1.
3. Volney Steele, "Fear in the Time of Infantile Paralysis: The Montana Experience," *Montana: The Magazine of Western History* 55 (Summer, 2005): 65.
4. Lynne M. Dunphy, "The Steel Cocoon: Tales of the Nurses and Patients of the Iron Lung, 1929-1955," *Nursing History Review* 9 (2001): 5.
5. Steele, "Fear in the Time," 65.
6. Ibid., 67.
7. Dunphy, "The Steel Cocoon," 8.
8. Edwin D. Neff, "Hope for Polio Victims," *Science Newsletter* (June 14, 1942): 378.
9. Arlene Keeling, *The Nurses of Mayo Clinic: Caring Healers* (Rochester, MN: Mayo Clinic, 2012): 72.
10. Ibid.
11. Ibid.
12. Sister Mary Brigh Cassidy, "Minutes of the Meeting of the Coordination Committee St. Marys Hospital," Mayo Historical Unit (hereafter MHU) MHU file: polio (August 9, 1949): 1.
13. Sister Mary Brigh, "Minutes of the Meeting of Hospital Coordinating Committee, St. Marys Hospital," MHU (September 5, 1949): 1.
14. Keeling, *The Nurses of Mayo Clinic*, 7.
15. Steele, "Fear in the Time," 67.
16. Dunphy, "The Steel Cocoon," 4.
17. Brigh Cassidy, "Minutes of the August Meeting."
18. Dunphy, "The Steel Cocoon," 17.
19. Ibid., 18.
20. Ibid., 21.
21. Marcia Meldrum, "'A Calculated Risk': The Salk Polio Vaccine Field Trials of 1954," *British Medical Journal* 317 (October 31, 1998): 1233.
22. Keeling, *The Nurses of Mayo Clinic*, 75.
23. "Nurses in the Korean War: New Roles for a Traditional Profession," https://www.Koreanwar60.com (accessed November 27, 2016): 1.

24. Booker King and Ismal Jatoi, "The Mobile Army Surgical Hospital: A Military and Surgical Legacy," *Journal of the National Medical Association* 97, no. 5 (May 2005): 648–656 (quote 650).

25. Ibid.

26. "Women in the Korean Conflict," http://userpages.aug.com/captbarb/femvets6.html (accessed November 27, 2016): 1.

27. Mary Sarnecky, "Army Nurses in the Korean War," https://www.Koreanwar60.com (accessed November 27, 2016): 1.

28. John C. Kirchgessner, *A Reappraisal of Nursing Services and Shortages: A Case Study of the University of Virginia Hospital, 1945–1965* (PhD dissertation, University of Virginia, 2006): 86.

29. Ibid., 87.

30. Joan Lynaugh and Julie Fairman, "New Nurses, New Spaces: A Preview of the AACN History Survey," *American Journal of Critical Care* 1, no. 1 (1992): 19–24.

31. Kirchgessner, *A Reappraisal of Nursing Services*, 90.

32. Ibid., 87.

33. Julie Fairman, "Watchful Vigilance: Nursing Care, Technology, and the Development of Intensive Care Units," *Nursing Research* 41 (January/February 1992): 56–58.

34. Julie Fairman, "Creating Critical Care: The Case of the Hospital of the University of Pennsylvania, 1950-1965," *Advances in Nursing Science* 22 (January 1999): 63–77.

35. Rosemary Stevens, *In Sickness and in Wealth: Hospitals in the Twentieth Century* (Baltimore, MD: Johns Hopkins University Press, 1999): 204.

36. "Analysis of Nursing Problems: Report from the Joint Commission for the Improvement of the Care of the Patient," *Hospitals* 27 (March 1953): 88.

37. Stevens, *In Sickness and in Wealth*, 203.

38. Kirchgessner, *A Reappraisal of Nursing Services*, 91.

39. Ibid.

40. Rebecca Bouterie Harmon, *Nursing Care in a State Hospital, 1950–1965* (PhD dissertation, University of Virginia, 2003).

41. Ibid., 74.

42. Stevens, *In Sickness and in Wealth*, 203.

43. George Bugbee, "Hospitals in the Public Eye," *Hospitals* 34 (1960): 55.

44. Stevens, *In Sickness and in Wealth*, 259.

45. Rebecca Bouterie Harmon, *Nursing Care in a State Hospital, 1950-1965* (PhD Dissertation, University of Virginia: 2003): 74.

46. Ralf Dahm, "Discovering DNA: Friedrich Miescher and the Early Years of Nucleic Acid Research," *Human Genetics* 122 (January 2008): 565–581.

47. By 1965, heart disease accounted for 39% of all deaths in the United States, followed by cancer at 15.7% and stroke by 11.1%. Signe Cooper, *Contemporary Nursing Practice: A Guide for the Returning Nurse* (New York: McGraw-Hill, 1970), 46.

48. Marijo Juzwiak, "Nursing Care Florence Nightingale Never Dreamed of," *RN* 27 (May 1964): 44.

49. U.S. Bureau of Census, "Characteristics of Population," *1980 Census Population, Volume 1* (Washington, DC: United States Printing Office, 1993): Table 45.

50. Stevens, *In Sickness and in Wealth*, 1233.

51. Robert Almack, "How Many Closed Beds?" *Hospitals* 21 (May 1947): 59.

52. Virginia H. Walker, correspondence Virginia H. Walker to Carlisle S. Lentz, November 12, 1945, University of Virginia Health Sciences Library Special Collections, University of Virginia Hospital Director's Office Collection, 1.

53. Esther Lucille Brown, *Nursing for the Future: A Report Prepared for the National Nursing Council* (New York: Russell Sage Foundation, 1948): 138.

54. Esther Lucille Brown, "Professional Education for the Nursing of the Future," *American Journal of Nursing* 47 (1947): 820.

55. Raymond B. Allen, Earl Lomon Koos, Frank R. Bradley, and Lulu K. Wolf, The Brown Report," *AJN* 48, no. 12 (December 1948): 736.

56. Brown, "Professional Education," 820.

57. Surgeon General's Consultant Group in Nursing, *Toward Quality in Nursing: Needs and Goals* (Washington, DC: U.S. Government Printing Office, 1963): 64.

58. Mildred L. Montag, *The Education of Nursing Technicians* (New York: G. P. Putnam's Sons, 1951): 3.

59. Ibid., 4.

60. Ibid., 7.

61. Ibid., 73.

62. Ibid., 79.

63. Edith S. Oshin, "Associate Degree Nurses at Work," *RN* 27 (March 1964): 80.

64. Joan E. Lynaugh and Barbara L. Brush, *American Nursing: From Hospitals to Health Systems* (Hoboken, NJ: John Wiley & Sons, 1996): 49.

65. M. Sturdavant, D. Hitt, and R. Jydstrup, "A Study of Turnover and Its Costs," *Hospitals* 29 (May 1955): 59–62.

66. Philip Kalisch and Beatrice Kalisch, *The Advance of American Nursing*, 2nd ed. (Boston: Little, Brown, 1986): 360.

67. Joint Commission on Improvement of the Care of the Patient, "Analysis of Nursing Problems," *Hospitals* 27 (March 1953): 87–88.

68. Barbara Brush, *Sending for Nurses: Foreign Nurse Immigration to American Hospitals, 1945–1980* (PhD dissertation, University of Pennsylvania, 1994).

69. Faye Abdellah and Eugene Levine, "Why Nurses Leave Home," *Hospitals* 28 (June 1954): 80–81.

70. Kalisch and Kalisch, *The Advance of American Nursing*, 463–464.

71. American Nurses Association, "ANA Board Approves a Definition of Nursing Practice," *AJN* 55, no. 5 (1955): 1474.

72. Arlene Keeling, *Nursing and the Privilege of Prescription* (Columbus: The Ohio State University Press, 2007): 96.

73. Faye Abdellah and E. Josephine Starchan, "Progressive Patient Care," *AJN* 59, no. 5 (May 1959): 649–655.

74. Ibid.

75. Fairman, "Watchful Vigilance."

76. Melissa McIntire Sherrod, "Nursing in West Texas: Trains, Tumbleweeds, and Rattlesnakes," ch. 8 in *Nursing Rural America*, eds. John C. Kirchgessner and Arlene W. Keeling (New York: Springer Publishing, 2015): 121–136.

77. Ibid., 124–125.

78. Ibid., 130.

79. Ibid.

80. Family members noted that when they went to church or were met in public, many would bow or try to kiss their hands, or touch their arms as a gesture of thanks. For some their presence in the community was seen as an omen of good fortune.

81. Sherrod, "Nursing in West Texas," 132.

FURTHER READING

Dunphy, Lynne M., "The Steel Cocoon: Tales of the Nurses and Patients of the Iron Lung, 1929-1955," *Nursing History Review* 9 (2001): 5.

Fairman, Julie, "Watchful Vigilance: Nursing Care, Technology, and the Development of Intensive Care Units," *Nursing Research* 41 (January/February 1992): 56–58.

Fairman, Julie, "Creating Critical Care: The Case of the Hospital of the University of Pennsylvania, 1950-1965," *Advances in Nursing Science* 22 (January 1999): 63–77.

King, Booker, and Jatoi, Ismal, "The Mobile Army Surgical Hospital: A Military and Surgical Legacy," *Journal of the National Medical Association* 97, no. 5 (May 2005): 648–656.

Kirchgessner, John C., *A Reappraisal of Nursing Services and Shortages: A Case Study of the University of Virginia Hospital, 1945–1965* (PhD dissertation, University of Virginia, 2006).

Lusk, Brigid, "Prelude to Specialization: U.S. Cancer Nursing, 1920-1950," *Nursing Inquiry* 12, no. 4 (2005): 269–277.

Lynaugh, Joan, and Brush, Barbara, *American Nursing: From Hospitals to Health Systems* (Cambridge, MA: Blackwell Publishers).

Lynaugh, Joan, and Fairman, Julie, "New Nurses, New Spaces: A Preview of the AACN History Survey," *American Journal of Critical Care* 1, no. 1 (1992): 19–24.

Numbers, Ronald L., "The Third Party: Health Insurance in America," in *Sickness and Health in America*, 2nd ed. (Madison: University of Wisconsin Press, 1985): 238–239.

Stevens, Rosemary, *In Sickness and in Wealth: American Hospitals in the Twentieth Century* (Baltimore, MD: Johns Hopkins University Press, 1989).

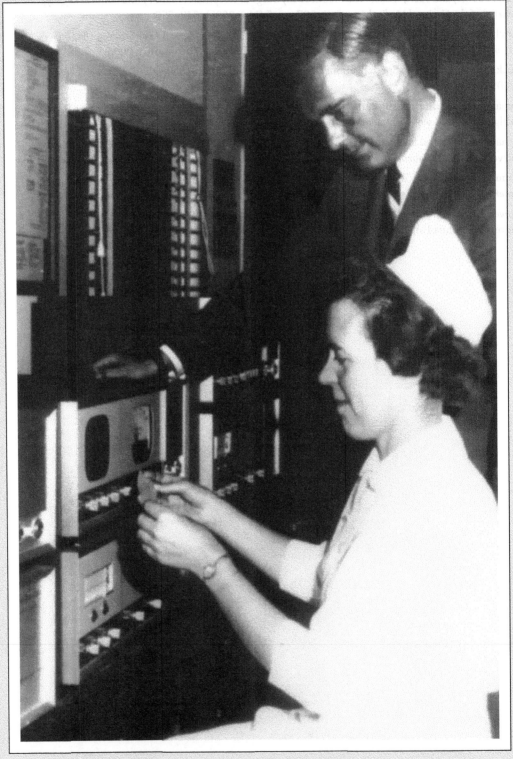

Dr. Lawrence Meltzer and Nurse Rose Pinneo reading EKG.

CHAPTER 13

Specialization, War, and the Expansion of Nursing's Scope of Practice

1961–1980

Arlene W. Keeling

"Why, after a century of modern nursing, do we feel compelled to confess that enough of us aren't clear about our own role in the vast complex of medical care? Nor are most nurses able to describe their primary role. They tend to believe that the only way for them to enhance their status is to develop great skill in the performance of straight medical tasks, or to move up into the administrative hierarchy. . . . There is no single approach to the matter of identifying the unique core of nursing. . . . We must have theorists . . . researchers . . . and those who have day-to-day contact with patients. The accumulated performance of thousands of nurses will bring us closer to understanding it than any single collection of words."[1]

Writing in the December 1961 issue of the *American Journal of Nursing,* editor Barbara Schutt tried to capture what she called "the greatest problem" facing nursing as the year came to a close. In the 1960s, the profession was grappling with its boundaries, its role in the health care system, its overall identity—one that would separate it from medicine and social work. For more than a century, the profession's scope of activity had merged with medicine and social work and nurse theorists and scholars had tried to identify exactly what it was that made nursing unique. Now the profession was faced with a decade of turmoil, and before the 1960s ended the context in which nursing existed would change dramatically. Political turmoil and racial unrest, President Johnson's Great Society legislative achievements supporting health care for seniors and the poor, and America's involvement in a war in Vietnam all contributed to the larger social context. Specific changes related to nursing would be the rise of coronary care units (CCUs), the introduction of new technology, the growth of medical specialization, and the inception of the nursing roles of clinical nurse specialist and nurse practitioner.

Each of these factors would challenge the profession to define itself. Central to that definition were two questions: whether nurses could expand their role within an increasingly high-tech and specialized hospital setting; and whether nurses could assume a larger role in primary care outside the hospital. The latter would expand the nursing role to include making medical diagnoses and prescribing treatments.

A NEW ERA OF SPECIALIZATION

In the mid-20th century, the nursing profession would be challenged once again with the enormity of change that was taking place in the United States, in medicine, in technology, and the growth of science. Within hospitals, new configurations of spaces and the ever-increasing nursing shortage demanded that nursing be done in unique and modern ways. Meanwhile, the continuous rise of subspecialty medicine increased the demands for nurses to acquire new specialty knowledge. A rise in subspecialties in nursing would soon follow.

Coronary Care Nursing

With the establishment of the Bethany Hospital CCU in Kansas City in 1962 and a second unit at Presbyterian Hospital in Philadelphia in 1963, coronary care nursing emerged as a new clinical specialty during the 1960s. Within a few short years, it spread rapidly throughout the nation, challenging the nurse's traditional role as a subservient caregiver—one who was "ordered to care."[2]

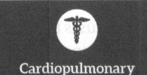

Cardiopulmonary Resuscitation (CPR)

In 1959, Johns Hopkins physicians William B. Kouwenhoven, James Jude, and G. Guy Knickerbocker did extensive research on the heart while they experimented with dogs. They discovered an effective method of "massaging the heart without thoracotomy"— that is, without surgically opening the chest. Over the next decade, CPR would become an effective way to save cardiac patients.[5]

The coronary care movement started in Bethany Hospital in Kansas in 1960. There, the chief of cardiology Hughes W. Day, MD, was concerned about the sudden deaths of his middle-aged cardiac patients.[3] Mortality in patients with acute myocardial infarction who were admitted to the community hospital was 30% to 40%. Moreover, the patients died suddenly and unexpectedly, usually while they were unobserved in their private rooms.

Determined to decrease that mortality rate and save patients whose hearts he considered "too young to die," Day initiated a new protocol for responding to patients who suffered cardiac arrest. His plan called for a "Code Blue" team composed of doctors, nurses, and an inhalation therapist to rush to the patient's room with a cart of emergency supplies, including a portable cardiac defibrillator. On arrival at the patient's bedside, the team would begin cardiopulmonary resuscitation (CPR), intubate the patient, and defibrillate his or her heart, if necessary. In addition, the team would insert intravenous (IV) lines into the patient and administer fluids and emergency drugs.[4]

Day's Code Blue team was an excellent idea—at least in theory. In reality, the protocol was used for 10 months without a significant decrease in patient mortality. Initial delays in recognizing that a patient had suffered a cardiac arrest and subsequent delays in getting the equipment and the Code Blue team to the bedside often meant it was too late to save the patient. As a result, of those in whom resuscitation was attempted, only 4% survived.[6]

Frustrated by the low success rate of the Code Blue procedure, Day decided to monitor all patients admitted for myocardial infarction by attaching them to cardiac monitoring equipment. The continuous monitoring, the same type that was being used in space, was meant to alert the nurse immediately when something was wrong.[7]

Having obtained the equipment, Day placed the cardiac monitor outside of the patient's room and set the arrhythmia alarms. That way, *theoretically*, the nurse caring for the patient could immediately observe a change in heart rhythm or respond to alarms signifying cardiac arrest. Nurse Judith Stuart at Bethany Hospital recounted what actually happened:

> *One of the engineers at Bethany, Johnny Walker, rigged up a cardiac monitor for Dr. Day. Originally the cardiac patients were just put in a room out on the floor and hooked to a monitor that sat outside the room. When the patient's heart stopped, the alarm would go off and the nurse would call Dr. Day at home so he could come to the hospital and try to resuscitate the patient. Usually it was too late because more than ten minutes had elapsed.*[9]

After 2 years of trying to monitor heart patients in their private rooms on a general medical unit and running into the hospital to respond to the nurses' requests for help, Day concluded that he needed to train a small group of nurses to interpret EKG rhythms, troubleshoot the monitoring equipment, and respond to emergencies. He explained:

> *We had no nurses who could correctly interpret the electrocardiographic patterns. . . . This was especially true at 3 a.m. Our crying need was for a group of specially trained nurses . . . who could . . . interpret signs of impending disaster and quickly institute cardiopulmonary resuscitation.*[11]

It was clear to Day that the new technology alone was not enough: nurses with specialized training in cardiology were the necessary link between the technology and the heart patients.

After Day discussed his idea for a special cardiac unit with Bethany's administrator, the pair developed a plan for combining a new intensive care unit (ICU) with a cardiac rehabilitation unit, calling it the Intensive Care–Cardiac Rehabilitation Unit. Funded by the Hartford Foundation, and supported by the director of nursing, Ruby Harris, the new unit became known as the "Hartford Coronary Care Unit."[12] The model unit was staffed by specially trained nurses who could handle two responsibilities—care for critically ill medical and surgical patients in the seven-bed, open ward, and monitoring of cardiac patients in the four private rooms.[13]

The plan to keep heart patients in private rooms separated from the open-ward ICU was based on the idea that cardiac patients needed a peaceful environment in which they could heal. The ICU was far from quiet. The open-ward ICU for critically ill patients had bright lights, emergency procedures, and late-night admissions. Even with private rooms, the reality of the new unit was less than peaceful. Each of the beds in the Hartford unit was equipped with an oscilloscope that had an audible signal to alert personnel of a cardiac arrest.[14] Each beeped on average 80 times a minute, every minute, day and night.

Furthermore, the four private rooms designated as the cardiac unit had a very limited bed capacity. Once the four beds in the private rooms were filled, a cardiac

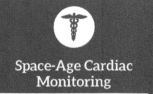

Space-Age Cardiac Monitoring

As Alan Sheppard and John Glenn voyaged into space in the early 1960s, the National Air and Space Administration developed new methods of monitoring the heart. They attached electrodes to the astronauts that beamed electronic information about their hearts' rhythms back to an oscilloscope on earth, where scientists could observe any irregularities.[8]

"Something Had to Be Done"

Dr. Day lived on North 17th Street. The hospital is on North 12th Street, and the floor nurses would call him all the time, just to turn the alarms off. . . . The patients were fine, but the electrodes had come off. . . . After many nights of lost sleep, Dr. Day said something had to be done.[10]

Penny Standish, 1963

"There were eleven different heartbeats audible at all times. It was confusing and noisy."[15]

Judith Stuart, Night Supervisor, 1963

patient might be admitted to the intensive care section where only a curtain separated the cardiac patient from the bustling environment. Soon the nurses questioned whether the new combined ICU–CCU environment was conducive to a patient's recovery. It would take years to separate the two units. Meanwhile, the nurses worked in the environment they had.

Although they were experienced in general medical–surgical nursing, the nurses who had been recruited to work in the CCU were novices in reading the EKG images that blipped across the screens.[16] Even head nurse Natalia Gill had no experience reading electrocardiograms. As she recalled, "all I knew about it was that everyone has a heartbeat, but I didn't know what else we would be looking for."[17] The nurses had only enough knowledge of cardiac rhythms to recognize one that was abnormal and then notify the physician. According to Judith Stuart, the only educational material the nurses possessed was a 12-page typewritten booklet that contained hand-drawn arrhythmias.[18] The nurses needed to learn how to interpret the cardiac rhythms—and that learning would have to occur on the job.

During their time spent in the Hartford unit, the nurses also had to learn to insert IV lines, a task that until the mid-20th century was performed only by physicians. Some nurses had inserted IV catheters in life-threatening emergencies during World War II. Usually, however, nurses assisted physicians with the task, setting up the IV pole, hanging the bottle of IV fluid, flushing the line, handing tape and dressings to the physician, and cleaning up the patient and the room after the IV was in place. Now, in the CCU, the nurse was expected to do the entire procedure by herself.

The problem was that starting an IV brought up questions about nursing's scope of practice. In the 1950s, a group of lawyers had addressed the issue and wrote about it in the *American Journal of Nursing*. In that article, they concluded that it was up to each state whether a nurse could legally insert an IV line:

The present legality of nurses' activities in this field is a matter of state law. Consequently . . . no one answer would be applicable to all states. The answer would depend upon the language of the nurse practice act and medical practice act in the particular state, and on the administrative rulings and judicial decisions interpreting such language.[21]

All that being said, the Hartford Unit nurses did not concern themselves with the law. When asked, the nurses responded: "We just did it."[22] To them, the practical aspects of patient care came first, and every patient needed a working IV line at all times in case of a sudden cardiac arrhythmia that required immediate IV medication.

Another question related to nursing's scope of practice had to do with the new procedure of CPR. The Hartford Unit nurses were expected to perform CPR if the patient had a cardiac arrest. To do so, they had to recognize ventricular fibrillation and/or asystole, correlate the arrhythmia with the patient's signs and symptoms, make a clinical judgment, and take action. When nurses were the only ones around—at 3 a.m., for example—they were authorized to do so. In the daytime, however, when physicians were available, the nurses deferred to the physician. In other words, the nurses' scope of practice expanded after midnight and contracted during the day.

From June 1962 to January 1963, seven patients who suffered cardiac arrests were successfully resuscitated in the CCU at Bethany. Eager to share those successes, Day presented a paper about the Hartford Unit at a national meeting. That presentation, along with publications about the unit and the nurses' role, had a major impact on the development of other CCUs.

Within a year after the Hartford Unit opened, other hospitals throughout the country established their own CCUs. Among these was one at Presbyterian Hospital in Philadelphia, where Drs. Lawrence Meltzer and J. Roderick Kitchell, assisted by nurse Rose Pinneo, conducted a research study to determine if nurses could take on the new, high-level responsibilities of cardiac monitoring, CPR, and cardiac defibrillation.[24] The experiment was a success—nurses could and *did* learn new skills. They expanded their scope of practice, achieved a new level of autonomy, and gained the respect of their physician colleagues.

Rose Pinneo, who participated in a study to prove that nurses could handle increased high-level responsibilities like cardiac defibrillation.

Because of Meltzer and Pinneo's presentations on the topic at national conferences, as well as their publications about coronary care nursing, their work soon received international acclaim. Thousands of nurses learned to interpret EKGs through reading the researchers' book: *Intensive Coronary Care for Nurses: A Manual for Nurses.*[25]

As CCUs materialized in hospitals throughout the United States, nurses and physicians gained increasingly specialized clinical knowledge in the field of cardiology. Together, these nurses and physicians discussed clinical questions and negotiated

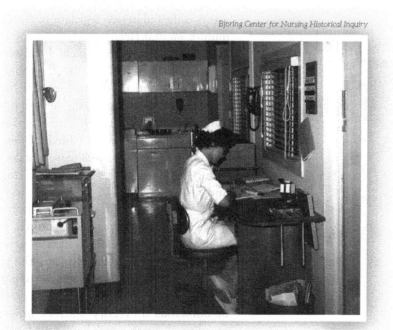

Presbyterian coronary care unit nurse Janice Lufkin at nurses' station.

"We really worked together as a doctor–nurse team."[26]

Rose Pinneo

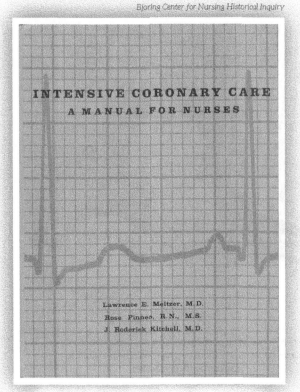

INTENSIVE CORONARY CARE

A MANUAL FOR NURSES

Lawrence E. Meltzer, M.D.
Rose Pinneo, R.N., M.S.
J. Roderick Kitchell, M.D.

Intensive Coronary Care: A Manual for Nurses,
written by Meltzer, Pinneo, and Kitchell who
pioneered expanding nurses' roles.

responsibilities, expanding nurses' scope of practice.[27] Janice Lufkin, head nurse in the Presbyterian Hospital CCU, recalled: "We soon got experience with the rhythm strips. The interns would even come up the stairs from the ER and ask if we could read the rhythm strip of an ER patient or interpret their EKG. They would ask if they should admit the patient . . . We would tell them what to do."[28]

Clearly, whenever nurses identified cardiac arrhythmias, administered IV medications, and took the initiative to defibrillate a patient's heart, they crossed the boundary of the physicians' customary territory. All were acts of diagnosis and treatment. The line between medicine and nursing was blurring, even though the nurses worked under guidelines provided by physicians through standing order sets.[29] The process was reminiscent of what nurses had done in earlier times and places in the absence of a physician.

Other Areas of Specialization

Coronary care nursing was not the only nursing specialization to develop in the 1960s. The decade was replete with the development of specialty practice in many areas, including renal nursing, oncology nursing, trauma and burn nursing, and psychiatric nursing. In 1965, nurse leader Hildegarde Peplau contended that the development of areas of specialization was preceded by three social forces: (a) an increase in specialty-related information, (b) new technological advances, and (c) a response to public need and interest. All of these factors converged in the 1960s.

Of these factors, a rise in public interest was manifested in new legislation. The Community Mental Health Centers Act of 1963 and the growing interest in child and adolescent mental health care directly enhanced specialization in psychiatric–mental health nursing. It also expanded the nurse's role in outpatient mental health care. The establishment of Regional Area Medical Centers under the "War on Heart Disease, Cancer and Stroke" increased the number of trauma and neurosurgical ICUs in addition to ICUs and CCUs. On a larger scale, the enactment of Medicare and Medicaid legislation in 1965 changed the health care system in general, providing care for the elderly and the poor. Specific to nursing, the federally supported 1964 Nurse Training Act led to the creation of numerous university master's programs for clinical nurse specialists, and later, for nurse practitioners.

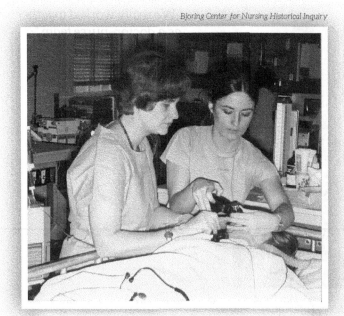

Intensive care unit nurses administering oxygen to a patient.

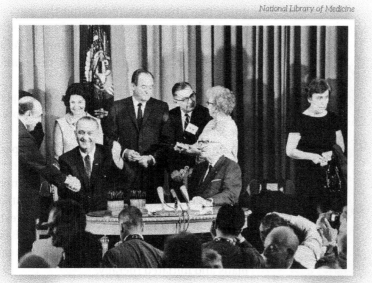

President Lyndon B. Johnson signing the Medicare Act.

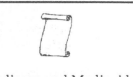

The Nurse Training Act, 1964

The Nurse Training Act of 1964 (H. B. 10042) authorized millions of dollars over five years to fund special projects and planning grants, student loans and scholarships, professional nurse traineeships, and nursing school construction. It was a "nationwide effort to alleviate critical shortages of nurses" to support "the health care of all citizens."[30]

Numerous nursing organizations representing different specialties soon emerged. In the late 1960s, the American Association of Critical-Care Nurses was organized to meet the continuing educational needs of new specialists in the areas of coronary care and intensive care nursing. Only a few years later, a group of oncology nurses met to discuss the need for a national organization to support *their* specialty.

NURSES AND ACCESS TO CARE

Coinciding with the rise of specialization in medicine in the late 1960s, fewer physicians were choosing to enter general practice. Instead, doctors chose to work in specialties such as cardiology, neurosurgery, nephrology, and oncology, clustering their practices near medical centers in cities and suburbs. As the trend drew more physicians away from general practice, particularly in rural areas of the country, the American Medical Association issued numerous reports decrying "the shortage of physicians in poor rural and urban areas."[32]

At the same time, Americans were demanding accessible and affordable care, while health care delivery costs were increasing at an annual rate of 10% to 14%.[33] Indeed, many considered the U.S. health care system to be "too specialized, too centralized and inaccessible, too impersonal and too disease oriented."[34] What people wanted was decentralized, accessible, primary health care that focused on the patient as a whole person. It was exactly what nurses were prepared to do.

Medicare and Medicaid Legislation, 1965

In 1965, President Lyndon B. Johnson signed legislation for Medicare and Medicaid (H. R. 6675), ensuring federal and state financial support for healthcare services for those older than 65 years of age and those who qualified for help because of insufficient income and resources. In previous decades, several administrations had established the basis of the law, but the national medical program proposed in the 1945 Wagner–Murray–Dingell bill was its strongest foundation.[31]

A Pediatric Nurse Practitioner Program

In response to the demand for health care in the rural areas of Colorado, nurse Loretta Ford and Dr. Henry Silver opened the first formal nurse practitioner program at the University of Colorado in 1965.[35] The demonstration project was designed to prepare professional nurses to provide comprehensive well-child care and to manage common childhood health problems. The 4-month program, which certified registered nurses as pediatric nurse practitioners *without* requiring a master's degree, emphasized the nurse's role in promoting health. Loretta Ford envisioned the development of the pediatric

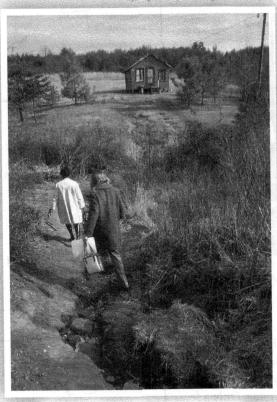

Nurses visiting rural home, providing access to care.

nurse practitioner as reclaiming the nurse's role in well-child care, a role that had been lost in the 1930s when the American Academy of Pediatrics claimed that well-child care was the domain of pediatricians.[36]

But the boundaries of the role of the pediatric nurse practitioner were blurry and nurse practitioners soon overstepped the invisible line separating nursing and medicine. In the Colorado pediatric nurse practitioner program, nurses learned to take health histories and conduct physical exams. They also learned how to devise a list of differential diagnoses, using the results of laboratory tests like EKGs, x-rays, and blood work to do so. Based on their clinical assessments, they made treatment plans and initiated therapy.

The Colorado program sparked the profession's interest, and soon certificate programs for nurse practitioners emerged in other states. In 1969, Wayne State University introduced a 2-year master's program for "health nurse clinicians" that would prepare nurses for practitioner roles in hospitals and public health agencies.[37] The development of nurse practitioner programs was not without controversy, however. Both nurses and physicians accused the nurse practitioners of practicing medicine when they made "medical" diagnoses and wrote prescriptions; both professions "skirmished over the status and power" of the nursing profession.[38] Because of this, some nurse educators and other nurse leaders, including those from the American Nurses Association (ANA), questioned whether the nurse practitioner role could be situated within the discipline of nursing or whether it was more appropriately a physician assistant role. Thus, the new role was controversial, especially in academia and in organizations like the ANA. In her history of the nurse practitioner movement, Dr. Julie Fairman commented on the issue, noting: "At best, the ANA was ambivalent about nurse practitioners during much of the last half of the twentieth century."[39]

The Proliferation of Nurse Practitioner Programs

While nursing leaders, nursing professors, and others debated the issue, policy makers supported the new role for nurses. They saw that nurse practitioners could fill a gap in providing health care to underserved communities. With government support and private funding, the idea spread. Some young nursing professors, eager to obtain funding and implement new programs that they considered "cutting-edge," opened nurse practitioner programs in universities.

Thus, by the 1970s Ford and Silver's idea had taken hold. It seemed logical to use the two major health care professions, medicine and nursing together, to expand primary care to the American public. People living in rural areas needed health care providers and overworked physicians needed help. The federal government was also interested. In the early 1970s, Health, Education and Welfare Secretary Elliot Richardson established the Committee to Study Extended Roles for Nurses to evaluate the feasibility of expanding nursing practice.[40]

The committee concluded that extending the scope of the nurse's role was essential to providing equal access to health care for all Americans. According to a 1971 editorial on the topic in the *American Journal of Nursing*: "The kind of health care Lillian Wald began preaching and practicing in 1893 is the kind the people of this country are still crying for.[41] The committee's report, published in November 1971, urged the establishment of innovative curricular designs for nurse practitioner education in health science centers and increased financial support for nursing education.[42] It also urged national certification for nurse practitioners, and developed a model nurse practice law that could be applied throughout the nation. In response, with mounting concern over the restrictive 1955 ANA definition of nursing practice, the ANA counsel suggested the following addendum to state nurse practice acts:

> *A professional nurse may also perform such additional acts, under emergency or other special conditions, which may include special training, as are recognized by the medical and nursing professions as proper to be performed by a professional nurse under such condition, even though such acts might otherwise be considered diagnosis and prescription.*[43]

Despite the cumbersome language, the addendum's meaning was clear—intensive care nurses (including coronary care nurses) could interpret EKGs, defibrillate, start IV lines, and give life-saving drugs according to standing orders; nurse practitioners could diagnose and prescribe—as long as these acts were done under "special" conditions. The addendum paved the way for nurses to take leadership roles in promoting access to primary care for people throughout the nation.

By the early 1970s, the University of Rochester, the University of Pennsylvania, and the University of Virginia all had programs for nurse practitioner education. In addition to the pediatric nurse practitioner program modeled after Ford and Silver's, programs for family nurse practitioners (FNPs) and emergency nurse practitioners also developed.

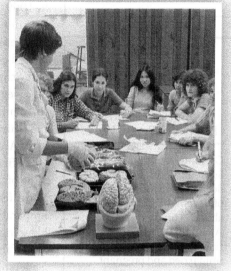

Nurse practitioner students at the University of Virginia in a dissection lab.

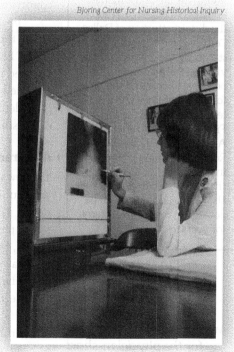

University of Virginia nurse practitioner student learning to interpret x-rays.

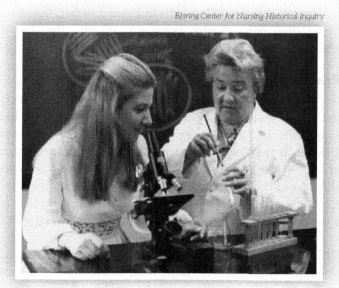

Nurse practitioner student learning from Dr. Phyllis Verhonick at the University of Virginia.

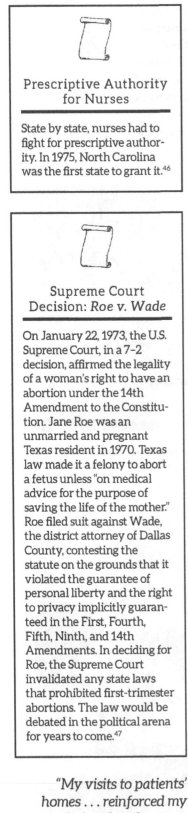

"My visits to patients' homes . . . reinforced my conviction that the nurse was an untapped resource for the physician-short Federal agency."[53]

Lorraine Duran, 1978

Despite the rapid growth of nursing programs, several questions remained unanswered. Among these were issues related to how nurse practitioners were to be defined, how they could "effectively and efficiently fit into the health care system to improve access to primary care, and how the nurse practitioner differed from the physician assistant."[44] Two specific issues needed to be addressed: (a) Would nurse practitioners have the authority to write prescriptions? And (b) how would nurse practitioners be reimbursed for their services?[45]

The Frontier Nursing Service Opens an FNP Program

In 1969, a consultant firm made an in-depth study of how nurses from the Frontier Nursing Service could play a larger role in providing health care in "inaccessible counties of Appalachian Kentucky." They concluded it was indeed possible and recommended that the "Frontier Nursing Service Graduate School of Midwifery" be "expanded and modified" to incorporate a master's degree program in "comprehensive family nursing." The consultants further recommended that the Frontier graduate program be affiliated with the University of Kentucky.[48]

Accepting the consultants' advice, leaders of the Frontier Nursing Service offered its FNP certificate program in 1970. The first class entered in June of that year, and the school changed its name to the Frontier School of Midwifery and Family Nursing to reflect the expansion of the educational preparation it offered. According to the school catalog, the "FNP would be a blending of nursing with selected medical and public health functions." The aim of the program was "to prepare nurses as colleagues of the physician for leadership positions in the delivery of family health services."[49] The traditional nursing role would be expanded to include basic diagnostic, treatment, and preventive skills "so that FNPs would be able to provide assistance to families, whether they be living in Appalachia, inner cities or developing countries."[50]

By 1974, more than 80 students had graduated from the program. By 1975, the Frontier staff included four physicians, seven nurse-midwives, seven FNPs, nine nurse-midwives/FNPs, 19 registered nurses, and five licensed practical nurses. Together they served a population of 15,000 and provided care to more than 66,000 patients in 1 year.[51] In fact, the new program left the Frontier nurses better prepared to do what they had been doing since 1925.

A Nurse Practitioner in the Indian Health Service

The new nurse practitioner role soon became a benefit to other remote rural communities. In the southwest, a Native American Indian public health nurse, Lorraine Duran, took advantage of the opportunity to become a nurse practitioner in the Colorado pediatric nurse practitioner program. Duran, born into the Ute tribe, had grown up near the Navajo reservation and was well aware of the dwindling number of physicians on the reservations. Later, while working as a public health nurse in Shiprock, New Mexico, she saw the potential for nurses to deliver primary care services in that area.[52]

In 1970, Duran was faced with the opportunity to succeed her mother as head of the Indian Health Service clinic on the southern Ute reservation. She accepted the job on one condition: that she could first become a pediatric nurse practitioner through the Colorado program.

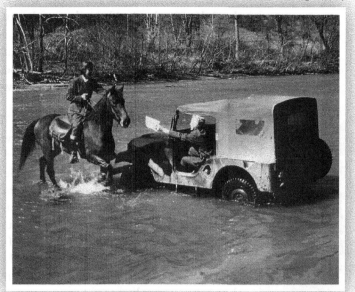

Frontier nurses provided care to more than 66,000 patients per year.

After graduating from the program, Duran worked with physicians in the Indian Health Service for the next 7 years, providing care to the Ute tribe. Working in a small, red brick clinic, Duran saw patients with respiratory and gastrointestinal problems, skin infections, sore eyes, lacerations, burns, and factures—in short, every type of illness that physicians saw in high-volume outpatient clinics. And, like Indian Health Service nurses who had preceded her, Duran also taught nutrition, hygiene, and pre- and postnatal care, and visited the elderly in their homes. Incorporating herbal medicines, sacred rituals, and input from the Ute medicine men was important to her work. "You have to remember," she commented, "that the American Indians got along nicely for thousands of years before Western medicine was introduced."[55]

"I knew that my Ute blood was a strong point in winning acceptance from the Indian people."[56]

Lorraine Duran, 1978

Other legislation in the 1970s benefited both rural clinics, in general, and Indian Health Service clinics, in particular. In 1976, Congress passed the Indian Health Center Improvement Act. Title I of that Act authorized funding to increase the number of Indian health professionals available to serve their own communities. It also allocated funds to improve inadequate, outdated clinics and hospitals on the reservations.[57] A year later, Congress passed the Rural Health Clinicians Act (Pub. L. No. 95-210), allowing some nurse practitioners to receive Medicare and Medicaid reimbursement for their services. The one condition the nurse practitioners had to meet was that they worked in freestanding, physician-directed *rural* clinics in areas where there was a shortage of health professionals. Payments were made to the nurses' physician employers.[58]

NURSING IN THE VIETNAM WAR, 1965–1973

In the mid-1960s and early 1970s, while numerous changes in nursing practice and nursing education were taking place within the boundaries of the United States, American nurses were involved in the Vietnam War halfway around the world. Since 1962, when the first U.S. military hospital was established there, about 15 Army nurses were in Vietnam. Even after President

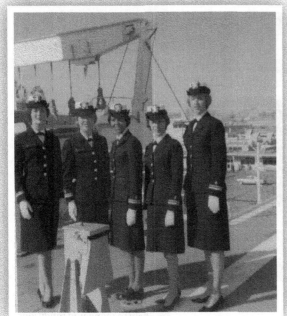

Female Navy nurses in Vietnam, all of whom enlisted, as women were never drafted.

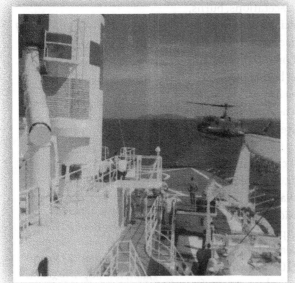

Hospital ship that provided care to wounded and sick soldiers during the Vietnam War, where nurses often worked around the clock.

"With each assignment, the war changed, the country changed, and I changed."

Rosemary Cox, USS Repose, 1966

Johnson mobilized ground troops in 1965 after the Gulf of Tonkin incident, the number of nurses assigned to Vietnam remained low. That number changed in 1966, when the growing number of American soldiers deployed to Vietnam fought and were wounded in battle. As the number of wounded increased, the demand for nurses rose.

In 1966, the government conscripted 700 male nurses for the Army and 200 for the Navy, while additional American nurses, both male and female, volunteered for service overseas. Female nurses were never drafted; they enlisted of their own accord. Many had been recruited to do so as part of "Operation Nightingale," an intensive educational assistance program that paid a portion of student nurses' tuition and a monthly wage in exchange for corresponding years of active service.[60] By 1968, there were more than 800 Army nurses stationed in Vietnam; by January 1969, there were more than 900.[61] Other military nurses served on airlift helicopters and airplanes with the Air Force, or on land and sea with the Navy Nurse Corps.

Many Navy nurses were assigned to hospital ships. In December 1965, 14 Navy nurses sailed aboard the USS *Repose,* arriving off the coast of the Hue-Phu-Bai area in January 1966. By late March, 15 other Navy nurses had joined the corps. On board the ship, the nurses worked day and night to care for casualties. Nurse Frances Buckley described her experience:

Amid the anguish, suffering, and tragedy of receiving casualties . . . a bonding developed among all crew members, unlike any I had ever experienced before or since Vietnam. Crew members, whether ship's company or hospital personnel, truly cared about the patients. Compassion and charity were every day norms.[62]

Other Navy nurses completed their tours of duty on the USS *Sanctuary,* in the station hospital at DaNang before it was turned over to the Army in 1970, or at naval hospitals in Guam, Japan, Europe, and the United States.

The Army nurses also did their share. Among these was nurse anesthetist Elwood Wilkins, who enlisted in the U.S. Army on June 2, 1966, the day he graduated from the nurse anesthetist program in the Mayo School of Health Sciences. In Vietnam, Wilkins administered anesthesia to patients in one of the Army's busiest evacuation hospitals, a less than ideal setting. Short of supplies and without access to running water, Wilkins improvised, doing what he could to save lives. Like other nurses, Wilkins worked 12-hour shifts, 6 days a week. During mass casualty events when "it was not uncommon to have 100 casualties at a time," Wilkins was in the operating room around the clock.[63]

For the Army nurses in particular, living conditions varied during the nurses' 12-month tour of duty. Until 1967, nurses lived in tents; afterwards, most all lived in tropical buildings, many of the Quonset hut variety, and a few in air-conditioned trailers. Most of the quarters were hot and humid, and infested with bugs.

In Vietnam, there were "no front lines and no safe areas"[65] and most U.S. military nurses feared for their physical safety at some time during their tour of duty.[66] During the Tet Offensive in 1968, when 70,000 enemy troops attacked hundreds of Vietnamese towns and American military installations, nurses at the 67th Evacuation Hospital "adjusted to sleeping under their beds with flak jackets on and helmets nearby."[67] Other nurses worried about being taken hostage like those who were captured in the Philippines during World War II.

Nurses worked whether they were on duty or off. While on duty, the nurses cared for patients with battlefield injuries that had occurred just hours before. The establishment of rapid aerial evacuation to MUST units (medical unit, self-contained, transportable) facilitated that care. "The average time interval from battlefield injury to hospital admission was 2.8 hours." As a result, for the most part nurses practiced emergency and trauma care, and surgical intensive care.[69] The nurses were horrified by the injuries they saw in Vietnam. Jeanne Rivera, an operating room supervisor in both Qui Nhon and Saigon during 1967 to 1968, wrote: "I remember one fellow didn't even know that when I took his boot off, I took his foot."[70] Other nurses cared for patients whose legs or arms had been blown off and those with severe head injuries. Afterward, the nurses would not talk about it. Lorraine Boudreau, who served two tours of duty in evacuation hospitals in Vietnam, was adamant about that: "We never talked about what was going on. Nobody ever did."[71] While off duty, Army nurses voluntarily cared for Vietnamese civilians, treating them in clinics, immunizing them, making sick calls at local orphanages, and conducting courses in child care for the villagers.[72]

Army and Navy nurses were not the only ones who were sent to Vietnam during the war. Air Force nurses also volunteered for assignments in Southeast Asia. In 1966, 16 female Air Force nurses arrived in Vietnam for duty at the U.S. Air Force (USAF) base at Cam Ranh Bay, where they filled the "full range of nursing specialties" in the new 12th USAF Hospital.[73]

Back in the United States, people began to question the value of the war and the U.S. involvement in it. When the evening news started to broadcast pictures of flag-draped coffins returning from Vietnam, American citizens demonstrated against the war in the streets and on college campuses. As young men approached the age at which they would be drafted, they were not willing to die in what they saw as a futile, endless conflict. The people's negative attitude had a devastating impact on returning soldiers and military nurses. They were stunned when they were advised

"In Vietnam we practiced jungle anesthesia. You make do with what you've got."[64]

Elwood Wilkins

The Tet Offensive

"The morning of the Tet Offensive, the telephone rang . . . the U.S. Embassy had been attacked, we were on red alert, report to the hospital. . . . Around eight in the morning, the casualties were coming into triage. Within an hour we were four hours behind."[68]

Lois Johnson, 629th Medical Detachment, 1968

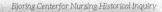
Bjoring Center for Nursing Historical Inquiry

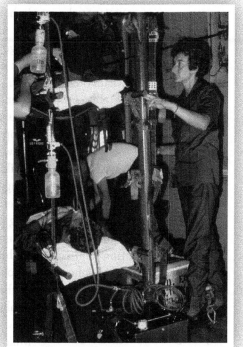

A nurse tending to wounded soldiers in Vietnam.

to change out of their uniforms as soon as they could to avoid being harassed. Some service members expressed feelings of being abandoned by their fellow citizens. Re-entry into civilian life proved difficult for retuning military nurses. The negative public attitude exacerbated their other difficulties of posttraumatic stress syndrome and moral distress about what they had witnessed in Vietnam.[74]

NURSING IN THE COMMUNITY IN THE 1960s

In a time of social and political unrest, the profession would grapple with the best way to provide care for not only individuals but also aggregates. Within the profession, there was a growing interest in the notion that the profession had to focus on the community as client. Underpinning that idea was a belief in connecting with the community to find out what their particular needs were before attempting to provide care. Nancy Milio, a public health nurse who worked to ensure care for underprivileged mothers and babies in Detroit, Michigan, did just that.

Nancy Milio and the Clinic on Kercheval Street

While military nurses struggled to save lives in Vietnam and to understand their role in the war when they returned, other nurses worked within a politically and socially charged environment within the United States. Demonstrations against the war in Vietnam, assassinations of political leaders, unrest on college campuses, and deadly race riots in inner cities filled the headlines.

In an inner-city Black neighborhood of Detroit, Michigan, where racial conflicts, poverty, and social inequities were the norm, one nurse tried to make a difference. Public health nurse Nancy Milio had seen these problems firsthand since she had grown up in the area and had worked for the Visiting Nurse Association. In Detroit, African Americans struggled to obtain jobs, housing, food, and medical care. Now, in the mid-1960s, Milio was determined to do something—at least make a change to their access to health care. As a 25-year-old White nurse doing graduate work in sociology, she saw her opportunity. She decided to design a new model of care for the disadvantaged patients she saw in her public health role. The model would be based on collaboration *with* the community and its members. Milio realized she would have to take several steps to achieve her goal. First and foremost, she wanted to help mothers and children: "I put on paper what women had told me in their homes . . . [and] my thoughts about what could be done. . . . It was the first of many drafts of what became the 'Maternity Satellite Project,' later known as the 'Mom and Tots Center.'"[75]

Milio's idea was to establish a community center that would have a nurse, but would be run, not "top down" by nurses and physicians, but by women in the neighborhood. Her main goal was "to address the care of inner-city, socioeconomically disadvantaged women and children." The community center would address issues from a holistic perspective, including services of day care and free transportation to the clinic. That way, women could get to the clinic with their children without having to rely on bus schedules or needing money to pay for public transportation. Once at the clinic, they could receive the immunizations and check-ups they needed and stay for health education seminars—all while their children were kept busy in the day-care center. Neighborhood volunteers, who understood the community's culture and health practices, would conduct the seminars on health topics. They could also translate advice given in medical terms into everyday language the women of the community could grasp.[76]

"The quest for funds for the project gave me my first gut-awareness of bureaucratic complexities."[77]

Nancy Milio, 1971

Milio's biggest problem was obtaining funding for the project. But, when President Lyndon Johnson signed the Economic Opportunity Act into law on August 20, 1964, her ideas gained traction. Johnson's "War on

Poverty" had hit Detroit, bringing with it funds for projects such as hers. In 1965, Milio heard "un-officially that funding was forthcoming." Those initial funds were just the beginning, however, of a long and complicated battle to obtain more resources. Later, when the Total Action on Poverty committee cut her support, Milio appealed to the Adult Community Movement for Equality (ACME), a politically active Black community organization. At first, ACME members were hostile to the fact that a White woman was leading the project. After months of a contentious relationship, however, members of ACME eventually supported Milio's efforts. They even moved furniture into the new clinic and helped to paint the rooms in the clinic before it opened.[78]

Milio staffed the renovated storefront center almost exclusively with people from the neighborhood since she knew the project "would be a failure" if it did not deliver what the community wanted. She hired the local people on a "first come, first served" basis, "no questions asked." Sometimes, Milio had to turn down free labor from volunteer nurses and student nurses in order to stay consistent with her promise. As she later explained: "The project, if it was to be, was to belong to the people it was intended to serve."[79]

Milio's plan worked. The innovative approach broke down the barriers that White middle-class professionals usually created when they developed health centers in poor, inner-city neighborhoods. Instead of managing the clinic with only White professionals, Milio ensured that the Kercheval Street community "owned"

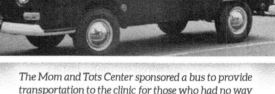

The Mom and Tots Center sponsored a bus to provide transportation to the clinic for those who had no way of getting there.

their clinic and took pride in it. Proof of its success and Milio's relationship with the neighborhood came during a race riot on July 23, 1967. The riot in the Kercheval Street neighborhood lasted 4 days, left 36 people dead, and more than 7,000 homeless. The rioters started fires that destroyed homes and business; hundreds of National Guard soldiers were called in to restore order. Afterward, Milio was certain that the Mom and Tots Center had been destroyed as were so many other neighborhood properties; in fact she was surprised to find that the clinic had been spared. Someone in the neighborhood had scrawled the letter "B" for "brother" on the storefront window during the riots, clearly indicating that the clinic belonged to the local community and was not to be harmed.

AN OFFICIAL VOICE FOR GRADUATE EDUCATION IN NURSING

While others dealt with racial conflicts and wars, more mundane matters also demanded the nursing profession's attention in the 1960s. Among these were questions about the educational requirements for entry into nursing practice as well as the question of who should make those decisions. With the steady growth of nursing programs in colleges and universities, deans of these schools saw the necessity of organizing themselves to address common concerns. They were particularly interested in problems specific to the world of academia—issues related to graduate education, and to the demands on university nursing faculty to conduct research and publish their findings. In short, a small group of deans

The Detroit Riots

"Throughout the first days and nights of the rioting, the Mom and Tots staff kept a watch on the Center and kept me informed by phone about what was happening on Kercheval. I waited for the message that said it was burning. I thought it would burn, if not by intention, then surely by accident . . . how could we begin all over again? But there was no damage."[80]

Nancy Milio, 1967

saw the need to establish a new organization, separate from the National League for Nursing, that would speak for *them*. It was well known that the League spoke for diploma and associate degree programs, and members did not always address issues that were important to professionals in higher education. In 1968, Dr. Ruth McGrorey of the State University of New York at Buffalo wrote a position paper on the subject, stating: "Vital to the promotion and development of graduate education in nursing is . . . an official voice."[81] According to McGrorey's paper, there was "a need for an educationally constituted group at the level of University graduate education to speak forcefully and effectively for the support and maintenance of graduate programs for nursing in institutions of higher education."[82]

Of particular concern to the deans was the fact that the ANA had published a position paper in 1965 on "professional versus technical" levels of nursing practice. Now the profession was divided. The ANA had declared that only nurses with a bachelor of science in nursing (BSN) degree should be called "professional nurses," and that nurses graduating from diploma programs and associate degree programs would become "technical" nurses.[84] In other words, educational preparation for professional nurses required a college degree. Many nurses disagreed with that position, insisting that the diploma-prepared nurse and the associate degree–prepared nurse (both RNs) should also be considered "professional." Others, particularly those who directed bachelor degree programs in colleges and universities, supported the BSN as the entry level for professional nursing practice. But, as the deans noted, their voice was lost in the League's meetings because the majority of the League's members were directors of diploma and associate degree programs. The deans were easily outvoted on many issues.

Meeting on May 19, 1969, 44 deans voted to form a new organization: the "Conference of Deans of Colleges and University Schools of Nursing."[85] The new Association would give the deans both the authority and the responsibility for leading collegiate and university nursing. Moreover, the "Conference of Deans" would serve as the official voice for baccalaureate, master's, and doctoral education across the country. Just 2 years later they had their chance to speak. In the spring of 1971, American Association of Colleges of Nursing (AACN) President Madeleine Leininger and a group of deans marched from their hotel rooms in Washington, DC, to Capitol Hill, determined to voice their opposition to the proposed reduction in funds for nursing education.[86] They planned to tell Congress what nurses were doing to promote access to health care services for all Americans.

The Association's march was timely. The Committee to Study Extended Roles for Nurses had just published their report, concluding that expanding the scope of nursing practice was essential if the United States was to provide equal access to health care for all Americans.[88] That report, *Extending the Scope of Nursing Practice*, justified the Association's request that Congress continue to appropriate funds for graduate nursing programs.[89]

With input from its constituents, Congress passed the Nurse Training Act of 1971, specifically stating that funds could be used "to develop training programs . . . for new roles, types or levels of nursing personnel."[90] Thus, with continued funding for graduate nursing education, programs for both the clinical nurse specialist and the nurse practitioner burgeoned in the 1970s. Moreover, specialty organizations grew in number and type, setting practice standards and developing certification examinations for their respective areas of practice. "The American College of Nurse-Midwives established exams in 1971, the American Association of Critical Care Nurses . . . began to certify practitioners in 1976, and the National Board of Pediatric Nurse Practitioners followed suit in 1977."[91] Others would soon follow.

THE NEONATAL NURSE PRACTITIONER

One of the first new nurse practitioner roles to emerge in the 1970s was that of the neonatal nurse practitioner. The role originated in response to a shortage of neonatologists, restrictions on the total time pediatric residents could devote to neonatal intensive care, and the subsequent expansion of the general staff nurse's role in the newborn ICU. Patricia Johnson, a nursing graduate student at the University of Utah, first investigated the possibility of the new role in her thesis work; after graduation she implemented it at Children's Hospital in St. Paul, Minnesota.[92] The new role was adopted in other neonatal ICUs, as neonatal nurse practitioners demonstrated that they gave "more consistent care and improved communications with families and with private doctors."[93]

These highly skilled, experienced neonatal nurse practitioners accepted a wide range of responsibilities formerly performed by pediatric residents. These included interhospital transport of critically ill infants, newborn resuscitation, lumbar punctures, and umbilical artery catheterization.[94] By 1983, more than half of the Level III newborn intensive care units in the United States were employing neonatal nurse practitioners. That year saw the beginning of national certification for these nurses.[95]

The next two decades would have exponential growth in specialty practice and nurse practitioner programs, as well as new legal challenges to nurse anesthetist and nurse-midwifery practice. Recognizing the wide variety of problems facing the profession as the 20th century came to a close, the AACN would propose two major educational programs for the future: the clinical nurse leader (CNL) and the doctor of nursing practice (DNP). Before that, the challenge for nursing would be to situate nursing practice and education within the context of an international AIDS crisis, rising medical care costs, proposals for health care reform, and a war in the Persian Gulf.

For Discussion

1. How did the inception and growth of coronary care nursing affect nurses' roles within the hospital?
2. Compare and contrast nursing in the Vietnam War with nursing in previous wars of the 20th century.
3. What social and economic factors influenced the rise of the nurse practitioner role? What changes in nursing and medicine supported the nurse practitioner role?
4. In what way did the neonatal nurse practitioner lay the foundation for the acute care nurse practitioner role that would develop later in the 20th century?

NOTES

1. Barbara Schutt, "Defining Nursing by Doing Nursing" (editorial), *American Journal of Nursing* (hereafter *AJN*) 61, no. 2 (December 1961): 49.

2. Susan M. Reverby, *Ordered to Care: The Dilemma of American Nursing, 1850-1945* (New York: Cambridge University Press, 1987).

3. Earl G. Dimond, "The First CCU: One Man's Effort," *The View from the Hill* (December 1990): 3.

4. Ibid.

5. William B. Kouwenhoven, James Jude, and G. Guy Knickerbocker, "Closed Chest Cardiac Massage," *Journal of the American Medical Association* 173 (July 9, 1960): 1064–1067 (quote 1064).

6. American College of Cardiology and Presbyterian/University of Pennsylvania Medical Center, "Current Status of Coronary Care Units," *Symposium Proceedings* (New York: Charles Press, July 15, 1966): 1.

7. Hughes W. Day, "History of Coronary Care Units," *American Journal of Cardiology* 30 (1972): 405–407.

8. Alan B. Shepard, "The Astronaut's Story of the Thrust into Space," *Life* (May 19, 1961): 25; and John Glenn, "Minute by Minute Story of the Flight," *Life* (March 9, 1962): 23.

9. Arlene Keeling, interview with Judith Stuart, RN (July 22, 1999), The Raphael Hotel, Kansas City, Missouri; transcript, Keeling Collection, Eleanor Crowder Bjoring Center for Nursing Historical Inquiry (hereafter ECBCNHI).

10. Day, "History of Coronary Care," 405.

11. Ibid.

12. Ibid.

13. Ibid.

14. Paul M. Zoll, Arthur J. Linenthal, Leona R. Norman, H. Paul Milton, and William Gibson, "Treatment of Unexpected Cardiac Arrest by External Electric Stimulation of the Heart," *New England Journal of Medicine* 254 (March 22, 1956): 541–546 (quote 544).

15. Judy Stuart, "Hartford Coronary Care Unit," in Judith Stuart papers, Keeling Collection, ECBCNHI, 1.

16. Ibid., 4.

17. Ibid.

18. Ibid.

19. Arlene Keeling, interview with Nida Brant, RN (July 22, 1999), Transcript, Keeling Collection, ECBCNHI.

20. Ibid.

21. "Nursing Practice and Intravenous Therapy," *AJN* 56, no. 5 (May 1956): 572–573.

22. Penny Standish, Judith Stuart, Nida Brant, Shirley Reubhausen interviews (July 22, 1999), Transcripts, Keeling Collection, ECBCNHI.

23. Arlene Keeling, interview with Shirley Reubhausen (July 22, 1999), Transcript, Keeling Collection, ECBCNHI.

24. Arlene Keeling, "Blurring the Boundaries between Medicine and Nursing: Coronary Care Nursing, Circa 1960s," *Nursing History Review* 12 (2004): 139–164.

25. Lawrence Meltzer, Rose Pinneo, and J. Roderick Kitchell, *Intensive Coronary Care: A Manual for Nurses* (New York: Charles Press, 1965).

26. Rose Pinneo, telephone interview with Julie Fairman, cited in Julie Fairman and Joan Lynaugh, *Critical Care Nursing: A History* (Philadelphia: University of Pennsylvania Press, 1998): 88.

27. Joan Lynaugh and Julie Fairman, "New Nurses, New Spaces: A Preview of the AACN History Study," *American Journal of Critical Care* 1, no. 1 (1992): 19–24.

28. Keeling, "Blurring the Boundaries," 163.

29. Ibid.

30. U.S. Congress, House Committee on Interstate and Foreign Commerce, Subcommittee on Public Health and Safety, *Nurse Training Act of 1964* (Washington, DC: Government Printing Office, 1964).

31. Wilbur Cohen, "Reflections on the Enactment of Medicare and Medicaid," *Health Care Financial Review*, Supplement (December 1985): 3–11.

32. Julie Fairman, "The Roots of Collaborative Practice: Nurse Practitioner Pioneers' Stories," *Nursing History Review* 10 (2002): 159–174 (quote 163).

33. F. M. Jones, "ANA Certification for Specialization," in *Current Issues in Nursing*, eds. J. C. McCloskey and H. K. Grace (Boston: Blackwell Scientific, 1981).

34. Joan Lynaugh, Patricia Gerrity, and Gloria Hagopian, "Patterns of Practice: Master's Prepared Nurse Practitioners," *Journal of Nursing Education* 24, no. 7 (September 1985): 291–295 (quote 291).

35. Julie Fairman, "Playing Doctor?: Nurse Practitioners, Physicians and the Dilemma of Shared Practice," *The Long Term View, Massachusetts School of Law, Amherst* 4 (1999): 27–35 (quote p. 44).

36. Loretta Ford and Henry Silver, "The Expanded Role of the Nurse in Child Care," *Nursing Outlook* 15, no. 8 (1967): 43–45.

37. Denise Geolot, "Federal Funding of Nurse Practitioner Education: Past, Present and Future," *Nurse Practitioner Forum* 1, no. 3 (December 1990): 159–162.

38. Julie Fairman, *Making Room in the Clinic: Nurse Practitioners and the Evolution of Modern Health Care* (New Brunswick, NJ: Rutgers University Press, 2008): 129.

39. Ibid., 115.

40. Philip Kalisch and Bernice Kalisch, *The Advance of American Nursing,* 2nd ed. (Boston: Little, Brown, 1986).

41. "Editorial," *AJN* (1971): 53.

42. Geolot, "Federal Funding."

43. Jerelyn P. Weiss, "Nursing Practice: A Legal and Historical Perspective," *Journal of Nursing Law* 2, no. 1 (n.d.): 17–35 (quote 28).

44. Fairman, *Making Room in the Clinic,* 91.

45. Arlene Keeling, *Nursing and the Privilege of Prescription* (Columbus: The Ohio State University Press, 2007).

46. Elizabeth Hadley, "Nurses and Prescriptive Authority: A Legal and Economic Analysis," *American Journal of Law and Medicine* 15, nos. 2–3 (1989): 245–299.

47. *Roe v. Wade,* 410 U.S. 113 (1973), landmarkcases.org/en/landmark/cases/roe_v_wade (accessed November 20, 2016).

48. Keeling, *Nursing and the Privilege,* 128.

49. Gertrude Issacs, "A Training Program for Development of the Family Nurse Practitioner," *FNS Quarterly Bulletin* 45, no. 1 (1970): 34–40.

50. Keeling, *Nursing and the Privilege,* 128.

51. Ira Moscovice, "The Influence of Training Level and Practice Setting on Patterns of Primary Care Provided by Nursing Personnel," *Journal of Community Health* 4, no. 1 (Fall 1978): 4–14 (quote 5).

52. Robert Isquith, "Pediatric Nurse Practitioner Succeeds Mother as Indian Health Care Provider," *Commitment* 3, no. 3 (Summer, 1978): 22–26 (quote 23).

53. Ibid., 24.

54. Ibid., 24.

55. Ibid., 25.

56. Ibid., 23.

57. Indian Health Center Improvement Act, 1976, https://www.ihs.gov (accessed October 28, 2016).

58. Fairman, "Playing Doctor?," 40.

59. Marlene Heffer, "Monthly Report, April 1979," Northern Arizona University, Cline Library 313, MS 269, box 7, folder 447.

60. Karen Vuic, "'Officer, Nurse, Woman': Army Nurse Corps Recruitment for the Vietnam War," *Nursing History Review* 14 (2006): 111–159.

61. Ibid., 111.

62. Maryanne Ibach, "Memories of Navy Nursing: The Vietnam Era," http://www.vietnamwomens memorial.org (accessed October 11, 2016): 1–6.

63. Elwood Wilkins, quoted in Arlene Keeling, *The Nurses of Mayo Clinic: Caring Healers* (Rochester, MN: Mayo Foundation for Medical Education and Research, 2014): 79–80.

64. Ibid.

65. Jennie Caylor, *End of Tour Report, U.S. Army, Vietnam, Feb 1967-1968*, ANC Historian Files, U.S. Center of Military History, Washington, DC.

66. Ibid.

67. Elizabeth Norman, *Women at War: The Story of Fifty Military Nurses Who Served in Vietnam* (Philadelphia: University of Pennsylvania Press, 1990).

68. Dan Freedman and Jacqueline Rhoads, *Nurses in Vietnam* (Austin: Texas Monthly Press, 1987): 47.

69. Iris West, "The Women of the Army Nurse Corps during the Vietnam War," U.S. Army Center of Military History (n.d.), http://www.vietnamwomensmemorial.org (accessed October 11, 2016): 1–6.

70. Freedman and Rhoads, *Nurses in Vietnam*, 65.

71. Lorraine Boudreau, quoted in Freedman and Rhoads, *Nurses in Vietnam*, 33.

72. Iris West, "The Women of the Army Nurse Corps," 3–6.

73. Jeanne Holm and Sara Wells, "Air Force Women in the Vietnam War," http://www.vietnam womensmemorial.org (accessed October 11, 2016): 1–8 (quote 2).

74. Norman, *Women at War* (page 1557 of 3561, Kindle).

75. Nancy Milio, *9226 Kercheval: The Storefront that Did Not Burn* (Ann Arbor: University of Michigan Press, 1971): 24.

76. Pamela DeGuzman and Arlene Keeling, "Addressing Disparities in Access to Care: Lessons from the Kercheval Street Clinic in the 1960s," *Policy, Politics and Nursing Practice* 12 (2011): 199–207 (quote 201).

77. Milio, *9226 Kercheval*, 25.

78. DeGuzman and Keeling, "Addressing Disparities," 204.

79. Ibid.

80. Milio, *9226 Kercheval*, 142.

81. Ruth T. McGrorey, *A Position Paper: Toward a Rationale for an Organization of Deans of Graduate Programs in Nursing*, prepared for the meeting of Tuesday, November 13, 1968, Phoenix, AZ. American Association of Colleges of Nursing, One DuPont Circle, Washington, DC (hereafter cited as AACN archives).

82. Mary Mullane, "Summary of the History of the Association of Colleges of Nursing," AACN archives (December 28, 1976): 2.

83. Ibid., 4–5.

84. American Nurses Association, "ANA's First Position on Education for Nursing," *American Journal of Nursing* 65 (1965): 106–111.

85. Ibid.

86. Madeleine Leininger correspondence to Rachel Booth (January 29, 1996), box 156, AACN archives.

87. Arlene Keeling, Barbara Brodie, and John Kirchgessner, "The Voice of Professional Nursing: A 40 Year History of the American Association of Colleges of Nursing" (Washington DC: AACN, 2010).

88. Geolot, "Federal Funding."

89. Fairman, *Making Room in the Clinic*.

90. Geolot, "Federal Funding," 160.

91. Fairman and Lynaugh, *Critical Care Nursing: A History*, 101.

92. Mary Honeyfield, "Neonatal Nurse Practitioner: Past, Present and Future," *Advances in Neonatal Care* 9, no. 3 (June 2009): 125–128.

93. Amy Farah, Amy Bieda, and Shyang-Yun Pamela Shiao, "The History of the Neonatal Nurse Practitioner in the United States," *Neonatal Network* 15, no. 5 (August 1996): 11–21 (quote 13).

94. Ibid., 13.

95. Ibid., 15.

FURTHER READING

American Nurses Association, "ANA's First Position on Education for Nursing," *American Journal of Nursing* 65 (1965): 106–111.

DeGuzman, Pamela, and Keeling, Arlene, "Addressing Disparities in Access to Care: Lessons from the Kercheval Street Clinic in the 1960s," *Policy, Politics and Nursing Practice* 12 (2011): 199–207.

Fairman, Julie, "Playing Doctor?: Nurse Practitioners, Physicians and the Dilemma of Shared Practice," *The Long Term View, Massachusetts School of Law* 4, no. 4 (1999): 27–35.

Fairman, Julie, "The Roots of Collaborative Practice: Nurse Practitioner Pioneers' Stories," *Nursing History Review* 10 (2002): 159–174.

Fairman, Julie, *Making Room in the Clinic: Nurse Practitioners and the Evolution of Modern Health Care* (New Brunswick, NJ: Rutgers University Press, 2008).

Fairman, Julie, and Joan Lynaugh, *Critical Care Nursing: A History* (Philadelphia: University of Pennsylvania Press, 1998).

Farah, Amy, Amy Bieda, and Shyang-Yun Pamela Shiao, "The History of the Neonatal Nurse Practitioner in the United States," *Neonatal Network* 15, no. 5 (August 1996): 11–21.

Freedman, Dan, and Jacqueline Rhoads, *Nurses in Vietnam* (Austin: Texas Monthly Press, 1987).

Geolot, Denise, "Federal Funding of Nurse Practitioner Education: Past Present and Future," *Nurse Practitioner Forum* 1, no. 3 (December 1990): 159–162.

Holm, Jeanne, and Sara Wells, "Air Force Women in the Vietnam War," http://www.vietnam womensmemorial.org (accessed October 11, 2016): 1–8.

Honeyfield, Mary, "Neonatal Nurse Practitioner: Past, Present and Future," *Advances in Neonatal Care* 9, no. 3 (June 2009): 125–128.

Keeling, Arlene, "Blurring the Boundaries between Medicine and Nursing: Coronary Care Nursing, Coronary Care Nursing in the 1960s," *Nursing History Review* 12 (2004): 139–164.

Keeling, Arlene, *Nursing and the Privilege of Prescription, 1893-2000* (Columbus: The Ohio State University Press, 2007).

Lynaugh, Joan, and Julie Fairman, "New Nurses, New Spaces: A Preview of the AACN History Study," *American Journal of Critical Care* 1, no. 1 (1992): 19–24.

Milio, Nancy, *9226 Kercheval: The Storefront that Did Not Burn* (Ann Arbor: University of Michigan Press, 1971).

Norman, Elizabeth, *Women at War: The Story of Fifty Military Nurses Who Served in Vietnam* (Philadelphia: University of Pennsylvania Press, 1990).

Smoyak, Shirley, "Specialization in Nursing: From Then to Now," *Nursing Outlook* 24, no. 11 (November 1976): 676–681.

Vuic, Karen, "'Officer, Nurse, Woman': Army Nurse Corps Recruitment for the Vietnam War," *Nursing History Review* 14 (2006): 111–159.

West, Iris, "The Women of the Army Nurse Corps during the Vietnam War," U.S. Army Center of Military History, http://www.vietnamwomensmemorial.org (accessed October 11, 2016).

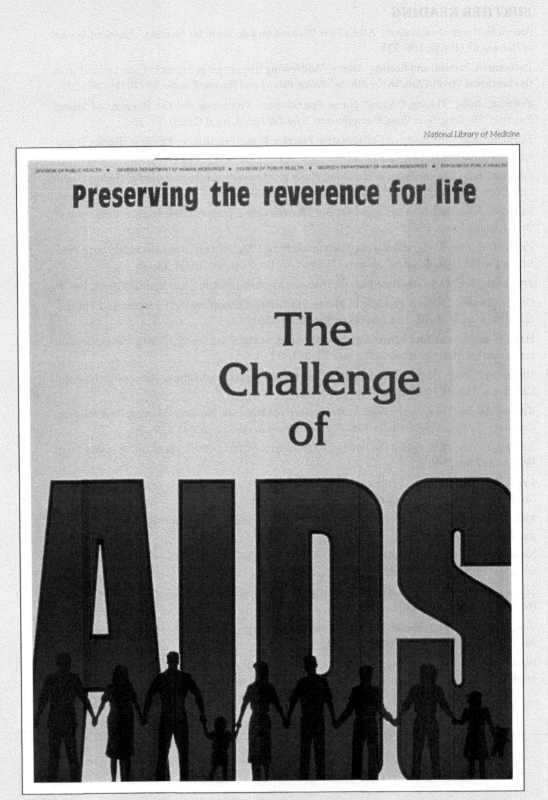

DIVISION OF PUBLIC HEALTH ♦ GEORGIA DEPARTMENT OF HUMAN RESOURCES ♦ DIVISION OF PUBLIC HEALTH ♦ GEORGIA DEPARTMENT OF HUMAN RESOURCES ♦ DIVISION OF PUBLIC HEALTH

Preserving the reverence for life

The
Challenge
of
AIDS

Challenge of AIDS.

CHAPTER 14

Caring in Crisis

1980–2000

Michelle C. Hehman

"There are no bunkers, no sidelines for nursing today. We find ourselves the center of attention. As the government and corporate America fight escalating health care costs, AIDS is wreaking havoc and technology swells unchecked. Underpaid, overworked and overstressed nurses are in the midst of the conflagration. Nursing is in greater demand than ever before." [1]

Speaking to the American Nurses Association (ANA) House of Delegates at the 1988 Convention, ANA President Margareta Styles highlighted the crucial role of nurses in dealing with the current and ongoing health care crises. More than simply drawing attention to the need for more nurses, Styles began her address with a call "to march," recalling Florence Nightingale's caution that "no system can endure that does not march."[2] Nearly 100 years earlier, Nightingale had warned nurses against complacency, arguing for the forward progress of the profession to continue. Following in Nightingale's footsteps, Styles challenged delegates to once again heed the call to action, saying: "We must organize, unite, go on the offensive."[3] In the last few decades of the 20th century, professional unity and purpose were needed more than ever for nurses to successfully endure the myriad of challenges facing the nation and their profession.

Between 1980 and 2000, nurses would witness major economic changes in the health care system. The United States faced a recession at the start of the 1980s, and the government implemented fiscally conservative policies to improve the economy. Total health care costs had risen exponentially, from just $27.2 billion annually in 1960 to more than $255 billion in 1980.[4] Health care spending far outpaced growth in the rest of the economy and comprised an increasingly larger percentage of the gross national product—from 5.3% in 1960 to almost 9% in 1980—making health care costs a serious economic issue.[5] The cause was complex but related to unrestrained

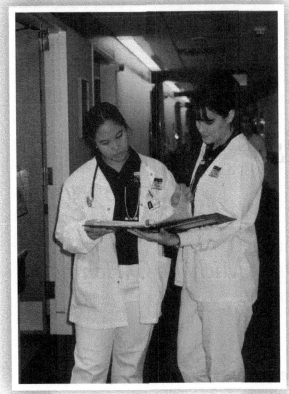

Nursing students review a patient's chart.

hospital spending, advances in technology, and an aging population. In response, the federal government began to reduce funding for many of the social programs of the 1960s like Medicare and Medicaid, and national organizations sought ways to promote health and prevent illness. The government's publication of the Healthy People initiatives demonstrated a shift in national understanding of health and wellness for all Americans.

In 1980, the ANA published *Nursing: A Social Policy Statement,* a declaration of nursing's value in and responsibility to society. Over the next two decades, the profession would continuously affirm these values and its commitment to promoting health in the face of numerous challenges in the provision of direct patient care. At the start of the 1980s, a new and deadly disease emerged: acquired immune deficiency syndrome (AIDS). It would become one of the largest public health emergencies in history. Changes to federal reimbursement for hospital services increased the acuity of inpatient care and demanded a greater number of nurses. As a result, another critical nursing shortage threatened hospitals' ability to meet patient needs and forced working nurses to do more with limited staffing. Public health funding for poor and rural areas decreased access to primary care services, pushing some nurses to find innovative solutions to combat growing health disparities in these underserved communities. Also, nurses would once again be sent to war when the United States entered the Gulf War in 1991. Throughout every crisis, nurses continued to offer quality care, compassion, and support to those in need.

POLICIES AND SOCIAL ISSUES
The First Social Policy Statement in Nursing

In 1980, the ANA published *Nursing: A Social Policy Statement*, which articulated the nature and scope of nursing practice. The report attempted to not only define the essence of nursing, but also convey a professional duty to improve the health of the nation. Ultimately, the document would serve as the foundation for the Association's social policy going forward.

According to the Association, nursing helped "to serve society's interests in the area of health," and was defined as "the diagnosis and treatment of human responses to actual or potential health problems."[6] The policy statement affirmed the core principles and scope of nursing practice while also recognizing a professional responsibility and commitment to serve humanity. Since the ANA admitted that definitions alone do not change important public policy, they urged individuals and groups who implemented policy to use the statement when they drafted new proposals.[7]

The social policy statement clearly stated that the goal of the nursing profession was to improve and maintain the health and well-being of all citizens. In this way, nurses would continue to alleviate suffering, prevent

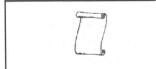

A "Decade of Decision"

"The 1980s have been identified as a decade of decision in nursing. The social policy statement has been so cast as to facilitate decisions through which nursing can consolidate achievements of the past and move with wisdom and courage into its future of service to society."[8]

ANA Social Policy Statement, 1980

disease, and promote health as they had been doing for years. Although economic forces had recently pushed U.S. health care leaders to recognize the importance of wellness and preventive service, the ANA noted: "Nursing practice has been health-oriented for more than half a century, partly because of its focus on individuals as persons and on the family as the necessary unit of service. In nursing so practiced, the current health movement was foreshadowed."[9]

The ANA understood that teamwork with different but likeminded professionals was required to achieve this objective. Thus, their key concern was to prioritize and nourish collaborative relationships with other health care providers. For the Association, collaboration meant a "true partnership, in which the power on both sides is valued by both, with recognition and acceptance of separate and combined spheres of activity and responsibility, mutual safeguarding of the legitimate interests of each party, and a commonality of goals that is recognized by both parties."[10] To clarify its position, the Association's statement outlined that the scope of nursing practice within the health care system would shift according to the changing needs and demands of the public. Through education and research, nursing would continue to grow and develop, as well as enrich and extend its core characteristics of nurturing and protecting the patient.[11]

The 1980 policy statement did more than simply offer a definition of nursing; it legitimized nursing's privilege as a true profession. The policy statement included a long history of nursing service, asserted that nurses required a complementary but specialized knowledge, declared an ethical foundation for the nurse–patient relationship, and claimed that nurses held a unique position within the health care system. In this declaration, the ANA logically and emphatically affirmed professional status for nursing, and demanded recognition in the policy sphere. Throughout the next 20 years, nurses would work to live up to the ANA's claims, amidst a number of unprecedented challenges. The first would begin almost immediately, with the emergence of the HIV/AIDS epidemic in 1981.

> "Nurses are committed to respecting human beings because of a profound regard for humanity . . . unaltered by the social, educational, economic, cultural, racial, religious, or other specific attributes of the human beings receiving care."[12]
>
> ANA Social Policy Statement, 1980

The HIV/AIDS Epidemic

On June 5, 1981, the Centers for Disease Control and Prevention (CDC) released a *Morbidity and Mortality Weekly Report* describing the "unusual" diagnosis of *Pneumocystic carinii* pneumonia (PCP) and other common infections in five young men in Los Angeles, California.[13] By press time, two of the men had already died. In these previously healthy individuals, the presence and high fatality rate of the disease proved alarming, as these types of diseases usually occurred in patients with compromised immune systems. Later these articles would be recognized as the first reports of the AIDS epidemic in the United States, but at the time, few clinicians recognized the impact and severity of the disease. As nurse Mary Foley recalled, "we didn't see the significance of what was to occur."[14]

Although outbreaks of unidentified contagious diseases have occurred throughout human history, the discovery of AIDS challenged clinicians and the public alike. The rapid spread of the disease was particularly troubling, as researchers struggled to identify its root cause and modes of transmission. In June 1981, five individuals had the disease; by the end of 1981, 259 patients with severe immune deficiency were reported to the CDC; and by July 1982, a total of 514 cases were diagnosed.[15] As the incidence of the disease doubled every 5 months and infected individuals experienced a near 40% fatality rate, investigators searched for commonalities among the identified patients.[16]

Fear and prejudice played a significant role in the early years of the AIDS epidemic. Virtually all of the initial cases had occurred in homosexual and bisexual men, with some found among intravenous drug users. Those associations led researchers to focus

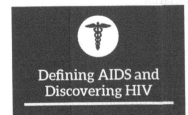

Defining AIDS and Discovering HIV

The CDC first used the term *acquired immune deficiency syndrome* (AIDS) in September of 1982 to describe "a disease at least moderately predictive of a deficit in cell-mediated immunity, occurring in a person with no known case for diminished resistance to that disease."[18] From 1983 to 1985 multiple research groups independently determined the causative agent, and in May 1986, the International Committee on the Taxonomy of Viruses determined that the identified retrovirus would officially be known as human immunodeficiency virus (HIV).

on lifestyle choices as potential risk factors. The general public responded unsympathetically to both groups, and the terms "gay cancer" and "gay plague" regularly appeared in mass media. Even the scientific community contributed to the stigma, as researchers initially referred to the disease as gay-related immune deficiency (GRID). Both responses contributed to perceptions that the disease was limited to specific populations and subsequently delayed the recognition of AIDS as a widespread public health issue.

Before the CDC and other researchers fully understood the disease, individuals suffering from AIDS still wanted and needed competent and compassionate care from nurses and other health care providers. Working against considerable obstacles—including a lack of knowledge regarding the disease process, no identified diagnostic test, no known treatment or cure, and questions about its communicability—nurses across the United States developed their own routines, participated in research and community outreach programs, and offered AIDS patients the dignity and comfort they desired. One of the first comprehensive programs for supporting and treating AIDS was developed in San Francisco. It would become a model for other health care systems throughout the country.

The San Francisco Model

Health care providers in the city of San Francisco saw some of the first patients with severe immune deficiencies in their local hospitals and clinics. As these numbers increased, researchers, clinicians, and social workers at the University of California San Francisco and San Francisco General Hospital responded by developing new programs to assist and treat individuals suffering from AIDS. Over time, these teams would partner with the San Francisco Department of Public Health and local community groups to cultivate a comprehensive medical, psychological, and social support program to help patients at all stages along the continuum of AIDS care.

The cooperation among hospitals and regional agencies in San Francisco was more important than ever, as the AIDS crisis began just as federal policies shifted the burden of responsibility for social programs to state and local governments. Interestingly, those involved in the process never set out to develop a coordinated multidisciplinary system of care. In fact, many of the programs were simply a logical response to new medical, social, and economic issues that surfaced as the AIDS epidemic spread across the city. As coordinator of the first specialty inpatient AIDS unit at San Francisco General Hospital, Clifford Morrison remembered:

The media reported the San Francisco model as if this was a very deliberate thing, that we had thought about it; we'd all planned it; there had been all these meetings and all this wonderful cooperation. Some of that was true, but none of it happened that way. What happened was that there were all these pieces, and everybody was working on a piece here or there, and luckily, because there weren't so many of us, there was coordination and communication. That was the important piece. There was never a conscious decision, "We're going to sit down and develop a San Francisco model."[20]

Since San Francisco was home to a large gay community, the San Francisco Health Department already had a coordinating committee in place to respond to health issues relevant to gay, lesbian, and bisexual citizens. As early as 1981, this committee began to compile what little information was known about the disease and developed a resource guide for patients and physicians.[21] As an increasing number of similar cases emerged throughout San Francisco, the Department of Public Health created a case registry system that compiled information gathered in patient interviews and provided follow-up care. By the end of 1981, city leaders recognized that if they were to adequately respond to the epidemic, they would need planning, communication, oversight, and much more funding. Responding to a request for local tax appropriations by the Health Department, the city's Board of Supervisors allotted nearly $200,000 to support AIDS programs in January 1982.

Just 1 year later, in January 1983, more than 130 cases of AIDS had been reported in San Francisco. To help patients navigate the complexity of an AIDS diagnosis and to create a central location for the delivery of health services, San Francisco General Hospital opened the first specialty AIDS outpatient clinic. The clinic, called Ward 86, provided patients with a multidisciplinary team of specialists who provided screening, diagnosis, education, and counseling all in one place. Housing a full range of specialties, including oncology, infectious disease, social work, and case management, Ward 86 increased the likelihood that patients would receive proper education, follow-up care, and access to available resources by eliminating the need to schedule and visit multiple offices. Case management services were incredibly important, since many AIDS patients dealt with complex social issues such as poverty and homelessness. Collaboration among health professionals became a necessity, without the traditional hierarchy evident in most hospitals and clinics. As nurse Gayling Gee remembered, "We were side by side with [physicians], learning about this new disease and attending many of the same conferences that they had. We were very interested and we worked well with the patients. So I think we did a great job of really maximizing the role of the nurse in assisting the process. It was innovative."[23]

Since inpatient care at San Francisco General Hospital for AIDS patients became the next priority for health officials, they discussed how best to develop a specialized unit in the hospital. Maryanne McGuire, the hospital's director of nursing, approached clinical nurse specialist Clifford Morrison to organize and run such a unit. After being given assurances that he could design the unit and direct care as he desired, Morrison took charge of opening Ward 5B that opened in the summer of 1983.

From the beginning, the staff on Ward 5B encouraged patient-directed holistic care, which required interprofessional collaboration. They gave patients the freedom and authority to make decisions about visitors, treatment options, and long-term plans. Patients alone identified their own "family" members, whether they were friends, lovers, or relatives, regardless of standard hospital policy. Patients also determined visiting hours, and the staff encouraged family members to stay overnight and assist in patient care activities.[25] All patients also had private rooms, a fact that not only satisfied policies regarding infection control but more importantly offered patients a measure of privacy during the advanced stages of their illness.

Before any definitive or effective treatment for HIV/AIDS emerged, nursing care was largely supportive, as nurses managed infections and eased suffering. As one nurse recalled: "In this high-tech world, the AIDS nurse spends a lot of time holding hands."[27] With the success of San Francisco's outpatient AIDS clinic, patients only ended up admitted to Ward 5B when they were seriously or terminally ill. By the end of the 1980s, the average

"What [AIDS] brought to nursing is a much stronger understanding of patient advocacy . . . of a need to take a holistic approach."[22]

Diane Jones, 1996

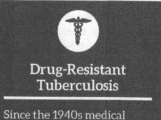

Drug-Resistant Tuberculosis

Since the 1940s medical professionals had studied the rise of resistance to antitubercular agents. Nonetheless, a resurgence of a strain of tuberculosis that was resistant to multiple drugs began in the late 1980s. Scientists largely attributed these outbreaks to the HIV/AIDS epidemic, but knew that poor adherence to TB treatments and worsening economic and social conditions played a part. In response, public health officials began to test for drug susceptibility in cultures they used to make a diagnosis. They also provided better education on controlling infection, and delivered medications directly to the patient while they observed.[24]

"These are patients shunned by society and they come here and it's an accepting environment. They're sponges for any sort of care."[26]

Dianne Jones, 1983

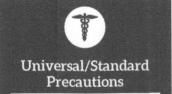
"For such a high profile disease, nursing certainly has kept a very low profile. As much as we do, we need to talk about it more."[30]

Gayling Gee, 1987

"It's one thing to reach the people who recognize the risk. It's another entirely to reach the people who think they have nothing to fear."[35]

Jo Ann Bennett, 1985

"What we know and what we do are not the same thing . . . how we feel keeps us from making decisions that are healthy."[36]

Dr. Richard Keeling, 1992

time between diagnosis and death for HIV/AIDS patients was only 18 months.[28] Case management became paramount, and staff on the unit encouraged patients to develop an individual hospice plan.

Because a medical standard of care for the disease did not exist, Morrison built Ward 5B upon a primary nursing model, in which each patient had one dedicated nurse who was involved in all aspects of their plan of care. Morrison insisted that the unit be exclusively staffed with registered nurses (RNs) rather than a mix of licensed practical nurses and unlicensed assistants. He also only offered positions to nurses who volunteered, as many health care workers worried about being exposed to the disease and transmitting the disease to others.

The success of Ward 5B and the increased inpatient admissions required the hospital to expand the unit from 12 to 20 beds. As the HIV/AIDS epidemic spread across the United States, other hospitals began to incorporate the San Francisco model of care as they developed comprehensive, coordinated AIDS services. Administrators in hospitals with dedicated AIDS units found that patients were more satisfied with the care provided and had a lower 30-day mortality rate than institutions without beds dedicated to AIDS patients.[29]

The Public Health Education Campaign

By the end of 1985, every major region of the world reported at least one HIV case. That same year, a teenager from Indiana with hemophilia contracted the disease through a contaminated blood transfusion. Ryan White's case awakened the medical community and the public at large to the widespread potential of the epidemic. By 1986, the surgeon general issued a report on AIDS, calling for a nationwide education campaign, early sex education

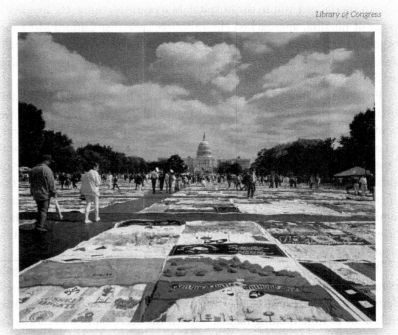

Library of Congress

The AIDS Memorial Quilt containing 1,920 names of AIDS victims displayed on the National Mall in 1987.

in schools, increased access to and use of condoms, and voluntary HIV testing. Public awareness continued to grow with the display of the NAMES Project AIDS Memorial Quilt on the National Mall in Washington, DC, during the National March on Washington for Lesbian and Gay Rights on October 11, 1987. At the time the quilt contained 1,920 panels, each containing the name of a victim of the AIDS epidemic; that number would grow to more than 48,000 panels and names by the beginning of the 21st century.[32]

Over time, the general public stigmatized the disease and believed that the risk of potential transmission was limited to members of the gay and bisexual community. These misunderstandings created significant disparities in other high-risk groups, and unfortunately had serious and tragic consequences, particularly for vulnerable Blacks and Hispanics, who experienced a disproportionately high incidence rate. Infants born to infected mothers became one of the fastest growing groups of AIDS patients, and accounted for nearly 80% of all pediatric cases by the end of 1990.[33] Health care providers recognized that the challenge was to "provide reliable information and support to two different publics: those with the disease and those at risk."[34] Most individuals outside of the homosexual or intravenous drug-using populations underestimated their risk for contracting AIDS. Thus, national educational programs focused on overcoming strong cultural beliefs and overt denial among at-risk groups.

In response to the surgeon general's call for early sex education, high schools and colleges across the nation began to enlist nurses to teach students about condom use and safe sexual practices. For AIDS prevention nurse Louise Davis, the goal was "striking just the right balance . . . [between] making them believe that having unprotected sex could easily lead to their death and scaring them so much they'll stop listening."[37] Universities also began to push the notion of safe sex as a vital component of student health. While the overall incidence of HIV/AIDS on universities remained lower than that found in the general population, the majority of campuses confirmed the presence of the disease in the student body and recognized the potential for transmission.[38] Fighting general perceptions of invincibility by adolescents and young adults, sexual health initiatives often encouraged peer education programs and honest risk assessment.

By December 31, 2000, the CDC reported a total of 774,467 HIV/AIDS cases in the United States; nearly 60% had died.[39] With the advent of successful antiretroviral combination therapy, the incidence of AIDS and death rates declined sharply. As the 21st century approached, health professionals focused on managing HIV/AIDS patients by detecting the disease early and providing access to medication. These actions suppressed the virus, decreased the risk of transmission, and transformed the treatment into a standard way to manage a chronic disease.

RISING COSTS AND UNEQUAL ACCESS

In response to an economic recession and continually rising health care costs, government policy makers focused on ways to control and reduce hospital spending throughout the 1980s. Federal agencies cut costs by evaluating the need to continue funding nurse education, and reducing reimbursements to hospitals not recognized by the Social Security Administration. However, the greatest change was how health care costs were reimbursed

<aside>

AIDS Care as Culturally Appropriate Care

"Because of all the denial around this, the AIDS epidemic quickly flung open a lot of doors. San Francisco had a reputation of being the gay mecca, but, in health care, we knew very little about gay lifestyle. . . . You've got a whole cultural system here that you need to be aware of, because you're not just treating or caring for a person. You've got to look at the person for where they're coming from, and in order to do that, you have to have some understanding."[31]

Clifford Morrison, 1999

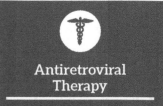

Antiretroviral Therapy

Once scientists uncovered the pathophysiology of HIV/AIDS, they focused their research efforts on developing treatments for the disease. Antiretroviral drugs prevented development of the disease by inhibiting a step in the viral life cycle. The earliest of these drugs—azidothymidine and zidovudine—were approved in the late 1980s, but had the potential of being highly toxic and were poorly tolerated by patients. In the mid-1990s, new classes of drugs led to the standardization of "highly active antiretroviral therapy" (HAART). This combination therapy changed HIV/AIDS into a manageable chronic illness for those with access to treatment.

</aside>

with the government-implemented Medicare's prospective payment system and the diagnosis-related group (DRG) classification structure. The shift to DRG reimbursement had profound effects on hospital nursing services and eventually exacerbated a nursing shortage.

Before the new reimbursement system went into effect, hospital costs had risen exponentially, and many government officials believed they could not continue to pay the increased costs, especially with Medicare funds. The passage of Medicare and Medicaid in 1965 had essentially granted hospitals and physicians complete authority to determine which services were required for each patient and to set their own cost that the government would reimburse. Hospital costs varied widely among patients with the same diagnosis, even within the same hospital. Standardization of costs for the same services across the country seemed nonexistent, with hospitals charging different prices for procedures irrespective of patient demographics or geographic location. Medicare had given hospitals a "license to spend," and had encouraged the hospitals to use more services than necessary because "the more expenditures they incurred, the more income they received."[40] As a result, Medicare payments had doubled nearly every 5 years, and private employers saw their insurance premiums rise upward of 15% to 20% each year.[41] As medical historian Paul Starr noted, the rising costs "brought medical care under more critical scrutiny, and the federal government, as a major buyer of health services, intervened in unprecedented ways."[42]

The idea for a new standardized payment system came out of a Yale University study in the 1970s that aimed to improve the quality of hospital services and encourage the responsible use of medical resources. Using data from 35 hospitals in Connecticut, the researchers developed an interactive computer program that grouped patients into a small number of categories, or DRGs, and then determined how many hospital services were used. The researchers had hoped to give hospital administrators a way to predict costs and possibly gauge how much they would be reimbursed. The premise behind this prospective payment system rested on the theory that medical costs could accurately be predicted based on patients' demographics, their diagnosis, and the average cost of the services they would require. Under the system, a patient's illness would be coded into a particular diagnostic group when he or she was admitted. The hospital would then be reimbursed for the predetermined, fixed cost associated with that diagnosis.

> "Medicare's traditional model of cost reimbursement was insanity. On the face of it, it encouraged people to do more; it paid them to do more and not in any particularly rational way."[43]
>
> Sheila Burke, 2002

While many hospital administrators were slow to recognize the benefits of the payment system, federal policy makers embraced its potential to curb health care spending. By using the new payment model, the risk of operating losses shifted to the hospital. If administrators could not figure out how to deliver care at or below the fixed reimbursement rates, they would have to increase efficiency and productivity, and/or lower costs for supplies and services in order to remain solvent.[44] The system also had the potential for the hospitals to make significant profits if hospital administrators could deliver services well below proposed standard reimbursement rates. The DRG payment system went into effect nationwide in 1983 for all hospitals that delivered services to Medicare recipients.

Almost immediately, hospital administrators looked for ways to cut costs as a way to increase profits, or at least break even. They found little success in persuading physicians to alter their practice, so they turned their attention to services over which they had complete control. As a result, they decreased the use of available laboratory and diagnostic tests, discharged Medicare patients from the hospital early, and transferred these patients to outpatient facilities, which were not regulated by DRG guidelines.[45] Ultimately, these actions resulted in a much higher acuity level on inpatient hospital units and increased the demand for outpatient facilities and services. Both options, however, required even more nursing staff.[46]

Cost Containment and the Nursing Shortage

Issues of nurse shortages had plagued the nation and the profession since World War II. The problem came to a head beginning in the late 1970s as part of the crisis in health care costs. Federal funding for nursing education came under fire, after a few studies suggested that a potential nursing surplus was on the horizon. In response, appropriations for the Nurse Training Act began to decrease annually, dropping from 125 million dollars in 1978 down to 50 million dollars in 1982.[47] Data compiled by the National League for Nursing suggested that a health care crisis was coming due to a nursing shortage.[48]

"The nation is entering what may be the biggest nursing shortage ever . . . The shortage of nurses in many states has hit crisis proportions among hospitals, nursing homes, and home health agencies."[49]

Carolyne K. Davis, 1980

Unfortunately, two federal research studies in the early 1980s downplayed the impact and severity of the nursing shortage. In 1981, the U.S. Department of Health and Human Services published *The Recurrent Shortage of Registered Nurses,* which evaluated potential factors behind a persistent scarcity of nurse labor. The study questioned why hospitals continually reported a relative shortage of available nursing staff while the number of nursing graduates had consistently outpaced population growth since 1960. Concluding that issues regarding the supply of nurses was a result of stagnant wages and a decline in women and men entering the profession, the study suggested that nothing could really be done to solve the problem, and that the current shortage simply reflected fluctuations in the labor market that would eventually self-correct.[50]

In 1983, the Institute of Medicine (IOM) published a study on federal expenditures for nursing education. In addition, the research looked at ways to encourage nurses to practice in "medically underserved areas," as well as keep nurses "active in their profession."[51] The study was well designed and provided thorough justification for its recommendations. The Institute, however, incorrectly concluded that the overall supply of RNs would be "in reasonable balance during this decade" and that perceived nurse shortages were simply a reflection of an improper distribution of nurses in undesirable areas and in institutions that served the poor.[52] As a result, the Institute recommended that federal money for nursing education be directed toward graduate students, as additional funding for entry-level programs seemed unwarranted.

"Not only is this the first time a nursing shortage has cut across all categories of nurses and all regions of the country, but it is occurring despite the fact that demand for inpatient hospital beds is declining."[56]

Connie Curran, 1987

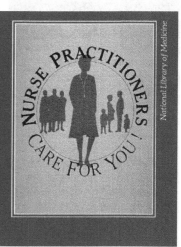

National Library of Medicine

Acute Care Nurse Practitioner (ACNP)

In the 1990s, hospital-based care became increasingly more complex, and many institutions had fewer residents in medical subspecialties. Nursing leaders saw an opportunity to develop an advanced practice nursing role to fill both these needs. The decision made sense in light of increased federal funding directed toward educating graduate nurses. The ACNP specialty was established to provide continuity and coordination of diverse medical services for patients in intensive care and specialty units in tertiary care facilities. Graduate programs offering ACNP classes proliferated in the early 1990s, growing to 43 programs nationwide by 1997.[53]

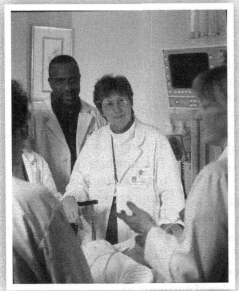

Acute care nurse practitioner students, whose program was created to organize diverse medical services for patients in intensive care and specialty units in tertiary care facilities.

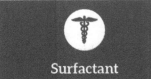

Surfactant

Surfactant is vital for an infant to successfully take his or her first breath. Unfortunately, many preterm babies are born before their lungs can naturally produce the substance, often leading to respiratory failure and death. Clinical trials in the 1980s evaluated the potential of administering natural and synthetic surfactant to premature infants. The results showed a substantial decrease in mortality. The widespread use of surfactant could reduce neonatal mortality by up to 50%, and decrease overall infant mortality in the United States by about 6%.[60] Surfactant is currently on the World Health Organization's Model List of Essential Medicines, those deemed most important in a basic health system.

Over the next few years, hospitals cited an increasing need for RNs. One survey found that the percentage of unfilled nursing positions in hospitals across the United States more than doubled between September 1985 and December 1986. Some institutions even had to shut down parts of or entire units as a result of inadequate nurse staffing.[54] Hospital industry leaders remained perplexed by the paradox of the issue—as the shortage worsened, the nursing workforce actually swelled while the use of hospital inpatient resources declined.[55] The issue appeared to be related to a demand for RNs that far outpaced any growth in the supply.

Even though the country saw 50 million fewer inpatient hospital days in 1987 than it had in 1981, a number of factors contributed to a greater need for nurses.[57] During that same time, the overall acuity of hospitalized patients increased as hospital administrators responded to the use of the Medicare prospective payment system. In addition, the elderly population—individuals most likely to consume health care resources—continued to grow. The rising HIV/AIDS epidemic also added to increased utilization of hospital services by acutely ill patients with a complex disease. Finally, the total number of critical care beds increased dramatically, which obligated hospitals to employ more nurses. The number of intensive care beds more than doubled between 1973 and 1989, with 17,000 beds added in the 1980s alone.[58] Patients being admitted into specialty critical care wards like neonatal intensive care units (NICUs) increased the percentage of overall inpatient days.

NICUs, in particular, demonstrated remarkable growth, with the number of NICU beds growing more than 130% between 1980 and 1995.[59] Infant mortality rates had decreased dramatically in the 20th century, but

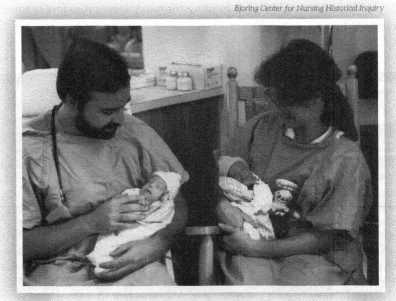

Nurses holding premature babies, whose survival rates increased with the discovery of prenatal corticosteroids and surfactant.

too many newborns continued to perish unnecessarily. Studies showed that infants with low birth weights were at the greatest risk of dying. The leading cause of low birth weight—prematurity—was not well understood, so the medical response to the problem focused on keeping premature infants alive rather than preventing preterm birth. Survival rates for extremely premature infants improved, however, as scientists discovered prenatal corticosteroids and surfactant, and the technology for respirators and mechanical ventilation advanced. By the mid-1990s, neonatologists were saving more babies at younger gestations than ever before, and these infants stayed in intensive care longer and required more expensive treatments. Hospital administrators who recognized the economic benefit of neonatal services expanded their bed capabilities in existing units while other hospitals established their own NICUs. More beds were easy to supply, but more specially trained nurses would be much harder to come by, as the complex environment of infant care required a higher ratio of nurses to patients.

A similar pattern emerged across other critical care units, as research on disease treatment often proved more straightforward and successful than research on prevention. Advanced treatment methods and technology were implemented, and hospitals reaped financial benefit through longer intensive care stays and utilization of more expensive resources. This reactionary approach offered greater economic incentive than prevention, but also increased demand for RNs. Hospitals began replacing licensed practical nurses and unlicensed aides with RNs, whose expertise was needed to adequately monitor critically ill patients and navigate the increasingly sophisticated equipment. By 1986, more than 80% of hospitals nationwide reported employment vacancies for RNs, with intensive care positions rated as the most difficult to fill.[61]

By 1988, the nationwide critical shortage of nurses prompted the Department of Health and Human Services to respond. The Department appointed the Secretary's Commission on Nursing to evaluate the situation. The Commission's Final Report emphatically proclaimed that the nursing shortage was "real, widespread, and of significant magnitude," and had affected all sectors of health care, including hospital, ambulatory, home health, and nursing home care.[62] Acknowledging that the problem was primarily the result of increased demand for RNs, the report also suggested that noncompetitive wages negatively affected nurse staffing.

Not only did the Commission legitimize the nursing shortage, it also offered suggestions for improving the situation. The report admonished hospitals for low wages for nurses. RNs received less pay than other occupations, including secretaries, accountants, and clerks. Because of poor salary increases, the nursing workforce lost workers, and deterred men and women from entering the profession. In addition, recent research proved that there was a correlation between stagnant compensation for nursing services and critical shortages of nurses. Over more than 25 years, a cyclical pattern developed: when compensation for nursing staff stalled or lagged behind other professions open to the female labor pool, a nursing shortage appeared or worsened.[63] The Commission called for employers to expand pay ranges for RNs and immediately increase their wages.

Recognizing the importance of the work environment, the Commission also recommended that RNs not be responsible for non-nursing job functions. It encouraged ways to promote professional growth, autonomy, and collaborative relationships, as well as ways to improve the use and application of technology—including electronic medical records—to increase nursing efficiency. Improving working conditions would allow hospitals to retain their current staff and attract new employees.

Magnet® Hospital Recognition Program

In 1990, the American Nurses Credentialing Center created the Magnet Hospital Recognition Program for Excellence in Nursing Services. Hospitals received a Magnet designation when they satisfied a set of criteria designed to measure the strength and quality of their commitment to nurses. The University of Washington Medical Center in Seattle, Washington, received the first Magnet recognition in 1994. Since then, research has proved that Magnet organizations have improved clinical outcomes, and score higher on patient and nurse satisfaction surveys.[65]

"It has become increasingly clear that work settings which foster a professional practice environment are fundamental to resolving the nursing shortage."[64]

American Nurses Association Resolution, 1988

The National Institute of Nursing Research

In the early 1980s, both the IOM and the National Institutes of Health (NIH) concluded that nursing research had a distinct and legitimate place in national biomedical and behavioral research. In response, the NIH established the National Center for Nursing Research in 1986, which was elevated to an institute with the passage of the NIH Revitalization Act of 1993. The mission of the National Institute for Nursing Research (NINR) was to "promote and improve the health of individuals, families, and communities" by supporting research on the nursing care of individuals across the life span.[66]

To Err Is Human

In 1999, the IOM published *To Err Is Human*, a report highlighting the impact of medical errors on the U.S. health care system. The report suggested that preventable medical mistakes accounted for up to 98,000 deaths annually, with a total national cost of up to $29 billion.[67] Hoping to break the cycle, the report called for heightened safety measures and the development of new protocols to try and reduce the incidence of errors.

In the late 1980s and throughout the 1990s, many hospitals did exactly as the Commission report advised. As a result, the shortage of nurses slowed down in the mid-1990s as wages and enrolled pre-licensure students increased. Still, critical shortages continued to plague the profession into the 21st century. Projections estimate that national and worldwide nursing shortages will increase as the current nurse labor force retires, and the number of elderly patients rises sharply as the baby boomer generation grows older.

Nurses and Access to Care

As federal policy makers focused on inpatient services in the 1980s, federal support for public health programs declined. In an effort to balance the health care budget, the government cut funding to rural health programs right as the need for services increased in these areas. Individuals and families now had to assume primary responsibility for their own health, and access to health care services became increasingly difficult in remote and/or economically disadvantaged regions. Few health care providers desired to practice in many rural areas, and the closure of public hospitals and clinics further decreased the availability of jobs and the ability of communities to access care. The total number and overall percentage of the U.S. population without health insurance increased dramatically in the face of rising insurance costs. By 1999, more than 42 million citizens—approximately 15% of the U.S. population—were without insurance.[68]

As national leaders grew more concerned over the uninsured, they commissioned the IOM to investigate the status of public health services in the United States. Two years later in 1988, *The Future of Public Health,* was published. The report highlighted the disorganization in public health agencies across the country and described how the political landscape had negatively affected any progress. Ultimately, the IOM concluded that public health was "currently in disarray."[69] Findings indicated wide fluctuations in service availability and an uneven distribution of technical expertise by public health providers, with economically disadvantaged regions suffering the most. The report stated that "both the mix and the intensity of services vary widely from place to place . . . in too many localities, there is no health department."[70] In addition, the IOM presented

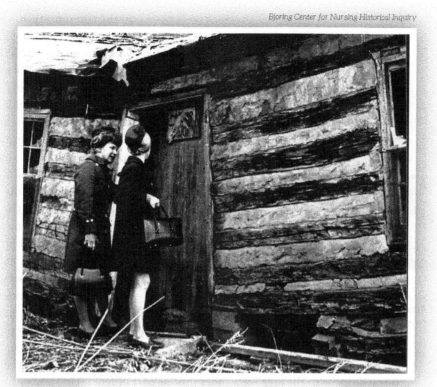

Nurses visiting patients in rural America, who had very little access to care as the government cut funding for rural health programs throughout the 1980s.

a new mission statement and outlined responsibilities for federal, state, and local public health departments. The report issued a bold statement by asserting that: "No citizen from any community, no matter how small or remote, should be without identifiable and realistic access to the benefits of public health protection."[71]

Unfortunately, many communities continued to suffer significant health disparities related to diminishing access to health services, particularly in areas of Appalachia. In this region, some health care providers refused to wait for outside help, and took it upon themselves to assist communities in need.

Mobile Nursing Care in Appalachia

Appalachia covers a large rural region of the eastern United States, stretching from the southern tip of New York and down to northern areas of Alabama, Georgia, and Mississippi. The area traditionally faces a shortage of public health clinics, hospitals, and experienced health care providers. Many Appalachian residents also live in isolated mountain regions and experience a higher rate of poverty when compared to overall national data.[73] Beginning in 1980, residents of the region began to suffer from increasing health disparities. Appalachian counties saw a higher overall mortality rate, a higher infant mortality rate, and a lower life expectancy than the rest of the country. One such county—Dickenson County in southwest Virginia—had some of the poorest health statistics of the entire state.[74] For this reason, the Catholic Church and Saint Marys Hospital sent medical missionary Sister Bernadette Kenny to serve Dickenson County beginning in 1980.

A trained nurse-midwife, "Sister Bernie" moved to Virginia and began working part-time doing quality assurance with a local nursing home. After living and working

"The wonder is not that American public health has problems, but that so much has been done so well, and with so little."[72]

Institute of Medicine, The Future of Public Health, 1988

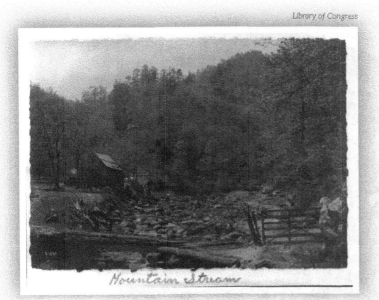

A cabin in rural Appalachia, where residents experienced higher mortality and poverty rates than the rest of America beginning in 1980.

in the community, Kenny began to recognize a great need for public health services but no one to fill the role. Packing supplies in the trunk of her own Volkswagen Beetle, Kenny decided to volunteer herself, providing home health services to area residents.

At the time, residents of Dickenson were without any home health agency, and the nearest hospital was located an entire county away. For many, transportation to the lone clinic in Dickerson proved too difficult, as the area lacked any public transportation system. In addition to geographic and transportation barriers, cultural norms in Appalachia also hindered care. Despite high rates of poverty, residents expressed pride in self-sufficiency and an aversion to receiving free care. The people of the community also had difficulty trusting outsiders, particularly public health workers who came to the area for a short time as part of federal initiatives to send physicians to underserved populations. Most felt that these physicians never made an effort to understand the true needs of the community, and left the area as soon as their contract was fulfilled.[75]

Kenny took a different approach. She drove the mountainous roads to individual homes to assess community needs, bringing supplies and expertise. Aware of the county's high infant mortality rate, Kenny focused on providing early prenatal care and maternal education, activities well within her scope of practice as a midwife. Her efforts proved successful. From 1970 to 1982, Dickenson County had an average infant mortality rate of 6.69 per 1,000 live births; that rate dropped to only 1.86 per 1,000 between 1983 and 1989.[76]

After visiting people in their homes, many of them multigenerational families living together, Kenny began to realize that residents needed a full range of primary care services. As she recalled: "I wanted to offer whatever was needed for the people."[77] Since practice regulations prevented her from offering such comprehensive care, Kenny enrolled in a family nurse practitioner program at the Medical College of Virginia, designed specifically for rural outreach.

"You have to be willing to address and listen to each person in the family. Sit on the couch and listen."[78]

Sister Bernadette Kenny, 2012

In 1982, Sister Kenny purchased a recreational vehicle from the Catholic Church in Richmond, Virginia. She collaborated with emergency room physicians at Saint Marys Hospital to develop a protocol book and ensure backup medical supervision should the need arise. Armed with medications and donated supplies, Kenny brought the roving Health Wagon RV back to the community. Despite her Boston accent and ties to the Catholic Church, she slowly gained acceptance among residents once they recognized the services she offered and her willingness to reach out and listen.

After a few years, local organizations and Saint Marys Hospital began to appreciate the value of the Health Wagon. A coal miner's strike in 1989 also increased its recognition, as Kenny offered services and medicine to protesters during the dispute. The hospital paid for two part-time RNs to assist Kenny on the Health Wagon. In addition to their traditional nursing duties of taking vital signs, providing patient education, and giving vaccines, Kenny expected the nurses to know how to drive, maintain, and repair the RV.[79] Over the years, the nurses developed partnerships with local health departments, participated in immunization clinics and health fairs, and helped with community outreach. These partnerships eventually expanded beyond the region. In 1999, the Health Wagon began to help in Remote Area Medical (RAM) clinics.[80]

Sister Kenny and the mobile Health Wagon offered beneficial primary and preventive care services to underserved communities in Appalachia. By providing comprehensive, compassionate, and quality nursing care free of charge, the Health Wagon filled a much-needed gap in health services for the poor, uninsured residents of the community. Today, the Health Wagon continues its mission of providing culturally sensitive health care and education to rural Appalachia, visiting 11 sites in southwest Virginia on a weekly, biweekly, and monthly basis.[81]

WAR IN THE PERSIAN GULF

Nurses would soon be involved in areas far from the United States. On August 2, 1990, the Iraq Army invaded and annexed Kuwait. The international community immediately condemned the action, and the United States initiated Operation Desert Shield. Its purpose was to build up the defense of Saudi Arabia and liberate Kuwait. A coalition of more than 35 nations joined the military alliance, offering money, troops, and military supplies. However, the United States carried the largest portion of the military and economic burden. A 5-month diplomatic effort to liberate Kuwait from Saddam Hussein ensued, leading to the initiation of Operation Desert Storm, a month-long air war beginning January 17, 1991. A failed ultimatum by President George H.W. Bush in late February led to a ground war, when U.S. armed forces moved into Iraq and Kuwait. A ceasefire was ordered just 5 days later, ending what some have called the "one hundred hour war." Of the 533,608 troops who served in the Gulf War, 148 died in combat; another 145 died of noncombat–related injuries.[82] As they had in so many other conflicts, nurses deployed during the Gulf War served a pivotal role in providing specialized care to American troops in wartime.

Right after the initiation of Operation Desert Shield, the Navy readied and deployed two hospital ships, the USNS *Comfort* and the USNS *Mercy*, both manned and ready to receive casualties by September 30, 1990. By the time Operation Desert Storm began in 1991, 2,000 army nurses were already stationed in the Persian Gulf and more than 900 Air Force nurses had deployed for active duty. Most of the latter had trained as flight nurses.[83] These military nurses served in a variety of capacities and in numerous locations.

By the start of the Gulf War, medical plans had progressed to support a more fluid operation, with the goal of creating small, mobile facilities that followed the battlefront. When an injury occurred, a field medic immediately treated and triaged the soldier for

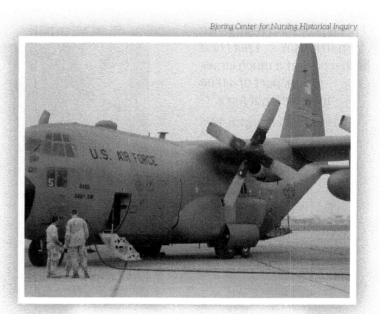

Bjoring Center for Nursing Historical Inquiry

A transport plane, which brought wounded soldiers to battalion aid stations outside of conflict zones during the Gulf War.

transport to the battalion aid stations outside of the conflict zone. Once there, the patient received a thorough assessment, and if necessary was sent to a medical battalion surgical support company or casualty receiving and treatment ship, both of which had more personnel, more sophisticated equipment, surgical capabilities, and pharmacy and lab facilities. Any casualty requiring more intensive care was transported to a combat zone fleet hospital or a hospital ship. Both were as well staffed and well equipped as any major hospital facility in the United States.[84]

Nurses serving in the Gulf War conflict relied on teamwork and dedication to handle the multitude of injuries and illnesses they treated. While injured soldiers came in with battlefield and combat-related wounds, a significant portion of the patients suffered from accidents or common illness. As one nurse described:

> We were very busy with broken bones, twisted ankles, lacerations. . . . We had construction site injuries; deep lacerations, and skin evulsions. . . . We had patients who needed limbs put back on, facial, chest, abdominal injuries from truck accidents, crushing injuries from vehicles colliding, head traumas like shots in the head, people who fell from helicopters. . . . We saw acute respiratory infections and a lot of diarrhea, nausea, vomiting.[86]

As another nurse explained, "We saw the things you see everywhere. People actually have normal health problems when they're at war."[87]

Depending on the timing of a deployment and the medical unit nurses were stationed in, total patient census and acuity level varied tremendously. Some nurses complained that they had nothing to do for most of their deployment, while others dodged Scud missiles and dealt with the difficulty of triaging during mass casualty situations. Frequently working 12-hour shifts, 5 days a week, these nurses dealt with challenging environmental conditions and sometimes serious safety risks.[88]

Throughout the conflict, these military nurses demonstrated a deep commitment to their patients and a strong sense of teamwork and unity. As one nurse explained: "All

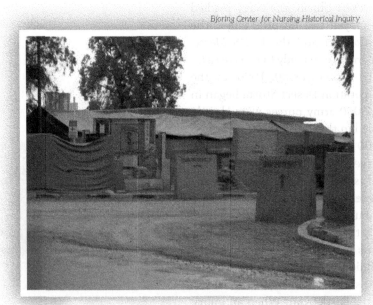

Bjoring Center for Nursing Historical Inquiry

Signs pointing to a hospital tent, where military nurses treated combat-related injuries as well as everyday health problems from soldiers.

of the nurses had such ownership that none of us would leave if there was a casualty. . . . We were very selfless when it came to that because it's 'what we're here for.'. . . We're here for the guys."[89]

NURSES AND HEALTHY PEOPLE
The Surgeon General's Report

In 1979, the U.S. Department of Health Education and Welfare published *Healthy People: The Surgeon General's Report on Health Promotion and Disease Prevention*, which outlined broad national goals for improving the health of all Americans. This report began the Healthy People initiative, a government-sponsored program offering quantitative goals to help reduce preventable death and injury. Intended as a guide for health care providers, educators, community organizations, and leaders in industry and labor, *Healthy People* aimed to provide a unified vision for ensuring a beneficial future for generations to come.

Healthy People took a definitive stance on the importance of prevention to improve health for a lifetime. The report broke down goals into five major life stages—infants, children, adolescents and young adults, adults, and older adults—with different priorities for each age group. Actions for health were broken down into three categories: prevention, such as family planning services and immunizations; protection, like occupational safety and water fluoridation; or promotion, like smoking cessation and proper nutrition. As the health care circumstances of American citizens changed, so did the content of the initiatives. In fact, the initiatives were updated every decade. With each new publication, the number of Healthy People initiatives increased, growing from 15 priority areas in 1979 to 22 priority areas in 1990. By 2000, there were 28 focus areas, each with a specific number of quantifiable objectives to achieve the initiatives.[91] Healthy People 2010 and 2020 continued this pattern.

What began as a largely expert-driven analysis and action plan evolved into a joint effort between government agencies and the public. With each iteration of the *Healthy People* publication, the development process involved more community engagement and feedback. One of the greatest criticisms of earlier *Healthy People* publications was that selected priorities focused on overall national averages, neglecting the racial and class discrepancies that resulted from lack of access to care or poor living conditions. *Healthy People 2000* aimed to improve the specificity of its objectives, and asserted that: "The correlation between poor health and lower socioeconomic status has been well documented, but that does not make it right or inevitable. Good health should not be seen, or, for that matter, be permitted to exist in fact, as a benefit for only those who can afford it; it should be available and accessible to every citizen."[93]

As the government moved national health goals toward strategies of prevention rather than reacting with medical intervention, they significantly changed the approach to health and wellness. Nurses, however, had embraced this viewpoint for decades. Unfortunately, members of the Healthy People Advisory Committee—the small group of industry leaders tasked with creating new objectives each decade—lacked a nursing perspective. Although nurses had been invited to attend advisory meetings and participate in smaller working groups, no nurse had been appointed to an Advisory Committee position. For many nursing leaders, the omission ran counter to the profession's pledged duty and responsibility to society. As Rita Carty, president of the American Association of Colleges of Nurses, asserted: "It is our front-lines

> "Further improvements in the health of the American people can and will be achieved—not alone through increased medical care and greater health expenditures—but through a renewed national commitment to efforts designed to prevent disease and to promote health."[92]
>
> *Surgeon General*
> *Dr. Julius B. Richmond, 1979*

> "As the nation's largest health profession, as the primary provider to long-term care, and as the largest component of the hospital labor force, nursing is health care."[95]
>
> *Rita Carty, 1991*

expertise in patient care, case management, patient education, healthcare administration, health outcomes research, and health promotion that puts nursing in a leadership position to shape a new healthcare system for the future."[94]

Years passed before a nurse was elected to an Advisory Committee position, but finally Therese S. Richmond was appointed to serve on the committed for the Healthy People 2030 initiative. While the delay may have baffled many nurses, the appointment reflected an increasing awareness by national and international agencies, including the World Health Organization, the United Nations, and the IOM, regarding the important role of the nursing profession in promoting health across the world.

Health Disparities and Ethics

Nurses were not without fault when it came to providing access to care for minorities. In fact, from the 1930s to the 1960s, nurse Eunice Rivers worked for the U.S. Public Health Service to recruit volunteers for the Tuskegee Syphilis Study in Alabama. During her tenure, Rivers functioned as the liaison between the men in the study and Public Health physicians. Whether she was to blame for carrying out the orders given by a group of White physician scientists is still a matter of debate. As an African American woman, some historians have questioned her dedication to the unethical experiment, while others have pointed to her status as a Black woman and nurse, using expectations of obedience to explain her actions. Nonetheless, she played a key role. Not until the 1990s did the federal government accept responsibility for racial discrimination and medical disregard for subjects participating in the research project. On May 16, 1997, President Bill Clinton issued a formal apology for the "Tuskegee Study of Untreated Syphilis in the Negro Male." The 40-year-long research project was deemed "ethically unjustified" for operating without informed consent, misleading study participants, and denying men adequate treatment for syphilis even after the discovery and widespread use of penicillin. In his remarks, President Clinton admitted: "The United States government did something that was wrong—deeply, profoundly, morally wrong. It was an outrage to our commitment to integrity and equality for all our citizens . . . and I am sorry."[96]

With new regulations in health care, including HIPAA, nurses' roles would become increasingly complicated in the 21st century. Indeed, nurses would be needed more than ever to continue providing holistic care in numerous social, economic, and political contexts. The first of these would involve preparation for disasters. As the new millennium opened, the United States would be attacked and once again embroiled in war.

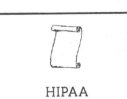

HIPAA

On August 21, 1996, the United States Congress enacted the Health Insurance Portability and Accountability Act (HIPAA). The act carries two main provisions: the first protects health insurance coverage for workers and their families in the event of a job change or loss, and the second established national standards for protecting the privacy and security of an individual's identifiable health information; it also set civil and criminal penalties for any violations. These rules apply to "covered entities" under HIPAA and include health plans, health care billing services and community health information systems, and individual health care providers transmitting data. The enactment of HIPAA caused major reform in clinical operations and research capabilities.

For Discussion

1. Describe how the publication *Nursing: A Social Policy Statement* asserted professional status for nursing. Do you feel it is important for a profession to define itself? Why or why not?
2. Describe the San Francisco model for AIDS care. How did stigma around HIV/AIDS contribute to discrimination and health disparities in treating the disease?

(continued)

3. Why was the national nursing shortage in the 1980s and 1990s particularly perplexing? How did prospective payment and the DRG reimbursement plan worsen the shortage?
4. What factors worsened access to care for rural communities starting in 1980? How did Sister Kenny and the mobile Health Wagon instill trust among Appalachian residents?
5. Describe the experience of nurses serving in the first Gulf War.
6. What did the *Healthy People* initiative demonstrate about our national approach to illness? Do you think the lack of a nursing perspective on the Advisory Council was important? Why or why not?

NOTES

1. "ANA '88: Pay Us More and Let Us Nurse," *American Journal of Nursing* 88 (1988): 977.

2. Florence Nightingale, "Sick Nursing and Health Nursing," in *Nursing of the Sick 1893: Papers and Discussions from the International Congress of Charities, Correction, and Philanthropy, Chicago, 1893* (New York: McGraw-Hill, 1949): 35.

3. "ANA '88: Pay Us More," 977.

4. Centers for Medicare and Medicaid Services, "National Health Expenditure Data: Historical," https://www.cms.gov/Research-Statistics-Data-and-Systems/Statistics-Trends-and-Reports/NationalHealthExpendData/NationalHealthAccountsHistorical.html (accessed September 19, 2016).

5. Thomas A. Hodgson and Andrea N. Kopstein, "Health Care Expenditures for Major Diseases in 1980," *Health Care Financing Review* 5 (1984): 1–12.

6. American Nurses Association, *Nursing: A Social Policy Statement* (Kansas City, MO: American Nurses Association, 1980): 5, 9.

7. Ibid., 2.

8. Ibid., 2.

9. Ibid., 5.

10. Ibid., 7.

11. Ibid., 18.

12. Ibid.

13. Centers for Disease Control and Prevention, "*Pneumosystis* Pneumonia—Los Angeles," *Morbidity and Mortality Weekly Report* 30 (June 5, 1981): 250–252.

14. Charles Mayer, "Nursing and AIDS: A Decade of Caring," *American Journal of Nursing* 91 (1991): 26.

15. Jerry D. Durham and Felissa L. Cohen, *The Person with AIDS: Nursing Perspectives* (New York: Springer Publishing, 1987): 2.

16. Centers for Disease Control Task Force on Kaposi's Sarcoma and Opportunistic Infections, "Epidemiologic Aspects of the Current Outbreak of Kaposi's Sarcoma and Opportunistic Infections," *New England Journal of Medicine* 306 (1982): 248–252.

17. Clifford L. Morrison, "The AIDS Epidemic," an oral history conducted in 1995 and 1996 by Sally Smith Hughes, in *The AIDS Epidemic in San Francisco: The Response of the Nursing Profession, 1981-1984, Volume III*, Regional Oral History Office, The Bancroft Library, University of California, Berkeley (1999): 86.

18. Centers for Disease Control and Prevention, "Current Trends Update on Acquired Immune Deficiency Syndrome (AIDS)—United States," *Morbidity and Mortality Weekly Report* 31 (1982): 507–508.

19. Brian Budds, "How Do You Do It?" *American Journal of Nursing* 92 (1992): 38.

20. Morrison, "The AIDS Epidemic," 120.

21. Mervyn Silverman, "AIDS Care: The San Francisco Model," *Journal of Ambulatory Care Management* 11 (1988): 16.

22. Diane Jones, "First Wave of the Nursing Staff on the AIDS Ward, San Francisco General Hospital," an oral history conducted in 1995 and 1996 by Sally Smith Hughes in *The AIDS Epidemic in San Francisco: The Response of the Nursing Profession, 1981-1984, Vol. III*, Regional Oral History Office, The Bancroft Library, University of California, Berkeley (1999): 56.

23. Gayling Gee, "The AIDS Clinic, Building 80," an oral history conducted in 1995 and 1996 by Sally Smith Hughes in *The AIDS Epidemic in San Francisco: The Response of the Nursing Profession, 1981–1984, Volume IV*, Regional Oral History Office, The Bancroft Library, University of California, Berkeley (1999): 19.

24. Salmaan Keshavjee and Paul E. Farmer, "Tuberculosis, Drug Resistance, and the History of Modern Medicine," *New England Journal of Medicine* 367 (2012): 931–934.

25. Charles Mayer, "Nursing and AIDS: A Decade of Caring," *American Journal of Nursing* 91 (1991): 26–31.

26. Ibid., 27.

27. Ibid., 31.

28. "AIDS and Life Insurance," *Lancet* 8597 (1988): 1293.

29. Linda Aiken, Douglas Sloane, Eileen T. Lake, Julie Sochalski, and Anita L. Weber, "Organization and Outcomes of Inpatient AIDS Care," *Medical Care* 37 (1999): 760–772.

30. Jo Anne Bennett, "Nurses Talk about the Challenges of AIDS," *American Journal of Nursing* 87 (1987): 1152.

31. Morrison, "The AIDS Epidemic," 84–85.

32. "The AIDS Memorial Quilt Archive," http://www.aidsquilt.org/about/the-aids-memorial -quilt (accessed November 28, 2016).

33. Bill Barrick, "Light at the End of a Decade," *American Journal of Nursing* 90 (1990): 36–40.

34. Jo Ann Bennett, "AIDS: Epidemiology Update," *American Journal of Nursing* 85 (1985): 972.

35. Ibid.

36. Elisabeth Dexter, "Keeling Gives Details of AIDS at Colleges: Doctor Points Out Problems with Attitudes," *The Cavalier Daily*, November 3, 1992, 1.

37. Valerie Hart, Susan Henderson, Juliana L'Heureux, and Ann Sossong, *Maine Nursing: Interviews and History on Caring and Competence* (Charleston, SC: The History Press, 2016): 112.

38. Helene D. Gayle, Richard P. Keeling, Miguel Garcia-Tunon, Barbara W. Kilbourne, John P. Narkunas, Fred R. Ingram, Martha F. Rogers, and James W. Curran, "Prevalence of the Human Immunodeficiency Virus among University Students," *New England Journal of Medicine* 353 (1990): 1538–1541.

39. Centers for Disease Control and Prevention, "HIV and AIDS—United States, 1981-2000," *Morbidity and Mortality Weekly Report* 50 (2001): 430–434.

40. Rosemary Stevens, *In Sickness and in Wealth: American Hospitals in the Twentieth Century* (Baltimore, MD: Johns Hopkins University Press, 1998): 284.

41. Rick Mayes, "The Origins, Development, and Passage of Medicare's Revolutionary Prospective Payment System," *Journal of the History of Medicine and Allied Sciences* 62 (2006): 22.

42. Paul Starr, *The Social Transformation of American Medicine: The Rise of a Sovereign Profession and the Making of a Vast Industry* (New York: Basic Books, 1982): 379.

43. Sheila Burke, oral history interview with Rick Mayes, October 2, 2002, as quoted in Mayes, "The Origins, Development, and Passage of Medicare's Revolutionary Prospective Payment System," 43.

44. Mayes, "The Origins, Development, and Passage of Medicare's Revolutionary Prospective Payment System," 50.

45. Rick Mayes and Robert Berenson, *Medicare Prospective Payment and the Shaping of U.S. Health Care* (Baltimore, MD: Johns Hopkins University Press, 2006): 54.

46. Joan E. Lynaugh and Barbara L. Brush, *American Nursing: From Hospitals to Health Systems* (Cambridge, MA: Blackwell Publishers, 1996): 57.

47. Institute of Medicine, *Nursing and Nursing Education: Public Policies and Private Actions* (Washington, DC: National Academies Press, 1983): 231.

48. Claire M. Fagin, "The National Shortage of Nurses: A Nursing Perspective," in *Nursing in the 1980s: Crises, Opportunities, Challenges*, ed. Linda H. Aiken (Philadelphia: J.B. Lippincott, 1982): 23–24.

49. As cited in U.S. Department of Health and Human Services, *The Recurrent Shortage of Registered Nurses: A New Look at the Issues* (Washington, DC: Government Printing Office, 1981): 7.

50. Ibid.

51. Institute of Medicine, *Nursing and Nursing Education*, xv.

52. Ibid., 2–3.

53. Anne Z. Cockerham and Arlene W. Keeling, "A Brief History of Advanced Practice Nursing in the United States," in *Advanced Practice Nursing: An Integrative Approach*, eds. Ann B. Hamric, Charlene M. Hanson, Mary Fran Tracy, and Eileen T. O'Grady (St. Louis, MO: Elsevier, 2014): 21.

54. Connie R. Curran, Ann Minnick, and Joan Moss, "Who Needs Nurses?" *American Journal of Nursing* 87 (1987): 444–447.

55. Linda Aiken, "The Hospital Nursing Shortage: A Paradox of Increasing Supply and Increasing Vacancy Rates," *Western Journal of Medicine* 151 (1989): 87–92.

56. As quoted in John K. Inglehart, "Health Policy Report: Problems Facing the Nursing Profession," *New England Journal of Medicine* 317 (1987): 647.

57. Aiken, "The Hospital Nursing Shortage," 87.

58. Ibid., 88.

59. Embry M. Howell, Douglas Richardson, Paul Ginsburg, and Barbara Foot, "Deregionalization of Neonatal Intensive Care in Urban Areas," *American Journal of Public Health* 92 (2002): 120.

60. H. L. Halliday, "Surfactants: Past, Present and Future," *Journal of Perinatology* 28 (2008): S47–S56.

61. American Hospital Association, *Report of the Hospital Nursing Personnel Survey: 1987* (Washington, DC: American Hospital Association, 1987).

62. *Secretary's Commission on Nursing: Final Report* (Washington, DC: U.S. Department of Health and Human Services, 1988): 3.

63. Linda Aiken, Robert Blendon, and David Rogers, "The Shortage of Registered Nurses: A New Perspective," *Annals of Internal Medicine* 95 (1981): 365–371.

64. "ANA '88: Pay Us More," 977.

65. See Linda H. Aiken, Sean P. Clarke, Douglas M. Sloane, Eileen T. Lake, and Timothy Cheney, "Effects of Hospital Care Environment on Patient Mortality and Nurse Outcomes," *Journal of Nursing Administration* 38 (2008): 223–229; and Colleen J. Goode, Mary A. Blegen, Shin Hye Park, Thomas Vaughn, and Joanne Spetz, "Comparison of Patient Outcomes in Magnet and Non-Magnet Hospitals," *Journal of Nursing Administration* 41 (2011): 517–523.

66. National Institute for Nursing Research, "Mission," https://www.nih.gov/about-nih/what -we-do/nih-almanac/national-institute-nursing-research-ninr (accessed November 18, 2016).

67. Institute of Medicine, *To Err Is Human: Building a Safer Health System* (Washington DC: National Academies Press, 2000): 1–2.

68. U.S. Census Bureau, "Health Insurance Coverage, 1999: Table A, People without Health Insurance for the Entire Year 1998 and 1999," http://www2.census.gov/programs-surveys/ demo/tables/p60/211/hi99ta.txt (accessed November 23, 2016).

69. Institute of Medicine, *The Future of Public Health* (Washington, DC: National Academies Press, 1988): 3.

70. Ibid., 3.

71. Ibid., 9.

72. Ibid., 2.

73. Dan A. Black, Mark Mather, and Seth G. Sanders, *Standards of Living in Appalachia, 1960 to 2000* (Washington, DC: Appalachian Reference Bureau, 2007).

74. Audrey Snyder and Esther Thatcher, "From the Trunk of a Volkswagen Beetle: A Mobile Nursing Clinic in Appalachia," *Family and Community Health* 37 (2014): 239.

75. Ibid., 244.

76. Centers for Disease Control and Prevention, "Compressed Mortality Data," https://wonder .cdc.gov/mortsql.html (accessed November 26, 2016).

77. Interview with Bernadette Kenny by Audrey Snyder, March 30, 2012, as quoted in Snyder and Thatcher, "From the Trunk of a Volkswagen Beetle," 241.

78. Ibid., 240.

79. Snyder and Thatcher, "From the Trunk of a Volkswagen Beetle," 242–243.

80. Ibid., 246.

81. The Health Wagon, "History," http://thehealthwagon.org/hwwp/history (accessed November 26, 2016).

82. Patricia Rushton, Lynn Clark Callister, and Maile K. Wilson, *Latter-Day Saint Nurses at War: A Story of Caring and Sacrifice* (Provo, UT: Brigham Young University, 2005): 199.

83. Elizabeth Scannell-Desch and Mary Ellen Doherty, *Nurses in War: Voices from Iraq and Afghanistan* (New York: Springer Publishing, 2012): 15–16.

84. Ibid., 17.

85. Patrick Amersbach, "Patrick Amersbach," in *Gulf War Nurses: Personal Accounts of 14 Americans, 1990-1991 and 2003-2010*, ed. Patricia Rushton (Jefferson, NC: McFarland, 2011): 18.

86. Patricia Rushton, Jared E. Scott, and Lynn Clark Callister, "'It's What We're Here For': Nurses Caring for Military Personnel During the Persian Gulf War," *Nursing Outlook* 56 (2008): 181.

87. Ibid.

88. Rushton, Callister, and Wilson, *Latter-Day Saint Nurses at War*, 200.

89. Rushton, Scott, and Callister, "It's What We're Here For," 181.

90. Rushton, Callister, and Wilson, *Latter-Day Saint Nurses at War*, 200.

91. U.S. Department of Health and Human Services, "Phase I Report: Recommendations for the Framework and Format of Healthy People 2020," http://www.healthypeople.gov/2010/ hp2020/advisory/PhaseI/sec3.htm (accessed November 20, 2016).

92. U.S. Department of Health, Education and Welfare, *Healthy People: The Surgeon General's Report on Health Promotion and Disease Prevention* (Washington, DC: U.S. Government Printing Office, 1979): 1–1.

93. U.S. Department of Health and Human Services, *Healthy People 2000: National Health Promotion and Disease Prevention Objectives* (Boston: Jones and Bartlett Publishers, 1992): v.

94. American Association of Colleges of Nurses, *Annual Report*, 1991, 4.

95. Ibid.

96. Office of the Press Secretary, "Remarks by the President in Apology for Study Done in Tuskegee," May 16, 1997, http://www.cdc.gov/tuskegee/clintonp.htm (accessed November 18, 2016).

FURTHER READING

American Nurses Association, *Nursing: A Social Policy Statement* (Kansas City, MO: American Nurses Association, 1980).

Institute of Medicine, *To Err Is Human: Building a Safer Health System* (Washington, DC: National Academy Press, 2000).

Keeling, Richard P., *Effective AIDS Education on Campus: New Directions for Student Services* (San Francisco, CA: Jossey-Bass, 1992).

Lynaugh, Joan E., and Barbara L. Brush, *American Nursing: From Hospitals to Health Systems* (Cambridge, MA: Blackwell Publishers, 1996).

Mayes, Rick, and Robert Berenson, *Medicare Prospective Payment and the Shaping of U.S. Health Care* (Baltimore, MD: Johns Hopkins University Press, 2006).

Reverby, Susan M., "Rethinking the Tuskegee Syphilis Study: Nurse Rivers, Silence, and the Meaning of Treatment," *Nursing History Review* 7 (1999): 3–28.

Rushton, Patricia, Lynn Clark Callister, and Maile K. Wilson, *Latter-Day Saint Nurses at War: A Story of Caring and Sacrifice* (Provo, UT: Brigham Young University, 2005).

Scannell-Desch, Elizabeth, and Mary Ellen Doherty, *Nurses in War: Voices from Iraq and Afghanistan* (New York: Springer Publishing, 2012).

Shilts, Randy, *And the Band Played On: Politics, People, and the AIDS Epidemic* (New York: St. Martin's Press, 1987).

Snyder, Audrey, and Esther Thatcher, "From the Trunk of a Volkswagen Beetle: A Mobile Nursing Clinic in Appalachia," *Family and Community Health* 37 (2014): 239–247.

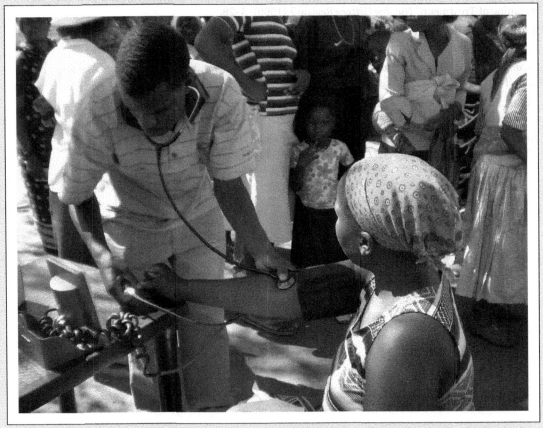

Nursing Students without Borders, South Africa.

CHAPTER 15

Toward a Culture of Health: Nursing in the 21st Century

Arlene W. Keeling

"Nurses will be called upon to lead efforts to build a Culture of Health and to ensure that people in this country get and stay as healthy as possible.... The Campaign's efforts to make sure that nurses have the right to practice to the full extent of their training means more nurses are able to provide primary care in more settings; in turn Americans will have better access to affordable care." [1]

Susan Hassmiller, 2011

Responding to questions during an interview about the "Culture of Health" initiative launched by the Robert Wood Johnson Foundation earlier in the decade, Dr. Susan Hassmiller emphasized the central role that nurses would play in the plan. As the senior advisor for nursing at the Robert Wood Johnson Foundation and director of nursing's "Campaign for Action," Hassmiller had been involved in implementing strategies for the Culture of Health initiative for several years. As a nurse herself, she not only understood the central role nurses played in the health care system in the 21st century, but was also familiar with their long history in health promotion.

From 1607 when the English colonists settled in America to 2016, the United States had made significant progress toward achieving a culture of health. At the turn of the 21st century, new medical technologies, scientific discoveries in epigenetics, targeted cancer chemotherapies, noninvasive surgeries, joint replacements, and advances in cardiology, nephrology, and other subspecialties all played a role in increasing life expectancy and quality of life. In addition, a growing

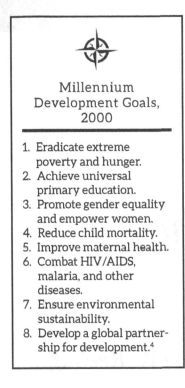

Millennium
Development Goals,
2000

1. Eradicate extreme
   poverty and hunger.
2. Achieve universal
   primary education.
3. Promote gender equality
   and empower women.
4. Reduce child mortality.
5. Improve maternal health.
6. Combat HIV/AIDS,
   malaria, and other
   diseases.
7. Ensure environmental
   sustainability.
8. Develop a global partnership for development.[4]

awareness of the environmental causes of disease, a focus on access to care and the social determinants of that care, an interest in emergency prepared-ness, and an emphasis on the prevention of disease had turned the nation's attention to the promotion of health. The widespread use of the Internet, the development of electronic medical records, advances in cell-phone tech-nology, capabilities in telemedicine, the growth in online education pro-grams, and other technological advances in communication also promoted access to information and care.

Indeed the nation was making progress, and Hassmiller made a good point: nurses had an important role to play in moving the country toward a culture of health. Building on their past, nurses were uniquely positioned to adapt to new social, political, and economic contexts, restore sick people to health, encourage Americans to take steps toward healthy living, and teach them to be proactive in preventing disease.

The initiative had the support of the global community. In 2000, the United Nations drafted the Millennium Declaration enshrining "global health as one of the, if not *the*, centerpiece issues in global development."[2] That year, 189 nations voted to support the Millennium Goals—several of which addressed global health. The goals were developed to relieve poor health conditions around the world and to establish positive steps for improv-ing living conditions by the year 2015.[3] Nurses' participation would be cru-cial. However, it would not be the first time that nurses took positive steps to reduce child mortality, improve maternal health, or work with others to combat disease. As professionals they had been doing so for more than a century. As *lay nurses* and *lay-midwives*, they had been doing so for centuries.

NURSING'S RESPONSE TO HISTORIC EVENTS

Before the profession could embark on any campaign for health, it would have to respond to a series of unforeseen historic events. Some were man-made disasters—like the attack on the World Trade Center on September 11, 2001, and the Flint Michigan water crisis later in the century. Others included war, nursing shortages, hurricanes and pandemics, and the growth of a rapidly aging population. Once again the profession would respond, sometimes as individuals traveling to the scene of a disaster and at other times collaborating with other professions to meet the larger need.

Nursing and September 11, 2001

For Americans, the traumatic events of September 11, 2001—just a year after the United Nations voted on the Millennium Goals—made thoughts of developing a healthy, thriv-ing world seem a far cry from reality. The morning of September 11 changed everything, and nurses, like everyone else in the United States, could focus only on the threat of terrorism. That morning nurses throughout the country stopped what they were doing and listened to the news. It was only 8:45 a.m. on a beautiful autumn day, and Al-Qaeda terrorists had just crashed a jetliner into the North Tower of the World Trade Center in Lower Manhattan, New York City.

What the nurses and other Americans saw and heard was horrifying. A second jet-liner crashed into the South Tower just minutes after it was reported that a third plane had attacked the Pentagon, and that a fourth was in the air over Pennsylvania, headed for Washington, DC. The nation was under attack.

Minutes after the attacks, hospitals in Washington, DC, New York City, and New Jersey activated emergency plans. In New Jersey, just across the river from Lower Man-hattan, director of Patient Care Services Frank Hickey was on duty in Union Hospital, a

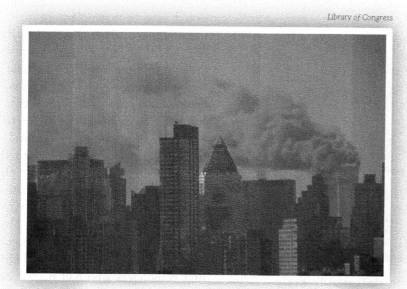

The collapse of the World Trade Center in New York City, September 11, 2001, where 3,000 people lost their lives.

The Pentagon Attack

"I was in a cab on Pennsylvania Avenue, right next to the White House, [headed to Capitol Hill to testify] when I heard an explosion and saw a huge cloud of black smoke rise from the area of the Pentagon. My cab driver turned on the radio and we then realized what was happening. In the meantime, hundreds of people were pouring out of every federal building around. . . . It was terrifying to see the rapid response of what seemed like hundreds of soldiers with AK-47s appear!"[5]

Jean Bartels, 2001

200-bed community hospital. Having just had coffee, Hickey was beginning to make rounds when he noticed that the nurses were clustered around televisions, watching the news. Before he could find out what happened, he was paged on the overhead speaker system to report to the administration offices. There, he and Chief Executive Officer Kate Coyne were told to secure the hospital and to implement the disaster plan. It was expected that hundreds of casualties would be ferried to Union Hospital from across the Hudson River.

Working under orders from the New Jersey State Department of Health, both Hickey and Coyne immediately began to collect data about the number of medical, surgical, and critical care beds they had available. They also recorded the current emergency department capacity, the operating room capacity, the number of available staff at all skill levels, the number of days' food the hospital had on hand, and the number and acuity level of all patients. In addition, the pair opened the hospital command center, briefed key leaders, and assigned duties as outlined in the disaster plan.[6]

Hickey and Coyne then made rounds throughout the hospital to reassure the staff, discovering that a number of nurses had family members who worked at the World Trade Center, and that no one was able to make contact with their relatives. Cell phones were down—or no one was answering. Realizing that these nurses could not work effectively, Hickey activated the emergency call list, bringing in replacements for the nurses who needed to leave.[7]

Having attended to the staffing concerns, Hickey turned his attention once again to the disaster plan. First he ordered tents to be set up outside the hospital to receive casualties. Then he saw to it that nurses prepared stretchers and intravenous lines so that the hospital would be ready for the anticipated onslaught of victims. The staff then waited. However, few trauma patients arrived.[8]

Instead, the hospital received an onslaught of friends and relatives of the thousands who had died or were missing after the Towers collapsed. Many who came to the makeshift emergency room were in shock and disbelief, and nurses and doctors at Union Hospital helped them in their despair. Responding to their distress, Hickey summoned priests and chaplains to the scene. He also directed the staff to prepare basic paper and pencil psychological assessment tools to use for triage. Then he set to work providing emotional support, food, and comfort for staff and survivors alike. Later that day Hickey

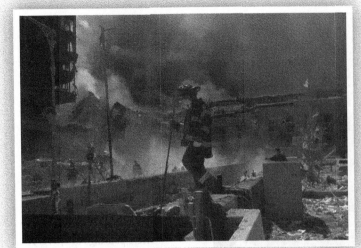

Firemen and other rescue workers worked around the clock to unearth survivors and remains from the rubble while they sustained multiple injuries and casualties themselves.

would have to make plans to care for the orphans of those who had died in the World Trade Center—orphans brought into the hospital by people in the neighborhood; children who were terrified and wanted their parents.[9]

Meanwhile, across the river in New York, personnel in every hospital in Manhattan rallied to respond to the crisis. In every facility, nurses and physicians saw more injured rescuers than people who had been in the World Trade Center when it collapsed. More than 3,000 people died in the disaster, including police, firefighters, and other first responders who had rushed into the Twin Towers just as they imploded.

At New York's Bellevue Hospital, patients came through the emergency room sporadically, and not in the numbers expected. Instead, rescue workers presented with fractures, burns, respiratory difficulties, and eye injuries from the smoke and dust that blanketed Lower Manhattan. Bellevue's first disaster victim arrived on his own. After debris from one of the collapsing towers injured his knee, he simply hailed a taxi to take him to the hospital. Bellevue's second patient, however, was more representative of what was to come: he was a firefighter who had died at the scene when a falling body hit him. The next patient was a chaplain who had been administering last rites to the firefighter on the scene. The chaplain was "dead on arrival." More patients soon arrived. From the time of the disaster until midnight that night, the Bellevue emergency room staff treated close to 220 patients.

Nurses and physicians at St. Vincent's Medical Center, the trauma center closest to the World Trade Center, saw more patients than did staff in other hospitals. Three hundred and sixty-one patients arrived at St. Vincent's in the first 24 hours after the attack. Fifty-eight of the 361 patients were paramedics, firefighters, and police officers.[10] Four died. Emergency room nurse Nancy Issing later recalled: "I had never seen the volume of patients that came into the ER that day. . . . It was one patient after another after another. It was overwhelming."[11]

At New York University Medical Center, nurses and physicians also responded. Hundreds lined up on the hospital steps, expecting thousands of trauma victims to deluge the hospital. Few came. Instead, like nurses and doctors elsewhere in the city, the staff did whatever they could to help in the disaster response. Some treated firefighters, rescue squad workers, police officers, and other first responders who were trying desperately to recover people from the disaster scene. Others, like Clinical Associate Professor Elizabeth Ayello, worked with her students to organize blood donations. Recalling that day, Ayello said: "Almost immediately, people started walking into the lobby of the hospital wanting to help. Soon there was a two and a half hour wait to give blood and there wasn't enough staff to draw it."[14] Later Ayello and her nursing students helped at Chelsea Piers, a waterfront sports complex set up as an emergency treatment center. There they treated about 200 people, "most of whom were rescue workers who were combing the site." As Ayello recalled, she and the students "washed out

"So many of the injuries I saw were so severe. Some patients had burns over 90 percent of their bodies."[12]

Nancy Issing, 2001

The Nurses Respond

"From the beginning, staff nurses just showed up ready to work, even staff who no longer were Saint Vincent's Hospital employees and RNs from other hospitals who could not get to their regular jobs."[13]

Suzanne Pugh, 2001

irritated eyes, gave breathing treatments, took EKGs, and treated minor burns and injuries."[15]

Nurses and physicians were needed to care for the rescuers for the weeks and months that followed. In the meantime, the world situation changed dramatically. In an unprecedented move, the U.S. government immediately shut down all civilian air travel. President George W. Bush later declared a war on terror and established a department of Homeland Security. The nation's focus—and the focus of nurses, physicians, and hospital administrators—turned to disaster response and preparedness.

Ensuring a safe environment for all Americans was critical to the survival of the nation and the health of its citizens. In the first days after the attack, nurses played an important role in promoting health. Just as they had done in response to other disasters earlier in the century, nurses provided physical comfort and psychological support to caregivers. St. Vincent's Medical Center was one of many hospitals that set up a Support Center. As director of nursing for behavioral health, Susan Castello later explained: "There was such a need in the community—so many people just needed someone to listen to them."[16]

Like the ongoing treatments for physical ailments that resulted from the collapse of the Towers and the polluted air, psychological support would be needed for years.[17] Healing would take time, and nurses, like other Americans, faced a new normal: a world threatened by random acts of terror, changes in national security, and the continuous threat of bioterrorism. Disaster planning, drills, and preparedness would become a focus of health departments, hospitals, and every health agency in the country. As part of that response, nurses would participate on disaster planning committees at the federal, state, and local levels. Meanwhile, military nurses would be called for active duty.

Nurses in the Iraq War

By November 2001, the United States was at war in Afghanistan, and full-time members of the Army, Air Force, and Navy Nurse Corps, as well as those in the Reserve, were activated. When the U.S. invasion of Iraq began in late March 2003, signaling the beginning of Operation Iraqi Freedom, even more nurses were called to service. Some came from the "plains of west Texas," others from "the commuter suburbs of New York City, or the heartland of Iowa."[18] All of them took an oath to support and defend their country. Within days of receiving orders, some headed overseas, some to American military bases in Europe, others to locations in the Middle East. Hundreds deployed to Kuwait.

After landing in Kuwait, nurses assigned to mobile hospitals moved into Iraq and set up their equipment, working with nurses and other hospital personnel from other countries in a multinational response.[20] One nurse anesthetist, Rita, recalled how her team joined the Forward Surgical Team Charlie in Iraq, and together they moved forward. Later she said: "We were like a well-oiled machine. Everyone knew their job, how to put up the tent hospital and all the equipment and gear that went into it. . . . We took people from bases up and down the eastern U.S. who had never worked together and threw them into a horrific environment. We were so well rehearsed, it was like a symphony."[21]

Commander Cheryl Ruff, a Navy nurse, was stationed with Bravo Surgical Company just south of the Iraqi border when the fighting began in 2003. At first the staff members were told that they had "little more than forty-eight hours" before they were to "board convoy trucks and begin a 30-hour journey to an area expected to experience heavy and major casualties." Instead, the company experienced several days and nights of delays—packing

The Flight to Kuwait

We boarded a United Airlines charter flight . . . all red, white and blue on the inside. We stopped in Germany to refuel and the Red Cross was set up to give us little packets with snacks and toothbrushes and some cold drinks. As we were flying into Kuwait, they had all the lights off and the sun visors down because they didn't want us to be a target. We landed in the middle of the night.[19]

Nurse anesthetist, 2003

and unpacking hospital equipment and waiting for orders.[22] Finally, the company flew on marine cargo planes to Camp Hasty, "a desolate place offering very little security, no shelter, and no bathroom facilities." From there trucks transported the group to Camp Anderson, another remote area that Ruff labeled "the other side of hell."[23] There, under the scorching sun, Bravo Surgical Company set up a triage tent, two operating rooms, and an intensive care unit. According to Ruff: "We scarcely had an opportunity to eat a snack from our MRE [meals ready-to eat] packs when the first choppers landed at the camp, carrying the first of the many wounded and dead who would arrive that day."[24]

What Ruff saw at Camp Anderson haunted her. Over the next 3 days Bravo Company treated 106 casualties. During that time she and her colleagues witnessed an "overwhelming degree of human destruction." As Ruff later recalled: "The sights we witnessed were haunting, and the smells of this hell invaded our senses and penetrated deep into our very souls."[25]

In addition to full-time military nurses, reservists were also activated. Debora Jonas and Charles Peworski, both from Mayo Clinic, were among those who were deployed. Jones was sent to Balad, 40 miles north of Baghdad, where she worked in the 332nd Air Force Theater Hospital. The tent hospital consisted of "three operating rooms, three ICUs, an ER, and five intermediate care wards," as well as a radiology department, a clinical lab, and a pharmacy. There the dust, heat, and sun were "incredible," and Jones had to protect herself as well as she could, all the while trying to "provide the best nursing care possible in those conditions."[28] As was the case for other nurses in previous wars, Jones had to make do with what she had. She later noted: "The oxygen and suction didn't just come out of the wall, you had to go and get the tank and the suction machine and make sure everything was in working order."[29]

Reservist Charles Peworski also served in Iraq, later receiving the 2004 Arizona Military Nurse of the Year award for his heroic actions. On Easter Sunday 2004, a blinding desert dust storm resulted in a three-vehicle high-speed crash, leaving the unit's medic injured and unable to perform his duties. Peworski, relying on his triage experience, ignored his own fractured arm and took control, collaborating with other nurses "to start three IVs, apply pressure dressings, stabilize fractures, treat for shock, and triage those who needed immediate care."[31]

As the war dragged on, hundreds of military nurses were deployed time after time to Iraq and Afghanistan. According to Major General Melissa Rank, the 14th chief nurse of the Air Force Nurse Corps, because of the duration of the war "a new set of issues was emerging related to steady-state deployments." Indeed, military nurses were experiencing difficulties in sustaining "a high level of personal readiness, finding inner resilience to sustain the mission despite its wartime tragedies, enduring prolonged exposure to secondary trauma, and most importantly, finding the ability to rejuvenate" when they returned home.[32]

Some nurses never returned. On July 10, 2007, 40-year-old Captain Maria I. Ortiz was killed in Iraq. Deployed as head nurse of Intermediate Care with the 28th Combat Support Hospital, Ortiz died as a result of a mortar attack on her unit. She was the first army nurse to be killed in action since the war in Vietnam.[33]

Geriatric Nursing and a Nursing Shortage

At home in the United States, civilian nurses soon discovered that what had been predicted in the 1990s was becoming a reality. Large numbers of Americans, the baby boomers, were aging, and their health care needs were both unique and complex. In response, health care agencies retooled to address the care of an aging population. Home health agencies opened and hospitals developed programs for nurse follow-up for discharged elderly patients. Meanwhile, faculty in schools of nursing added geriatric nursing courses to the curriculum; a new generation of nurses needed to be prepared to care for the elderly.

A second prediction made in the 20th century was also proving to be true: the profession was facing another shortage of nurses. Many nurses, baby boomers themselves, were retiring from full-time employment. Of particular importance, faculty and deans in schools of nursing were retiring in unprecedented numbers. Developing new leaders for nursing education was essential for nursing's future.

The profession, however, would get the support it needed. In 2003, the Helene Fuld Health Trust provided funding to extend the American Association of Colleges of Nursing's leadership program, ensuring that mentoring for new nursing school deans would be mentored. The Institute of Medicine further backed the initiative in 2003 when it released a report, *Health Professions Education: A Bridge to Quality*. That report advocated patient-centered care, and the use of interdisciplinary teams, evidence-based practice, quality improvement, and informatics. Each of these recommendations offered a unique and unparalleled opportunity for nursing to participate in and lead their profession.[34]

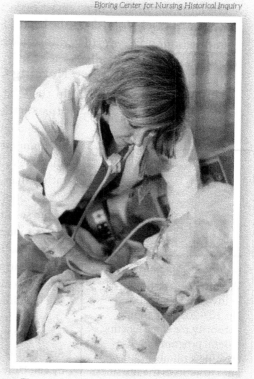

The number of geriatric nursing courses rose in the 1990s to address the growing elderly population of baby boomers who were aging.

The profession needed to consider alternate ways to create leaders for the future. In May 2003, the American Association of Colleges of Nursing released a white paper proposing a new master's degree for a clinical nurse leader (CNL). Calling for a "new nurse" to better meet the needs of a dramatically changing health care system, the CNL paper advocated for a nurse prepared with a master's degree who could manage care at the "point-of-care to individuals, families, and communities." The Association also appointed a task force to consider a practice-focused doctorate degree: the doctor of nursing practice (DNP). This degree would provide an alternative doctoral degree to the doctor of philosophy (PhD), a degree that focused on research.

Implementing two new degree programs would take time. First, the Association would hold numerous regional conferences to secure support from nursing faculty from across the country, some of whom were resistant to change. Then, college and university faculty who wanted to offer the new degrees would have to present detailed plans for the programs to their faculty curriculum committees, university boards of visitors, and regional oversight groups for approval. Finally, they had to interview applicants and admit students.

Meanwhile, the student response to the new degree programs was positive. Registered nurses who had graduated from bachelors' programs, as well as those who had graduated from diploma programs, were interested in the CNL master's degree. College graduates with degrees in other fields were also interested. Through the CNL program, nurses could pursue a "second degree" in nursing. Advanced practice nurses, particularly nurse practitioners and nurse anesthetists, were interested in obtaining the practice doctorate degree. Due to this high level of interest, the programs expanded rapidly. By the end of 2005, 25 schools in the United States offered the DNP degree, and an additional 150 schools were in the process of developing a DNP program.[35] By 2008,

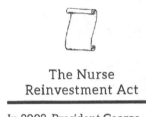

The Nurse Reinvestment Act

In 2002, President George W. Bush signed the Nurse Reinvestment Act (Pub. L. No. 107-205), expanding authority for some existing federal programs and creating a number of new ones to address the nursing shortage in the United States. Specifically, the law established scholarships for nursing students who committed "to working in a health care facility deemed to have a critical shortage of nurses." It also gave scholarships to nurses seeking an advanced degree.[38]

practice doctorate programs were available in colleges and universities across the United States. What had started only a few years earlier was resonating with students, practicing nurses, and nursing faculty.[36]

Nursing Clinics

In the 21st century, nurses continued what they had started at Henry Street Settlement in the 1890s, established in Appalachia in the 1920s, and launched on Indian reservations and in migrant camps in the 1930s. They set up nurse-managed clinics to meet the health care needs of the poor and underserved. This time, however, the clinics employed nurse practitioners rather than general registered nurses.

Nonetheless, the problems remained much the same as the problems of nurse-run clinics in the 20th century: the nurse practitioners could not get reimbursement for their services without a physician making a medical diagnosis. In order to remain viable, the nurse-run centers would have to collaborate in a multidisciplinary approach to care—just as they had in earlier times. To meet Medicare and Medicaid eligibility requirements for a Federally Qualified Health Center (FQHC), nursing clinics had to hire physicians. They also had to be governed by community boards.[39]

In 2003, several nurse-run clinics did exactly that. Others simply closed. Among the clinics that changed direction was the Health Annex Clinic run by the University of Pennsylvania School of Nursing. Because the nurse faculty had other obligations besides running the clinic, the Health Annex was open only 12 hours a week, not nearly enough to meet the needs of the vulnerable population it served. To expand those hours and qualify for payment for services, the clinic turned itself over to the Family Practice and Counseling Network, a group that had FQHC designation. Another clinic, the 11th Street Family Health Services, run by Drexel University College of Nursing and Health Professions, did the same. In contrast, La Salle Neighborhood Nursing Center closed entirely when its application for FQHC designation was denied.[40]

Still other nursing clinics pursued grant funding and explored innovative methods of health care delivery in order to stay open and continue their work. The School of Nursing of the University of Mississippi Medical Center launched The Mercy Delta Express, a state-of-the-art mobile clinic to "bring community health programs to rural communities" in the state. That initiative, developed by nursing professor Peggy Hewlett, was "made possible through a donation of the van and a $50,000 grant by the Sisters of Mercy in Vicksburg.[42]

Nurses and Hurricane Katrina, 2005

In August 2005, while nursing schools across the United States were preparing for the start of the fall semester, those in Louisiana had larger, more pressing problems to address. A hurricane was headed for the Gulf Coast. Day after day, the predictions grew worse: the storm would be a category four or five in strength and would devastate the area. Both coastal Louisiana and New Orleans residents were told to evacuate. Years earlier, New Orleans had been hit by another hurricane and that experience showed that the Superdome, used as a shelter for thousands, had not worked. Therefore, residents of New Orleans were told to go to the dome only as a last resort. Moreover, those who went to the Dome were to bring everything they needed with them—food, water, medicines, and clothes.

In preparation for the storm, Louisiana National Guard reservists were summoned to help. On Saturday, August 27, the National Guard called 4,000 troops, including nurses, to active duty. One of these was Colonel Patricia M. Prechter, state chief nurse and deputy commander of the Louisiana Army National Guard. Her assignment was to activate at least 71 Guard members to report to the Superdome the next day—Sunday, August 28. Their mission was to establish a "special medical-needs unit in the Superdome"—an area for the disabled and elderly who could not care for themselves and needed help with daily activities. To be permitted entry, the "special needs" person had to be accompanied by a caretaker. He or she also had to bring to the dome "anything they might need."[44] The unit would have only minimal supplies on hand.

By Sunday morning, thousands of people had gone to the Dome for shelter. The plan was to have "special needs" patients check in on the loading dock on the ground floor of the dome, after which they would be sent to the special needs area. This check-in procedure quickly broke down, however. As Colonel Prechter described:

> I went to the loading dock to survey what was happening. I was overcome. I will never forget the feeling, because the loading dock area in the Dome was like mass chaos. Jammed with people in no particular order, the New Orleans Health Department group became overwhelmed. They told me they had run out of check-in slips so were just sending everyone upstairs to the medical-needs unit. People with intravenous infusions (IVs), tracheostomies, those needing suctioning—all were being directed to the special-needs unit.[45]

As the population in the dome grew to nearly 10,000, security was required at the general population check-in area. When darkness descended and the storm predictions grew grave, people continued to arrive. To complicate the situation, the only medical supplies were those a National Guard physician had obtained from Charity Hospital.

In the early morning hours of August 29, 2005, the category-four hurricane slammed into the city of New Orleans. With winds of 150 miles per hour, Hurricane Katrina caused a storm surge of 25 feet. Water breached the city's levees and 80% of the city flooded. People were stranded on their rooftops, waiting for help. More than 1,800 people died and 1 million people were displaced.[48]

When the storm hit, the dome's roof was damaged and the electricity failed. Loss of the electricity also meant the loss of sanitation; by the next morning, a half-inch of wastewater had accumulated on the floors of the restrooms. All through the night rainwater poured in through the roof. Chaos ensued as more and more people streamed into the Dome seeking shelter and help. According to Prechter:

> There were patients with IVs, patients needing medications that we did not have. The new patients were kept in the loading dock area that became a makeshift emergency room. We would put any of the patients that had to be bagged (for ventilation) there. All day Monday, people came . . . Babies in the special-needs area had no formula or bottles.[49]

Security problems became worse Monday evening as darkness and a shortage of military presence affected people's behavior. Guard members arrived, bringing radios and M16 rifles.

"Very few nursing clinics are designated FQHCs [Federally Qualified Health Centers] and must rely on support from nursing schools, universities, and a patchwork of grants."[43]

American Journal of Nursing, 2003

"The loading dock was mass chaos."[46]

Colonel Prechter, 2005

Triage

"I quickly set up an Army-system triage with two ER physicians and some medics. Those being triaged were divided into the ones who could not stay at the Dome because of their conditions and needs, and those who could remain for shelter. No tags were available to delineate these groups, so sections of the loading dock area were designated for the various groups."[47]

Colonel Prechter, 2005

"I requested soldiers with M16s in my area for security, because theft became an issue."[50]

Colonel Prechter, 2005

The situation in the Superdome medical area was slightly better organized by Tuesday, August 30, but the crowds continued to swell. With the electricity still out, the interior Dome temperature rose; the heat and humidity became unbearable. Moreover, the flooded city was in chaos and it was not going to improve. The National Guard continued to rescue people from rooftops; many others had drowned. Martial law was declared as desperate survivors looted stores for food; others for whatever they could salvage. People had lost everything.

With conditions deteriorating in the Superdome, Prechter's mission now was to move 1,500 special needs patients to the neighboring Arena, where the Federal Emergency Management Agency (FEMA) had set up a hospital. However, with increased security problems, FEMA withdrew its civilian staff, leaving the hospital and supplies. The National Guard alone was left to police the area, guard the medications, and care for the victims of the disaster. The situation was overwhelming, and there were simply not enough nurses.

Outside the Dome, other nurses also responded to the disaster. Many were on duty in various hospitals throughout the city and surrounding area and could not leave. Replacement staff never came; streets were flooded, and there was nowhere to go since their homes were destroyed. The nurses also had an ethical obligation to stay with their patients—the "duty to care." At Memorial Medical Center, where conditions were "nightmarish" due to power outages and flooding, nurses faced the very difficult moral dilemma of what to do for critically ill patients: allow them to die slowly due to nonfunctioning equipment and no hope of rescue from outside, or provide a quick and painless death with intravenous medications. It was a "no win" situation; the patients would die either way.

In other areas of Louisiana, civilian nurses and the Red Cross worked under different, less chaotic circumstances, addressing the needs of disaster refugees who had fled New Orleans. Nurse Tess O'Neil worked in Gonzales, Louisiana, at the Lamar-Dixon Exposition Center, where she had been asked by the Red Cross to organize a medical unit. Evacuees from New Orleans streamed into the Center. Many needed help for minor ailments, others needed prescription medications; O'Neil's first task was to set up a system for dispensing medications and "some type of documentation . . . to keep track of what was occurring."[52]

When the National Red Cross disaster nurse, Janice Springer, arrived at Lamar-Dixon, she asked that O'Neil continue to assist her. Springer then negotiated with officials for supplies, requesting that they deliver "tables, storage cabinets, and other equipment," including a cooler to refrigerate insulin. Additional medical equipment also appeared, including kits for glucose testing and a nebulizer for treating asthma attacks.[53]

By Friday 1,700 people were at Lamar-Dixon, a shelter designed for 1,200. As the population soared to 1,900, the prevention of disease became the nurses' priority. According to O'Neil: "Soon large gallon size sanitizer dispensers were in place throughout the Center with periodic exhortations over the system announcements to 'wash your hands.'"[54] Meanwhile, the kitchen became the "baby bottle cleaning and sanitizing station."

At Lamar-Dixon, volunteer nurses helped to organize and staff the medical unit. The specialized expertise of the nurses helped the diverse group of patients who were presenting for help. Those with diabetes could speak with diabetic nurse educators and receive counseling. Pediatric nurses could effectively manage children suffering asthma attacks.[56]

Difficult Choices in Extreme Conditions

Some doctors and nurses at Memorial Medical Center in New Orleans faced ethical dilemmas in the care of critically ill patients under nightmarish conditions of heat, power loss, and flooding. For patients who would die regardless of what they did, the staff wondered if they should administer drugs to ease that process. Later a physician and two nurses would be accused of "administering a lethal combination of sedatives and painkillers to four critically ill patients."[51]

Addressing Patients' Needs

"Several evacuees needed chemotherapy. In addition to determining specific chemotherapy protocols, challenges were complicated by the implications of immunosuppression in an emergency shelter environment."[55]

Tess O'Neill, 2005

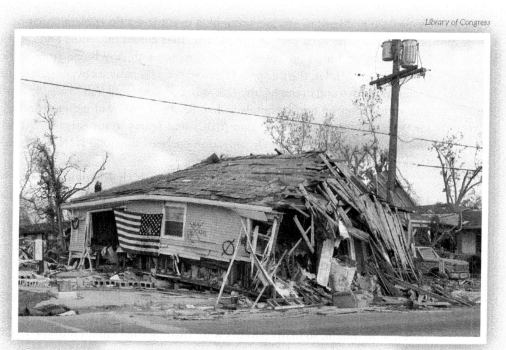

The aftermath of Hurricane Katrina, which left more than 1,800 dead and a million displaced.

During the following days, weeks, and then months, hundreds of medical and nursing volunteer teams from all over the United States traveled to Louisiana to help. On September 9, Mayo Clinic sent a team of health care providers, including nurses, to help in the aftermath. The team, led by Dr. John Black, and nurses Debra Hernke, Beth Borg, and Naomi Woychick, traveled to Lafayette, Louisiana, to assist evacuees from New Orleans. Their effort was part of "Operation Minnesota Lifeline"—a health care relief team led by the Minneapolis-based American Refugee Committee, and done in conjunction with colleagues from the University of Minnesota and the College of St. Catherine.[57] Mayo center was one of 30 centers established in Region IV, under the direction of Dr. Tina Stefanski, the region's medical director. Their mission was to assess the needs of evacuees in sanctioned and unsanctioned shelters; to evaluate chronic health conditions and provide immunizations; and to establish primary care options for those who were unable to access health care within the overloaded system in Louisiana.[58]

Mayo's first team of volunteers included everyone from program analysts to security supervisors and photographers, from physicians and nurse practitioners to patient care assistants. Operating out of a makeshift emergency clinic set up in the Heymann Performing Arts Center in Lafayette, they worked together to meet patients' needs. Mayo team provided care for thousands of evacuees in the area. They screened patients, checked blood pressures, renewed prescriptions, and immunized more than 1,400 people for "tetanus, hepatitis A, and measles, mumps and rubella."[59] The process of care would be repeated again and again as hundreds of volunteers from other hospitals and organizations across the United States traveled south to help.

Nurses and Influenza, 2009

Only a few years later American nurses were involved in another crisis, this one due to the spread of H1N1 influenza from Mexico to the United States. The flu was not an ordinary one—it would turn out to be the same strain that had devastated the world in 1918.

In April 2009, Mexican officials scrambled to control a flu epidemic that had killed 61 people during the early part of the month. They closed museums and schools around Mexico City and urged people with flu symptoms to stay home from work. Despite attempts to control it, the flu spread rapidly; soon flu patients overwhelmed emergency rooms in Mexico and in the nearby U.S. states of Texas and California. By April 25, hospital officials set up tent hospitals to handle the overflow of patients and the Centers for Disease Control and Prevention (CDC) sent teams to investigate. Within days the director of the World Health Organization declared the 2009 H1N1 outbreak a Public Health Emergency of International Concern.[60]

About the same time, a school nurse from a high school in Queens, New York, reported an acute outbreak of illness; she had just sent over a hundred students home "for symptoms that included fever, headache, dizziness, sore throat and cough."[61] The nurse's report prompted the CDC to investigate, and by April 26 the CDC had confirmed that the illness was caused by H1N1, the same strain of influenza that had broken out in Mexico. That news prompted the school's principal to close the school for 9 days.[62]

A second wave of the H1N1 virus hit 5 months later in September 2009 and the news was grim; medical centers in Texas and Tennessee were inundated with sick patients. In Austin, so many parents were rushing their children to the Dell Children's Medical Center of Central Texas that hospital officials set up tents in the parking lot to cope with the onslaught of patients and to isolate those who were infectious. In Memphis, the Le Bonheur Children's Medical Center emergency room was so overcrowded with feverish, miserable youngsters that they too set up tents outside.[63]

Emergency room nurses and physicians were "on the front line" once again, closing schools and working in the tent hospitals—just as they had in 1918 when a deadly form of influenza struck the United States. As they had done in previous flu epidemics, nurses advised patients to stay home, rest and drink fluids, cover coughs and sneezes, wash hands, and wear masks in public places. Despite major changes in medical and nursing therapeutics—including the availability of H1N1 vaccines and antiviral medications—much of the national and community response to the epidemic remained unchanged.[64]

Fortunately, the actions of the public health officials stopped a worldwide spread of the virus in 2009. To prevent subsequent outbreaks of flu, nurses were charged with the ongoing responsibility of health education regarding handwashing, self-imposed isolation, and the need for vaccines. Moreover, it soon became clear that Americans needed access to primary care services and preventive health measures. Too many people were relying on hospital emergency rooms for their primary care services: a fact that drove up the cost of health care and resulted in lengthy delays in care for those with true emergencies. Health care insurance for all Americans became a major topic of discussion in government and medical circles. Insurance for all was not something new, in fact, it had been proposed more than half a century earlier.

Nurses in Remote Area Medical Clinics

Nowhere was the lack of access to health care services more apparent in the United States than it was (and still is) in the southwest region of Virginia, a poverty-stricken remote rural area that had few physicians. There, even in the 21st century, many residents had no health insurance or coverage for preventive health screenings, dental, or eye care. The residents of Wise County were isolated by geography and distance from access to clinics in urban areas of the state, and lived in a vicious cycle of poverty and poor health. They had little money to begin with, and paying for food, clothing, and shelter took priority over any treatment of chronic diseases and dental problems.[65]

To address the lack of health care services, doctors and other health care providers from a variety of medical centers, hospitals, and other organizations conceived of a new clinic idea. They collaborated in a community outreach project, the Remote Area Medical (RAM) Clinic, led by the University of Virginia. Each year a group of health professionals traveled to southwest Virginia to provide free health care. At first, the Clinic focused only on dental care and vision screenings. But once the group became aware of the dramatic needs for care of patients with chronic conditions such as coronary disease, diabetes, and hypertension, they added medical care to the clinic's services. Patients came from all over the region to receive medical and dental care. Many came from the coal counties of

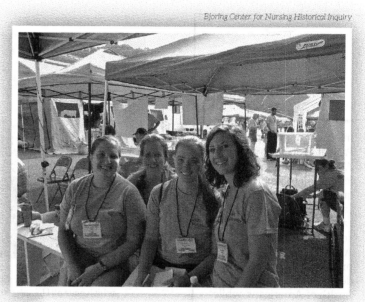

The Remote Area Medical Clinic, which traveled to southwest Virginia to provide free medical care to populations that sometimes could only seek primary care once a year.

southwest Virginia, getting "on the road before sunrise" to seek help for their "aching teeth and ailing kidneys."[66] For many patients, the clinic provided the only primary care they received all year.

At the RAM Clinic, patients received help from doctors, dentists, ophthalmologists, student nurses and medical residents, nurse practitioners, and registered nurses. In fact, the Clinic became a model of interprofessional education and practice as hundreds of volunteers learned and worked together to treat patients. At the RAM event, they saw for themselves the need for services in rural counties and why health insurance mattered. As one student nurse reported: "All students should attend a RAM event. The clinical experience is excellent and eye opening. It is an opportunity to practice skills, assessments, experience a different culture, and look at health care reform issues first hand."[67]

Healthy People 2020 and the Affordable Care Act

In 2010, nurses received major support for their roles in the U.S. health care system, particularly related to their role in nurse-managed clinics. That year the Institute of Medicine published its report *The Future of Nursing: Leading Change, Advancing Health,* writing that: "Nurse-managed health clinics offer opportunities to expand access; provide quality, evidence-based care, and improve outcomes for individuals who may not otherwise receive needed care . . . These clinics also provide the necessary support to engage individuals in wellness and prevention activities." The report had profound implications for the nursing profession, as it also advocated that nurses should work at "the full extent of their training."[69] That same year, the U.S. Department of Health and Human Services presented its plan for "Healthy People 2020," a plan focused on attaining "high quality, longer lives free of preventable diseases, achieving health equity, creating healthy environments, and promoting healthy behaviors across all life stages."[70] Federal legislation passed in 2010 also supported Americans' access to health care.

"The Woodstock of Health Care"

"This was my first year to participate and it was truly an amazing and inspiring experience . . . I know that we did a great job; you could see it on the faces of the patients. I was describing this experience to my coworkers as "the Woodstock of health care—complete with the rain!"[68]

Carol Hendrickson, 2009

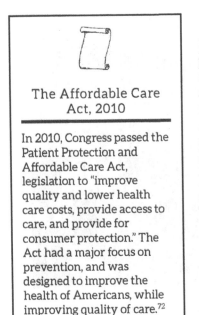

The Affordable Care Act, 2010

In 2010, Congress passed the Patient Protection and Affordable Care Act, legislation to "improve quality and lower health care costs, provide access to care, and provide for consumer protection." The Act had a major focus on prevention, and was designed to improve the health of Americans, while improving quality of care.[72]

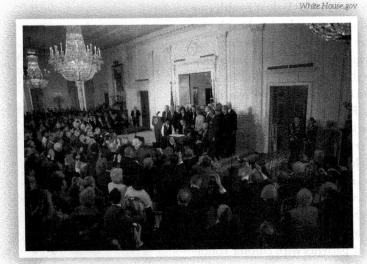

White House.gov

President Barack Obama signing the Affordable Care Act in 2010, which gave all U.S. citizens the opportunity to buy affordable health insurance.

That year Congress passed the Patient Protection and Affordable Care Act (ACA), to provide millions of citizens with the ability to obtain health insurance plans. It was legislation that moved the nation from "a focus on sickness and disease to a health care system based on wellness and prevention."[71]

The ACA took years to implement fully and did not solve all the issues of access to care for all Americans. However, the Act raised public awareness of the facts that disparities in access to quality health care existed and that many Americans did not have health insurance.[73] By October 2013, all U.S. citizens had the opportunity to purchase affordable health insurance through the Health Insurance Marketplace. That insurance had some benefits: young adult children could stay on their parents' plans until they were 26 years old. In addition, patients with chronic conditions such as cancer, heart disease, or renal failure could not be denied coverage. Over the next 3 years, more than 2 million Americans obtained health care insurance: insurance that paid for preventive services, primary care, and hospitalization. Despite that success, the Affordable Care Act (also called "Obamacare") would be a source of political contention for years.

American Nurses in Haiti

In 2010, a devastating earthquake in Haiti drew Americans' attention to their responsibility to the global community. The magnitude 7.0 quake happened in January; by mid-February 230,000 people had died, 700,000 were displaced, and 511,400 refugees had departed the capital city of Port-au-Prince. Altogether, more than 3 million people were affected.[74] Many of those who had survived major wounds, amputations, and blunt trauma injuries.

The country was in shambles. Damaged and collapsed buildings (including hospitals and government facilities), destroyed communications services, and disrupted water and sewage lines were wreaking havoc in the poverty-stricken country. Thousands of homeless Haitians set up refugee camps in tent cities, where food and water were scarce. Grief-stricken survivors wandered aimlessly in the wreckage.

Thousands of health care professionals from all over the world responded to the calls for emergency assistance.[75] American nurses were among them. Many nurses rotated for tours of duty on board the United States Navy Ship (USNS) *Comfort*, a thousand-bed floating hospital that had deployed to Haiti in the early days after the earthquake. Others worked on the ground, doing the best they could as they traveled from place to place or set up clinics in any building left standing. Some nurses traveled alone; others went in teams from universities, churches, and other organizations. Among these were acute care nurse practitioner Audrey Snyder and emergency medicine physician Scott Syverud from the University of Virginia. The two joined a group working in Jacmel, a quaint, historic Caribbean Port city about 25 miles from Port-au-Prince and not far from the epicenter of the earthquake.

Like Port-au-Prince, Jacmel had been devastated. Makeshift cloth tents lined the streets and an odor of human decomposition hung over the city. By the time Snyder and Syverud arrived at the improvised clinic in a Lutheran church, the townspeople and volunteer response teams were trying to restore some semblance of "normalcy" for the earthquake survivors. During the night, the church provided a place for people to sleep; in the day, it served as a temporary medical clinic. The church was also a source of food: during the day, patients and their families were fed lunch; later they were given bags of food to take with them.[76]

Working in the church in 90-degree heat, Snyder and Syverud worked with other health care providers, seeing more than 120 patients a day. They treated patients for anything from malnutrition, dehydration, worms, lice, and scabies to wound infections, respiratory illnesses, malaria, and dengue fever. Some problems were the result of trauma, lack of clean water, and the squalid living conditions in the refugee camps; others were typical diseases of tropical third-world countries. Using bottled water and improvised bandages, Snyder and Syverud cleaned and dressed patients' wounds, applying antibiotic creams when necessary. They also gave tetanus shots, typhoid and other vaccines, and dispensed medications.[77]

The two worked in spite of difficulties. Language barriers and a lack of translators complicated their communication with their patients, and their makeshift paper medical records curled in the heat and humidity. Snyder and Syverud made rounds morning and evening to improve communication. Without patient charts on which to record the time of the last pain medication, they wrote the information on the patient's forehead instead.

As was true in other disasters, Snyder and Syverud had to address the survivors' psychological needs. Patients were grief stricken and many presented with blank stares,

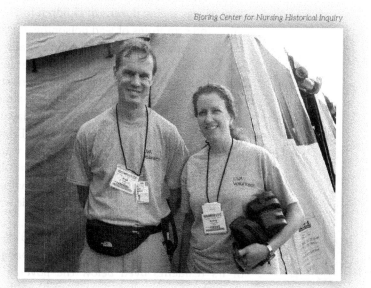

Bjoring Center for Nursing Historical Inquiry

Syverud and Snyder in Haiti, where they cared for patients despite high temperatures, inadequate supplies, and language difficulties.

Support for Survivors

"We tried. We asked patients to "identify what they liked to do before the earthquake and to focus on their ability to do that activity again. We also asked them to create a good dream to replace the nightmares and flash backs they were experiencing. And third, we asked them to create a plan to do one thing each day that would help them the next."[79]

Audrey Snyder, 2010

evidence of their distress. Without sufficient numbers of social workers and psychologists to meet the patients' needs, local and visiting health care teams did their best to intervene. Often nurses were the only support.[78]

The inability to provide follow-up care was especially hard for the nurses and other health care providers who gave emergency treatment on the ground in Haiti. A retired nurse who was working with the organization "Forward in Health" traveled throughout the country with a team, going "from place to place, to the mountains and to tent cities, providing care." The care they provided was "drastically different" from what they provided at home. Follow-up care was impossible; the team moved on.[80]

The School Nurse and the Flint, Michigan, Water Crisis

Five years later, American nurses were involved in another crisis, this one a man-made disaster rather than an act of nature. In September of 2015, news broke about a crisis in Flint, Michigan. The people of Flint had been complaining about discoloration and foul-smelling water since 2014, shortly after city officials had switched the source of the city's water from Lake Huron to the Flint River to cut costs. Within months the residents also experienced skin rashes and hair loss.[82] Marc Edwards, a Virginia Tech civil engineering professor, brought attention to the problem when his team of students tested Flint's water. Each of the professor's water tests of individual households came back staggeringly high for lead levels. The government's response was the household pipes were to blame.

To further their investigation, the Virginia Tech team tested the water directly from the Flint River and found that its corrosion levels were 19 times higher than those of the Detroit water system.[83] The team made their findings public, hoping that adding undeniable scientific results would finally urge the government to become involved. Both the local government and the state had been denying and ignoring the problem for over a year.

In addition, in 2015 local pediatrician Mona Hanna-Atisha publically announced her research findings that showed that many of Flint's children had lead poisoning. By this time school nurse Eileen Tomasi was seeing dozens of children in Flint with signs and symptoms of lead poisoning. As the only nurse in Genesee County, she rotated daily among the 11 schools, and saw the problem everywhere.[84] Indeed, the percentage of young children showing elevated levels of lead in their blood had almost tripled in Flint since April 25, 2014, the day officials had changed the city's source for water. Eventually, it became known that the Flint River water had eroded the pipes throughout the city, resulting in lead levels almost twice as high as the Environmental Protection Agency standards for "toxic waste" in drinking water.[85]

Statistically, Flint was 57% Black, 37% White, 4% Latino, and 41% mixed race. Forty-one percent of its residents lived below the poverty level.[86] One U.S. representative serving the Flint area described the problem clearly: "While it might not be intentional, there's this implicit bias against older

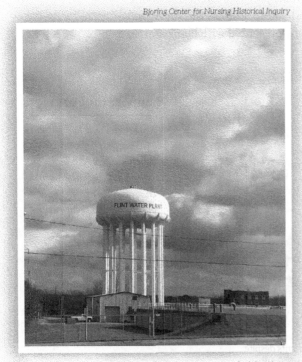

Bjoring Center for Nursing Historical Inquiry

The Flint, Michigan, water tower became a symbol for the crisis in water pollution.

cities—particularly older cities with poverty and majority-minority communities. It's hard for me to imagine the difference that we would have seen exhibited if this had happened in a much more affluent area."[87]

On September 25, 2015—days after Professor Edwards' research grabbed the attention of the public, Flint's mayor issued a warning about lead in the water. A few weeks later, Michigan's governor announced that Flint would return to purchasing water from the Detroit system. The switch was made a week later.[88] It was too late, however. All the city's pipes were corroded and were leaking lead. Moreover, Flint residents would not be granted bottled water from the government until January 2016, almost 2 years after the problem started.

For the citizens it was a crisis. For the school nurse, it was a problem of unprecedented need for more help. Tomasi was responsible for testing both the blood lead levels and the mental and physical development of each child who was affected—a herculean task. Tomasi was working long hours, doing everything she could to help the community, going far beyond testing students' blood lead levels in her office during the 8-hour school day. One of her main concerns was the education of both the students and their families about what was happening and how they would be affected.

On January 5, 2016, Michigan's governor finally issued a State of Emergency for Flint. Eleven days later President Obama declared the situation a Federal State of Emergency.[89] This Federal State of Emergency status came with a $5 million emergency relief fund, almost all of which was spent supplying bottled water to families via the Red Cross and the National Guard.

On January 29, the governor signed a $28 million bill to further address the problem and provide aid to Flint residents. Included in the spending plan were water filters and repairs of the damaged pipes. The top priority, however, was for school nurses. Because of the high demand for medical monitoring and care, hiring more school nurses was critical. The state, like other states from across the nation, had been reducing the number of school nurses for years. In fact, from the last decades of the 20th century to 2015, the entire public health nursing infrastructure in the United States had been corroding.[90]

Meanwhile, in Flint, nurses volunteered to help. Until new nurses could be hired, organizations like the American Red Cross and Quest Diagnostics held numerous clinics to provide free blood tests for lead poisoning. In those clinics, volunteer nurses educated the public and provided people in the community the medical attention that they deserved.[92] Organizations like *Show Me Your Stethoscope*, *Hirenurses.com*, and the Henry Ford College Student Nursing Association also helped, collecting and delivering bottled water, water filters, and home water test kits to anyone who needed them.[93]

Caring for the Caregivers

Creating resilient practitioners is a critical first step toward creating a culture of health, and in 2009 University of Virginia's Dean Dorrie Fontaine launched a Compassionate Care Initiative (CCI). Her purpose was to "reclaim

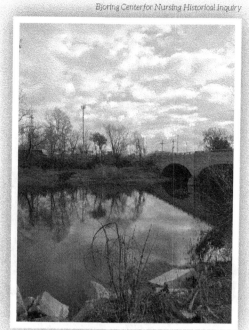

Polluted water in the Flint River was corrosive enough to erode pipes throughout the city and cause lead poisoning in the children.

"The one very good thing about all this is the state is going to provide us with money to hire some nurses."[91]

Eileen Tomasi, 2016

Reflections on Compassionate Care

"In 2008 when I first became Dean of the School of Nursing at the University of Virginia, I began to focus on a healthy work environment where students, faculty and staff all could flourish. This transformed into a Compassionate Care Initiative (CCI) to assist nurses and physicians to develop the resilience, reflection, and relationships necessary to enhance patient care with a sense of compassion."[94]

Dean Dorrie Fontaine, 2015

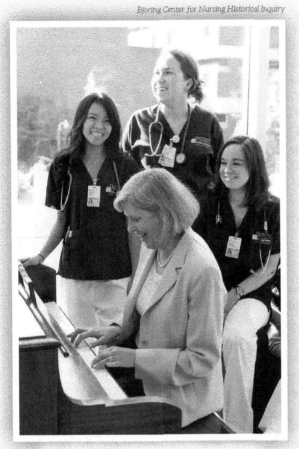

Dean Fontaine, who launched a Compassionate Care Initiative (CCI) to encourage compassion and resilience in nursing students to help them care for themselves as well as their patients.

the soul of compassion for seasoned nurses and physicians" and "ensure that the fire of empathy and compassion burned brightly in the students, the next generation of nurses."[95]

One of the innovations that resulted from the Initiative was "the Pause," a moment of reflection after a death in an acute care setting. One University of Virginia nurse, Jonathan Bartels, noticed that typically after a patient's death in the busy emergency department, staff members quickly left the room to go on to the next patient. Instituting "the Pause" became a compassionate intervention due to this nurse's empathy for his colleagues. As Bartels described it:

I noted that when people die after a traumatic incident, a code, often I would see surgeons and docs and nurses walk away in frustration, throw their gloves off in a defeatist attitude, not recognizing that the patient was a human being we worked on saving. So after these deaths I decided it would be a good thing to stop, pause and do a moment of silence—just stopping: honoring the patient in your own way, in silence. We have even had family members participate.[96]

Initially implemented at the University of Virginia Medical Center, this practice has spread to hospitals throughout the United States.[97] It is one way in which nurses can care for themselves as they strive to create a culture of health for others. Today, the CCI is a highly integrated program that touches students, faculty, and staff across the university, the broader community, and beyond.

> "'Caring for self to better care for others' is our value. This is not selfish but essential to protect the current and future workforce in their mission."[98]
>
> Dean Fontaine, 2015

LOOKING TOWARD THE FUTURE

Today, nurses, like all citizens, are faced with a myriad of issues. Many issues are either not new or are a variation on the problems that preceded them. A few of these issues include an increase in drug-resistant antibiotics; the return of lead poisoning; threats from emerging viruses (Zika and Ebola) and recirculating viruses (H1N1 influenza); an epidemic of childhood obesity; the continued problems of child abuse, bullying, and intimate partner violence; an increase in drug use and opioid-related deaths; and a burgeoning number of elderly patients with Alzheimer's disease and heart failure.[99]

For more than a century, nurses have been dealing with some form of each of these problems. For years nurses cared for critically ill patients without the benefit of antibiotics. Now they must address antibiotic resistance. In the past, nurses treated underweight, "sickly children" in the home and in preventoria. Now they are faced with an epidemic of childhood obesity. In the past, nurses cared for victims of polio, smallpox, yellow fever, and measles epidemics. Now they must teach Americans about the importance of vaccination.[101] In the past, nurses worked in psychiatric hospitals trying desperately to restore patients to mental health. Now they help mentally ill homeless patients in mobile clinics. In the past, nurses made "friendly visits" to the elderly at the

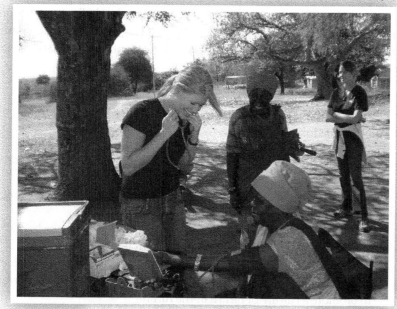

Nursing Students without Borders in South Africa.

end of a day in the tenement district; now geriatric nurse practitioners and registered nurses care for the elderly in nursing homes or in the patients' own homes.

Today nurses are focusing on outcome research related to their health initiatives. The American Academy of Nursing created an initiative called "Edge Runner" to identify nurses who have developed innovative models of care that have good clinical and financial outcomes. Recently, the Academy partnered with the RAND Corporation to collect and analyze data from those models of care. Their purpose is to identify what the nurses have learned that can help others in their efforts to promote a culture of health.

Nurses can also look to their history for outcome data. In Henry Street Settlement, nurses ran a "First Aid" Room, open on evenings and weekends to treat immigrants who spent long days in factories; in urban and rural areas, school nurses taught hygiene and disease prevention and screened children for vision and hearing problems; public health nurses taught well-baby care on Indian reservations and in remote rural counties; operating room nurses sterilized instruments and washed down walls to prevent infections; nurse anesthetists administered anesthesia to thousands of patients with few complications; military nurses saved lives during war. The time has come for nurses to claim that history and build on the good work nurses have done in the past. As historian Julie Fairman recently noted: "This is truly nursing's time to . . . move forward an agenda of reform and public engagement. The profession's historic

"Our past shapes everything we do, whether we explicitly acknowledge it or not."[102]

Julie Fairman, 2016

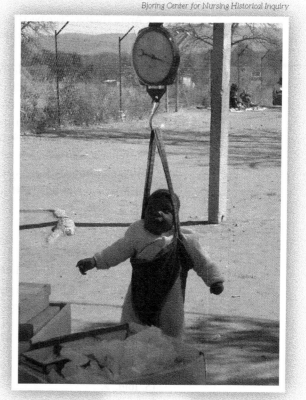

Weighing a baby.

paradigm of caregiving across time and place provides legitimacy."[103] Today, a new generation of professional nurses must rise to the challenge of promoting health in the 21st century. Meeting that challenge will take collaboration, innovation, resilience, compassion, competence, and determination—just as it did in the past.

For Discussion

1. What was the effect of the September 11, 2001, attacks on the World Trade Center on nursing and disaster preparedness?
2. What are the major social, political, and economic factors influencing nursing today?
3. Is nurses' involvement in a culture of health a new idea? Why or why not?
4. What role did race and class play in the Flint water crisis of 2014?
5. Discuss the implications of the corrosion of the public health infrastructure in the United States. How might that affect nurses' efforts to promote a culture of health in the future?

NOTES

1. Susan Hassmiller and Jennifer Mensik, *The Power of Ten: A Conversational Approach to Tackling the Top Ten Priorities in Nursing,* 2nd ed. (Indianapolis, IN: Sigma Theta Tau International Honor Society of Nursing, 2016).

2. Joshua Leon, *The Rise of Global Health: The Evolution of Effective Collective Action* (New York: SUNY Press, 2015): 38.

3. Anita Hunter, "Perspectives in Global Health Care," ch. 4 in *Public Health Nursing,* 9th ed., eds. Marcia Stanhope and Jeanette Lancaster (St. Louis, MO: Elsevier, 2016): 61–92 (quote 65).

4. United Nations, UN Millennium Development Goals, http://www.un.org/millenniumgoals (accessed November 7, 2016).

5. Arlene Keeling, Barbara Brodie, and John Kirchgessner, *The Voice of Professional Nursing Education: A Forty Year History of the American Association of Colleges of Nursing* (Washington, DC: AACN, 2010): 99. Bartels was president-elect, American Association of Colleges of Nursing in 2001 and was scheduled to testify before Congress on September 11.

6. Franklin Hickey, "Nursing Reflections on 9-11: A View from Across the River," Paper presented at the ECBCNHI History Forum, September 2016.

7. Ibid.

8. Ibid.

9. Ibid.

10. Hickey, "Nursing Reflections on 9-11."

11. Susan Trossman, "Nurses Share Accounts of 9-11 Aftermath," *The American Nurse,* November/December 2001, 1–6 (quote 3). http://www.nursingworld.org (accessed November 1, 2016).

12. Ibid., 3.

13. Ibid., 3.

14. Ibid., 3.

15. Ibid., 2.

16. Susan Costello, "Nurses Making a Difference," *American Journal of Nursing* (hereafter *AJN)* 101, no. 11 (2001): 94–95 (quote 94).

17. AJN Reports, "The Health Legacy of September 11," *AJN* 106, no. 9 (September 2006): 27–28.

18. Elizabeth Scannell-Desch and Mary E. Doherty, *Nurses in War: Voices from Iraq and Afghanistan* (New York: Springer Publishing, 2012): Preface.

19. Ibid., Kindle edition 30–31. No nurses' last names are recorded in this book.

20. Ibid., Kindle edition 19.

21. Ibid., 32.

22. Cheryl Ruff and Sue Roper, *Ruff's War: A Navy Nurse on the Frontline in Iraq* (Annapolis, MD: Naval Institute Press, 2005): Kindle edition 108.

23. Ibid., Kindle edition 117.

24. Ibid., Kindle edition 125.

25. Ibid., Kindle edition 125.

26. Ibid., Kindle edition 125.

27. Ibid., Kindle edition 128.

28. Deb Jones, RN, quoted in Arlene Keeling, *The Nurses of Mayo Clinic: Caring Healers* (Rochester, MN: Mayo Clinic, 2012): 117–118.

29. Keeling, *The Nurses of Mayo Clinic.*

30. Ibid.

31. Margarita Gore, "A Follow-Up Story," *Vital Link* 8, no. 1 (March 2005): 1. See also: "Winner: Arizona Military Nurse of the Year, 2004," Reprint, Mayo Clinic.

32. Scannell-Desch and Doherty, *Nurses in War,* 266 (Kindle edition).

33. Madison Park, "Nurse Killed in Iraq Remembered," *Baltimore Sun,* July 19, 2007, 1.

34. Keeling, Brodie, and Kirchgessner, *The Voice of Professional Nursing.*

35. Ibid., 112.

36. Ibid., 115.

37. Ibid., 108. Kathleen Long was president of AACN in 2003.

38. Washington Watch, "The Nurse Reinvestment Act," *AJN* 102, no. 11 (November 2002): 24.

39. AJN Reports, "How Healthy Are Nursing Clinics?" *AJN* 103, no. 11 (November 2003): 22–23.

40. Ibid.

41. Ibid. Denise Geolot was director of the Division of Nursing in 2003.

42. Ibid., 23.

43. Ibid.

44. Theresa O'Neill and Patricia Prechter, "A Tale of Two Shelters," ch. 12 in *Nurses on the Frontline: When Disaster Strikes, 1878-2010,* eds. Barbra Mann Wall and Arlene Keeling (New York: Springer Publishing, 2011): 231–253.

45. Ibid., 237.

46. Ibid., 237.

47. Ibid., 237.

48. Ibid., 237.

49. Ibid., 238.

50. Ibid.

51. "Post-Katrina Murder Charges," *AJN* 106, no. 9 (September 2006): 19.

52. O'Neill and Prechter, "A Tale," 244.

53. Ibid., 244.

54. Ibid., 247.

55. Ibid.

56. Ibid.

57. Mary Pattock, "Hurricane Katrina: When the World Changed . . . and SON Faculty Made a Difference," *Minnesota Nursing*, Spring 2006, 20–21.

58. Arlene Keeling and Adam Holland, interview with Debra (Hernke) Harrison, RN, Mayo Clinic, Jacksonville, Florida (September 2012).

59. Ibid.

60. Marc Lacey and Donald McNeil, "Fighting Deadly Flu, Mexico Shuts Schools," http://www.nytimes.com/2009/04/25/world/americas/25mexico.html?pagewanted=print (accessed October 10, 2013): 1–3.

61. Justin Lessler, Nicholas Reich, Derek Cummings, and the New York City Department of Health and Mental Hygiene Swine Influenza Investigation Team, "Outbreak of 2009 Pandemic Influenza A (H1N1) at a New York City School," *New England Journal of Medicine* 361 (December 31, 2009): 2628–2636 (quote 2629).

62. Ibid., 2629.

63. Pandemic Influenza News, September 2009, http://cmssolutionsinc.wordpress.com/2009 /09 (October 28, 2009).

64. Arlene Keeling, "Treating Influenza 1918 and 2010: Recycled Interventions," ch. 3 in *Nursing Interventions through Time: History as Evidence,* eds. Patricia D'Antonio and Sandra Lewenson (New York: Springer, 2011): 31–41 (quote 31).

65. Audrey Snyder, "Profile in Practice: Health Care Needs in Rural Appalachia," in *Conceptual Foundations: The Bridge to Professional Nursing Practice,* 5th ed., eds. Elizabeth Friberg and Joan Cresia (St. Louis, MO: Elsevier Mosby, 2001): 314–315.

66. Rex Bowman, "UVA Doctors Aid Appalachian Poor," *Daily Progress,* Sunday, July 28, 2002, B1.

67. Student nurse, "Post-Event Medical and Nursing Student Comments, RAM, 2009," in *2009 RAM Clinic, Virginia Event Summary* (2009): 4.

68. Ibid. Woodstock was a music festival held on an upstate New York dairy farm. The 4-day event in August 1969 attracted more than 400,000 people.

69. Institute of Medicine, *The Future of Nursing: Leading Change, Advancing Health* (October 5, 2010): 5. campaignforaction.org/resource/future-nursing-iom-report (accessed November 18, 2016).

70. "Healthy People 2020," https://www.healthypeople.gov (accessed November 18, 2016): 1.

71. Marcia Stanhope, "The Changing US Health and Public Health Care Systems," ch. 3 in *Public Health Nursing: Population-Centered Health Care in the Community,* 9th ed., eds. Marcia Stanhope and Jeanette Lancaster (St. Louis, MO: Elsevier, 2016): 56.

72. Ibid.

73. Ciro V. Sumaya, in *Rural Populations and Health: Determinants, Disparities, and Solutions,* eds. Richard A. Crosby, Monica L. Wendel, Robin C. Vanderpool, and Baretta R. Casey (San Francisco, CA: Jossey-Bass, 2012). See also: http://www.hhs.gov/healthcare/facts/factsheets/ 2013/09/rural09202013.html (accessed December 5, 2013): 1–3.

74. https://www.dec.or.uk/articles/haiti-earthquake-facts-and-figures. (accessed June 29, 2017): 1.

75. Laura Stokowski, "Nurses in Haiti: The Good, the Bad, and the Unthinkable," http://www.medscape.com (accessed November 16, 2016): 1–11.

76. Audrey Snyder, Fusun Terzioglu, and Arlene Keeling, "Striving for the New Normal": The Aftermath of International Disasters," ch. 13 in *Nursing on the Frontline: When Disaster Strikes, 1878-2010,* eds. Barbra Mann Wall and Arlene Keeling (New York: Springer Publishing, 2011): 253–263.

77. Ibid.

78. Ibid.

79. Audrey Snyder, personal communication, March 15, 2010.

80. Laura Stokowski, "Nurses in Haiti: The Good, the Bad, and the Unthinkable," 2–3. No nurses' last names are used in this article.

81. Ibid.

82. Rachel Friend, "The Flint Water Disaster: From Cost-Saving Measure to Crisis," Paper for requirements of University Seminar Course (USEM-1570): Nurses and Global Disasters, University of Virginia, Spring 2016.

83. Steven Mackay, "Engineering's Marc Edwards Heads to Flint as Part of Study into Unprecedented Corrosion Problem," *Virginia Tech University*, September 14, 2015, http://www.vtnews.vt.edu/articles/2015/09/091415-engineering-edwardsflint.html (accessed April 19, 2016).

84. Hillary Coker, "There's Only One Nurse for 5,500 Students in Flint, Michigan," *Jezebel*, January 29, 2016, http://jezebel.com/there-s-only-one-nurse-for-5-500-students-in-flint-mic-1756011390 (accessed April 17, 2016).

85. Christopher Ingraham, "This Is How Toxic Flint's Water Really Is," *Washington Post*, January 15, 2016, https://www.washingtonpost.com/news/wonk/wp/2016/01/15/this-is-how-toxic-flints-water-really-is (accessed April 15, 2015).

86. Friend, "The Flint Water Disaster."

87. Michael Martinez, "Flint, Michigan: Did Race and Poverty Factor into Water Crisis?" *CNN*, January 28, 2016, http://www.cnn.com/2016/01/26/us/flint-michigan-water-crisis-race-poverty.

88. Ibid.

89. Jessica Durando, "How Water Crisis in Flint, MI Became a Federal State of Emergency," *USA Today*, January 20, 2016, http://www.usatoday.com/story/news/nation-now/2016/01/19/michigan-flint-water-contamination/78996052 (accessed March 18, 2016).

90. Ibid.

91. Tomasi, quoted in Rachel Friend, "The Flint Water Disaster," 10.

92. Amanda Emery, "Hundreds Tested at Free Blood Lead Level Clinic during Flint's Water Crisis," *Michigan Live*, January 23, 2016, http://www.mlive.com/news/flint/index.ssf/2016/01/hundreds_tested_at_free_blood.html.

93. Rebecca Love, "Public Health Crisis Flint Michigan: Nurses Mobilizing to Help." https://hirenurses.com/tips-resources?tag=nurses-mobilizing-to-help-flint-michigan (accessed June 29, 2017).

94. Dorrie Fontaine and Arlene Keeling, "Compassionate Care through the Centuries: Highlights in Nursing History," *Nursing History Review* 25, no. 1 (2017): 13–25 (quotes 13–14).

95. Susan Bauer-Wu and Dorrie Fontaine, "Prioritizing Clinician Well Being: Organizational Case Report of the University of Virginia's Compassionate Care Initiative," *Global Advances in Health and Medicine* 4, 5 (2015): 16–22.

96. Jonathan Bartels, "The Pause," *Critical Care Nurse* 30 (2014): 74–75 (quote 74).

97. Ibid.

98. Fontaine and Keeling, "Compassionate Care."

99. President's Perspective: "Global Action for a Healthier World," *The American Nurse*, September/October 2016, 3.

100. Ibid.

101. Brigid Lusk, Arlene Keeling, and Sandra Lewenson, "Using Nursing History to Inform Decision-Making: Infectious Diseases at the Turn of the Twentieth Century," *Nursing Outlook* 64, no. 2 (March–April 2016): 170–178.

102. Julie Fairman, "Foreword," in *Nursing History for Contemporary Role Development*, eds. Sandra Lewenson, Anne Marie McAllister, and Kylie Smith (New York: Springer Publishing, 2017): 1.

103. Julie Fairman, "Afterward," in *The Power of Ten: A Conversational Approach to Tackling the Top Ten Priorities in Nursing*, 2nd ed., eds. Susan Hassmiller and Jennifer Mensik (Indianapolis, IN: Sigma Theta Tau International Honor Society of Nursing, 2016).

104. Fairman, "Foreword," 1.

FURTHER READING

AJN Reports, "How Healthy Are Nursing Clinics?" *American Journal of Nursing* 103, no. 11 (November 2003): 22–23.

AJN Reports, "The Health Legacy of September 11," *American Journal of Nursing* 106, no. 9 (September 2006): 27–28.

Brinkley, Douglas, *The Great Deluge: Hurricane Katrina, New Orleans, and the Mississippi Gulf Coast* (New York: HarperCollins Publishers, 2006).

D'Antonio, Patricia, and Sandra Lewenson, *Nursing Interventions through Time: History as Evidence* (New York: Springer, 2011).

Fontaine, Dorrie, and Arlene Keeling, "Compassionate Care through the Centuries, Highlights in Nursing History," *Nursing History Review* 25, no. 1 (2017): 13–25.

Hassmiller, Susan, and Jennifer Mensik, *The Power of Ten: A Conversational Approach to Tackling the Top Ten Priorities in Nursing,* 2nd ed. (Indianapolis, IN: Sigma Theta Tau International Honor Society of Nursing, 2016).

Keeling, Arlene, "Treating Influenza 1918 and 2010: Recycled Interventions," ch. 3 in *Nursing Interventions through Time: History as Evidence,* eds. Patricia D'Antonio and Sandra Lewenson (New York: Springer Publishing, 2011): 31–41.

Keeling, Arlene, Barbara Brodie, and John Kirchgessner, *The Voice of Professional Nursing Education: A Forty Year History of the American Association of Colleges of Nursing* (Washington, DC: AACN, 2010).

Keeling, Arlene, and Sandra Lewenson, "A Nursing Historical Perspective on the 'Medical Home,'" *Nursing Outlook* 61, no. 5 (September/October 2013): 360–366.

Keeling, Arlene, and Mary Ramos, "The Role of Nursing History in Preparing Nursing for the Future," *Nursing and Health Care: Perspectives on Community* 16, no. 1 (January/February 1995): 30–34.

Kulbok, Pamela A., Joan Kub, and Doris F. Glick, "Cornerstone Documents, Milestones, and Policies: The Changing Landscape of Public Health Nursing 1950–2015," *Online Journal of Issues in Nursing,* volume 20, no. 2, manuscript 3 (2017).

Lessler, Justin, Nicholas Reich, Derek Cummings, and the New York City Department of Health and Mental Hygiene Swine Influenza Investigation Team, "Outbreak of 2009 Pandemic Influenza A (H1N1) at a New York City School," *New England Journal of Medicine* 361 (December 31, 2009): 2628–2636.

Lusk, Brigid, Arlene Keeling, and Sandra Lewenson, "Using Nursing History to Inform Decision-Making: Infectious Diseases at the Turn of the 20th Century," *Nursing Outlook* 62, 2 (2016): 170–178.

Scannell-Desch, Elizabeth, and Mary E. Doherty, *Nurses in War: Voices from Iraq and Afghanistan* (New York: Springer Publishing, 2012).

Stanhope, Marcia, "The Changing US Health and Public Health Care Systems," ch. 3 in *Public Health Nursing: Population-Centered Health Care in the Community,* 9th ed., eds. Marcia Stanhope and Jeanette Lancaster (St. Louis, MO: Elsevier, 2016).

Wall, Barbra Mann, and Arlene Keeling, *Nursing on the Frontline: When Disaster Strikes, 1878–2010* (New York: Springer Publishing, 2011).

Index